trim healthy mama

trim healthy
table

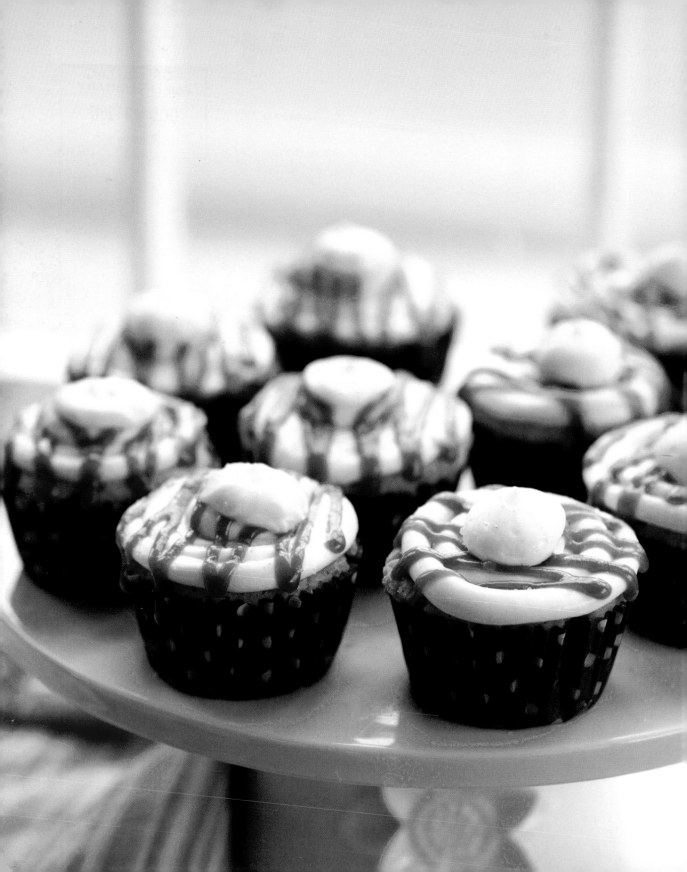

Gather the Family, Eat Up, and Trim Down

trim healthy *mama*

trim healthy table

More Than 300 All-New Healthy and Delicious
Recipes from Our Homes to Yours

PEARL BARRETT & SERENE ALLISON

HARMONY BOOKS

New York

Published in the United States by Harmony Books, an imprint of the Crown Publishing Group, a division of Penguin Random House LLC, New York.

crownpublishing.com

Harmony Books is a registered trademark, and the Circle colophon is a trademark of Penguin Random House LLC.

Library of Congress Cataloging-in-Publication Data is available upon request.

ISBN 978-0-8041-8998-9
Ebook ISBN 978-0-8041-8999-6

Printed in the United States of America

Photographs by Rohnda Monroy
Photograph on page 272 by Lauren Volo

Cover design by Jan Derevjanik

Cover photographs by Lauren Volo (front), Rohnda Monroy (back), and SalomeNJ/Shutterstock (spine)

10 9 8 7 6 5 4 3 2 1

First Edition

To our husbands and children—the biggest most heartfelt shout-out goes out to you for your patience during the past year as we were "pregnant" with this book. You heard us say at the start, "This time around, let's just do a smaller, more manageable book, perhaps 150 recipes . . . let's not kill ourselves this time." But you secretly knew we couldn't do small or manageable, so you were patient and forgiving when this book took over our lives. You endured our late nights, our four a.m. mornings, our days of repeating a recipe over and over again until we went insane or got it right, our meltdowns during deadlines. You loved us through it all. And when we ended up with more than 300 recipes and couldn't part with one, you just cheered us on rather than saying "I told you so." We love you all so much we can barely stand it!

To Rohnda—our amazing photographer and sister Mama. Once again you went above and beyond. Everyone wanted more of your beautiful pictures this time around, so your workload was insane. You had to make each recipe, photograph each recipe, feed each recipe to your family, and then give us your feedback. Oftentimes that sent us back to the drawing board. We'd start again, which meant you'd have to start again, too. Thank you for hanging in there with us and for loving our crazy selves even though we took your orderly life and shook it up so you barely knew what day it was. Lesser women would have quit on us! Thank you for the fact that even though you have such a rare talent for capturing joy and love in a plate of food, you still don't consider yourself a professional photographer. Well, we don't consider ourselves professional authors, so let's never change, huh?

To our recipe testers—our generous and tireless admins who gave of your valuable time to help us tweak these recipes so we could make them the absolute best they could be. Thank you so much. You'll never know how grateful we are for your precious hearts to help hundreds of thousands of women become trimmer and healthier. May God bless your socks off!

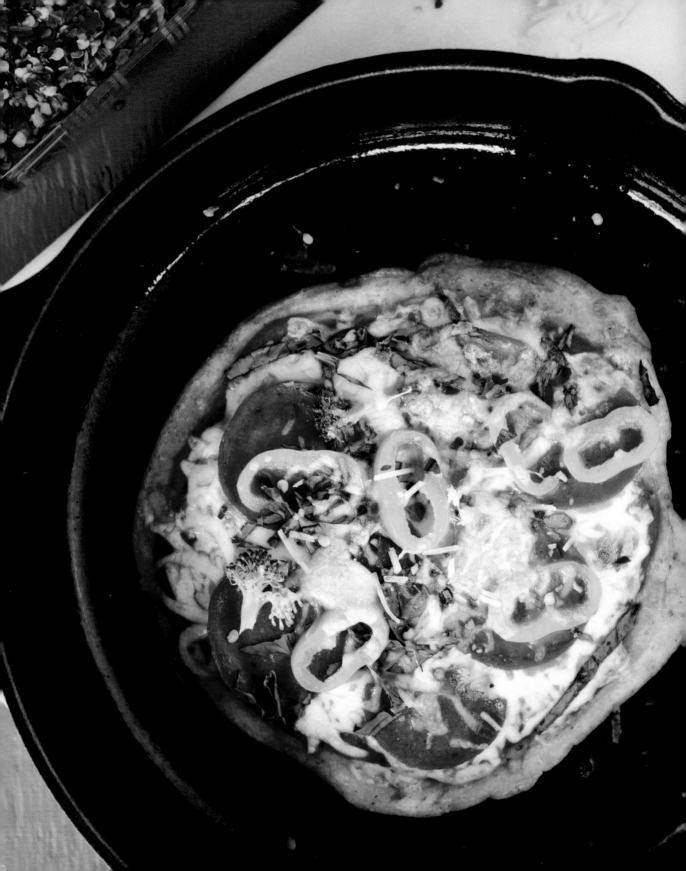

Contents

DELICIOUS DESSERTS AND TREATS

SLIMMING SIPS

CRACKERS, CRUSTS, TOPPINGS, AND MORE

The Power of Your Table

You don't have to look far—weight problems and degenerative diseases like type 2 diabetes are afflicting families everywhere. Now it's no longer just adults who are suffering. For the first time in history, children are being diagnosed with the same issues at an alarming rate. But this weight and health epidemic won't be solved in the doctor's office. It has to be fixed where it starts: in our homes and around our tables.

You and your family can trim down and gain health and you don't have to lose your mind doing it! You are going to fill your table with delicious, filling, Trimming meals that meet the needs of the whole family. This is not some out of touch fantasy that you can never attain—this is real-world stuff. It's you in the midst of your too-busy and crazy life, discovering health for you and your family little by little as you chow down on good stuff!

You have to eat, right? You're going to feed yourself and your family something, so while you are at it why not make your meals both scrumptious and slimming? The family-friendly, quick and flavorful skillet meals, hearty casseroles, comforting crockpot meals, filling stews, big bowls of soup, huge tasty salads—and of course, let's not forget desserts—in this book are going to bless your pants off, literally. You'll notice your pants become looser the more of these meals you eat! Our tricks, tips, and tweaks take the sort of meals your family already loves (the very ones that were exploding your waistline) and make them both trimming and healthy.

THE MAMA MOVEMENT

Just a few years ago, we wrote a self-published book and titled it *Trim Healthy Mama*, never guessing in our wildest dreams what would happen with it. Women began to discover the book and it resonated with a longing they had deep down in their souls. Like us, they felt "done" with diets and yearned for a doable way of eating that would enable long-term success rather than short-term, extreme results. Those women shared the plan with their friends, who shared it with their friends. Trim Healthy Mama became a grassroots movement and now close to a million people have slimmed down and gained better health eating this way.

It was not us who caused this movement, it was Mamas everywhere who couldn't keep the good news to themselves. Soon it was not just Mamas slimming down and gaining health, but also whole families, churches, and communities. Daily we hear stories and see pictures of men, children, and teens with incredible health and weight transformations. We have Trim Healthy Daddies (commonly known as Trim Healthy Hunks), teens, singles, grandparents, second cousins, and long-lost uncles, all coming on board.

This book is for all of you who took us two crazy sisters into your hearts and homes and who shared our plan with your family members and friends. You wanted more family style "get 'er done" recipes, and you wanted a simple start guide of the eating plan to share with others. Well, here they are.

The recipes in these chapters can fulfill the needs of all the different members of your household. At the bottom of each family recipe, you'll find how to make it work for the various challenges in your family so you don't have to cook two different meals. Some members in your family may need to slim down, others may need to actually gain weight, and still others may need to learn to maintain a healthy weight. These recipes can healthfully meet all those challenges. There are also a whole bunch of 5- to 10-minute single-serve meals in here, too, perfect for quick lunches or easy dinners . . . because you are not always going to be eating with your family, and we also have thousands of singles doing the plan.

A GENTLE CHANGE

If you are new to this whole Trim Healthy Mama thing, perhaps you're thinking this is impossible. You don't have the time. Your kids are too picky. Your husband (or wife, if you are a guy reading this) won't play along. You don't have the money. You've tried "healthy" in the past only to give up and gain the weight back (and more). You've got a feeling that dragging your whole family along for the

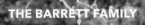
THE BARRETT FAMILY

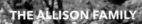
THE ALLISON FAMILY

ride will make that sort of repeat failure all the more miserable. Most of all . . . like us, you get hungry and don't want to feel deprived!

We know change can seem daunting, but the Trim Healthy approach is gentle. This is not a boot-camp lifestyle. You don't have to militantly preach this to your family (actually . . . we forbid that!). You're not about to put anyone in your family on a "diet." (And we're definitely not going to say the word "diet" to our kids!) You are simply going to bring food sanity to your home through tasty, healing meals that nurture and honor the lives that you are entrusted to raise. And eat? Oh boy, are you going to get to eat. None of this calorie-counting misery, thank you very much!

If at first your family doesn't join you perfectly on the minor details of this eating plan, that's okay. Give them grace. Certain family members (can we say stubborn hubbies?) learn these truths in their own time, which may be different from your time. Or they may never learn them at all. That's okay, too. Simply start making our family-friendly meals and soon your family will be eating healthier without even knowing it. This begins with you and trickles down.

These recipes are sneaky (in a good church attending way of course). There are times your family will scarf down your meal and ask for seconds, and you'll have to hide the smile that knows what's in it! We have a unique, God-given ability to hide veggies and other healing ingredients in undetectable ways. This is Sunday Service approved deception! Can we get an Amen? Cue the choir! (We are a preacher's kids after all, can't help ourselves.)

You are not going to have to stay chained to the kitchen or kill your grocery budget. We have plenty of level 1, insanely quick and simple meals for you to start with, then we have some that use a few more ingredients, that you'll grow into when you feel ready. It is a proven fact that if you cook more of your meals at home, you and your family become healthier and slimmer, but while we encourage home-cooked meals on your table, we also know there are plenty of times for eating out. You can do that with ease. Even if you are a traveling businessperson and have to eat most of your meals in restaurants . . . yes, you can do this! You also don't have to run straight out and buy a bunch of special ingredients. The majority of the recipes have an NSI sign, which means No Special Ingredients, or NSI Friendly, which means we give you easily found subs for any special ingredients. Lay down your fears and give us some baby step belief here.

And speaking of fear, let's address it for a minute. Most diets are fear based. They make you fearful of certain food groups. Take your pick. Carbs are evil! Or fats will do you in! Or grains aren't for human consumption! Or meat will give you cancer! Or more than 1,300 calories will cause weight gain. We embraced most of those fears, too, at one time or another. But the day we threw them all down and chose food peace and freedom . . . wow, it felt good! Fear and self-loathing are not part of this lifestyle. Don't do this plan because you hate your body and wish it were completely different. Do this because you are fearfully and wonderfully made by our Creator and because you want and *need* to honor this unique body He gave you. Stop self-loathing and start self-honoring!

These days it is so politically correct to tell people they should make only healthy changes when they feel ready and for nobody else but themselves. "Do it for you," is the politically correct mantra. We have a different take. You are your children's role model and your spouse's investment. Attaining a healthier, trimmer body is not just a gift to yourself . . . it sets a legacy for your children to follow. Your children (or grandchildren) need the healthiest and most vibrant you in their lives for as long as they can have you. Yes, absolutely do this for yourself, but also do it for "them."

Melissa Shattuck, one of our Trim Healthy Mamas who has lost 73 pounds through the Trim Healthy Plan and gone from a size 16/18 to a size 6/8, wrote this recently: "God showed me through this plan just how selfish I was being by not taking care of the body He gave me, even though I thought of myself as selfless, always putting my family first. I was robbing Him and my family of the best of me. I am free, satisfied, joyful, and thankful. You got this! Keep going, people!"

She's right. You CAN do this! Take this stand. This is a heart and mind change, a new way of thinking that you'll practice. Practice getting rid of the toxic thoughts that say you can't. When negative thoughts tell you to just give up, that this is not worth it, give them a quick shove, because if you let those thoughts stay around, then they will steal your joy and your success. Don't listen to the voice that says change is too hard, that you'll never be able to get this right, that your family doesn't support you, that you can't find the time, that destructive foods are your comfort during stress, or that your life is just too difficult to make the change. While you do have challenges, and while some of these things may even be your reality, don't surrender to them! If you have obesity, heart disease, or diabetes in your family . . . be the one who says "Enough is enough!" Generations can be changed because of your decision today to embrace a new way of thinking! Yes, "thinking." Your doing will come out of your thinking.

Of course, some diseases are beyond our control and only God knows why they happen; but so much illness is preventable. Obesity and the health complications that come from it, like type 2 diabetes, are curable and preventable. We see testimony after testimony of this every day with blood work to prove it.

DON'T FORCE THE "TRIM"

This is unlike any other diet plan you have ever done because you need to let the "trim" part happen in its own good time. We don't want you to focus solely on it or force it. This plan is called Trim Healthy Mama for a reason. The healthy part is just as important as the trim part, and healthy weight loss needs to take its own good time. Slow, steady, and long-term wins the race. Some lose more quickly than others. Everybody has his or her own pace, even if it is a snail's pace. Celebrate every tiny move forward toward better health rather than backward. This is for life.

Let this be a joyful journey, not a miserable one. To experience the joy, you must throw out the impatience. You are reading the wrong book if you intend to get all obsessed with the scale and determine to see new extreme lows on it every week. That is more of the "same ol' yo-yo danger-ous diet" approach you've done in the past, and it cannot heal you or be a healthy example to your family. The scale will start to smile at you as your body gets your blood sugar under control. Take your body measurements when you first start. You'll find that they continue to change even when the scale doesn't move for periods of time.

If you are a woman no longer in your teens or even twenties, please don't put near-unattainable high school or college weight goals on yourself! That was your Princess weight. You are a Queen now. You may have birthed children, experienced extreme life challenges, had some hormonal hiccups . . . you're in a different life season. Spring was lovely but summer, fall, and winter are all spectacular seasons, too! If you are in your fall season of life, embrace the vibrant beauty of it! Yes, be the best and healthiest you, but don't make yourself miserable trying to attain something that was another season. Find your Queen weight . . . it will fit you just right, and you'll wear it with grace and class!

WHY WAIT?

Don't wait to start until you feel perfectly ready or life's circumstances line up just so. They never will. You can start little by little in the midst of your crazy life. We know about crazy lives because we live them, too. This plan was birthed during challenging seasons in our own lives when money was tight and life was ridiculously chaotic.

Oh . . . and you don't have to be a certain type, either. Not the crunchy granola type? Come as you are. Don't change for us. If you love to cook from scratch . . . great! If you don't . . . no worries. Try some of the supereasy recipes to get you going like Whoop Whoop Soup (page 149) or Save My Sanity Chili (page 81).

We might be sisters, but we are far from twinsies, and although our core beliefs about the basics of the plan are the same, we have very different approaches to food and cooking. One of us (Serene) is a purist and loves to ferment foods, grow veggies, make stock from bones, milk cows, and thinks the microwave is the devil incarnate! The other of us (Pearl) is a Drive-Thru Sue or you could call her a Prepackaged Pam. She loves to find shortcuts for everything while still eating as healthfully as possible (she makes use of the microwave when Serene is not looking). You'll find us feuding and competing all the way through this book with our different approaches, but just know that we're doing it with smiles on our faces.

Not much of an exerciser? That's fine, too. Once you find your lost energy you'll naturally find yourself wanting to move more. But until then, you can still find your Trim without putting in a bunch of miserable hours at the gym. Just focus on the food plan at first. Don't overwhelm yourself with exercise. Choose something that you love once you feel ready and please, don't overdo it! Long exercise sessions can be harmful. Twenty minutes a few times a week is all you really need along with some brisk walking. Check out our Workins DVD for quick, effective, healing exercise sessions at www.trimhealthymama.com once you feel ready for some movement.

YOU NEED THE KNOWLEDGE

Before you jump into the recipes . . . read (no really, read it . . . don't skim it) the next chapter. It is a quick explanation of the eating plan and covers how to do it as a family. Once you have read that a time or two, you can start making some of the recipes. Please don't feel overwhelmed as you try to digest the information in the next chapter. It will teach you to look at food as fuel rather than just items on your plate, and that takes a little getting used to. Brain scientists have discovered that most of us need to read or hear new concepts about six times before we really grasp them. So give your-self lots of time and grace. As you get started you'll have a bunch more questions about the plan. For more details, and the scientific and Biblical background behind it, please check out *Trim Healthy Mama Plan* or our original 640-page encyclopedia that leaves no stone unturned . . . *Trim Healthy Mama*. Listen to our free weekly podcast for lots of encouragement (found at www.trimhealthy mama.com), or go to our membership site and watch some of our videos. Also, "like" our Facebook page and join one of the many official Trim Healthy Mama Facebook groups for wonderful support.

FOOD, GLORIOUS FOOD

Do you smell that deliciousness? Oh yeah, baby . . . that's a Trim Healthy meal about to be devoured! The more you put these meals on your table, the more you and your family will thrive! Or perhaps your kitchen island is your table. Sometimes even your car might have to become a hub of whole-some food. It doesn't matter, these recipes were made for real life . . . so if you have to grab one of our "to go" bars and eat in the car in the morning, we've got you covered. Whether you are a THM veteran or completely new to this lifestyle, we couldn't be more excited to bring you more than 300 new Trimming recipes to enjoy.

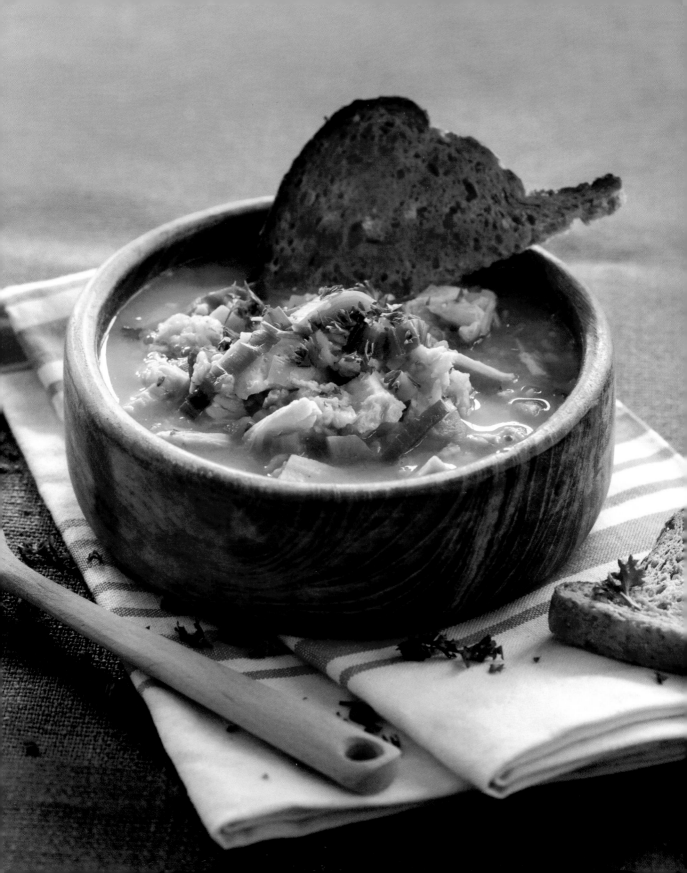

Trim Healthy Basics—
Your Simple Start Guide

Welcome to the nutshell explanation of how this way of eating works. This simple start guide will teach you first how to use it to shed weight. Following that, how to easily make it work to meet the needs of your whole family. Please don't skip this chapter and jump straight into the recipes. You need the knowledge if this is to be your long-term success story. Unlike most diets, we are not going to tell you exactly what to eat and take over your food life. That is more "diet mentality" nonsense, and it cannot help you in the long- term. We will hold your hand as you start, but our ultimate goal is for you to be able to stand on your own, fully equipped with the knowledge on how to eat healthy for the rest of your life, and how to raise a trimmer and healthier family. (To our Mama vets: use this as a little refresher course; you may learn something new or things may click in a new way.)

If you don't grasp these concepts immediately, don't get frustrated. The initial learning curve is usually a bit bumpy for everyone. Read this through, reread a couple of times if necessary, then start baby-stepping your way in with our Simple Start assignments, tips, and suggestions. Things will begin to click and become second nature over days and weeks, perhaps even months, as you apply the principles. Lightbulb moments will happen when they happen . . . no need to force them.

Throughout this chapter we refer to the plan as THM, which stands for Trim Healthy Mama, but if you are a guy reading this or if you are not a literal Mama (or if you are doing this with your family and you think they will be weirded out by the "Mama" word), then you can call it Trim Healthy Life or Trim Healthy Way. Some husbands proudly share with their guy friends that they are doing the Hot Mama Diet . . . (chuckle). Call it whatever you are comfortable with.

This Simple Start guide is just to get you going. We recommend you read *Trim Healthy Mama Plan* for more details (or check it out of your local library).

FIRST, STABILIZE YOUR BLOOD SUGAR

The first goal of THM is to bring your blood sugar into healthier balance. The Trimming part of this plan begins to happen once your blood sugar stops swinging from highs to lows. This means you'll eat foods that have mild rather than dramatic effect on your blood sugar. Goodbye to blood sugar drama, you won't miss it.

Choosing foods that are kind to your blood sugar is known as a low-glycemic approach to eating. Notice we said "low glycemic," not "low carb." You need carbs for the health of your thyroid, your adrenals, your brain function, your metabolism, your energy, and countless other bodily functions. Low-carb diets can mess with your entire endocrine system and eventually slow your metabolism. Your children need healthy carbs for growth and development, so don't kick them off your table! You will eat both carbs and fats on this plan, but if you have weight to lose, you simply won't eat them together (as we're soon to explain).

YES!

This is not a "No" plan . . . it is a "Yes" plan. You'll be so busy enjoying all your "Yes" foods all day long that you'll barely have time to dwell on the "No's." So, let's quickly get them out of the way. There are only a couple of them.

THE NO'S

Goodbye sugar and white flour (which is actually sugar in your bloodstream)! If you are an adult who needs to lose weight, then you will also be parting ways with white potatoes for a while since they tend to spike your blood sugar. We're not banning them; they can come back in a smaller way once you're at goal weight. (Since growing children have higher metabolic needs, they can still include them.)

SUGAR BONDAGE

While God made the sugarcane, it has been sorely abused and is a harmful addiction for most people. The more you eat, the more you want, and the more your fat cells multiply and your health suffers. We have a novel approach to help you overcome sugar bondage, and you sure don't have to cut out sweet treats to do it. In fact, you'll enjoy a lot of them . . . Chocolate Chip Pancakes (page 341) for breakfast? You bet!

While this is a sugar-free plan, that doesn't mean you're a miserable failure if sugar ever passes your lips again. Don't beat yourself up when you eat one of the "No's." We all mess up or even choose to go off-plan sometimes. Practice your comeback. Just pick yourself up with the knowledge that you are always only three hours from your next slimming meal. Don't stay down there in defeat and shame no matter how many cupcakes you caved to at that birthday party. The scriptures tell us God's mercies are new every morning, so give yourself the same beautiful grace and the same clean slate. And we're certainly not saying "STOP EATING SUGAR THIS INSTANT AND BANISH IT FROM YOUR HOME." That's a sure way to make you crave a candy bar. But slowly and surely you are going to break its hold over you.

DEFEAT SUGAR'S POWER!

Repeat after us: "You must fight chocolate with chocolate!"

That's right . . . the lure of chocolate and other sweet treats is not overcome by sheer will power. You can enjoy sweets without guilt; you'll just eat them slimming style! Start replacing destructive sweets with delicious, health-building, kind-to-your-waistline alternatives, such as Lemon Lime Burst Whip (page 442) or Brownie Batter in a Mug (page 405). One day you'll wake up to realize, "Hey, I haven't had sugar in a week and I'm not missing it!" Go you!

Sugar-free does not mean the use of artificial sweeteners. Those are not part of this plan. You will be sweetening your treats with natural sweeteners that have zero impact on your blood sugar. Pure stevia or blends of stevia mixed with erythritol or xylitol (which are blood sugar–friendly sugar alcohols) are the sweeteners we use. Stevia is simply the sweet part of the leaves from stevia plants and is not to be confused with artificial sweeteners. Monk fruit extract is another natural sweetener that is also plan-friendly.

If you have tasted stevia before and decided you hate it, give it another chance. Your taste buds need a few weeks to adjust as they wean off sugar. But the type of stevia you use and how you use it make all the difference. Check out page 38 for more info on how to use and learn to love stevia—

or what to use if you can't eat it, as that won't have to be a deal breaker. Growing children without weight issues can still use honey in moderation as they have less insulin resistance than we adults.

Any time you see the words "white or wheat flour" on a label, just replace those words with the word "sugar," since that is what most flour-based foods become once they hit your bloodstream. Don't worry, you don't have to give up bread altogether; we'll simply steer you to healthier sources. Whole-grain sprouted breads are "on plan," as are other gentle flours like oat flour. By "gentle," we mean they don't cause your blood sugar to skyrocket. If you are gluten-free, no worries . . . all our bread recipes in the Breads chapter (page 240) are gluten-free. You are going to love Wonderful White Blender Bread (page 242).

SIMPLE START RECAP 1:

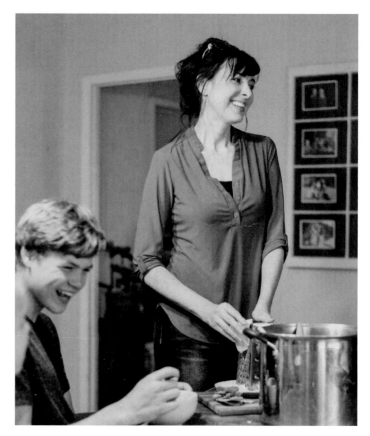

- You are going to steady up your blood sugar

- There are only two chief things you are saying "no" to: sugar and white flour. (You're not divorcing white potatoes, just separating while you work out your differences.)

- Fight chocolate with chocolate

SEPARATE YOUR FATS AND CARBS

Okay, time to learn the Trim Healthy magic. Here is the simple trick behind how the weight-loss part of this plan works:

DON'T EAT FATS AND CARBS IN THE SAME MEAL IF YOU WANT TO LOSE WEIGHT!

The beauty of eating this way is that you won't have to give up either of your body's main fuels (fats or carbs). You'll lose weight by metabolizing them one at a time. Your meals will feature either fats or carbs but not both. Your body burns through either the carbs or the fats alone in a faster time than if it has to burn both. You have to keep living, and that requires more fuel so your body must look around for something else to burn. The only thing left is your own body fat . . . just what we want to happen! You burn your own fat for fuel and you get trimmer . . . woo-hoo!

There are two main meal types on plan. One is called **S,** and the other is called **E.** They each feature a chief fuel. Don't mix them if you want to shed weight.

S MEALS (SATISFYING MEALS)

S stands for Satisfying because this type of meal includes yummy fats. Your innate craving for fatty foods need not be denied! **S** meals always include protein, either lean or fatty, but also allow for other yummy fats such as oils, cheese, or butter. **S** meals are filling and delicious. Think steak, chicken with skin, avocado, or creamy dressings on salads. Check out the food lists (see page 536) for more details on the foods that fit into an **S** meal.

THM is not a number-centric plan. We want you to start thinking of your food in terms of fuels rather than numbers. Think of fat as your fuel in your **S** meals. Fat-based meals make you lose weight, so long as you don't throw a bunch of carbs in them. Essentially, **S** meals are low-carb meals. If you are a numbers person, you can have a basic guideline of about 10 grams of net carbs with your **S** meals (net carbs are total carbs minus fiber and sugar alcohols). But this is only for those of you who love numbers. We didn't create this plan around numbers, but we had some number lovin' people beg us for them. Many of us, including your friendly neighborhood authors, rarely count anything doing THM and love the freedom that affords us. Rather than counting, we simply think thoughts like "Fat is my fuel in this **S** lunch so I'm pulling back the carbs." So please don't get all caught up in that 10-gram limit; it is not a law—just a guideline to keep your body from burning too many carbs along with your fat and stopping weight loss. Remember: single fueling not double fueling is the name of the game! We do want you to eat lots of veggies with your **S** meals, though, so don't ever bother counting those as part of your 10 grams . . . have at 'em!

E MEALS (ENERGIZING MEALS)

E stands for Energizing because this type of meal features carbs to boost your energy levels. There are harmful carbs (sugar and white starches) and there are helpful carbs. Helpful carbs are the ones that are gentle on the rise of your blood sugar. On THM, you'll be eating only the helpful ones like fruit, sweet potatoes, beans, and whole grains. Energizing meals always include protein (only the lean kind) and don't contain a bunch of fat (only about a teaspoon), but you'll learn to create them in such tasty ways you won't miss those fats.

Once again, don't get too caught up in the numbers. Think in terms of fuels. In **E** meals, carbs are your fuel. Let your body burn those carbs, then it can turn to your own body fat and start melting that. That's the Trim Healthy magic happening right there, baby! To ensure your **E** meal is a weight-loss meal, don't throw a bunch of fat in there with it or it will stop weight loss. One chief fuel per meal, remember?

E meals are low-fat meals, not "no-fat" meals. A little bit of fat is welcome. That 1 teaspoon of fat equals about 5 grams of fat for you number-loving people. And just to repeat (in case this number is going to take away your joy and freedom): 5 grams of fat is a guideline, not a law! If you have 6 grams of fat in your **E** meal you didn't blow it, you just colored outside the lines a tad. Cut yourself some slack! Just think in terms of a smear of mayo on your sandwich rather than a big dollop, or a teaspoon of peanut butter rather than a huge tablespoon or two with your apple . . . or a lean dressing on your salad rather than oodles of oil. Check out the food lists (page 538) for more details on foods that fit into **E** meals.

We do want you to be mindful of just one number in **E**. In order to protect your blood sugar from dangerous highs, you need to keep your total **E** meal at or under 45 grams total net carbs. But if you consult the food list for **E**-friendly carbs, you won't really have to count anything, as amounts are listed for you.

NEVER FORGET YOUR PROTEIN!

If you need to lose weight (or even if you don't), protein is crucial. Protein is one of the chief tools of THM that brings your blood sugar into balance. Protein will anchor every meal you eat, whether it is **S** or **E**. Don't worry, this is not a high-protein eating plan where you'll have to constantly count up your protein grams and stuff your face with chicken breast all day to make your goal. This is a beautifully balanced protein approach. Again, no need to focus too much on numbers, but if you prefer having a number to shoot for, most main meals are 20 to 30 grams of protein, and snacks can be less, starting around 10 grams. Sometimes meatless meals (such as bean-based meals or a bowl of oatmeal) contain less protein, but that's okay, as you'll probably have a higher-protein meal at another time during the day and it will all balance out. Don't stress the numbers.

SIMPLE START RECAP 2:

- **S** meals focus on fats for fuel

- **E** meals focus on carbs for fuel

- Separate fats and carbs for weight loss

- Make sure every meal contains protein

This will all start to sink in with time and practice. But if learning anything more today will make your head feel like it will explode, better to take a break at this point. Relax, let all this mull around in your head for a while, do the Simple Start assignment (see below) tomorrow morning, then come back to some more reading later.

SIMPLE START ASSIGNMENT 1: Get up in the morning and make your first **S** breakfast. You don't even need a recipe from the book (because we are not up to those yet). While sipping your coffee with cream, make two to three eggs any style. You can have grated cheese with them if you want. Add either a side of nonstarchy veggies like spinach or peppers or mushrooms sautéed in butter or a breakfast meat like bacon or sausage. If you like a bigger breakfast, feel free to add ½ cup berries. Feels nothing like dieting, right? Told ya.

FP MEALS (FUEL PULL MEALS)

Now back to learning more about the plan. You're not going to put only carbs or fats and hunks of protein on your plate of course. You'll also fill your plate with other foods that match both **S** and **E** fuels. These are nonstarchy veggies, berries, and lean forms of meat and dairy. On THM, we call these sorts of foods Fuel Pulls (**FP**) because they don't offer your body ample fuels of fats or carbs; you're literally pulling those fuels out. Just like your khaki skirt or pants, these Fuel Pull foods match every meal, whether it be an **S** or an **E**. Adding them to any meal does not result in that head-on collision of fats (**S**) and carbs (**E**) together, which causes weight gain for most people.

What are nonstarchy veggies? Thankfully these include pretty much all veggies except white potatoes, sweet potatoes, corn, parsnips, rutabaga, and carrots (in large amounts). That leaves you with literally hundreds of options. These veggies are a huge part of this plan. We predict you'll eat more veggies than you ever have before and you'll eat them in succulent ways, such as broccoli tossed with butter and Mineral Salt or asparagus roasted with garlic and coconut oil . . . delish!

Did you know that meat contains all essential vitamins except vitamin C? Leafy greens are chock-full of vitamin C, so they are perfect to pair with any meal that contains meat for optimum nutrition.

SIMPLE START TIP

Another question to ask yourself daily is, "Where are my greens?"

Not every single meal needs greens. You don't have to have them with oatmeal in the morning of course, but so many meals are made healthier and "Trimminger" with greens. It is even a great idea to sometimes throw some of your dinner meals over a plate of leafy greens. For example, look at Taco Pie (page 119). It is rich and cheesy and a family favorite. You don't have to be afraid of rich foods like this on plan, but you will find the best balance with these sorts of meals by pairing them with veggies. Put a big pile of greens on your dinner plate, then put your pie over top. You'll fill up more and detox your body while you eat. The more you do this little trick, the more you will trim!

If you are not much of a salad eater, it might be because you've been trying to choke salads down in dry and boring ways. We celebrate salads and make them beyond appealing. Try Ranch Hand Taco Salad (page 200) or Ten-Minute Chinese Chicken Salad (page 199). If you're still salad leery, we have lots of yummy ways to hide greens in your foods. We even eat them in cake and you'd never know. (Check out the Trimtastic cakes starting on page 388.) So don't throw down the book yet if you think we're forcing you to become a salad cruncher . . . you can do the plan in your own unique way and baby-step your way into salad loving somewhere in the future.

Fuel Pulls can be part of your meal or snack or be a full meal sometimes, too. They will still always be protein-centered of course, but you'll keep both fats and carbs lower. Essentially, they are both low-carb and low-fat. While **FP** meals are ultra-weight-loss-friendly, they should not be overdone. They are much lower in calories than **S** and **E** meals (since they contain very little carbs or fats) and you don't want your body to adjust to a too-low-calorie state and shut down your metabolism. Allow **FP** meals to help rather than harm you. Sure, you can have a Mocha Secret Big Boy (page 479), which is a **FP**, a few times a week as your breakfast or lunch, but don't eat more full **FP** meals than **S** and **E** meals. They are fantastic options for snacks and desserts, though. Check out the food lists (see page 540) for foods that fit into **FP** meals.

PROTEIN'S LEADERSHIP ROLE

Protein anchors all the three meal types (**S**, **E**, and **FP**) we just mentioned. Let's break these meals down into Simple Start bites and look at how protein leads every charge in each of them.

SIMPLE START BREAKDOWN:

S = Lean or fatty Protein + FATS + nonstarchy veggies

(this is a lower-carb meal)

E = Lean Protein only + CARBS + nonstarchy veggies

(this is a lower-fat meal, although not fat-free)

FP = Lean Protein only + nonstarchy veggies or berries

(this is both a lower-carb and lower-fat meal)

We know . . . at first this feels like you are learning a new language, but what feels confusing at first will soon become second nature! Let's do another little summary of what we have learned so far to help:

- You're ditching sugar and white flour and taking a time-out with white taters

- You're eating both fats and carbs but not in the same meal

- **S** meals are your fats meals. **E** meals are your carb meals. **FP**'s match everything.

- Protein anchors your meals

JUGGLE YOUR MEALS

There is no set order for eating **S** or **E** meals. You will change them up throughout the week, however you wish. This is called freestyling. You don't need to eat an **S** then an **E** then an **S** and so forth. Start tuning in to what your body is telling you. Need a filling, hearty meal to help curb sugar cravings? Go with an **S** meal or a couple in a row. Dragging and need some more energy? Go with an **E** for a meal or two. You can do a whole day of **S** meals if you want, or even two days, but that is about the limit for staying with one fuel only. After that, add some healthy-carb **E** meals; your body needs them. The main thing to keep in mind is that you don't stay with just one fuel. You can do more **S** meals than **E** meals, but be sure to include at least five **E** meals per week (with some **E** snacks, too). Many successful Trim Healthy Mamas include one **E** meal per day.

Fuel your body with a snack or a meal every three to four hours. Of course life is not perfect . . . on some days, life will get in the way and you won't get to eat anything for five or six hours. You're forgiven, but generally try not to go longer than four hours without some protein so your body does not fall into a catabolic state and break down your muscle.

Did you notice that "three-to-four-hour" range? We didn't say "have a few bites of something every thirty minutes to one hour." Constantly nibbling is not a wise habit. You might think you are only having a "little" or a "bite," but it is interfering with your body's natural rhythm of taking in fuel and then burning that fuel, which is key to you being a healthy weight.

If you are changing from an **S** to an **E** meal, you need to leave two and a half to three hours between those different fuels of carbs and fats. That length of time is needed so the carbs in an **E** meal won't be digested with the fats in an **S** meal and inhibit weight loss. **FP** snacks are great when the timing between meals doesn't work out perfectly for you. Perhaps you have to run errands. You come home starving, it has been four hours since your last meal, and you are less than two hours away from dinner. You are HANGRY and need to eat! A cup of Greek yogurt with some berries is perfect, and since it is **FP** it won't interfere with your next meal, whether that be **S** or **E**.

Your afternoon snack is very important to help avoid that afternoon crash, keep your metabolism revved, and stop you from making all sorts of crazy, off-plan choices because you are so ravenous. Your afternoon snack is not optional . . . have it! If you eat breakfast very early in the morning, you may also want to include a midmorning snack. But some of us are later breakfast eaters so not everyone on plan eats a morning snack. Midmorning snacks are optional.

CONGRATULATIONS!

You just learned the basics of weight loss with THM.

SIMPLE START ASSIGNMENT 2: Make your first **E** lunch. You don't even have to use a recipe from the book (since we are not up to those yet). Make a sandwich with two pieces of sprouted whole-grain bread.* Include lean turkey, mustard, lettuce, and a very thin smear of mayo (or in place of the mayo use a wedge of Light Laughing Cow cheese or some 0% Greek yogurt). Enjoy a side of fruit (1 cup of fresh cherries or a piece of cantaloupe) and to fill up further, have ½ cup 1% cottage cheese or chocolate milk made with unsweetened almond milk blended with 1 teaspoon unsweetened cocoa and a stevia-based sweetener to taste.

*If you are gluten-free, try Wonderful White Blender Bread (page 242).

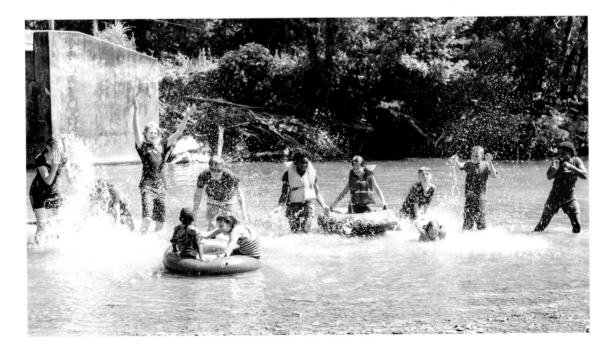

NOW GET STARTED!

You can start slowly by just trying breakfasts for a week. Go to the Breakfast chapter (page 325) and try different **S** or **E** breakfasts to help you get your feet wet. Or if you love a big smoothie or shake for breakfast, check out the Shakes and Smoothies chapter (page 468). Muffins are another delicious breakfast option. Check out the Muffins chapter (page 362). Or yes, even cake can be a breakfast on THM (page 372). Bless yourself with cake and coffee for breakfast with no guilt! Once you feel like you have a handle on breakfasts, work your way up to lunches, then dinners. Take your time, little by little, no pressure from us to get this perfect within your first month.

If you are the "jump in full force" person, that's okay, too. You can start making all your meals either **S** or **E** with the occasional **FP** thrown in if you want. Just know you are going to make some mistakes as you start, so don't let that throw you off and defeat you. Make use of the recipes here (or from *Trim Healthy Mama Cookbook*), but you probably have some favorite family recipes that you can already use for this lifestyle.

As you start, don't try to get all diet-y and eat less. Fill up until you are satisfied. This satisfaction will help you beat the sugar monster! Don't stuff yourself, but eat. You'll be surprised at how protein-centered meals leave you feeling complete. We know life is fast paced but try to slow down, sit down (if possible), and savor your meals. Eating too fast can cause a release of your stess hormone cortisol, which works against weight loss. Eating more slowly lowers cortisol. But even if you don't lose weight in your first month or so, you'll be getting your blood sugar into line. Wise portion sizes are different for everyone and you will learn to tune in and trust your body as you mature into this lifestyle.

You may go through a detox period at first. Not everyone does, but it hits some hard, especially if you are coming off soda. This may feel like the blahs, with general fatigue and perhaps some headaches. You'll make it through this rough start and feel so much better on the other side. Ditching soda is a big deal but you can do it! Thankfully there are many on-plan sodas and other drinks popping up on the market these days, which can be great replacements. Look for sugar-free drinks sweetened with stevia or erythritol (avoid ones with aspartame or Splenda). Our original all-day sipper drink Good Girl Moonshine (found free on our website or in *Trim Healthy Mama Cookbook*) can help you kick the soda habit. Or try some of the drinks in our Drinks chapter (page 450).

SIMPLE START ASSIGNMENT 3: Try your first THM dinner tonight. You don't even have to make a recipe from this book yet. For an easy **S** supper, how about roasted chicken (you can use rotisserie chicken or any baked, grilled, or roasted chicken without breading or a sugar-based sauce) and steamed broccoli (or another veggie that you like) tossed in butter and seasoned up well with Mineral Salt and black pepper. Add a side salad with a creamy, sugar-free dressing or olive oil and vinegar. You can toss a little cheese on your salad if desired. There are no special ingredients required in this hearty dinner and it is probably not too different from meals you already have. If you get a sweet tooth afterwards, have a couple squares of 85% dark chocolate (since you won't have made any of our desserts in this book yet).

DIFFERENT NEEDS IN YOUR FAMILY

Now let's get to the bigger picture of the plan and see how it can work for every member of your family. There's more to health than a number on the scale or a dress size. Some members in your family may not have weight to lose, or perhaps they are an intense athlete. Or you may be pregnant or nursing. We have two other meal types that cover these issues. They are Crossovers (**XO**) and S Helpers (**SH**).

XO–Crossovers put **S** and **E** back together again. They merge the gentle carbs from **E** meals with the healthy fats from **S** meals and of course are always centered on protein. Growing children (without weight issues) or high-metabolism, "skinny type" adults don't need to be separating fats and carbs or they will lose weight, so **XO**'s are the blood sugar friendly answer. Pregnant and nursing women also have higher metabolic needs, as do those who do serious, intense exercise for long periods of time. (Check out *Trim Healthy Mama Plan* for lots more in-depth info on how to do the plan while pregnant or nursing.) Crossovers are also used along with **S** and **E** meals for those who are at goal weight to ensure they don't get too skinny. They are the perfect solution for weight-loss maintenance.

As you first start your Trim Healthy journey, you may eat some accidental Crossovers. Don't worry about that. Even though we tell you to separate your carbs and fats for weight loss, Crossovers are still healthy meals and are an integral part of the plan as your journey progresses. Having a Crossover or two here and there when you start sure won't harm anything.

SH–S Helpers are the final meal type on plan. Most adults don't have to worry about this type of meal as they are starting out (you won't see any recipes marked this way in this cookbook), but understanding the S Helper can be useful for different seasons of life. Remember **S** meals use fat and have minimal carbs aside from veggies or some berries? **SH** meals bring in a few more carbs but not as many as a full-blown Crossover. For example, a regular **S** meal might be a couple of fried eggs and some breakfast sausage. An **SH** meal would include a piece of sprouted-grain toast; by contrast, a Crossover would include two pieces of toast. S Helpers are great for pregnant women struggling with gestational diabetes and are a wonderful and gentle approach for children who need to drop weight. If you want to learn more details about S Helpers, see page 542 in the appendix.

MAKE THIS WORK FOR YOUR FAMILY

You won't have to become a short-order cook and make completely different meals for every member in your family. While you may sometimes prefer to have your own quick "alone" lunch or breakfast or dinner (find those in the Hangry Meals chapter on page 293), the evening meal is usually the perfect time to nourish the whole family at your Trim Healthy Table. The core protein part of the meal will be the same for everyone; it is only the edges that will differ according to the needs of each person. If you have an **S** meal for dinner, you will just provide a healthy-carb option side for your children to turn their meal into a Crossover. If you have an **E** dinner, you will simply provide a healthy fat for your children so they can have a Crossover. Very simple. We give Crossover ideas for every family dinner recipe in this book, but you can choose your own, too.

CHILDREN WITH WEIGHT ISSUES

If you have a child with excess weight, it's best not to make their health journey all about the scale. Let them know you'll be getting healthy together as a family. Some growing children can make great progress shedding excess weight just by eating Crossovers alone. Simply getting all the sugar, soda, and whites out of their meals does wonders without the need to focus exclusively on **S** or **E** meals (of course they don't have to be perfect, and some sugar may slip in now and then). Other children may need to incorporate a nice mixture of pure **S** and **E** meals along with some Crossovers and some S Helpers in order to find their Trim. All children are different, so there is no set amount of **S** and **E** meals versus Crossovers they should eat to lose weight, but we don't ever see a reason why any child should be completely deprived of Crossovers while he or she is growing. Growing children have higher metabolic needs, and the combination of both gentle carbs and good fats in some meals will still be important.

While we urge you not to be impatient with your own weight-loss journey, we double-urge you not to be in a rush for your child to shed pounds. Place the focus on healthy, protein-centered meals and getting rid of the sugar, then the weight will take care of itself in its own good time. Please don't allow your child to get into a daily weighing habit (that is not good for you, either).

GUYS ON PLAN

Men usually need bigger portions than us Mamas do, even if they need to lose weight. Men have more natural muscle, so their metabolisms are naturally faster. Trim Healthy Daddies (or Trim Healthy Dudes . . . younger guys) will need to enjoy heartier servings of **S** and **E** meals. They can even usually eat more Crossovers than we women can and still lose weight, too. Doesn't sound fair but it's the way it goes. If you are a Trim Healthy Mama and want your man on board, entice him to the table with meals like Taco Cornbread Bake (page 139) or Meatball Casserole (page 128). Don't get stingy with portions and he won't feel a bit sorry for himself.

SIMPLE OR NOT . . . YOUR CHOICE!

You can make your Trim Healthy journey as simple or as involved as you want it to be. You don't have to use any special ingredients or you can enjoy plenty of them . . . all up to you (more on that on pages 38 to 45). We have alternatives for most special ingredients listed in the recipes. Look for the NSI label. Start with those recipes as you get your feet wet.

If you start getting overwhelmed, take a deep breath and regroup. **All you really need to do is start separating your carbs and fats and ask yourself, "Where's my protein?"** Don't make it more complicated than it is.

The same applies when you are eating out. It is so easy to stay on plan. Even most fast-food burger joints are accommodating the Trim Healthy crowd these days. Ask for your favorite burger to be bunless. They'll wrap it in lettuce leaves and it is an absolutely delicious **S**. Grab a side salad for extra greens and you're set. Have salmon, chicken, or steak at a sit-down restaurant and instead of having the starchy mac and cheese, baked potato, or fries, ask for steamed broccoli or other nonstarchy veggies of your choice tossed in butter.

Want menu plans? Our trimhealthymembership.com site has a custom menu builder that takes the recipes you've saved from the database and spits out a menu and shopping list for you. We also have lots of premade menus to give you ideas, or you can find many premade menus on THM blogger sites. But you don't have to turn into Mrs. Menu Maker, either. Some of us don't follow menus and just wing it. Be who you are and don't force another sort of personality onto your own. You sure don't have to join our member site or buy our products to be successful. All you really need is the knowledge to do the plan and any old grocery store.

Now turn to the next page for the simple Trim Healthy Breakdown.

TRIM HEALTHY BREAKDOWN

- Always ask yourself, "Where's my protein?"

- Eat every three to four hours

- Choose from your two main meals: **S** for fats, **E** for carbs (don't mix 'em for weight loss)

- **FP**'s round out your plate and make sure you eat your veggies (you can also eat some full **FP** meals, but don't overdo and stall your metabolism)

- Children, pregnant and nursing Mamas, and those at goal weight need some Crossovers

- See the **S**, **E**, **FP**, **XO**, and **SH** food lists (beginning on page 536) to help you out

- Done!

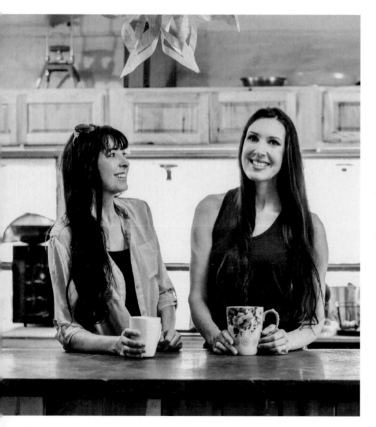

You're all set. Don't forget our Facebook groups for support and our weekly Trim Healthy Podcast for encouragement. Or you can go to trimhealthymembership.com for a printout of this breakdown along with printables of the food lists and lots of other aids, including heaps of cooking and question-and-answer videos from us. If you feel like you simply can't do this alone and need a total hand hold, you can find a certified Trim Healthy Coach at www.trimhealthy mama.com who can help you with meals, menus, tips, encouragement, and whatever else it is you feel you need to get you firmly on your feet.

You Need to Know This Stuff!

SERVING SIZES

There are two main recipe sizes in this book: large family serve and single serve. If any recipe yields a different amount than these two main sizes . . . it will be noted.

FAMILY SERVE (FEEDS 6 TO 8 HUNGRY PEOPLE)–We have large families so we need to make at least this much. Serene actually makes a double large serving for her huge crowd. If your family is smaller (or if you're single), simply cut the recipe in half or a third. Or make the full amount and freeze what you don't need for easy future meals.

SINGLE SERVE–These are our Hangry Meals, which of course means Hungry/Angry . . . HAVE TO EAT NOW!!! Sometimes you just want a quick-to-make, single-serve lunch or dinner. We've got you covered. (There are also plenty of breakfast and sweet treat single serves.)

DON'T MISS THE ABBREVIATIONS

You'll notice the letters **NSI** or **DF** at the tops of the recipes, followed by more information at the ends of the recipes, if needed.

NSI STANDS FOR NO SPECIAL INGREDIENTS. If there are special THM brand ingredients that you'd rather not use, that's fine. We almost always try to offer ways for you to make the recipe without them. Please note that more and more stores will be carrying the Trim Healthy brand in future months and years so what we mark as special now, may not be in the near future.

DF STANDS FOR DAIRY-FREE. There are lots of families following this plan with sensitivities and allergies, so sprinkling in plenty of DF recipes is important to us. Also, dairy balance is important for success on plan. While dairy can be a fantastic and, yes, trimming part of the plan, you don't want to include pasteurized dairy at every single meal, even if you are not intolerant. It can get to be too much of a good thing and cause weight loss stalls for some.

We don't use **GF** (gluten-free) as a label since almost all our recipes are naturally gluten-free.

WHAT IS A DOONK?–You'll notice some of our recipes calling for a doonk of pure stevia extract. A doonk is the name Serene came up with for the tiny ⅟₃₂ teaspoon measurement. You get a doonk spoon in your packet of THM Pure Stevia Extract or you can purchase our butterfly measuring spoons that have a stainless-steel doonk spoon attached. Sometimes you can find other measuring spoon sets that have them, too, using names like "smidgen," so once again, if you don't want to buy our brand, we'll get over it.

KITCHEN TOOLS

You can start today if you have a pot and a skillet and a kitchen knife. But as you continue making close friends with this book, you'll notice we use several THM tools over and over again. Each one needs its own little write-up.

BLENDER–The more powerful the better. You can get by with any ol' cheapo blender (we did for years when we were strapped for pennies), but the best, creamiest, and quickest results come from high-powered blenders, especially when it comes to blending okra.

HAND BLENDER–Not crucial but very helpful. They are only about 12 to 15 bucks at places like Walmart or Target.

FOOD PROCESSOR–You don't have to shell out a lot of money for one, but it will get a bunch of use. Even Goodwill finds usually work well.

CROCKPOT–This is a sanity saver. Come home to a ready dinner. 'Nuff said.

ELECTRIC PRESSURE COOKER–While not necessary for the plan, lots of Trim Healthy Mamas are loving their Instant Pots (or other brands) and we have included directions in the Crockpot chapter.

TROODLE–This is the THM brand of spiralizer, which turns zucchini into Trimming noodles. You can buy versions similar to the Troodle at some stores. Look soon for our Super Troodle–a battery-operated version for even faster troodling.

GARLIC PRESS–Whenever we call for fresh garlic in recipes, we use the word "minced." Really this is the same as pressed, or crushed; you can interchange those words. You'll want a heavy-duty garlic press, one that you can put unpeeled garlic in and squeeze to get all the good garlic meat out. This makes mincing garlic a quick cinch.

LOAD UP ON . . .

There are three produce ingredients you will want to keep as constants, so load up when you find them! Perhaps, if you are kind, you will leave a bag or two for other Trim Healthy Mamas in your area. (To the Trim Healthy Mamas who shop in Dickson, Tennessee . . . how's about leaving some frozen cauliflower for us! Seems to be a shortage in these parts. We're glad you're getting your veggies in, but if we spy you in the grocery store, keep an eye on your cart 'cause you might just find a bag or two disappearing from it . . .)

FROZEN DICED OKRA (it may be called cut or sliced–same thing)–This is a special, hidden ingredient in many of our recipes. It has incredible slimming and health-promoting powers! You can read all about how this superstar veggie balances your blood sugar, heals your gut lining, and powerfully trims you down in *Trim Healthy Mama Plan* or read more here about how and why the okra craze started on page 478. If you are a gardener, grow lots of okra, then cut, blanch, and freeze.

FROZEN SEASONING BLEND–This is simply a small-cut blend of diced onion, celery, and green or red bell pepper. It makes prep work for recipes far less time consuming. Sometimes it is called seasoning blend on the package, sometimes it is called other names such as onion and pepper blend or recipe starter blend, but it is all the same thing. In some of our recipes we also call for large-cut seasoning blend, which is a similar deal, although it usually doesn't have celery, just larger sliced onions and peppers. Again, it won't be called "large-cut seasoning blend" in grocery stores . . . it might be called pepper and onion mix or fajita mix. Just look for pictures of the veggies on the packet.

If you can't find seasoning blend, no worries, you don't need it; simply dice up a fresh onion and green and/or red bell pepper and throw it into the recipe. Or cut up a bunch of your own seasoning blend ahead of time and freeze.

FROZEN CAULIFLOWER FLORETS AND FROZEN CAULIFLOWER RICE–These are frequent ingredients in our recipes and thankfully cauliflower is usually inexpensive. If you can't find frozen cauliflower rice you can make your own by processing fresh cauliflower in your food processor until rice-size, then freezing it in quart-size baggies in batches of 10 to 12 ounces each. Some of our recipes also call for "cauliflower rice medley." This is just "cauli rice" mixed with a few finely chopped carrots and some peas. You can easily make your own version of that, too.

EGGS AND EGG WHITES–While free-range eggs are certainly the best option, don't stress if all you can afford are regular old eggs. All eggs contain beneficial vitamins, minerals, and nutrients. We love the inexpensive eggs from Aldi, as the yolks are golden, and did you notice the scripture when you open your carton of Aldi eggs? Blessed eggs! Can't beat that! Carton egg whites are another handy grocery item; on the THM plan, we often mix whole eggs with egg whites for a lovely balance. However, you can use fresh egg whites if preferred.

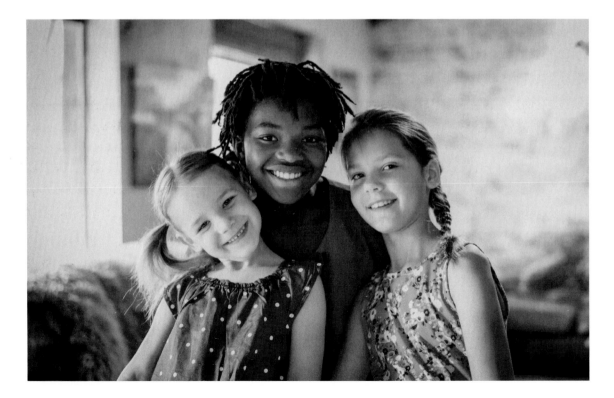

SALT, SEASONINGS, CONDIMENTS, AND EXTRACTS

Before we get into specifics here, we need to mention that when we list ingredients like soy sauce or rice vinegar, it is always best to try and find organic versions to ensure you are not getting a bottle of GMO. However, some of us care less about all that than others. You certainly don't have to go out and buy all organic condiments. If you can't afford organic, you are still making healthy strides and this is not an "organic only" sort of plan, but if you have a couple extra bucks, organic is preferred. Serene also wants you to know that in her recipes when black pepper is mentioned she uses freshly cracked. Pearl doesn't care about "fresh" or "cracked," so that is all up to you. There is one item we do urge you to find in a raw, unfiltered, and organic form if possible . . . that is apple cider vinegar (ACV). Raw and unfiltered ACV contains many more nutrients than regular apple cider vinegar and can be a huge boon to your health and weight-loss journey. You will sometimes notice the phrase "with the mother" on the label.

MINERAL SALT–This is the salt we use in our recipes because it is helpful rather than harmful to your body. You can read more about its health benefits in *Trim Healthy Mama Plan*. Salt has a reputation for raising blood pressure, but that is because table salt has been refined and devitalized, and natural important minerals such as potassium have been removed. Unrefined salt such as our THM brand of Mineral Salt has roughly 400 percent more potassium than table salt, so it helps protect your blood vessels from sodium imbalance and offers many other health benefits. If you'd rather not buy our brand, look for unrefined, ground versions of gray (Celtic) or pink (Himalayan) salt.

SPICES AND SEASONINGS–These don't just make your food taste great, they are also pure medicine for your body. While organic herbs and spices are always best, just use whatever you can afford, as even nonorganic spices like cumin, turmeric, cayenne, and black pepper and herbs of all kinds bring you benefits. Stock up on the following: dried oregano, cumin, paprika, chili powder, chipotle powder, onion powder, garlic powder, cinnamon, turmeric, Italian seasoning, thyme, cayenne pepper, red pepper flakes, parsley flakes, curry powder, dried minced onion, and your other favorites.

EXTRACTS–We use lots of them in recipes to bring great flavor. We list our new and pure Trim Healthy Natural Burst extracts in our recipes to replace artificial ones, but if you don't care about natural extracts, you can use any extract from your grocery store to make the recipes.

NUTRITIONAL YEAST–This used to be a superspecial ingredient that was hard to find in stores. Now even stores like Walmart have it. We use it in recipes because it has a wonderful cheesy flavor and is full of vitamins and minerals. Just shake it on! We can't eat eggs without it, and our children think popcorn without nutritional yeast is a crime! We offer it on our website because we wanted a version without synthetic B vitamins (most grocery-store versions have synthetic vitamins added). You can use store-bought versions (we did for years), but if you want a more natural form, we now carry it.

WHAT'S WITH THE SPECIAL INGREDIENTS!

Don't freak out thinking you are going to have to spend hundreds of dollars on special ingredients. Yes, you will sometimes see some ingredients listed that you are not used to, but always remember to look for our **NSI** alternatives. After a while though, some of these new ingredients won't seem so special anymore. They will be your new norm, and your old norm of white flour, packaged foods, and boxes of processed, refined foods will seem strange to you.

If you are just starting the plan, you certainly don't have to buy every special item mentioned. Start making the **NSI** recipes first, then buy a couple special items at a time, only when you are ready. And please know that if you are a newbie just starting on the plan . . . you are blessed! It used to be rare for stores to carry some of the items we urged people to try. Now many (like nutritional yeast or apple cider vinegar with the mother) are easy to find. Feel free to join our official THM No Special Ingredients Facebook group for more encouragement and ideas. Be sure to listen to Trim Healthy Podcast 17 about our top 10 least expensive foods to make you trim and healthy.

Below is a very brief write-up on some ingredients that might stump you at first. They can boost your health and help make incredible recipes but there are ways around them. If you have a sweet tooth, the first special item you'll want to get is a sweetener.

STEVIA SWEETENERS–We list Trim Healthy sweeteners in our recipes, but you can use any other brand from your grocery store, including monk fruit extract sweeteners. Just be sure not to use anything that has maltodextrin, dextrin, sugar, or maltitol as a listed ingredient. Also, please know that all stevia sweeteners on the market are not the same, and often ingredient lists don't give the full picture. Many stevia products lining grocery shelves have been through an "enzyme modified" process. This means maltodextrin was used in the processing. Yes, even if these sweeteners are labeled "organic," many have still been processed this way. While maltodextrin won't be listed on the actual ingredient list, it was used to obtain the final result.

This modified stevia is far less expensive for companies to buy. We have had multiple opportunities to import this type of stevia but have always turned it down, as it doesn't meet the high standards our brand sets. You can use other brands processed this way—we don't call them "off plan," but we just want you to know what you may be getting. If our sweeteners seem slightly higher in price, it is because quality is more important to us. Feel free to go to our website, www.trimhealthy mama.com, and find our sweetener chart to see how to convert different sweeteners for our recipes.

We use three different sweeteners: Gentle Sweet, Super Sweet Blend, and Pure Stevia Extract Powder. You can purchase just one to start and that would likely be Gentle Sweet, as it tastes the most like sugar to newbies starting on the plan. (We also have a new xylitol-free Gentle Sweet for families worried about their doggies snatching their treats.) But eventually having some Super Sweet Blend and Pure Stevia Extract on hand can save your budget (a tiny, one-ounce bag of extract will likely last you six months). Using Super Sweet Blend or the extract in recipes where they shine (like drinks, smoothies, and shakes) can save you from going through too much Gentle Sweet, as they are much sweeter and it takes only a little to get 'er done.

There are a rare few people who cannot use stevia due to allergies or who simply choose not to. If this is you, you can use erythritol and xylitol alone without added stevia or a monk fruit extract blend. Or if you don't have much of a sweet tooth and don't care to have sweet treats daily, you can use raw honey or coconut sugar for a rare treat, or simply enjoy wonderful fruit for daily sweetness! Just please know that using honey or coconut sugar on a daily basis can interfere with weight loss, as these sweeteners have a far greater impact on your blood sugar (they are acceptable options for growing children without weight issues, though).

TRIM HEALTHY MAMA BAKING BLEND—If it frustrates you to see us list THM Baking Blend in our recipes . . . hear us out. Our Mamas begged us to create an all-purpose flour blend since many of our early baked goods recipes required the combination of different flours to get the right texture and taste. Our readers wanted the ease of having a prepackaged blend, with all the work done for them. Back in the "very early days" of Trim Healthy Mama, the main baking flour options were either almond flour or flax meal. Almond flour was the favorite, but it is simply ground nuts. While nuts are on plan, they are best used in moderation, so constantly eating almonds in the form of almond flour can work against your weight-loss goals. We don't have to count calories but we shouldn't abuse them, either! Too much almond flour can become calorie abuse; it is like pouring cups of almonds down your throat! Also, almond flour is expensive. Generally it will cost you quite a bit more than our Baking Blend.

We worked for months, with much trial and error, to put together the flours that would make the best all-purpose, Fuel Pull baking flour. It had to be gluten-free, superfood protein-rich, low in carbs and fat, not too calorie heavy, and kind to blood sugar. We finally nailed it, released it to the

Trim Healthy Mama community, and it created a storm! Mamas got to eat fluffy cake again . . . they got to make breaded chicken again . . . they wanted more and more.

At first, we simply could not keep up with demand and there were terrible shortages for months on end (growing pains for our young business, which we have felt compelled to do debt-free). So some people came up with their own copycat baking mix recipes while they waited for us to get our act in gear. We did eventually get our act in gear and can now supply demand, but if you don't want to purchase THM Baking Blend you can google some of those copycat recipes online. We have heard back from many, though, that making your own version is not necessarily less expensive. Our blend uses super high-quality items like grass-fed collagen, and that is not cheap anywhere! But we want you to be able to make this plan work within your own budget and lifestyle, no matter how tight. So if you are very strapped financially, the simplest and least expensive substitute is this frugal flour option:

FRUGAL FLOUR–MIX TOGETHER EQUAL PARTS GOLDEN FLAX MEAL AND COCONUT FLOUR. Those two flours are easily and rather inexpensively found at most grocery stores, and this blend can be used for many recipes where we call for THM Baking Blend. The combination is not **FP** like our Baking Blend is. It is an **S**. This blend won't contain as much protein, be quite as smooth, or make for quite as fluffy a crumb in baked goods, but it can suffice. If you don't want to use coconut flour, you can mix the flax meal with equal parts oat fiber, which is also very inexpensive but is usually found only online.

The following is more expensive, so not really a frugal option, but some people like this mix better, and it is convenient because most grocery stores have the following three ingredients these days.

MIX TOGETHER EQUAL PARTS GOLDEN FLAX MEAL, ALMOND FLOUR, AND COCONUT FLOUR. Once again, be mindful this is an **S** blend not an **FP** blend, but it is a bit lighter than straight almond flour and can work for many recipes such as our cakes. (If you are on a tight budget, though, this one makes less sense because of the price of almond flour.)

COLLAGEN AND GELATIN–You'll see Just Gelatin and Integral Collagen mentioned in some of our recipes. Both are forms of gelatin, but one gels and thickens (Just Gelatin) and the other doesn't (Integral Collagen). While they shine in different ways to boost health, they are both fantastic sources of fat-busting protein. They contain high amounts of the amino acid glycine, which is sadly lacking in our modern culture due to a lack of bones and skin in meat items. Glycine helps your body shed fat more powerfully than other amino acids, but it also performs a host of other beneficial things.

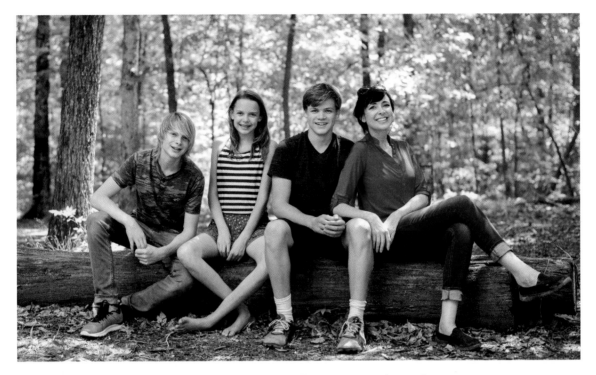

Gelatin and collagen bring healing to the lining of your intestinal tract, boost your immune system, aid healthy hair growth, smooth your skin, detoxify your liver, soothe anxiety, strengthen bones, remineralize teeth, help prevent heart disease, and help reduce cellulite . . . just for a start.

We don't have room or time to list all of collagen's and gelatin's benefits. But more important, they also make wonderful creamy recipes or thicken things up without the need for fattening starches. The Trim Healthy brand of collagen and gelatin are from pure, grass-fed sources. If you want to use grocery store unflavored gelatin in your recipes, you can, just know that it is from pork, not a pure grass-fed source. You can find collagen online, but please use a grass-fed source for health's sake. (You can certainly just make your own bone stock at home to receive the same glycine benefits . . . these powders are just more convenient.)

(You'll notice quite a few of our soup recipes call for an optional 3 to 4 tablespoons of gelatin or collagen added with the broth or water. Simply add either powder to the pot right after adding broth or water, then stir—the powder will dissolve well once the soup starts heating. Adding either of these powders will turn your store-bought broth into more of a nutritious bone stock and will amp up protein. These additions help bring more glycine to your meal and balance the amino acid profile of the recipe. If you are on a tight budget, however, you don't have to include them.)

BAOBAB BOOST POWDER—This powder is like a daily "multivitamin" that is 100 percent real food. We call it Baobab Boost, because this amazing fruit from the baobab tree boosts your nutrition in every area. Its citrusy tasting dried flesh has five times the fiber of oats, and get this . . . it has the highest amounts of disease-fighting antioxidants of all foods! Nothing beats it. That means eight times the antioxidant levels of açai berries and more than both blueberries and pomegranates combined! It has more than twice the calcium of milk, double the magnesium and iron of spinach, and is loaded with six times the amount of potassium than bananas. Mind-blowing stuff! Once we learned about its merits, we started using it in as many recipes as we could.

But now for the most important news . . . baobab boasts one of the highest vitamin C contents of foods on this planet. It has ten times the amount of oranges! Vitamin C is crucial when eating a protein-centered diet. We've shared with you how this plan is anchored around protein for ultimate blood sugar control. We add glycine-rich gelatin and collagen to bring a beautiful, safe balance to your protein intake. Those gelatin powders (or homemade bone stock) ensure your body does not become imbalanced with certain amino acids (such as methionine), which when unchecked can be harmful. They also heal, repair, and beautify your body. But they can do none of this protective, healing work without high levels of vitamin C.

Your body cannot produce vitamin C. It must get it from your foods. While a severe vitamin C deficiency, which would result in scurvy, is uncommon these days, very few Americans have optimal levels of vitamin C according to a study published in August 2009 in the *American Journal of Clinical Nutrition*. It takes high levels of vitamin C to synthesize proper collagen production. As we age, our bodies are able to retain less and less vitamin C according to a study published in 2012 in Japan's *Journal of Nutritional Science and Vitaminology*. We need to increase our intake!

Vitamin C is crucial for the health of your adrenals and it is a HUGE game changer when it comes to losing weight. Vitamin C–depleted people are resistant to fat loss. According to a study published in a June 2005 issue of *Journal of the American College of Nutrition*, those with adequate vitamin C levels oxidize 30 percent more fat during exercise than individuals with low levels. Plainly put, vitamin C helps prevent weight gain and makes it easier to lose weight.

Another way baobab helps with weight loss is it helps you better digest starches and lowers glycemic response to your meals. A study published in the journal *Nutrition Research* found that baking baobab extract into white bread significantly reduced the glycemic response in participants compared with those who had the bread without it. Meals that trigger a lower glycemic response promote weight loss by keeping your fat-storing hormone insulin under control.

You are going to love this powder in our recipes (or just mix some with water and drink) and love what it does for your body. If you don't want to buy our brand, we have started to spy baobab powder at some grocery stores lately, so we doubt it will be a special ingredient for much longer. And if you're thinking, why not just supplement with vitamin C powder itself? You can. However, your body absorbs vitamin C much more efficiently when in a whole-food form and some purists don't like ascorbic acid. And to our newbies in case you are feeling overwhelmed . . . you can certainly do the plan without baobab, just be sure to eat lots of the leafy greens and berries we encourage, as those are all high in vitamin C and should always anchor any protein-centered diet. (Note: Due to baobab's high fiber content, some may find they need to start with lower doses and work up to greater amounts as their bodies become accustomed to it.)

PRISTINE WHEY PROTEIN POWDER–If you are a shake and smoothie lover, this stuff will become your best creamy friend. It boosts glutathione production in your body (which enhances your immune system), helps your mood, and aids your slimming process. We use a cross-flow microfiltered whey isolate, which is the most undenatured whey available. If not using our brand, that's okay, but be careful about using a concentrate form (which easily oxidizes) and avoid any harshly processed isolate. Try to find a microfiltered isolate if you can, which is second best to cross-flow microfiltered. Look for carbs no more than 1 gram.

GLUCCIE–That's our nickname for it, short for glucomannan. It is a natural powder derived from the konjac root. It is our starch-free thickener of choice. One bag will last you close to a year, so while it costs around twenty bucks, it is very inexpensive long-term. We thicken up sauces, gravies, smoothies, and puddings with this stuff without adding a calorie or a carb! It powerfully helps your body shed fat (read more about it in *Trim Healthy Mama Plan*). You can sub xanthan gum (easily found at grocery stores) for thickening needs as it is starch-free, too; however, it doesn't boast the same weight-loss benefits.

TRIM HEALTHY NOODLES OR NOT NAUGHTY NOODLES AND RICE–These noodles (or rice) are so weight-loss friendly! They are both made from glucomannan (konjac root) and are used the same way as each other, the only difference being that the Trim Healthy version has a tiny bit of oat flour added so they are a little more "regular noodle" looking and tasting. Konjac noodles have been used in Asian countries for hundreds of years and incredibly are very close to being fat-, carb-, and calorie-free! At first you may find them a bit chewier than normal noodles, but once you start embracing them for what they are and make some of our recipes with them—such as Smoked Sausage Noodle Stir-Fry (page 312) or Sesame Lo Mein (page 71)—you'll wonder how you ever lived life without their yumminess. If you don't want to use our brand, you can sometimes find konjac noodles in grocery stores in the refrigerated section of the produce department, near the

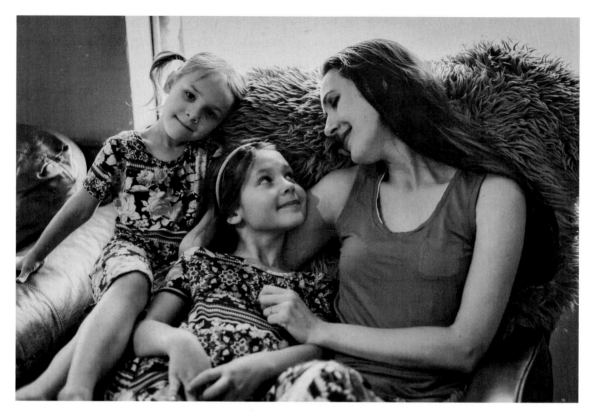

tofu. Just look for konjac as the main ingredient, although sometimes they add potato starch. While not perfect with that included, you can still use them.

PRESSED PEANUT FLOUR—This is simply ground peanuts with a lot of the oils pressed out. Sugar-free natural-style peanut butter is on plan, but you can easily overdo it and head into fat abuse if you heap spoonful after spoonful into your recipes. Peanut flour has all the flavor without the "over-doing it" part, so you can use it in **FP** or **E** recipes. Check out the Incredible Peanut Butter Cookie Muffins (page 371), which are **FP**. We sometimes pair both peanut butter and the peanut flour together in an **S** recipe for a nice balance. If you don't want to buy our brand, find one in grocery stores that is sugar-free and defatted.

WHOLE HUSK PSYLLIUM FLAKES—Not a "rush out and buy straightaway" ingredient, but at some point you may like to make our Wonder Wraps 2 (page 251) or the crust for Butterfly Pizza (page 282) or Beat the Cheat Pizza (page 283). If you don't want to buy our brand, you can find this stuff inexpensively at natural foods stores or online, but don't buy the fine powder. The flakes work better; they are just a much more coarsely ground powder.

SUNFLOWER LECITHIN—This is last on the list of ingredients you may not have heard of before. Once again, don't rush out and buy it when you first start. You can easily do the plan without it. But it helps make sauces, soups, and some smoothies creamier and helps them not separate. Usually we list this as optional in recipes, though if you start making Serene's Trimmy Bisque soups, she wants you to know that the lecithin makes them better (read her rant on page 163). Lecithin has many health benefits, including brain-boosting power, which you can read about in *Trim Healthy Mama Plan*. One bag will last you at least six months, probably more, so it's not an expensive, repeat-buy item.

GET PREPPED

CHICKEN BREAST PREP: Some of our recipes call for precooked chicken breasts (but both white and dark chicken meat can work for S recipes). It is a great idea to take one day each week to prepare a whole bunch of breasts ready for your week. That way you can not only use them for our recipes, but they'll be handy for quick salads and sandwiches, too. Pick any cooking method from below, then dice up your chicken and place in zippy bags. If you didn't get the chance to precook a bunch of chicken and need some quickly for a recipe, the fast-poach or electric pressure cooker methods will be your best options.

FAST-POACH: Add desired number of chicken breasts (fresh or frozen) to a pot of water. Bring to a quick boil, then simmer until tender, 10 to 15 minutes for fresh, 15 to 20 minutes for frozen.

ELECTRIC PRESSURE COOKER: Put desired number of fresh or frozen chicken breasts in the pressure cooker with seasonings of choice. Add 1 to 2 cups water or chicken broth and cook on high pressure for 10 to 15 minutes (or simply press the poultry button). Use natural pressure release.

CROCKPOT: Put desired number of fresh or thawed (if from frozen) chicken breasts in the crockpot seasoned with salt and black pepper. Add ¼ to ½ cup water, cover, and cook on low heat for 4 to 5 hours.

SLOW-BAKE: One of our favorite ways to precook chicken breasts is to bake long and slow. Covering the breasts while they cook is key for tenderness. Place frozen or fresh chicken breasts in a baking dish, sprinkle on a little Mineral Salt and black pepper, cover, and bake at 220°F for 2 to 3 hours, depending on whether frozen or fresh.

DON'T KNOCK 'EM!: And let's not sneer at rotisserie or even canned chicken. Sometimes these items can be lifesavers for Drive-Thru Sue's or Prepackaged Pam's.

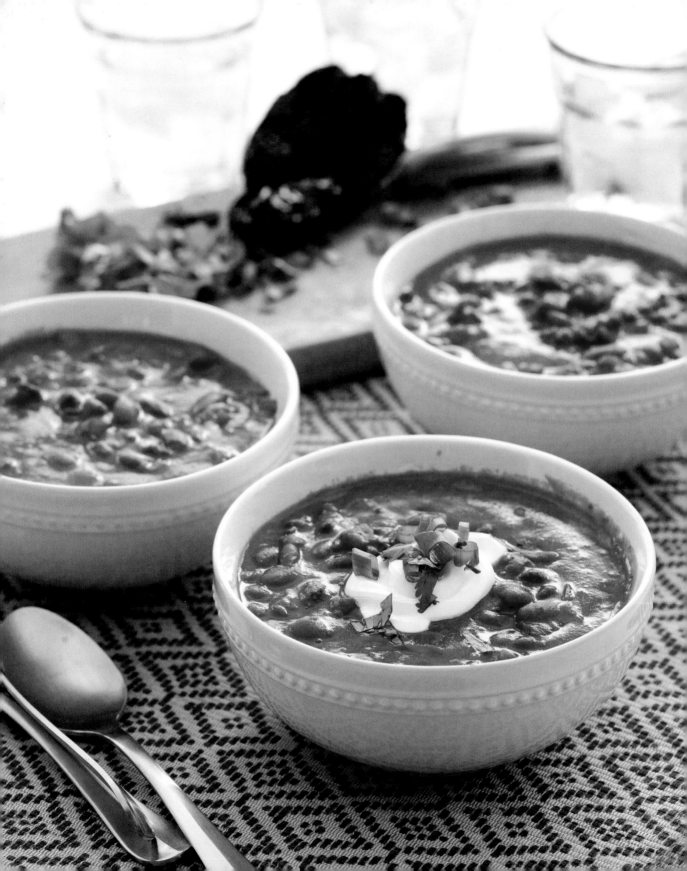

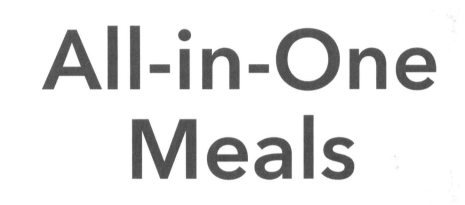

All-in-One Meals

Speedy Skillet Meals

Grab your big skillet and let these speedy, tasty, one-dish meals save your day!

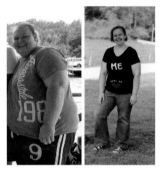

"Take delight in the Lord, and He will give you your heart's desires" (Psalm 37:4). I've been reminded of this scripture so many times lately. When I think about my Trim Healthy Mama journey, this is the scripture for me that describes it well. From one year ago, I've lost 100 pounds on this plan. But being able to say the words "I'm healthy'" are the most important to me. God has given me and continues to give me the desire of my heart. The desire to be healthy. That had been my desire for too many years to count, but a sustainable way to be healthy always seemed to escape me.

Last summer/fall, I was at a very miserable place when my best friend introduced me to Trim Healthy Mama. I had lots of health problems that had plagued me for a long time . . . PCOS (polycystic ovary syndrome), stomach issues, fatigue, etc. My health was declining quickly, and I knew that without a change it wasn't going to lead to anything good. I wanted to be active again, to feel good again. To my amazement, after starting, I started to feel amazing. Six weeks in, I was able to go off the medication for PCOS. My insulin levels are normal again! Several months ago I was able to stop the stomach meds that I've taken for near twenty years! I have more energy than I ever remember having in my life. I'm able to be as active as I want. Recently I've been running again, something I love and have missed. I give God all the glory! I'm humbled and amazed at His faithfulness, His mercy, His grace, and His love that He would continue to allow me to see the desires of my heart come to pass. **–PATRICIA**

(Note–Patricia sent this exciting update to us just before we handed this book to the printers. See the words "Mini Me" on the bottom of the T-shirt of her "now" picture? Patricia: "I'm pregnant!!!! My due date is October 27. I'm continuing THM through my pregnancy; it's just a normal way of life for me now.")

dreamy chicken lazone

S

FAMILY SERVE–FEEDS 6 TO 8 (HALVE IF YOUR FAMILY IS SMALLER, OR MAKE FULL AND FREEZE HALF)

1½ teaspoons Mineral Salt

1 tablespoon chili powder

1 tablespoon onion powder

1 tablespoon garlic powder

2 teaspoons paprika (smoked or regular)

⅛ teaspoon cayenne pepper (optional; add only if you like heat)

2½ pounds chicken tenderloins, thawed if frozen

6 tablespoons (¾ stick) butter

1 cup chicken broth

½ cup heavy cream

½ teaspoon Gluccie*

This sauce is the stuff dreams are made of . . . so flavorful! How can you eat this and lose weight you wonder as you take your first bite? Just trust us and enjoy. This is one of those quick and easy satisfying meals that you can serve up to family or even expected (or unexpected) company. The creamed up flavors will make them think that you spent hours in the kitchen rather than minutes.

1. Mix the salt, chili powder, onion powder, garlic powder, paprika, and cayenne (if using) in a small bowl. Sprinkle half the seasoning over tops of the chicken then turn the tenderloins over and coat the other side.

2. Melt 3 tablespoons of the butter in a large skillet over medium-high heat. Add all the chicken and cook for 6 minutes, turning once.

3. Reduce the heat to medium, add the chicken broth, cream, and the remaining 3 tablespoons butter. Once the butter has melted, move the chicken to one side, sprinkle in the Gluccie a little at a time, and whisk it well into the sauce. Toss the sauce around the skillet and cook for 8 more minutes.

4. Remove the pan from the heat. The sauce will thicken a little more as it cools but it is not supposed to be a thick sauce. Serve the chicken, then spoon more sauce on top.

MAKE A FAMILY MEAL: For the weight-loss plan, this is fabulous over sautéed shredded cabbage (cut into noodles as thin as angel hair pasta), spaghetti squash, or Troodles (page 264). Or have it with any nonstarchy veggie you desire! Add a side salad, and you're set. Be sure to add a healthy carb for growing children or others at Crossover stage, such as steamed potatoes with butter, brown rice, or even buttered sprouted-grain bread.

* FOR NSI: SUB XANTHAN GUM FOR THE GLUCCIE.

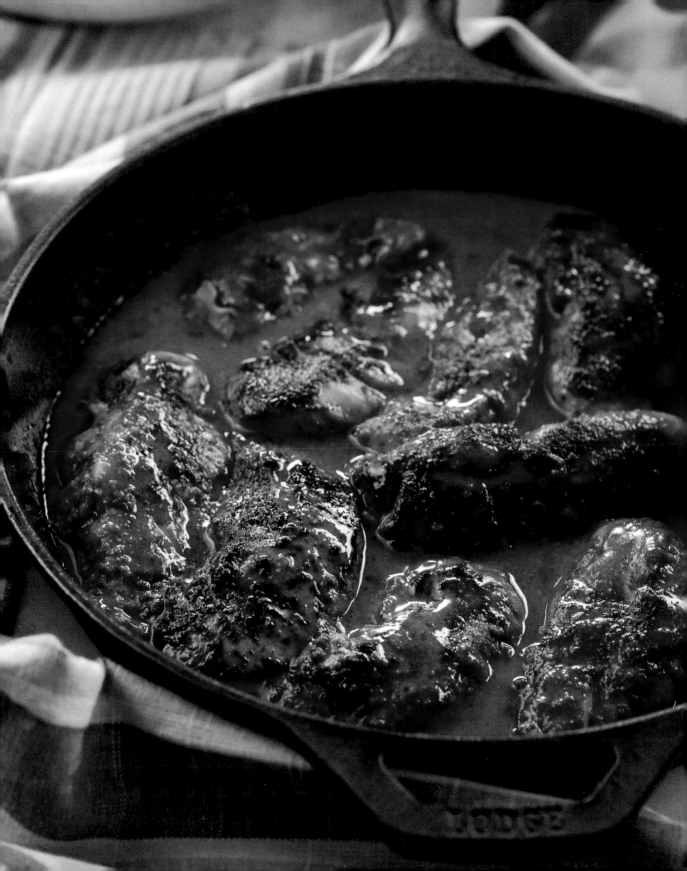

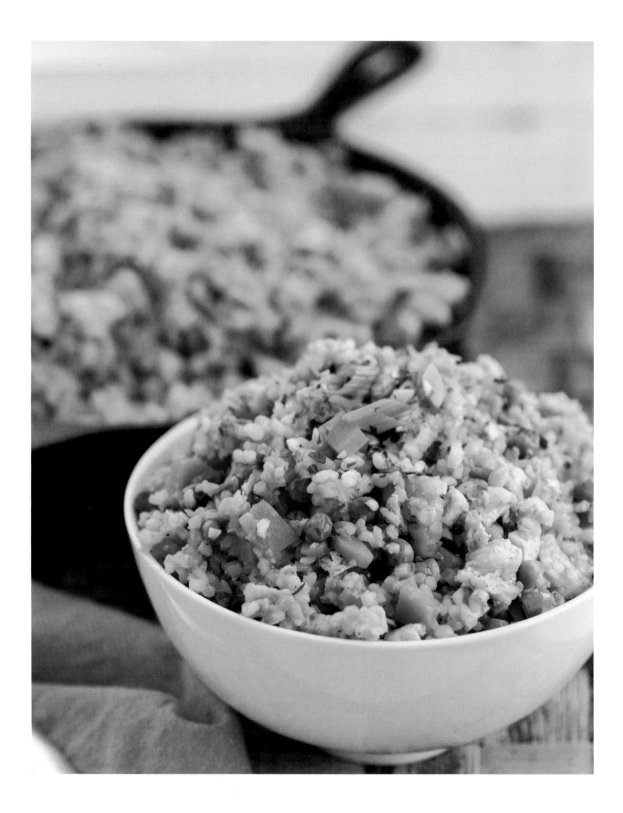

chicken fried double rice

(E)

Coconut oil cooking spray

1½ cups egg whites (carton or fresh)

Mineral Salt and black pepper

Nutritional Yeast (optional)

2 tablespoons toasted sesame oil

1 cup frozen peas

2 carrots, finely chopped

1 (12- to 16-ounce) bag frozen riced cauliflower (see page 263 for making your own)

6 to 8 green onions, finely diced

3 or 4 garlic cloves, minced

1½ pounds boneless, skinless chicken breasts (thawed if frozen), cut into ¼-inch pieces (easily done with kitchen scissors)

3½ to 4 cups cooked brown rice

¼ to ⅓ cup soy sauce

Red pepper flakes to taste (optional)

This is a hearty E meal with a secret, disguised veggie ingredient your children won't know they are eating. It is the perfect way to eat fried rice if you have any blood sugar issues because cauli rice is tossed with regular brown rice for double the rice! This makes you feel as if you have a lot of hearty rice on your plate, but almost half of it is a veggie not a grain. Mixing in cauli rice like this helps lower the impact of carbs on the amount of insulin your body has to make. Nobody is the wiser . . . just healthier!

1. Heat a large skillet over medium-high heat and spray with coconut oil. Pour the egg whites into the pan and season with a sprinkle of salt, pepper, and nutritional yeast (if using). Let the egg whites sit for a couple minutes until they set. Once set, turn the whites over, then chop into pieces. Remove from the skillet and set aside.

2. Increase the heat under the skillet to high and add 1 tablespoon of the sesame oil. Add the peas, carrots, cauli rice, green onions, and garlic. Season with a sprinkle of salt and pepper and toss in the hot oil for 3 to 4 minutes.

3. Push all the veggies to one side of the pan, add the remaining 1 tablespoon sesame oil to the other side of the pan, and add the chicken pieces. Sprinkle lightly with salt and pepper and cook without stirring for 2 minutes, then flip and allow to cook on the other side for another 1 to 2 minutes.

4. Return the egg whites to the skillet and add the brown rice and soy sauce. Reduce the heat to medium and toss all the ingredients for another couple minutes. Taste and add red pepper flakes (if using) and more seasonings if desired to "own it."

MAKE A FAMILY MEAL: For the weight-loss plan, this is fantastic all on its own in a bowl. Or add a side salad with a lean, E-friendly dressing to get even more veggies in. Growing children need a fat to make this a Crossover. That's easy—they can simply use a fattier dressing and grated cheese on their salad or a pat of butter or more sesame oil in their fried rice.

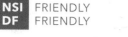
deconstructed stuffed peppers

S

FAMILY SERVE—FEEDS 6 TO 8 (HALVE IF YOUR FAMILY IS SMALLER; ONLY MAKE IN FULL AND FREEZE EXTRA IF USING THE CAULI RICE OPTION, AS KONJAC RICE DOES NOT FREEZE WELL)

2 pounds ground beef or venison, thawed if frozen

2 single-serve bags Trim Healthy Rice or Not Naughty Rice,* rinsed well and drained

1 tablespoon Worcestershire sauce

2 tablespoons soy sauce, or
  2 generous squirts Bragg liquid aminos or coconut aminos

1½ teaspoons Mineral Salt

1 teaspoon black pepper

1 teaspoon onion powder

1 teaspoon garlic powder

Cayenne pepper to taste (optional)

2 tablespoons Nutritional Yeast (optional)

3 to 4 green bell peppers, roughly chopped

1 onion, finely chopped (optional; only use if all family members are onion lovers)

1 (14.5-ounce) can diced tomatoes, drained

1 (14-ounce) jar sugar-free pizza sauce (we use Walmart Great Value brand), or 1 batch Perfect Pizza Sauce (page 516)

8 ounces cheddar cheese,* grated

Love stuffed peppers but hate the time they take to prepare? This is a supertasty way to eat them without all the fuss. (Remember to check out the no special ingredient options if you don't have the listed rice. Cauli rice is an easy replacement.)

1. Brown the beef in a large skillet over medium-high heat. Drain off any excess grease, then add the Trim Healthy Rice. Add the Worcestershire sauce, soy sauce, salt, black pepper, onion powder, garlic powder, cayenne (if using), and nutritional yeast (if using). Toss well, increase the heat to high, and cook the rice with the beef for several minutes, tossing frequently.

2. Add the bell peppers and onion (if using) and sauté for another 8 to 10 minutes. Pour in the tomatoes and pizza sauce, toss well, cover, reduce the heat to low, and simmer for another 3 to 4 minutes. Top with the cheddar, cover for another 2 to 3 minutes to melt the cheese, and you are ready to serve.

MAKE A FAMILY MEAL: For the weight-loss plan, enjoy with a side salad with an oil/vinegar or creamy dressing, and if desired a nonstarchy veggie like steamed buttered broccoli. Crossover stage family members need a carb side like brown rice with the meal or perhaps fruit to end the meal.

* FOR NSI: FIND KONJAC NOODLES (SEE PAGE 43) AT YOUR GROCERY STORE AND PULSE TO PROCESS INTO RICE IN A FOOD PROCESSOR, OR USE 1 OR 2 (10- TO 12-OUNCE) BAGS FROZEN RICED CAULIFLOWER.

* FOR DF: SIMPLY OMIT THE CHEDDAR—IT'S STILL FANTASTIC WITHOUT IT.

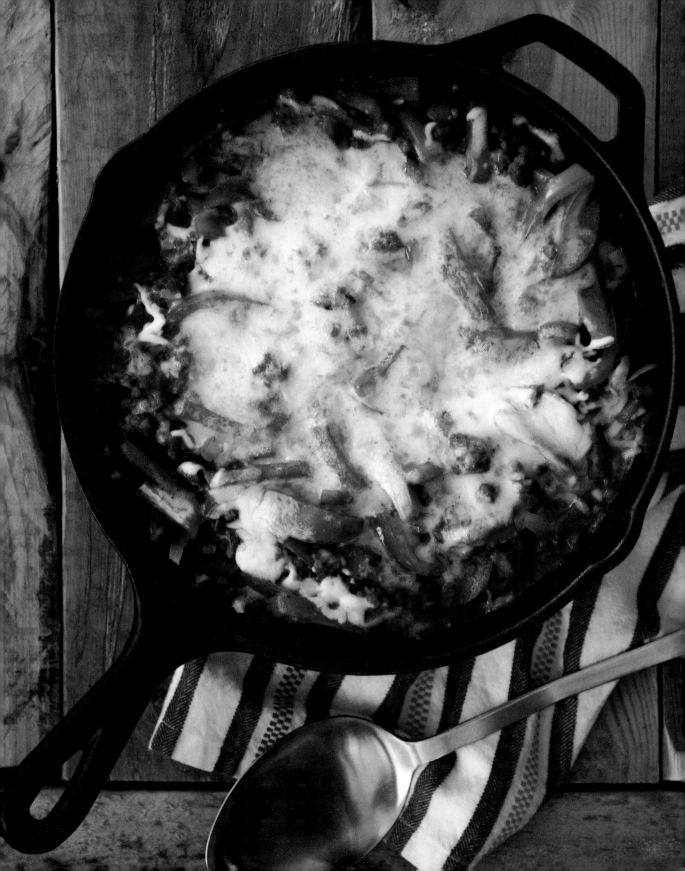

deconstructed fajitas

FP WITH **S** AND **E** OPTIONS

··

FAMILY SERVE—FEEDS 6 TO 8 (HALVE IF YOUR FAMILY IS SMALLER, OR MAKE FULL AND FREEZE HALF)

2 tablespoons coconut oil or butter
(can use more for S)

2 (12-ounce) bags frozen large-cut
seasoning blend (see page 35), or
1 large onion and 2 to 3 green or
red peppers, sliced

4 to 6 cups sliced precooked
chicken breast (can include dark
meat for S)

2 teaspoons chili powder

1 teaspoon onion powder

1 teaspoon ground cumin

¼ teaspoon cayenne pepper
(optional for heat lovers)

1 teaspoon Mineral Salt

1 teaspoon paprika (smoked
or regular)

2 fresh tomatoes, sliced, or
1 (14.5-ounce) can diced,
fire-roasted tomatoes, drained

Lots of cut lettuce (e.g., a couple
hearts of romaine at least)

Greek yogurt* (optional for FP or E)

Sour cream* (optional for S)

Sliced avocado (optional for S)

Grated cheese* (optional for S)

Brown rice or quinoa (optional
for E)

This is such a quick no-brainer for busy nights when you need dinner on the table in ten minutes. We enjoy this on dinner plates over a bunch of cut lettuce, but if you prefer you can stuff into Wonder Wraps 2 (page 251) or low-carb tortillas.

1. Heat a large skillet over medium-high heat and add the coconut oil. Add the seasoning blend or peppers and onions, tossing frequently for a few minutes until they begin to soften. Add the chicken, sprinkle on the chili powder, onion powder, cumin, cayenne (if using), salt, and paprika, and toss with the veggies for a couple more minutes. Add the tomatoes. Cook for 2 to 3 more minutes.

2. Serve on generous beds of lettuce and add toppings according to which fuel you decide on.

MAKE A FAMILY MEAL: For the weight-loss plan, you can add brown rice and dollops of Greek yogurt for E or toppings like avocado, sour cream, and cheese for S. Growing children can enjoy avocado, cheese, and sour cream plus brown rice for a Crossover.

* FOR DF: LEAVE OFF THE CHEESE, GREEK YOGURT, AND SOUR CREAM.

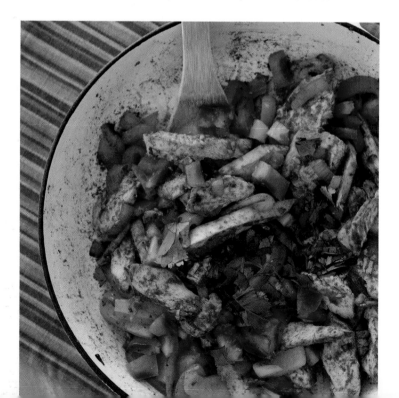

cabbage roll in a bowl

FAMILY SERVE–FEEDS 6 TO 8 (HALVE IF YOUR FAMILY IS SMALLER, OR MAKE FULL AND FREEZE HALF)

2 pounds ground beef or venison,
 thawed if frozen

⅔ cup beef or chicken broth

⅔ cup frozen diced okra

2 tablespoons coconut oil
 (use 3 to 4 for S)

1 large onion, sliced

3 to 4 garlic cloves, minced

½ large head cabbage, finely sliced,
 or 1 (16-ounce) bag very finely
 sliced cabbage or coleslaw

2 (14.5-ounce) cans petite diced
 tomatoes

1 (8-ounce) can tomato sauce

1 teaspoon black pepper

1½ teaspoons Mineral Salt

1 teaspoon onion powder

2 teaspoons paprika

2 tablespoons Worcestershire sauce

⅛ teaspoon cayenne pepper
 (optional if you like a hint of heat)

Squirt or 2 of Bragg liquid aminos
 or coconut aminos (optional)

All the flavor of stuffed cabbage rolls but way less work!

1. Brown the meat in a skillet over medium-high heat. Transfer the meat to a colander and rinse well under very hot water until all the fat is released. Set the meat aside on a plate.

2. Put the broth and okra in a blender and blend on high until completely smooth . . . blend the heck out of it until no pieces of okra are visible.

3. Add the coconut oil to the skillet and sauté the onion and garlic for a couple minutes over medium-high heat. Add the cabbage and toss with the onion and garlic. Cover, reduce the heat to medium, and cook for 4 to 5 minutes, until slightly wilted. Uncover, add the diced tomatoes, tomato sauce, blended okra, pepper, salt, onion powder, paprika, Worcestershire sauce, cayenne (if using), and liquid aminos (if using). Return the meat to the skillet, increase the heat to medium-high, and allow the dish to bubble and simmer for another 8 to 12 minutes.

MAKE A FAMILY MEAL: For the weight-loss plan, grab some on-plan bread (and generous butter for an S option; see the Breads chapter, page 240) or half of a Joseph's pita and have on the side to soak up some of the yummy sauce. You can always add a salad, if you want. Growing children or Skinny Jimmy husbies can have it with buttered sprouted-grain bread for a Crossover.

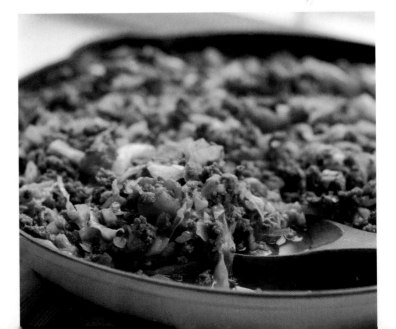

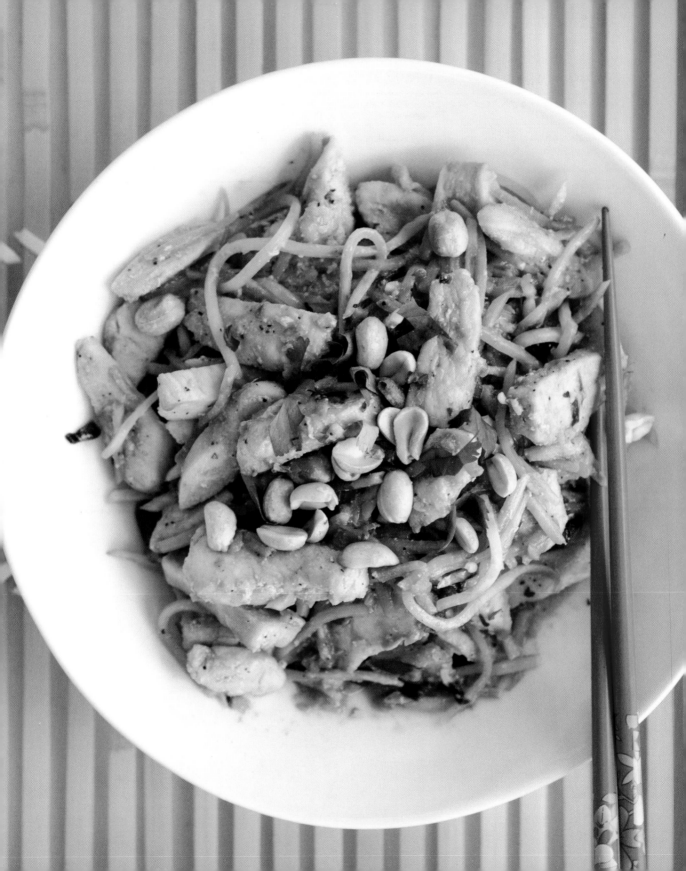

chicken satay in a bowl

S

FAMILY SERVE–FEEDS 6 TO 8 (HALVE IF YOUR FAMILY IS SMALLER, OR MAKE FULL AND FREEZE HALF)

1 cup chicken broth

¼ cup Pressed Peanut Flour*

¼ cup sugar-free natural-style peanut butter

¼ cup soy sauce

Black pepper

¾ teaspoon onion powder

¼ to ½ teaspoon cayenne pepper (reduce if you don't want too much heat)

1 to 1½ teaspoons Super Sweet Blend (optional if you like sweetness in your satay)

2½ pounds boneless, skinless chicken breasts or thighs (thawed if frozen), cut into small pieces (quickest way to do it is to use kitchen scissors)

Mineral Salt, for sprinkling

2 tablespoons coconut oil

2 garlic cloves, minced

2 (12-ounce) bags broccoli slaw

½ cup dry-roasted peanuts

Broccoli slaw makes for a healthy, quick, and easy rice or pasta sub. You can easily find it in bags in the produce section of your grocery store, already cut and ready to go. It is chock-full of powerful, disease-fighting nutrients and adds a great filling factor to this tasty recipe.

1. Whisk together the chicken broth, peanut flour, peanut butter, soy sauce, ½ teaspoon black pepper, the onion powder, cayenne, and sweetener (if using) in a bowl. Set the satay mixture aside.

2. Sprinkle the chicken with a light dusting of salt and pepper. Melt 1 tablespoon of the coconut oil in a large skillet over high heat, then add the chicken and garlic and cook for 4 to 5 minutes, tossing occasionally.

3. Remove the chicken. Add the remaining 1 tablespoon coconut oil and the broccoli slaw. Toss for 3 to 5 minutes, then add the satay mixture. Return the chicken to the skillet, toss all the ingredients, and simmer until the chicken is cooked fully through but the veggies do not lose their crisp . . . another few minutes.

4. Top each bowl with a sprinkling of peanuts.

MAKE A FAMILY MEAL: For the weight-loss plan, enjoy in a bowl. Growing children and others at Crossover stage can have brown rice or another healthy carb.

* FOR NSI: USE A GROCERY STORE SUGAR-FREE DEFATTED PEANUT FLOUR.

blackened fish tacos in a bowl

E WITH **S** AND **FP** OPTIONS

FAMILY SERVE—FEEDS 6 TO 8 (HALVE IF YOUR FAMILY IS SMALLER, OR MAKE FULL AND FREEZE HALF)

1½ pounds tilapia or other thin whitefish fillets, thawed if frozen

Chili powder, black pepper, and Mineral Salt, for blackening

2 tablespoons coconut oil or butter

1 (10- to 12-ounce) bag frozen large-cut seasoning blend (see page 35)

1 (10- to 16-ounce) bag very thinly sliced cabbage or coleslaw, or ½ head cabbage, finely sliced

2 (15-ounce) cans black beans, rinsed and drained

½ to ¾ teaspoon Mineral Salt

½ teaspoon red pepper flakes, or more to taste (optional)

½ to 1 bunch fresh cilantro, finely diced

4 tablespoons lime juice (fresh or bottled), plus lime wedges for serving (optional)

From start to finish, this ultraslimming meal is done within fifteen minutes. You need to eat more fish and you need to eat more E meals, so we have you covered here. This meal doesn't have to be expensive, either. We're landlocked here in Tennessee, but we buy inexpensive frozen fish fillets from Aldi or Walmart, then just thaw 'em out . . . easy peasy.

1. Generously sprinkle one side of the fish with chili powder, pepper, and salt.

2. Melt 2 teaspoons of the coconut oil in a large skillet over medium heat. Add half the fillets, seasoned side down. Sprinkle salt, pepper, and chili powder on the top side. Brown for 2 minutes on each side, then transfer to a plate. Do the same with the other half of the fillets, using 2 more teaspoons oil. Set the fish aside for now.

3. Put the last 2 teaspoons coconut oil into the pan and add the seasoning blend, cabbage, black beans, the ½ to ¾ tea-spoon salt, and the red pepper flakes (if using). Toss for 2 to 3 minutes, then add the cilantro and lime juice. Remove from the heat. Serve in bowls with pieces of lime if desired.

MAKE A FAMILY MEAL: For the weight-loss plan, enjoy as an E in a bowl with an optional side salad or have with Wonder Wraps 2 (page 251) or a low-carb tortilla. Make it an S by reduc-ing the beans to 1 can (or leaving the beans out altogether), then adding more coconut oil to cook the fish and veggies. Top with avocado pieces or guacamole. For FP keep the oil amount the same and reduce to 1 can of beans. Growing children can enjoy it with lots of beans plus any of the fats like avocado, sour cream, or cheese for a Crossover.

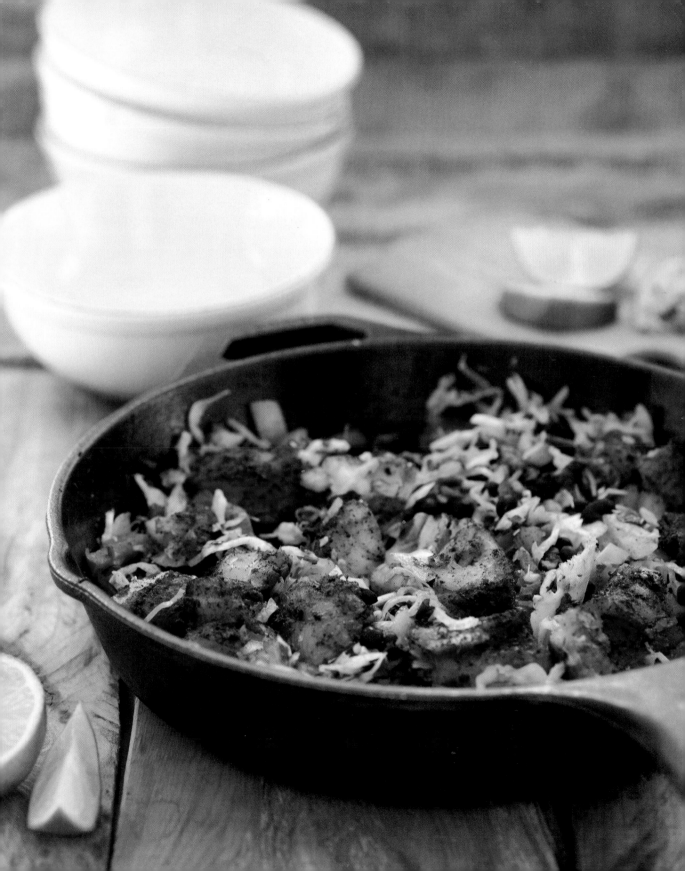

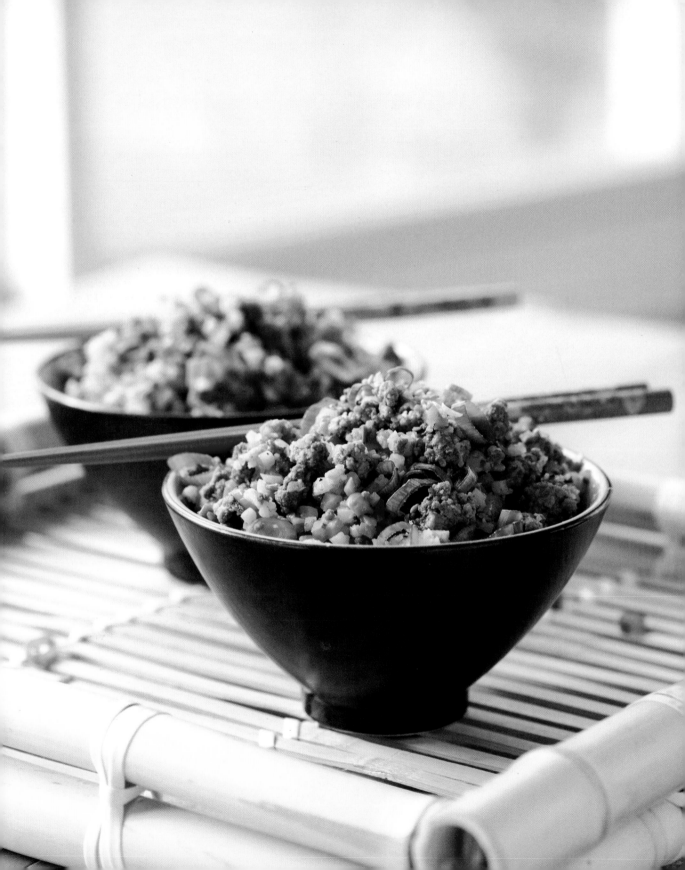

egg roll in a bowl part deux

S WITH **E** AND **FP** OPTIONS

FAMILY SERVE—FEEDS 6 TO 8 (HALVE IF YOUR FAMILY IS SMALLER, OR MAKE FULL AND FREEZE HALF)

2 pounds ground meat of any kind

3 tablespoons toasted sesame oil

1 large onion, chopped

⅓ cup soy sauce, or a few generous squirts Bragg liquid aminos or coconut aminos

2 to 3 (10- to 12-ounce) frozen bags riced veggies (either cauliflower medley or plain cauli rice)

4 garlic cloves, minced

2 teaspoons ground ginger, or 2 to 3 teaspoons finely grated or minced fresh ginger

Mineral Salt, black pepper, and red pepper flakes to taste

4 green onions, finely chopped

Another fast and yummy way to use riced veggies! The original Egg Roll in a Bowl was one of the biggest hits in *Trim Healthy Mama Cookbook.* Now we bring you part deux. Let's change things up, nix the cabbage, and make use of our new best friend riced cauliflower. You can get a frozen riced cauliflower medley at most grocery stores these days, which is a mix of cauliflower with a few riced carrots and peas added (read about how to make your own on page 36). Can we take a minute to let you know that you live in a very blessed time? When we first started Trim Healthy Mama there was nothing like riced veggies filling frozen shelves at grocery stores. Now they are practically everywhere (thanks to all our enthusiastic Trim Healthy Mamas and yes, thanks also to the Paleo crowd). You got it good!

1. Brown the meat in a large skillet over medium-high heat until fully cooked. Drain any excess fat.

2. Add the sesame oil, onion, soy sauce, riced veggies, garlic, and the ginger, and toss around the skillet with the meat for a couple minutes. Cover the skillet, reduce the heat to medium, and cook for 8 to 10 minutes, uncovering to stir periodically. Check that the veggies are tender and if not cook for a couple more minutes. Season with salt, pepper, and pepper flakes, then add in the chopped green onions and stir to combine. Taste to "own it" by adding more seasonings if needed, then serve.

MAKE A FAMILY MEAL: For the weight-loss plan, you can enjoy this as an S in a bowl or make this an E meal by having it over whole grain rice or quinoa. If having it as an E, make sure to use extra-lean meat (at least 96% lean) or if you don't have meat that lean, brown the meat, then rinse it well under hot water to release the fat before returning it to the skillet. Use no more than 2 tablespoons oil. If there is a lack of juiciness, add ¼ cup chicken broth or water to the skillet. To make this an FP meal, eat it in a bowl on its own following the E directions for cooking. Growing children can enjoy it with whole grain rice and a dollop of melty butter for a Crossover.

good grub

S

FAMILY SERVE—FEEDS 6 TO 8 (HALVE IF YOUR FAMILY IS SMALLER, OR MAKE FULL AND FREEZE HALF)

2 pounds ground meat of any kind

2 to 3 (10- to 12-ounce) bags frozen riced veggies (known as cauliflower medley)

2½ teaspoons Creole seasoning (we use MSG-free Tony Chachere's)

½ cup heavy cream

½ cup grated Parmesan cheese (the green can kind is fine)

Red pepper flakes

Once again, we're using riced cauliflower here. This meal is so insanely simple and so good we predict it will come to your rescue countless times as the years go by. Just two main ingredients: riced veggies and ground meat . . . it comes together in minutes! If you are lucky enough to have leftovers it is great as the next day's lunch or makes a yummy hash to go with eggs for breakfast.

This recipe calls for two bags of the riced veggies (commonly called cauliflower medley, which is simply riced cauliflower with a few peas and finely diced carrots added), but you can even add a third bag to the skillet (we do) if you want to get in more veggie power or stretch out the meal to feed a larger crowd. Just go a little heavier on the seasonings to balance it out. If you don't live in the United States and can't find frozen bags of riced veggies, go to page 36 to find out how to make your own.

1. Brown the meat in a large skillet over medium-high heat until fully cooked. Drain the excess fat if needed.

2. Add the veggies, Creole seasoning, cream, and Parmesan and stir until well combined. Cover the skillet, reduce the heat to medium, and cook for 8 to 10 minutes, uncovering to stir periodically. Uncover and shake in some pepper flakes to taste. Taste test to check that the veggies are tender and if not, cook for a couple more minutes. Taste again to "own it" with your seasonings, then serve.

MAKE A FAMILY MEAL: For the weight-loss plan, simply put it in a bowl and top with a little cheese if desired or put it inside any on-plan, S-friendly wrap or pita. Side salads are always welcome. For growing children who need Crossovers—ours love this stuffed into buttered whole-grain pitas with grated cheese. They're the ones that named it "Good Grub."

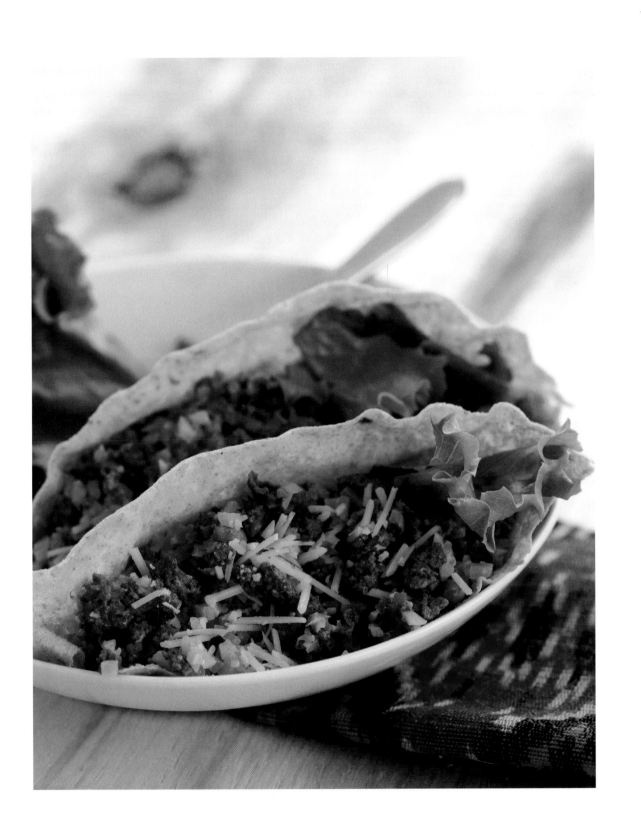

power skillet

Ⓢ

FAMILY SERVE—FEEDS 6 TO 8 (HALVE IF YOUR FAMILY IS SMALLER, OR MAKE FULL AND FREEZE HALF)

4 small or 3 medium to large
zucchini

3 pounds ground beef, venison,
or turkey, thawed if frozen

4 to 6 garlic cloves, minced

1½ teaspoons Mineral Salt

1½ teaspoons black pepper

Red pepper flakes to taste

3 tablespoons Nutritional Yeast
(optional)

24 to 32 ounces fresh spinach
(basically 2 large bags)

½ cup grated Parmesan cheese*
(the green can kind works best)

PEARL CHATS: Greens build up your blood with oxygen, detoxify your body, offer high amounts of vitamin C, and fight powerfully against disease. The whole family gets a double dose of healthy greens in this tasty, hearty dish (both spinach and zucchini), but they won't know it. Funny thing . . . in my house, I struggle to get my children to eat zucchini when they know it is in a dish, but they don't have the same problem with spinach, and they wolf it down like professional Popeyes! They have no clue there is zucchini in this yummy stuff. My boys go back for second helpings, and I just smile and serve them up.

1. Top and tail the zucchini. Don't bother peeling. Cut them into large chunks. Put half in a food processor and pulse until they look like tiny pieces (like cooked rice) but not mush. Transfer to a bowl. Repeat with the remaining zucchini. (If your processor is large enough, just do it all at once.)

2. Brown the meat in a large skillet over medium-high heat. Drain off any fat, then add the garlic and cook for 2 minutes, tossing the garlic through the meat. Add all the zucchini pieces, the salt, black pepper, pepper flakes (we use at least a teaspoon of the flakes, but you may want to start with less if you're not a heat lover), and nutritional yeast (if using). Cook over medium-high heat for 3 to 5 minutes, tossing well with the meat. Once the zucchini has wilted, add the spinach in 3 to 4 batches, as it will overflow if you add all of it at once. As you add each batch you may think "this is too much!" Be not afraid! Soon it will cook down and lose almost all its volume. Stir in the spinach well and allow it to wilt for a minute or two before adding the next batch. Once all the spinach is in, increase the heat to high, add the Parmesan, and cook while stirring for just a few more minutes.

MAKE A FAMILY MEAL: Enjoy this in a bowl as is or pair it with any on-plan, S-friendly bread such as Wonderful White Blender Bread (page 242) or buttered Joseph's pita. Growing children or others who need Crossovers can enjoy it with a buttered whole-grain pita, sprouted-grain bread, or even a baked white or sweet potato with butter.

* FOR DF: LEAVE OUT THE PARMESAN CHEESE.

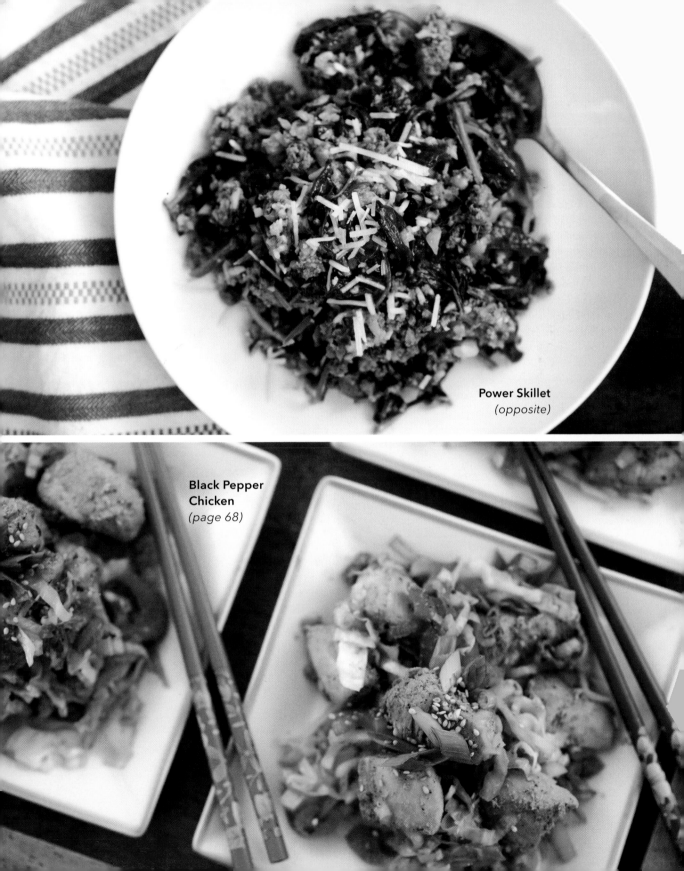

Power Skillet
(opposite)

Black Pepper Chicken
(page 68)

black pepper chicken

FAMILY SERVE—FEEDS 6 TO 8 (HALVE IF YOUR FAMILY IS SMALLER, OR MAKE FULL AND FREEZE HALF)

2½ pounds boneless, skinless chicken breasts or thighs (use breasts for FP), thawed if frozen, cut into ½-inch pieces (easily done with kitchen scissors)

¼ cup plus 2 tablespoons soy sauce

½ teaspoon ground ginger

1 teaspoon onion powder

1 teaspoon garlic powder

2½ teaspoons black pepper, or 3 teaspoons if you like more heat

1 tablespoon rice vinegar

4 tablespoons coconut oil (use only 2 tablespoons for FP)

1 onion, sliced

6 celery stalks, finely sliced

½ large head cabbage, finely sliced, or 1 (16-ounce) bag presliced cabbage or coleslaw

Think Chinese takeout . . . but ultrahealthy and made in a jiffy! Here's a time-saving tip—the night before, or the morning of, you can put the chicken in the marinade in a gallon-size baggie and refrigerate so it is all ready to go right before dinnertime. While you are at it, you may want to make double the amount of chicken and marinade. Put one of the bags in the freezer for a no-think, no-fuss dinner another night.

1. Place the chicken pieces in a bowl and add ¼ cup of the soy sauce, the ginger, onion powder, garlic powder, pepper, and vinegar. Allow to marinate for 10 minutes or so while you chop the vegetables (or do as described above and start marinating the night before or in the morning).

2. Melt 2 tablespoons of the coconut oil in a large skillet over high heat. Once hot, add the marinated chicken. Allow the chicken to cook for a couple minutes on one side, then toss periodically in the hot oil for 3 to 4 more minutes or until just done. Transfer the chicken to a plate.

3. Add the remaining 2 tablespoons coconut oil and all the veggies to the skillet. Add the remaining 2 tablespoons soy sauce and toss the veggies for 3 to 4 minutes, or until slightly wilted but still a bit crispy. Return the chicken to the pan, toss through, and serve.

MAKE A FAMILY MEAL: For the weight-loss plan, enjoy a big bowlful, no sides needed unless you want a salad or want to enjoy with some sautéed cauli rice or sautéed Trim Healthy Rice or Not Naughty Rice. If you prefer to make this as an FP, be sure to use a total of only 2 tablespoons oil. You can enjoy this in a bowl like the S version or over ¾ cup brown rice for an E. Children and others needing Crossovers can enjoy the S version over brown rice.

world's laziest lasagna skillet Ⓢ

FAMILY SERVE—FEEDS 6 TO 8 (HALVE IF YOUR FAMILY IS SMALLER, OR MAKE FULL AND FREEZE HALF)

2 pounds ground beef, turkey, or venison, thawed if frozen

20 ounces no-sugar-added pizza or spaghetti sauce, or 1½ batches Perfect Pizza Sauce (page 516)

1½ tablespoons dried oregano

½ teaspoon Mineral Salt

1 teaspoon onion powder

1 teaspoon garlic powder

⅛ teaspoon cayenne pepper

1 to 2 doonks Pure Stevia Extract Powder, or 1 to 2 teaspoons Super Sweet Blend* (optional)

16 ounces fresh spinach

1 (8-ounce) package ⅓ less fat cream cheese

1 (14-ounce) container 1% cottage cheese

8 ounces part-skim mozzarella cheese, grated

We gave you Lazy Lasagna, one of the most popular recipes in *Trim Healthy Mama Cookbook*, but now we have an even lazier version. No baking time . . . just throw it all in your skillet, then scoop into your mouth. Kids love this, too, and it makes sure they get a good dose of healthy greens in their dinner!

1. Brown the meat in a large skillet over medium-high heat, then drain off any excess fat.

2. Add the pizza sauce, oregano, salt, onion powder, garlic powder, cayenne, and stevia powder (if using). Add the spinach (you may need to add half the spinach, stir until it wilts a little, then add the rest). Reduce the heat to medium-low and allow to simmer.

3. Place the cream cheese and cottage cheese in a food processor and process until smooth. Add to the skillet. Allow all the ingredients to simmer a few more minutes, then you're done.

4. Top each plate with grated mozzarella.

MAKE A FAMILY MEAL: For the weight-loss plan, enjoy ladling this over a buttered piece of Wonderful White Blender Bread (page 242) or make WWBB Garlic Bread (page 245) and have a lovely salad on the side dressed with a vinaigrette. Or change it up and have it over Troodles (page 264), Cauli Rice (page 263), or spaghetti squash. Growing children love it over whole-grain noodles or buttered sprouted-grain bread for a Crossover.

* FOR NSI: USE YOUR FAVORITE GROCERY STORE ON-PLAN SWEETENER, OR LEAVE THE SWEETENER OUT.

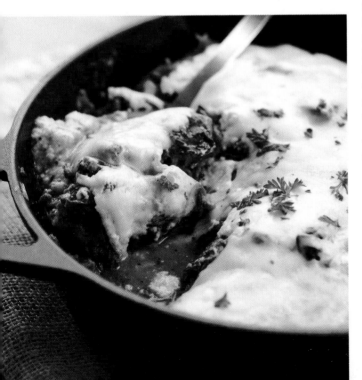

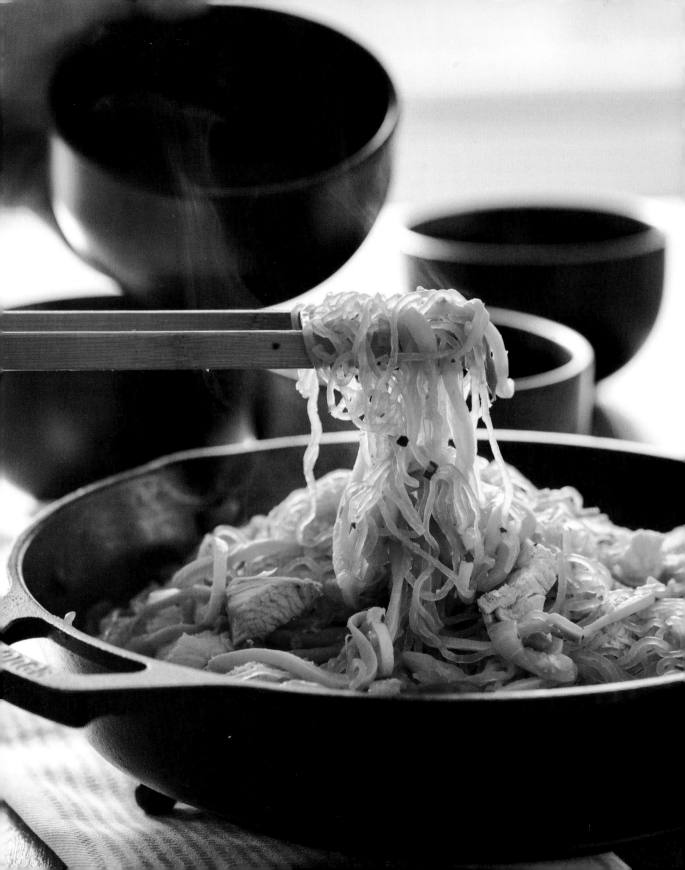

sesame lo mein

S WITH FP OPTION

FAMILY SERVE—FEEDS 6 TO 8 (HALVE IF YOUR FAMILY IS SMALLER, OR MAKE FULL AND FREEZE HALF).

2 teaspoons butter or coconut oil

3 to 4 garlic cloves, minced

1 (10- to 12-ounce) bag frozen large-cut seasoning blend (see page 35), or 2 cups of any chopped veggies you have lying around such as onion, red bell peppers, zucchini, radishes, and carrots (stick to a small amount of carrots for S); you can also include a few tablespoons frozen peas

3 single-serve bags Trim Healthy Noodles or Not Naughty Noodles,* well rinsed and drained

1 to 2 tablespoons Nutritional Yeast (optional)

¼ cup soy sauce, or a few good squirts Bragg liquid aminos or coconut aminos

Red pepper flakes or cayenne pepper to taste

2 to 4 medium zucchini or yellow squash, spiralized into Troodles (zucchini noodles)

4 large eggs (or use 1 cup egg whites for FP)

2 to 3 cups precooked or canned meat, such as diced chicken breast, salmon, or ground meat (use only chicken breast, lean salmon, or at least 96% lean ground meat for FP)

3 to 4 tablespoons toasted sesame oil (use only 4 to 5 teaspoons for FP)

3 to 4 green onions (optional), diced

Load your plate high with scrumptious noodles and slim down! Bet nobody has told you that before. Before you even have time to make a phone call for Chinese takeout, you can have this deliciousness ready for your table within 15 to 20 minutes. You'll save time *and* you'll save your waistline! We use two kinds of noodles in this dish for double the slimming power. It has konjac-based noodles, which are so fat-blasting and wonderful (read about them on page 43), and zucchini or yellow squash noodles, which we call "Troodles." If you are not yet a fan of konjac-based noodles, you can use all Troodles, just double up on the zucchini.

1. Melt the butter in a large skillet over medium-high heat. Add the garlic and toss in the butter for about a minute. Add the seasoning blend or chopped veggies and toss for another 2 to 3 minutes, or until softened. If using frozen veggies, toss on high.

2. Add the Trim Healthy Noodles or Not Naughty Noodles to the pan, increase the heat to high, and stir with a fork as they cook. While they are cooking, add the nutritional yeast (if using), soy sauce, and red pepper flakes. Toss them over high heat for a couple minutes, then add the Troodles and allow to cook for few minutes, tossing well. At first you think there are too many Troodles . . . have faith, they will wilt.

3. Push the noodles and veggies to one side of your skillet. Reduce the heat to medium and crack the eggs into the skillet. Stir and cut the eggs with your spatula, flip a few times while they cook, then toss them with all the other ingredients in the skillet. Add your precooked protein, continuing to heat the ingredients until the meat is warmed through. Top with the sesame oil and green onions (if using). Stir and lift the noodles so that they get coated with the sesame oil. Taste, then add more soy sauce, pepper, or other favorite Asian seasoning until it makes you say "Yeah Baby!"

MAKE A FAMILY MEAL: For the weight-loss plan, fill up on the big bowl of noodles then add on a baby-size shake (see pages 469 to 490). Growing children can have this as a Crossover with a glass of whole milk or another healthy carb.

* FOR NSI: LOOK FOR KONJAC NOODLES (SEE PAGE 43) AT YOUR LOCAL GROCERY STORE, OR USE DOUBLE THE AMOUNT OF TROODLES (ZUCCHINI NOODLES).

tuscan cream chicken

S

FAMILY SERVE—FEEDS 6 TO 8 (HALVE IF YOUR FAMILY IS SMALLER, OR MAKE FULL AND FREEZE HALF)

1 tablespoon garlic powder

2 teaspoons Italian seasoning

1½ teaspoons dried oregano

1 teaspoon Mineral Salt

2½ pounds chicken tenderloins, thawed if frozen

3 tablespoons butter or coconut oil

1½ cups chicken broth

½ cup heavy cream

½ cup grated Parmesan cheese (the green can kind is fine)

¾ to 1 teaspoon Gluccie*

5 to 6 ounces fresh spinach

½ (7-ounce) jar sun-dried tomatoes, roughly chopped

The insanely good smell that wafts from your kitchen as you prepare this dish will draw family members straight to the table! Once you've made this a time or two you can get 'er done in 15 minutes or less so it's perfect for busy nights when you are strapped for time.

1. Mix the garlic powder, Italian seasoning, oregano, and salt in a small bowl. Place the chicken in a large bowl, sprinkle with the seasonings, and toss with your hands so all pieces are coated well.

2. The recipe moves fast now, so line up everything on your counter that you'll need: butter, chicken broth, cream, Parmesan, Gluccie, spinach, and sun-dried tomatoes. Melt the butter in a large skillet over medium-high heat. Add all the chicken and cook for 6 minutes, turning once.

3. Reduce the heat to medium, then add the chicken broth, cream, and Parmesan. Move the chicken to one side of the pan and sprinkle in ¾ teaspoon Gluccie a little at a time, whisking well into the sauce while you sprinkle so it doesn't clump. Toss the sauce around the skillet. Allow it to simmer for another couple minutes and add only an extra ¼ teaspoon Gluccie if you like a thicker sauce. Add all the spinach (it will quickly wilt into the sauce as you toss it around the pan), then add the sun-dried tomatoes. Cook for 5 to 6 more minutes.

MAKE A FAMILY MEAL: For the weight-loss plan, this is fabulous with a nonstarchy veggie side like green beans or broccoli or enjoy with Troodles (page 264), Cauli Rice (page 263) or spaghetti squash and perhaps an S-friendly bread item such as WWBB Garlic Bread (page 245). Children can enjoy with whole-grain rice or noodles for a Crossover.

* FOR NSI: SUB XANTHAN GUM FOR THE GLUCCIE.

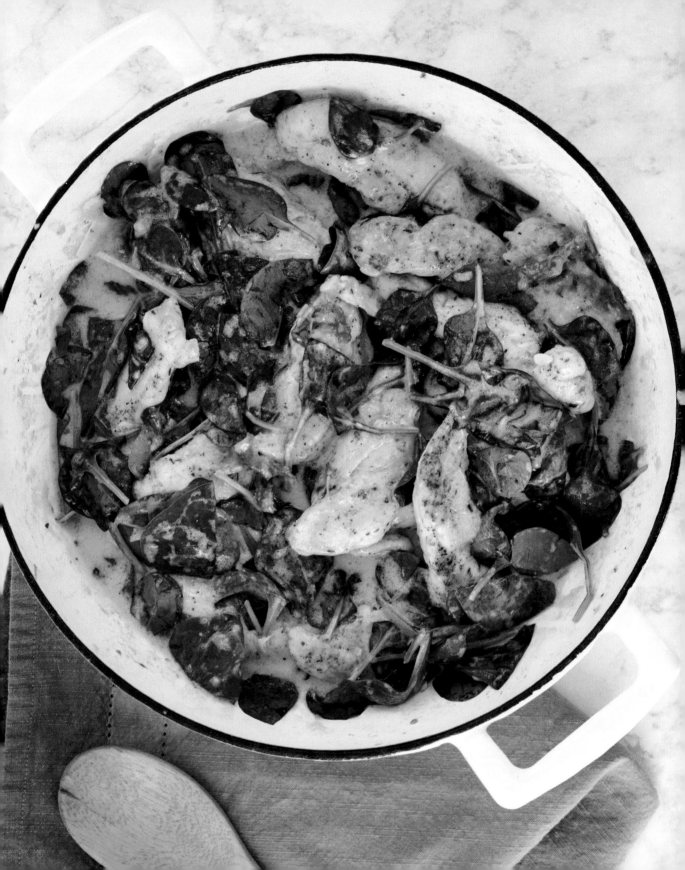

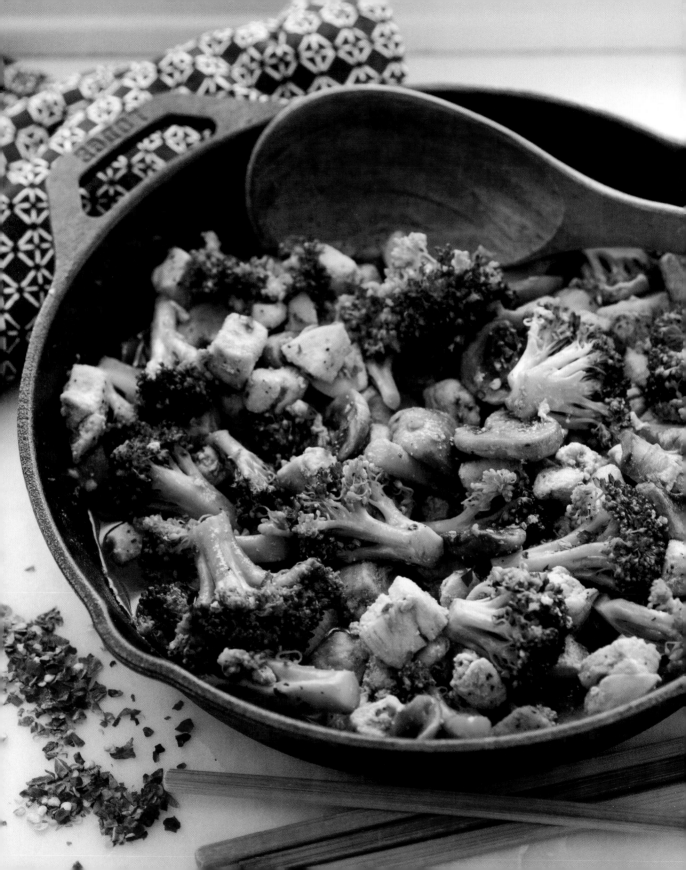

chicken, broccoli, mushroom stir-fry FP WITH S AND E OPTIONS

FAMILY SERVE—FEEDS 6 TO 8 (HALVE IF YOUR FAMILY IS SMALLER, OR MAKE FULL AND FREEZE HALF)

1 cup chicken broth

1 cup frozen diced okra

⅓ cup soy sauce, or several generous squirts Bragg liquid aminos

2½ teaspoons Super Sweet Blend*

½ teaspoon Gluccie*

2 tablespoons coconut oil or sesame oil

2½ pounds boneless, skinless chicken breasts (thawed if frozen), cut into ½-inch pieces (quickest with kitchen scissors)

Mineral Salt and black pepper

3 to 4 garlic cloves, minced

1 generous teaspoon finely grated or minced fresh ginger

2 (12-ounce) bags frozen broccoli, or fresh broccoli florets from a large head

8 ounces fresh mushrooms, sliced

1 teaspoon red pepper flakes (optional)

Your house will smell as wondrous as a Japanese restaurant when you make this. Watch your family wolf it down, never knowing there is a healthy secret ingredient in the sauce (so long as you don't tell!).

1. Prepare the sauce in advance. Put the chicken broth, okra, soy sauce, sweetener, and Gluccie in a blender and blend on high until completely broken down . . . we mean blend the daylights out of it so no bits of okra are left.

2. Melt 1 tablespoon of the oil in a skillet over high heat. Season the chicken pieces with salt and pepper, add them to the skillet, and cook for 4 minutes, turning once. Remove them from the pan and set aside.

3. Reduce the heat to medium. Add the remaining 1 tablespoon oil, the garlic, and ginger. Toss in the oil for about 30 seconds, then stir in the frozen broccoli. Increase the heat to medium-high, cover, and cook for about 2½ minutes. Stir in the mushrooms, cover, and cook for another 2½ minutes (if using fresh broccoli, add later with the mushrooms and cook without covering for several minutes, tossing often).

4. Uncover, pour in the sauce, and cook on high for 5 to 6 more minutes, returning the chicken for the last 3 minutes and adding the pepper flakes (if using).

MAKE A FAMILY MEAL: For the weight-loss plan, this dish is perfect with brown rice for an E, or have it with any nonstarchy veggie with seasonings and added sesame oil for an S, or just eat it as is for an FP. Children can enjoy it as an S with whole-grain rice or noodles for a Crossover.

* FOR NSI: USE GROCERY STORE ON-PLAN SWEETENER AND SUB XANTHAN GUM FOR THE GLUCCIE.

Sanity-Saving Crockpot & Electric Pressure Cooker Meals

Whether you want to cook your meal slowly in a crockpot or quickly in a pressure cooker, use these simple, family-friendly recipes to take the stress out of "what's for dinner."

A quick note about electric pressure cooker directions: electric pressure cookers come in a variety of sizes and each manufacturer's recommendations will be different. The directions listed here are what have worked for us and our Mama testers but may vary for you. Please always follow the procedures in your owner's manual.

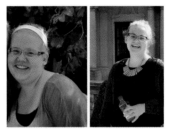

I am a nineteen-year-old Trim Healthy Teen, and I started this plan a year ago after I watched the amazing results that my mom had doing THM! Before starting, I weighed 210 pounds, was a size 18/20. I had low energy (I could barely handle a six-hour shift at my job), bad acne, as well as PCOS (poly cystic ovary syndrome). I had constant highs and lows, and I was as addicted to sugar/carbs as it gets, to the point where I could down seven or eight cookies or half a pizza at a party without batting an eyelash. Although I never had severe self-esteem struggles, I knew that my weight and habits affected me in more ways than my appearance.

Within a few months of doing THM, my acne cleared up, and I was shrinking out of my clothes! However, eight months into my journey, I moved to Northern California, where the stress of moving and my new environment stressed me to the point where I fell HARD off the bandwagon. For a few months, I had high carbs, and even had sugar occasionally (okay, quite a bit, LOL). My acne and sugar highs and crashes came back, along with some of the lost weight, and made me miserable, which really motivated me to get back on track!

Even though I went through that phase, I didn't let it discourage me or get to my head. And it didn't last long! Now I am solidly back on track. I spend only $130/month on food, and that includes fun stuff like Whey Protein Powder, Integral Collagen, almond milk, and on-plan sweeteners! Today, I am a size 10/12, have crazy high energy (I WANT to work out after my work shift!!), beautiful skin, and I don't suffer from most of the PCOS symptoms. Sugar and carbs don't rule me like they used to. It has been an amazing year, and I am so grateful for Serene and Pearl, who stepped out and shared the wisdom and knowledge given to them by the Lord, even though it wasn't what was popular at the time. My mom has also been such a huge support; I love doing this with family! <3 My life is forever changed, and I am excited to live the THM lifestyle for the rest of my life! —ABI R.

creamy verde chicken chili

S

FAMILY SERVE—FEEDS 6 TO 8 (HALVE IF YOUR FAMILY IS SMALLER, OR MAKE FULL AND FREEZE HALF)

2½ to 3 pounds boneless, skinless chicken breasts, thawed if frozen

1 (16-ounce) jar salsa verde (hot, medium, or mild)

1 (15-ounce) can white beans, rinsed and drained

1 (10-ounce) can Ro-tel-style diced tomatoes and green chilies (medium, mild, or hot)

1 (10- to 12-ounce) bag frozen riced cauliflower (see page 36)

1 (10- to 12-ounce) bag frozen small-cut seasoning blend (see page 35)

1½ (8-ounce) packages ⅓ less fat cream cheese

1½ cups frozen diced okra

3 cups chicken broth

1 teaspoon Mineral Salt

2 teaspoons ground cumin

1 teaspoon chili powder

1 teaspoon onion powder

1 teaspoon garlic powder

PEARL CHATS: The creaminess and flavor of this chili make you sorry for anyone else not eating the Trim Healthy way! It uses salsa verde, a green salsa that can be found in almost any grocery store and is an excellent sauce to enjoy on the Trim Healthy Plan, as it has only one net carb per serving. There are not one, but two, secret veggies in this chili. They are completely undetectable; all they'll do is sneakily improve the health of your family. The cauliflower softens so much it melts into the creamy sauce and the blood sugar–regulating okra is hidden in the beautiful, creamy color of this chili. Don't worry about the one can of beans here. It is not enough to mess with S mode.

1. Place the chicken, salsa verde, beans, canned tomatoes, cauliflower rice, and seasoning blend in the bottom of a crockpot.

2. Put the cream cheese, okra, 2 cups of the broth, the salt, cumin, chili powder, onion powder, and garlic powder in a blender and blend until smooth. Blend, baby, blend until no green specks are left!

3. Add the contents of the blender to the crockpot along with the remaining 1 cup broth and stir. Cover and cook on low for 6 to 8 hours. When done, shred the chicken with 2 forks right inside the pot.

ELECTRIC PRESSURE COOKER DIRECTIONS: Add everything to the pressure cooker (including the blended sauce and remaining cup of broth). Seal and cook at high pressure for 25 minutes. Use natural pressure release. Shred the chicken.

MAKE A FAMILY MEAL: For the weight-loss plan, you can top this S chili with grated cheese or diced avocado, but avoid corn chips. Growing children or those at goal weight can enjoy it with baked corn chips or toasted sprouted-grain bread with butter for a Crossover.

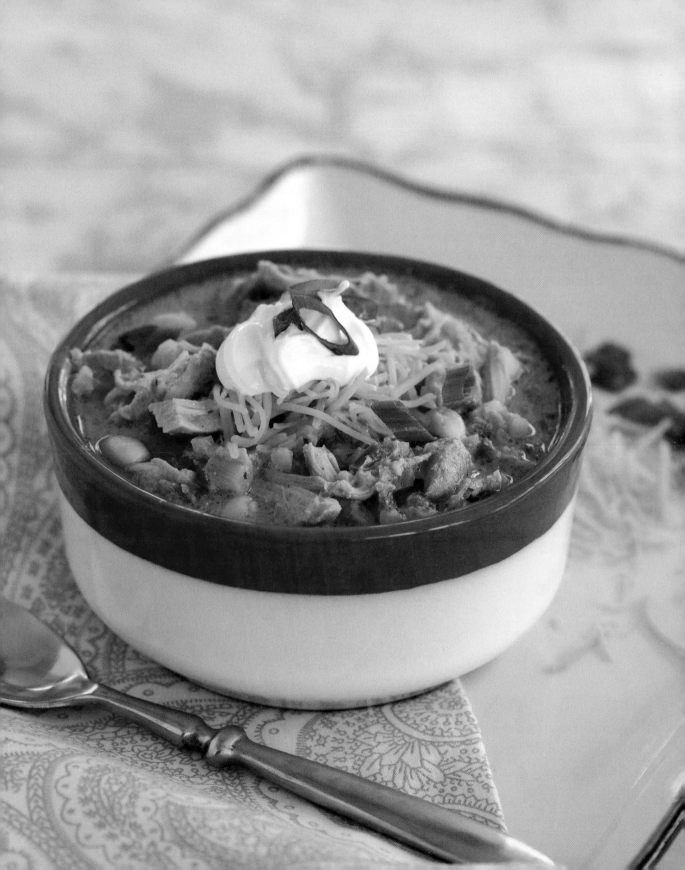

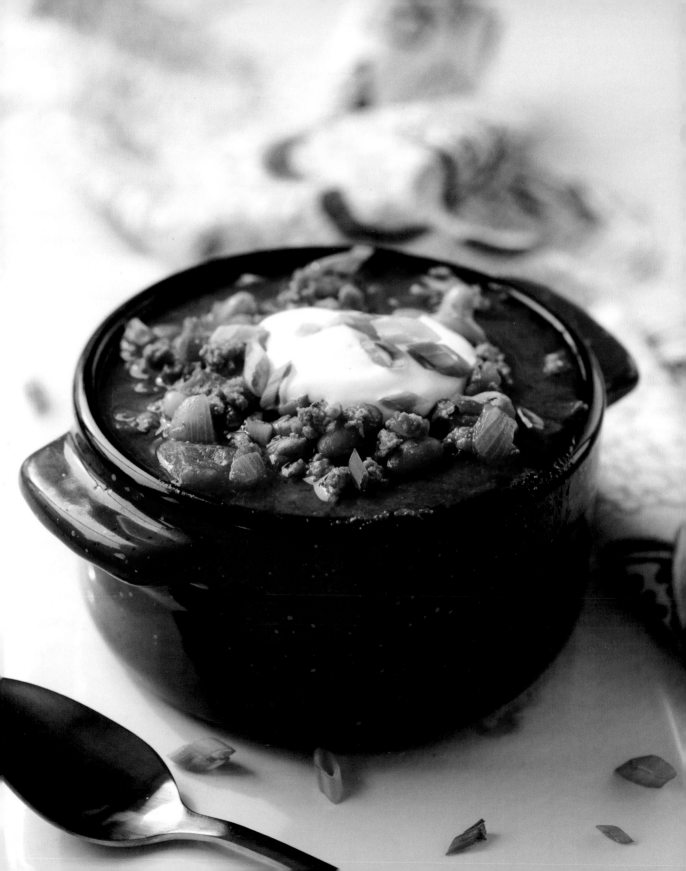

save my sanity chili

E

FAMILY SERVE–FEEDS 6 TO 8 (HALVE IF YOUR FAMILY IS SMALLER, OR MAKE FULL AND FREEZE HALF)

2 pounds ultralean (96%) ground turkey or venison, thawed if frozen (see Note)

2 (10- to 12-ounce) bags frozen small-cut seasoning blend (see page 35)

2 (14.5-ounce) cans diced tomatoes

1 (10-ounce) can Ro-tel-style diced tomatoes and green chilies (hot, medium, or mild)

2 (15-ounce) cans pinto beans, rinsed and drained

2 (15-ounce) cans white beans, such as cannellini or Great Northern, rinsed and drained

1 quart chicken broth

3 tablespoons chili powder

2 teaspoons ground cumin

1 teaspoon onion powder

1 teaspoon minced garlic

1 teaspoon dried oregano

1½ teaspoons Mineral Salt

1½ to 2 teaspoons Super Sweet Blend (optional, but gives a great hint of sweetness to balance flavors)

¼ teaspoon cayenne pepper (optional, depending on your heat preference)

We gave you an S chili on the previous page. Change it up and give E chili its turn! When life gets chaotic, this meal can come to your rescue. Throw it in the crockpot in the morning and you'll be able to breathe a sigh of relief knowing that supper is taken care of (or make it in a jiffy in your pressure cooker). This tasty chili is a no-brainer since it saves you a whole prep step. Most chili recipes that call for ground meat ask you to brown the meat and onions first, but we know life can be crazy busy and sometimes that just might be the 10 to 15 minutes you don't have! We don't want you giving in and considering picking up drive-thru food because you don't have time to cook! So no more excuses . . . extra steps are outta here! Throw all the ingredients in your trusty crockpot and come back in the evening to deliciousness! Now, let's say your life is extra crazy and you forget to prepare your crockpot meal in the morning but you don't have an electric pressure cooker. No worries—this can be made in a pot on the stove in about 30 minutes—just brown your meat and onions, add all the other ingredients, and let it bubble away.

1. Place the meat in the bottom of a crockpot and break up with a fork to spread around the bottom of the crock. Add all the other ingredients and mix well.

2. Cover and cook on low for 5 to 7 hours. Once the chili is ready, break up any larger chunks of meat.

ELECTRIC PRESSURE COOKER DIRECTIONS: Cook the meat on sauté mode, then add all the other ingredients. Seal and cook at low pressure for 10 minutes. Use the quick pressure release.

MAKE A FAMILY MEAL: For the weight-loss plan, garnish with just a sprinkle of grated cheese to stay within E fat guidelines and add a dollop of Greek yogurt if desired. You can also sprinkle on a few crushed baked corn chips. Growing children or those at goal weight can have this as a delicious Crossover with grated cheese, sour cream, and baked corn chips.

NOTE: If you use ground turkey it must be ultralean (at least 96%) to avoid a Crossover, since this is an E meal and you are not browning then rinsing the meat to release any extra fat. Venison is always lean enough for E recipes if not mixed with other meats, if you would prefer to use that.

teriyaki beef and broccoli

S WITH **E** AND **FP** OPTIONS

FAMILY SERVE–FEEDS 6 TO 8 (HALVE IF YOUR FAMILY IS SMALLER, OR MAKE FULL AND FREEZE HALF)

2½ to 3 pounds boneless beef chuck roast (thawed if frozen), sliced into thin strips or diced (use diced chicken breast for FP)

1 onion, sliced

4 to 5 garlic cloves, minced

1-inch cube fresh ginger

¼ to ½ teaspoon red pepper flakes

⅓ to ½ cup soy sauce

⅓ cup rice vinegar

⅓ cup Gentle Sweet, or
  2 tablespoons Super Sweet Blend*

2 tablespoons toasted sesame oil

¼ cup water

¾ to 1 teaspoon Gluccie* (optional)

2 (16-ounce) bags frozen broccoli florets, or the same amount of fresh broccoli

1 tablespoon sesame seeds

6 green onions, chopped

1. Place the beef in the bottom of a crockpot. Add the onion and garlic.

2. Put the ginger, pepper flakes, ⅓ cup soy sauce, the vinegar, Gentle Sweet, sesame oil, and water in a blender and blend well until the ginger is fully broken down. Pour over the beef. Cover and cook on low for 4 to 6 hours.

3. In the last hour, decide if you'd like your sauce thicker. If so, move some of the meat aside and slowly add ¾ teaspoon Gluccie (if using) by tapping the measuring spoon on the side of the crockpot, allowing a little at a time to fall in. Whisk like mad with your other hand so it doesn't clump. Whisk extremely well so the Gluccie can start to activate and thicken the sauce. Add the broccoli, toss well in the sauce, and continue cooking (another 45 minutes to 1 hour). Taste the sauce and see if it needs more soy sauce or sweetener, or if it is just right for you. Add the remaining ¼ teaspoon Gluccie if you would like the sauce thicker. Finally, top with the sesame seeds and chopped green onions.

ELECTRIC PRESSURE COOKER DIRECTIONS: Blend the sauce and place it in the pressure cooker with all the other ingredients except the broccoli. Seal and cook at high pressure for 10 minutes. Use natural pressure release. Either cook the broccoli separately and add it before serving, or add it in at the end and bring to pressure again for 1 minute.

MAKE A FAMILY MEAL: For the weight-loss plan, have the S version using beef over either Cauli Rice (page 263), Troodles (page 264), sautéed cabbage, or sautéed Trim Healthy Noodles or Not Naughty Noodles. Feel free to drizzle with a little more sesame oil if desired. You can have the chicken version with cauli rice without extra oil for an FP or over regular brown rice for an E. Growing children and others needing Crossovers can have the S version over whole-grain rice.

* FOR NSI: USE A GROCERY STORE ON-PLAN SWEETENER AND SUB XANTHAN GUM FOR THE GLUCCIE.

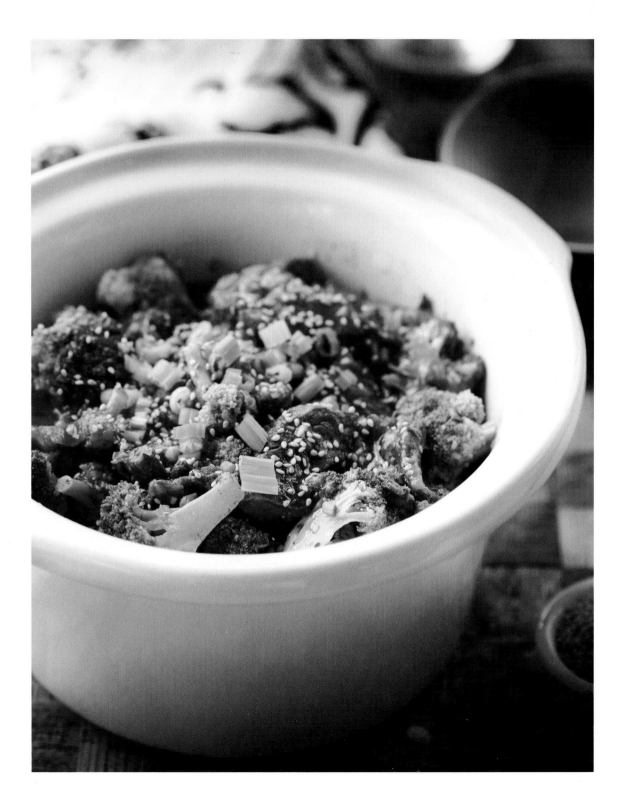

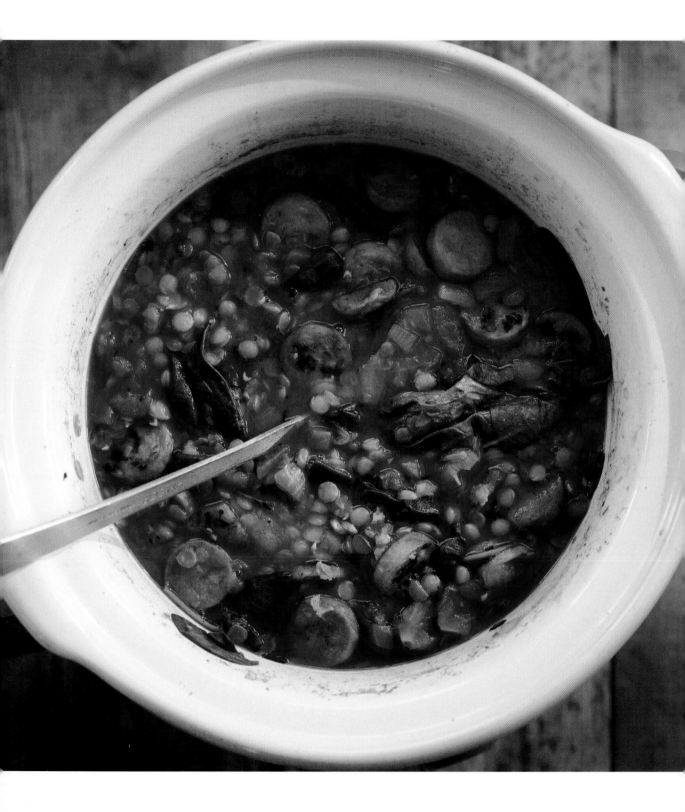

hearty lentil, chicken sausage, and spinach soup Ⓔ

FAMILY SERVE–FEEDS 6 TO 8 (HALVE IF YOUR FAMILY IS SMALLER, OR MAKE FULL AND FREEZE HALF)

1 pound dried lentils

1 (10- to 12-ounce) bag frozen small-cut seasoning blend (see page 35)

3 to 4 garlic cloves, minced

1 quart chicken broth (with an optional 4 tablespoons Just Gelatin or Integral Collagen, see page 40)

5 cups water

2 (14.5-ounce) cans fire-roasted tomatoes

1 (6-ounce) can tomato paste

4 fully cooked chicken sausage links (see Note), thinly sliced

2 teaspoons Mineral Salt

¼ teaspoon black pepper

½ teaspoon dried oregano

⅛ to ¼ teaspoon cayenne pepper (optional)

4 to 5 cups fresh spinach or kale

This is soul-warming, tummy-filling stuff! Lentils are super budget-friendly little powerhouses of health. They are perfect for the crockpot or electric pressure cooker since they are one of the only legumes that doesn't have to be soaked, so you can just throw them into the crockpot dry, add your other ingredients, and forget about them until dinnertime. That's right, for most people, they won't cause all those gassy problems that happen when you don't soak your beans or legumes. Yay for lentils making your life easier and for being such an inexpensive, health-giving food!

1. Place all the ingredients (except the spinach) in a crockpot. Cover and cook on high for 5 to 6 hours. During the last 30 minutes, add the spinach or kale.

ELECTRIC PRESSURE COOKER DIRECTIONS: Put all the ingredients except the spinach in the pressure cooker. Seal and cook at high pressure for 20 minutes. Use natural pressure release. Add the spinach or kale and stir until wilted.

MAKE A FAMILY MEAL: Enjoy this with a side salad with an E-friendly, lean dressing and/or an FP bread such as Wonderful White Blender Bread (page 242) with a thin smear of butter. Growing children can enjoy this topped with grated cheese for a Crossover.

NOTE: Get lean chicken sausage links that have 7 grams of fat per link, such as Al Fresco fully cooked sausage links—Sweet Italian or Sun-Dried Tomato. If you can find only chicken sausage with 9 grams of fat per link, use 3 links (unless you want a Crossover, which is fine, too).

save your waistline crockpot lasagna ⓢ

FAMILY SERVE—FEEDS 6 TO 8 (HALVE IF YOUR FAMILY IS SMALLER, OR MAKE FULL AND FREEZE HALF)

Coconut oil cooking spray

2 pounds ground meat, thawed if frozen (see Time-saving Tip)

2 (14-ounce) jars no-sugar-added pizza sauce (we use Walmart Great Value brand), or a double batch Perfect Pizza Sauce (page 516)

1 tablespoon garlic powder

1 tablespoon dried parsley flakes

1 tablespoon dried oregano

½ teaspoon Mineral Salt

Red pepper flakes

2 doonks Pure Stevia Extract Powder, or 1½ teaspoons Super Sweet Blend* (optional, but gives a richer, fresher tasting sauce)

2 large eggs

2 cups (16 ounces) 1% cottage cheese

1 (8-ounce) package ⅓ less fat cream cheese

4 medium zucchini or yellow squash, sliced ⅛ inch thick (sliced lengthwise or crosswise, but don't bother peeling)

2 cups (8 ounces) grated part-skim mozzarella cheese

⅓ cup grated Parmesan cheese (green can kind is fine)

Come home to a delicious smell in the air promising you lasagna—the ultimate comfort food. Yes, you can eat it without exploding your waistline! We took all the great flavors of Lazy Lasagna, one of the biggest hits in *Trim Healthy Mama Cookbook,* and tweaked it for the crockpot. With much trial and error, we found out spinach doesn't work so well cooking all day in a crockpot as a noodle layer but zucchini slices do! Just an FYI, slow-cooking lasagna does create more liquid. Just make sure you let your lasagna rest after cooking for about an hour before eating, and it won't be soupy. The liquid will stay at the bottom so your lasagna can set properly and you can cut pieces to serve.

TIME-SAVING TIP: It is a great idea to take one day every week (or perhaps every month) where you brown up a lot of ground meat, then freeze it for quick prep meals. For this recipe, take your cooked meat out the day before to thaw in the refrigerator so that in the morning you can mix it with the sauce and seasonings right in the crockpot! No extra pans to wash!

1. Coat a crockpot with coconut oil spray.

2. Brown the meat in a large skillet, then drain off any excess fat. Add the pizza sauce, garlic powder, parsley, oregano, salt, pepper flakes, and stevia powder (if using) to the meat (or combine prepped browned meat with the above listed ingredients in a bowl).

3. Put the eggs, cottage cheese, and cream cheese into a food processor or blender and process until smooth.

4. Layer half the meat sauce in the bottom of the crockpot. Top with half the cottage cheese mixture, then layer on half of the sliced zucchini. Follow with half the mozzarella. Repeat layers, ending with mozzarella, then the Parmesan on top.

5. Cover and cook on low for 5 to 6 hours. Turn off the crockpot and allow the lasagna to settle for 1 hour before cutting it into pieces and serving.

ELECTRIC PRESSURE COOKER DIRECTIONS: Prepare the recipe according to the directions for the crockpot, except add ½ cup water or chicken broth to avoid possible scorching. Leave off the last layer of mozzarella and the Parmesan. Seal and cook on high pressure for 7 minutes. Use quick pressure release.

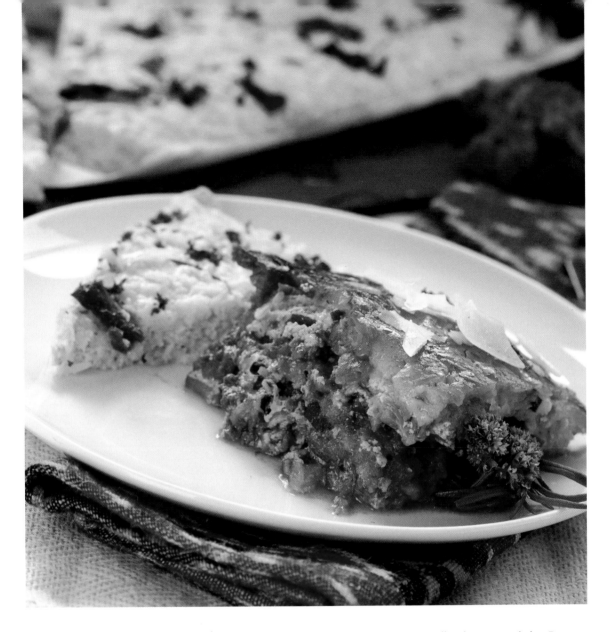

Sprinkle with the remaining mozzarella cheese and the Parmesan. Let it set for at least 15 to 20 minutes before serving.

MAKE A FAMILY MEAL: For the weight-loss plan, this lasagna is perfect with a very large salad, topped with an Italian-style oil and vinegar dressing and perhaps WWBB Garlic Bread (page 245). Growing children can have a healthy carb on the side, such as whole milk or a sprouted-grain bread item.

* FOR NSI: USE A GROCERY STORE ON-PLAN SWEETENER, OR LEAVE OUT THE SWEETENER.

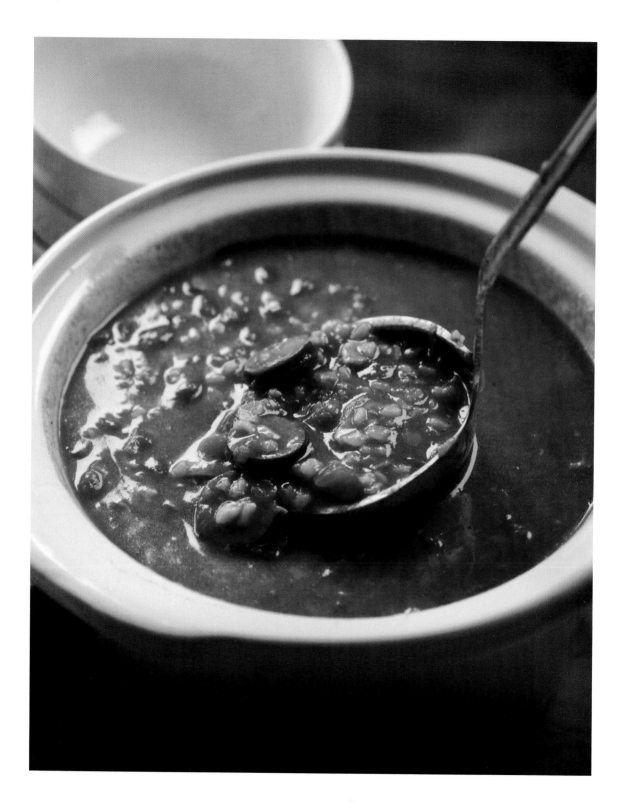

chicken sausage gumbo Ⓔ

FAMILY SERVE—FEEDS 6 TO 8 (HALVE IF YOUR FAMILY IS SMALLER, OR MAKE FULL AND FREEZE HALF)

2 cups frozen diced okra (plus
  1 to 2 more cups if you are an
  okra-loving household)
1 quart chicken broth or stock
4 cooked chicken sausage links
  (see Note), sliced small
1½ pounds boneless, skinless
  chicken breast, thawed if frozen
1 (6-ounce) can tomato paste
2 cans (14.5-ounce) stewed
  tomatoes
1 quart plus 2 cups water
1 (10- to 12-ounce) bag frozen
  small-cut seasoning blend
  (see page 35)
3½ teaspoons Creole seasoning
  (we use MSG-free Tony
  Chachere's)
2 teaspoons mesquite liquid smoke
4 to 5 garlic cloves, minced
¾ teaspoon black pepper
¼ to ½ teaspoon cayenne pepper
  (optional but wonderful)
3 bay leaves
1 cup uncooked rice

We present a gumbo without the need for a roux! Roux is the white flour/butter mix that is the usual beginning to a gumbo, but it is a huge meanie to your blood sugar and fattens you right up! You're going to love the flavors of this tomato-based gumbo and how healthy it is for you and your family. Gumbo traditionally uses okra as one of the featured veggies—go ahead and add as much visible diced okra as you want, if your family loves it. But we have some okra-despising kids in our families, so we hide it in this recipe. They have no idea, yet reap all the benefits.

TIME-SAVING TIP: Put all the ingredients in your crockpot the night before and place it in the refrigerator. All you have to do the next morning is turn it on and go about your day.

1. Put the 2 cups diced okra and 2 cups of the broth in a blender and blend on high until completely smooth. By this we mean blend the heck out of it until no little pieces of okra can be seen. Pour into the bottom of a crockpot.

2. Add the remaining 2 cups broth (along with the optional extra diced okra) and all the other ingredients and stir well. Cover and cook on low for 5 to 6 hours (if the gumbo gets too thick, feel free to add more liquid). Remove the bay leaf before serving.

ELECTRIC PRESSURE COOKER DIRECTIONS: Add all the ingredients, including the blended okra/broth, to the pressure cooker. Seal and cook on low pressure for 30 minutes. You can choose to use quick or natural pressure release.

MAKE A FAMILY MEAL: For the weight-loss plan, enjoy a big bowlful or two. Our children pile grated cheese on this E meal as they do just about any E meal for a yummy Crossover.

NOTE: Find a brand of lean chicken sausage with 7 grams of fat per link such as Al Fresco fully cooked sausage links—Sweet Italian or Sun-Dried Tomato. If you can't find those, most other chicken sausage brands have 9 grams of fat per link, so to fit within E guidelines it's best to use just 3 links in this recipe (unless you want a Crossover, which is also fine). Slice them finely and you'll still feel like you have enough.

chicken fajita soup

FP WITH **S** AND **E** OPTIONS

FAMILY SERVE—FEEDS 6 TO 8 (HALVE IF YOUR FAMILY IS SMALLER, OR MAKE FULL AND FREEZE HALF)

2½ pounds boneless, skinless chicken breasts or thighs (use breasts for FP and E), thawed if frozen

2 quarts chicken broth (with an optional 4 tablespoons Just Gelatin or Integral Collagen see page 40)

1 (10-ounce) can Ro-tel-style diced tomatoes and green chilies

1 (14.5-ounce) can diced, fire-roasted tomatoes

1 (10- to 12-ounce) bag frozen small-cut seasoning blend (see page 35)

1 teaspoon Mineral Salt

1 teaspoon black pepper

1 teaspoon onion powder

1 teaspoon garlic powder, or 4 to 6 garlic cloves, minced

1 teaspoon chili powder

¾ to 1 teaspoon chipotle powder (optional for an extra-awesome kick)

1 (8-ounce) package ⅓ less fat cream cheese* (optional)

Lime wedges (optional), for serving

This simple, flavorful soup lends itself perfectly to the crockpot or electric pressure cooker. This is level 1 cooking—you can't mess this up, so go ahead and wow your family! You have the option of making this more of a cream-based soup by adding in cream cheese, which makes it an S . . . your choice. It is great either way, so change things up! A time-saving and flavor-boosting tip is to put all the ingredients except the broth in a gallon-size baggie in the fridge to marinate, either the night before or whenever you get a chance, then just plop it into your pot when ready to cook and add the broth.

1. Put all the ingredients (except the cream cheese and lime wedges) in a crockpot. Cover and cook on high for 6 hours. If using the cream cheese, remove 1 cup of the hot broth and place it in a blender with the cream cheese. Blend until smooth, then stir into the crockpot.

2. Remove the chicken and shred on a plate with 2 forks. Return to the pot, stir well to combine, and serve with a squirt of lime (if using).

ELECTRIC PRESSURE COOKER DIRECTIONS: Add all the ingredients except the cream cheese and lime wedges to the pressure cooker. Seal and cook at high pressure for 25 minutes. Use natural pressure release. If including optional cream cheese, follow the crockpot directions. Shred the chicken.

MAKE A FAMILY MEAL: For the weight-loss plan, enjoy as is in a bowl for an FP or have the FP version with sprouted-grain toast or baked corn chips on the side and a garnish-size amount of cheese for an E. Want to have it as an S? Include the cream cheese. Or else leave it out and top with options of grated cheese, diced avocado, or perhaps a dollop of sour cream. Try one of the S-friendly bread sides in the Breads chapter (page 240) with butter. Growing children can enjoy this with cheese and baked corn chips or another healthy carb such as buttered sprouted-grain bread for a Crossover.

* FOR DF: LEAVE OUT THE CREAM CHEESE.

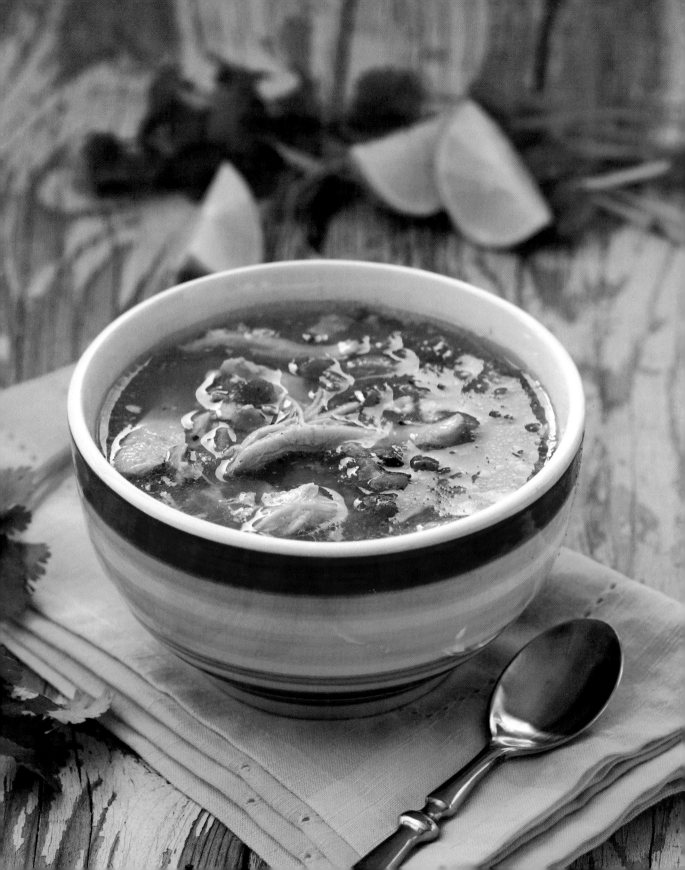

crockpot buffalo chicken

S

FAMILY SERVE—FEEDS 6 TO 8 (HALVE IF YOUR FAMILY IS SMALLER, OR MAKE FULL AND FREEZE HALF)

2½ pounds boneless, skinless chicken breasts or thighs, thawed if frozen

4 tablespoons (½ stick) butter

1¼ cups Frank's original hot sauce (reduce if you don't like heat)

1 (10- to 12-ounce) bag frozen small-cut seasoning blend (see page 35)

2 tablespoons apple cider vinegar

2 teaspoons dried parsley flakes

1 teaspoon dried oregano

½ teaspoon garlic powder

½ teaspoon onion powder

½ teaspoon Mineral Salt

½ teaspoon black pepper

½ cup sour cream* (optional)

This is flavorful, hearty eats and so versatile! Please don't be scared if you are not a spice lover. Just be sure to buy the original Frank's hot sauce, not the "hot" kind. And if you're still timid, pull back the amount of sauce to 1 or even ½ cup. That will give you a very mild heat level but still lots of flavor.

1. Put the seasoning blend at the bottom of a crockpot. Add all the other ingredients except for the sour cream. Cover and cook on low for 6 hours. Shred the chicken with 2 forks (it will fall apart easily). If using sour cream, stir it in well.

ELECTRIC PRESSURE COOKER DIRECTIONS: Add all the ingredients except the sour cream to a pressure cooker. Seal and cook at high pressure for 12 minutes. Use natural pressure release for at least 10 minutes, followed by quick pressure release. Stir in the sour cream and shred the chicken.

MAKE A FAMILY MEAL: For the weight-loss plan, enjoy this over Cauli Rice (page 263), stuffed into hollowed-out zucchini and baked for 15 minutes at 400°F, or wrap this (see Note) in lettuce wraps or Wonder Wraps 2 (page 251) or stuff it into low-carb tortillas or pitas with sour cream and grated cheese . . . or it can be the tasty protein to jazz up a big salad! Ways to enjoy this dish are endless! Growing children can have a healthy carb side like a piece of fruit, whole milk, or a whole-grain bread item for a Crossover.

NOTE: When wrapping or stuffing this into lettuce or tortillas, use a slotted spoon or tongs to remove the chicken from the crockpot and try not to get too much of the broth so it won't be too messy.

* FOR DF: LEAVE OUT THE SOUR CREAM—THIS RECIPE WORKS GREAT WITHOUT IT.

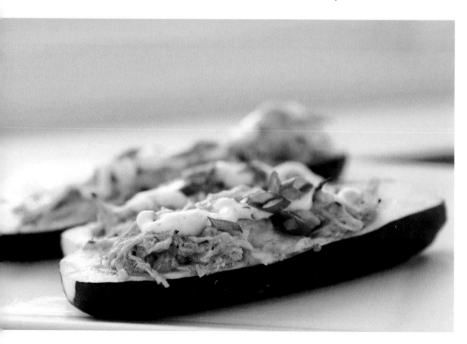

sweet lime taco joes

FP WITH S AND E OPTIONS

FAMILY SERVE—FEEDS 6 TO 8 (HALVE IF YOUR FAMILY IS SMALLER, OR MAKE FULL AND FREEZE HALF)

2½ pounds boneless, skinless chicken breasts, thawed if frozen

1½ cups salsa verde (mild, medium, or hot)

¼ cup Gentle Sweet*

¼ cup lime juice

2 teaspoons chili powder

¾ teaspoon smoked (or regular) paprika

¾ teaspoon ground cumin

1½ teaspoons Mineral Salt

¼ teaspoon black pepper

1 teaspoon onion powder

1 teaspoon garlic powder

This is some tasty eats . . . a chicken version of Sloppy Joes bursting with Mexican flavors with a twist! A handy jar of salsa verde once again makes a great meal here. The explosion in your mouth happens when you add sweetness to the spice of salsa verde, then a tart burst of lime!

1. Put all the ingredients in a crockpot. Cover and cook on low for 5 hours. Once finished, shred the chicken with 2 forks right inside the crock.

ELECTRIC PRESSURE COOKER DIRECTIONS: Add all the ingredients and cook at high pressure for 30 minutes. Use natural pressure release. Shred the chicken.

MAKE A FAMILY MEAL: For the weight-loss plan, stuff this into low-carb soft tacos or Wonder Wraps 2 (page 251). Or top a big plate of leafy greens with it and you'll have a meal experience you won't forget. For an S, add Mexican fixin's like avocado or sour cream. For an E meal, add beans or brown rice. Children can enjoy with fat like sour cream and carbs like beans or rice for a Crossover.

* FOR NSI: USE A GROCERY STORE ON-PLAN SWEETENER.

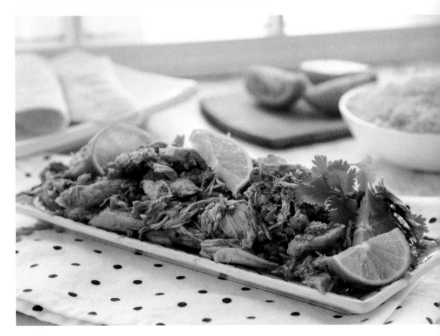

brown gravy stew

S

FAMILY SERVE–FEEDS 6 TO 8 (HALVE IF YOUR FAMILY IS SMALLER, OR MAKE FULL AND FREEZE HALF)

2½ to 3 pounds diced stew meat

2 carrots, sliced

1 pound radishes, trimmed and halved

8 celery stalks, sliced

1 quart beef broth (with an optional 3 to 4 tablespoons Just Gelatin or Integral Collagen, see page 40)

1 teaspoon onion powder

1 teaspoon garlic powder

2½ teaspoons Mineral Salt

1 teaspoon black pepper

⅛ to ¼ teaspoon cayenne pepper (or more to taste)

¼ cup Nutritional Yeast

A couple generous squirts Bragg liquid aminos (optional but makes it yummier)

2 to 2¼ teaspoons Gluccie*

2 handfuls of peas, either frozen or canned

If you are craving hearty, hot, comforting, wrap yourself in a blanket on a rainy night sort of food, this is it! The radishes look just like little potatoes once cooked and taste similar, too (especially when made in the crockpot), from soaking in all that good gravy. Don't be afraid of that bitter bite that comes to mind with radishes—all bitterness goes away after cooking. You'll sigh . . . feel your stress levels go down, and dig into goodness in a bowl without a trace of guilt.

1. Put all the ingredients (except the Gluccie and peas) in a crockpot and stir. Cover and cook on low for 7 to 8 hours.

2. During the last half hour, take out about 1½ cups of the broth and place it in a blender with the 2 teaspoons Gluccie. Blend well for about 1 minute, holding the lid on tightly. Vent hot air. Let the blender rest for 30 seconds, then seal again and blend for another minute. Return the thickened broth to the crockpot. Add the peas and cook for another 15 minutes. If the gravy doesn't get quite as thick as you like it, take a little more of the broth out, add another ¼ teaspoon of Gluccie to it, and blend again. Taste and adjust the flavors to "own it!"

ELECTRIC PRESSURE COOKER DIRECTIONS: Add all the ingredients (except the Gluccie and peas) to a pressure cooker. Seal and cook at high pressure for 35 minutes. Use natural pressure release. Add the peas to soften in the piping hot sauce and follow the directions in the crockpot version to thicken the gravy with Gluccie.

MAKE A FAMILY MEAL: For the weight-loss plan, make up some Fifteen-Minute Focaccia Bread (page 247) and put it on the side of this stew . . . mmmm, or eat the stew ladled over Mashed Fotatoes (page 264). Growing children can have a healthy carb on the side, such as buttered sprouted-grain bread or whole milk, or they can enjoy their stew over regular mashed potatoes.

* FOR NSI: SUB XANTHAN GUM FOR THE GLUCCIE.

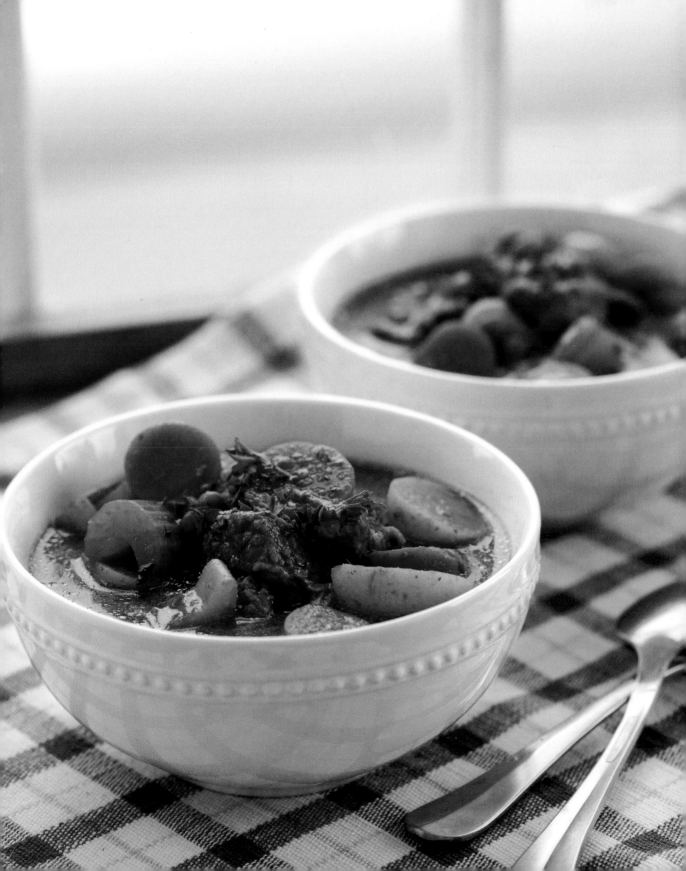

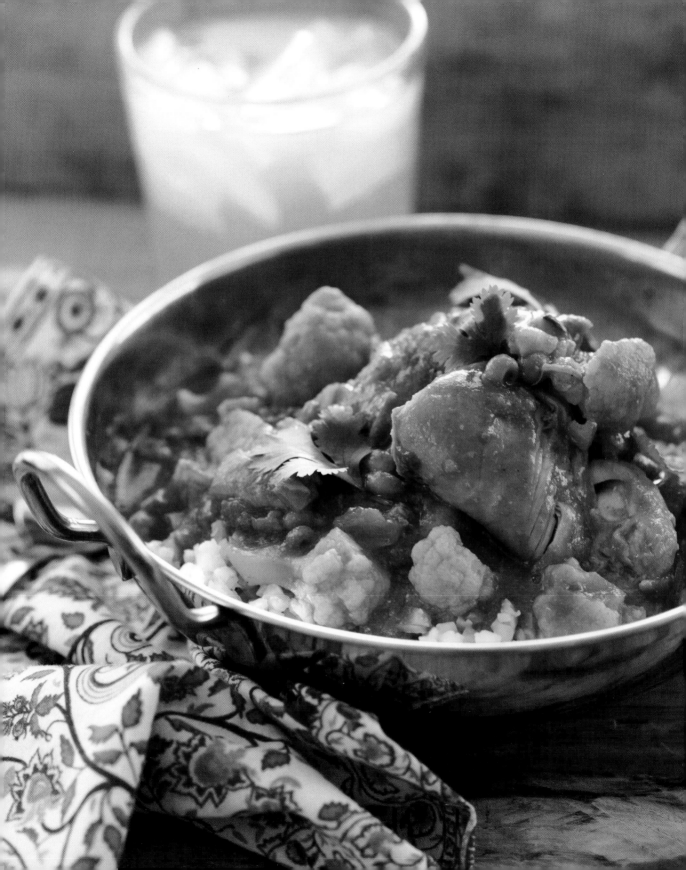

crazy easy curry

S

FAMILY SERVE–FEEDS 6 TO 8 (HALVE IF YOUR FAMILY IS SMALLER, OR MAKE FULL AND FREEZE HALF)

2½ pounds chicken tenderloins or boneless, skinless breasts or thighs, thawed if frozen

1 (10- to 12-ounce) bag frozen small-cut seasoning blend (see page 35)

2 (15-ounce) cans full-fat coconut milk

2 (6-ounce) cans tomato paste

1 rounded tablespoon yellow curry powder (see Note)

1 teaspoon garam marsala, or another 1 or 2 teaspoons curry powder

2½ to 3 teaspoons Mineral Salt

1 teaspoon red pepper flakes (add more if you love heat like we do, or pull back if you're a heat wimp . . . lol)

4 or 5 garlic cloves, minced

1 (16-ounce) bag frozen cauliflower florets (optional)

A couple handfuls of frozen peas (optional)

¼ to ⅓ cup heavy cream (optional)

This is the easiest curry you will ever make. It won't fail you! If you are not sure whether you love curry, we got a feeling this just might turn you on to the curry-loving side of life. Not a spicy food lover? Don't be put off by the word "curry"—simply use half the amount of pepper flakes called for or leave them out altogether, and you'll get all the delicious flavor without the heat. The creaminess of this Indian dish comes from the metabolism-revving coconut milk. This makes it a wonderful dairy-free meal since the heavy cream is not necessary at all but does shoot the yum factor through the roof!

1. Place all the ingredients (except the cauliflower, peas, and heavy cream) in the crockpot and stir. Cover and cook on low for 5 to 6 hours. If adding the cauliflower and peas, add them in the last hour.

2. Break up the chicken just a little (don't shred). If including the heavy cream, stir it in at the end. Taste and adjust the seasonings until you smile and say, "Serene and Pearl . . . you rock!" (Sorry, couldn't help it.)

ELECTRIC PRESSURE COOKER DIRECTIONS: Open the cans of coconut milk from the bottom and pour only the liquid into the pressure cooker. Set the coconut cream aside to add later. Mix together the remaining ingredients (except the cauliflower, peas, and heavy cream). Seal and cook at high pressure for 8 to 10 minutes. Use natural pressure release for 5 minutes. Stir in the peas and/or cauliflower (if using). Bring to pressure again for 1 minute. If including the heavy cream, stir it in just before serving.

MAKE A FAMILY MEAL: Enjoy this over Cauli Rice (page 263) or sautéed Not Naughty Rice, or just have it in a bowl alone with a side salad. Growing children or others at Crossover stage can enjoy this over whole-grain rice.

NOTE: Some curry powders are milder than others, so you may need another tablespoon or so if you taste this toward the end of cooking and the flavor is not "curryish" enough for your preference.

creamy bean, bacon, and butternut soup

E

FAMILY SERVE–FEEDS 6 TO 8 (HALVE IF YOUR FAMILY IS SMALLER, OR MAKE FULL AND FREEZE HALF)

1 pound dried white beans of any kind

1 teaspoon butter or coconut oil

4 garlic cloves, minced

5 to 6 slices turkey bacon, diced

1 (10- to 12-ounce) bag frozen riced cauliflower, or a similar amount fresh or frozen cauliflower florets

1 (12- to 16-ounce) bag frozen cut butternut squash (see Note)

1 onion, quartered

10 cups just off the boil water (with an optional 4 to 5 tablespoons Just Gelatin or Integral Collagen, see page 40)

A few squirts Bragg liquid aminos or coconut aminos (optional)

1 teaspoon black pepper

1 teaspoon onion powder

½ teaspoon mesquite liquid smoke

A few dashes hot sauce or cayenne pepper to taste

1¼ teaspoons Gluccie*

2 to 2½ teaspoons Mineral Salt

This beautiful thick and creamy soup will fool your taste buds into thinking you are eating plenty of fat. Nope, what you have here is a nurturing E meal with healthy, slow-burning carbs to soothe your adrenal glands and keep your metabolism in good working order. The little bit of fat in this soup comes from the tiny 1 teaspoon of butter and the turkey bacon, which is leaner than regular bacon but brings lots of wonderful flavor to the soup. You do start from scratch with the beans here, but don't be intimidated if you are a Drive-Thru Sue; this soup is a no-brainer.

1. Right before you go to bed the night before, put the beans in a large bowl and fill the bowl with water. Cover and allow the beans to soak for at least 7 hours. You can do this during the day if you'd rather cook the soup all night. Once soaked, rinse then drain the beans and place them in a crockpot.

2. When ready to make the soup, heat the butter in a skillet over medium-high heat. Add the garlic and sauté for about a minute, then add the bacon. Toss around the skillet until the bacon starts to crisp.

3. Add the bacon and garlic to the crockpot along with the riced cauliflower, butternut squash, onion, water, liquid aminos (if using), black pepper, onion powder, smoke seasoning, and hot sauce or cayenne. Cover and cook on high for 6 to 7 hours.

4. During the last 30 minutes of cooking, grab a ladle and transfer about one-third to one-half of the beans to a blender. Add the onion pieces, whatever cauliflower that is still showing (much of it will have turned to mush already), and a couple cups of the broth. Try to leave the bacon and butternut squash pieces in the pot to look beautiful. Add the Gluccie to the blender along with 2 teaspoons of the salt. Hold the lid on tightly and blend for 30 seconds. Turn off, vent the hot air, then blend for another minute until thickened. Return the puree to the pot, stir gently to combine (try not to smash the butternut, which at this point is supersoft), and keep cooking for another 30 minutes or so. Now "own it!" Taste and adjust the seasonings (perhaps you'll need more salt or black or cayenne pepper) until you love it.

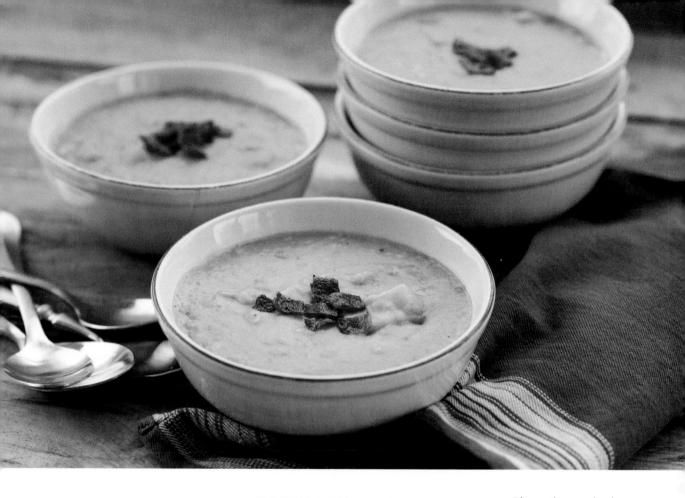

ELECTRIC PRESSURE COOKER DIRECTIONS: Place the soaked beans in a pressure cooker (some believe it is not necessary to use soaked beans in a pressure cooker—we still soak them, but it's up to you). Add all the other ingredients (except for the Gluccie and salt). Seal and cook at high pressure for 25 minutes. Use natural pressure release for 10 minutes, followed by quick pressure release. Then follow the crockpot instructions for thickening the soup and adding salt.

MAKE A FAMILY MEAL: Enjoy with a side salad with an E-friendly, lean dressing and/or an FP bread such as Wonderful White Blender Bread (page 242) or Nuke Queen's Cornbread (page 246) with a thin smear of butter to stay in E mode. Growing children can have this topped with grated cheese for a Crossover.

NOTE: You can find bags of cut squash in your frozen veggie section. If not, you should be able to find frozen cut sweet potato, which works great, too. Or cut up some fresh squash or sweet potato by hand.

* FOR NSI: SUB XANTHAN GUM FOR THE GLUCCIE.

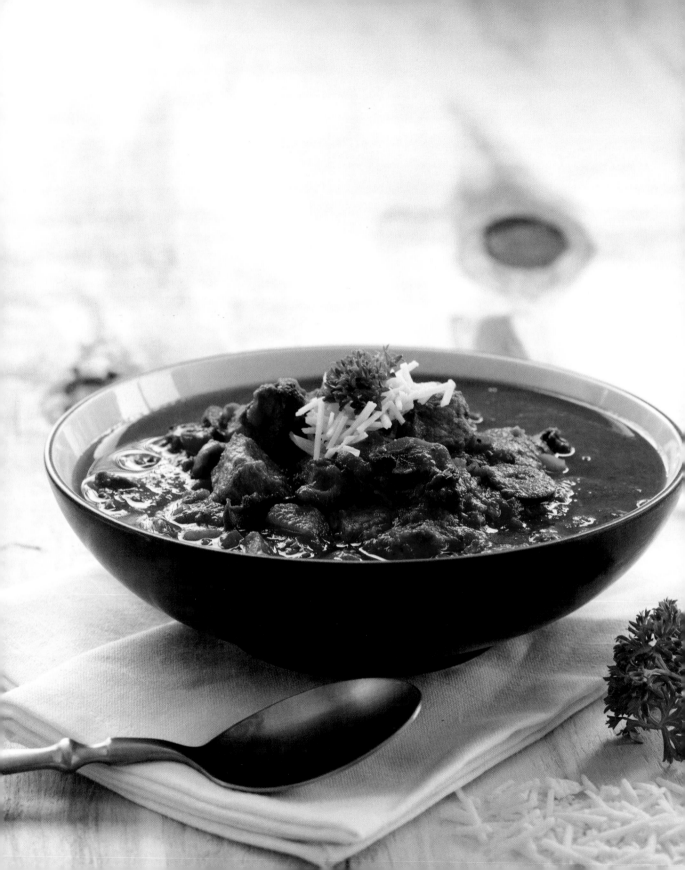

stew of love

S WITH **E** AND **FP** OPTIONS

FAMILY SERVE–FEEDS 6 TO 8 (HALVE IF YOUR FAMILY IS SMALLER, OR MAKE FULL AND FREEZE HALF)

2½ to 3 pounds diced beef stew meat (or use boneless, skinless chicken breasts for FP)

4 to 6 garlic cloves, minced

2 (14.5-ounce) cans fire-roasted or regular diced tomatoes

3 to 4 ounces sliced black (or other) olives

1 (10- to 12-ounce) bag frozen small-cut seasoning blend (see page 35)

8 ounces fresh mushrooms, sliced

1 (6-ounce) can tomato paste

1½ tablespoons smoked or regular paprika

2 to 2½ teaspoons Mineral Salt

1 teaspoon black pepper

1 teaspoon onion powder

½ teaspoon dried oregano

¼ teaspoon dried rosemary

1½ cups beef broth or water

¼ to ⅓ cup heavy cream* (optional)

This is *amore*. You can't help but fall in love with this rustic Italian stew inspired by the flavors of cacciatore. Now, if you have an Italian Mama who made cacciatore for you, you'd remember a bone-in chicken dish with incredible seared-in flavors. This is not exactly that. We can't compete with Italian Mamas who spent hours over the stove infusing flavor. But this dish is wonderful in its own right and so much quicker and easier for your fast-paced life. You can easily make this with chicken breasts instead of beef and even use the FP option of no cream. And yes, you can certainly take the time to use bone-in chicken here and sear it before putting it in the pot if you'd rather. However you "own" this dish, you'll feel the love in every bite of this soul-warming stuff!

1. Place all the ingredients (except the heavy cream) in the bottom of a crockpot and stir well. Cover and cook on low for 6 to 8 hours. If using the cream, pour it in at the end before serving.

ELECTRIC PRESSURE COOKER DIRECTIONS: Place all the ingredients (except the heavy cream) in a pressure cooker. Seal and cook at high pressure for 1 hour. Use quick pressure release. Add the cream (if using) and serve.

MAKE A FAMILY MEAL: For the weight-loss plan, enjoy with the cream for an S option or without (using chicken breasts) for an FP. Have a big bowlful or two alone, or spoon it over Troodles (zucchini noodles) and it becomes almost like a kicked-up spaghetti sauce. Add an on-plan bread from the Breads chapter (page 240) such as WWBB Garlic Bread (page 245) if desired. If making the FP version, you can enjoy it over whole-grain rice for an E. Children or others needing Crossies can enjoy the S version with whole-grain rice or noodles for a Crossover.

* FOR DF: LEAVE OUT THE CREAM.

slimming secret spaghetti

S WITH FP OPTION

FAMILY SERVE—FEEDS 6 TO 8 (HALVE IF YOUR FAMILY IS SMALLER, OR MAKE FULL AND FREEZE HALF; HOWEVER, DON'T FREEZE IF USING NOT NAUGHTY NOODLES OR TRIM HEALTHY NOODLES)

2½ to 3 pounds 85% lean ground beef (or use an even leaner meat for FP), thawed if frozen

1 (10- to 12-ounce) bag frozen small-cut seasoning blend (see page 35)

2 to 4 garlic cloves, peeled but whole

3 (14.5-ounce) cans diced tomatoes

1 (6-ounce) can tomato paste

2½ cups frozen diced okra

2 teaspoons dried oregano

1½ to 2 teaspoons Mineral Salt

½ teaspoon dried basil

½ teaspoon dried thyme

¼ teaspoon cayenne pepper (or more for us heat lovers)

½ to ¾ teaspoon Super Sweet Blend* (optional; it brings out sweetness in the tomatoes)

½ cup water

½ cup powder-style Parmesan cheese* (from the green can)

3 to 4 single-serve bags Trim Healthy Noodles or Not Naughty Noodles,* well rinsed, drained, and snipped a bit smaller, or 4 large zucchini, spiralized into Troodles

We managed to create a smashing spaghetti that doesn't require browning the meat first for crockpot cooking to save you that extra step on crazy days. For this reason, you need to use 85% lean ground meat. Using a fattier meat will make the sauce feel too greasy since you are not draining off the fat after browning. If you'd prefer to use an even leaner meat (like venison or 96% lean ground turkey), that would make this an FP and that's fine, too, but we prefer this as an S.

Now, time for a lecture. Tut-tut . . . we don't want to hear any fretting about the amount of okra here. It is part of the slimming magic of this sauce. Give us some faith! All fears about okra sliminess will be alleviated when you taste the final result . . . no okra detected. And here's a direct command from yours trulies . . . DO NOT TELL YOUR KIDS (OR PICKY HUSBAND) ABOUT THE OKRA IN THIS SAUCE! It is our little secret and we must keep it forever. Our okra-despising teenage boys love this meal, but only because they have no idea of our secret shenanigans. What if you don't have okra? Okay, leave it out. This recipe still works without it.

If you'd rather make this in a regular pot on the stove . . . go ahead and brown the meat with the seasoning blend first. It still works great. However, if you choose to use the Trim Healthy Noodles or Not Naughty Noodles, they get wonderfully soft after cooking in the crockpot all day. Slow-cooking konjac-based noodles all day like this is a fabulous way to develop a taste for them, and they can be a powerful tool in your weight-loss belt.

1. Put the meat in the bottom of a crockpot and break it up well with a fork. Add the seasoning blend and mix well with the meat.

2. Add the garlic, 1½ cans of the diced tomatoes, the tomato paste, okra, oregano, salt, basil, thyme, cayenne, and sweetener (if using) to a blender. Blend the dickens out of this until it is all perfectly smooth, then add to the crock. Add the water, Parm, and, if using, the Trim Healthy Noodles or Not Naughty Noodles and stir well. (If using Troodles, don't add these yet.)

3. Cover and cook on high for 5 to 6 hours. If using Troodles, add them during the last 15 minutes of cooking.

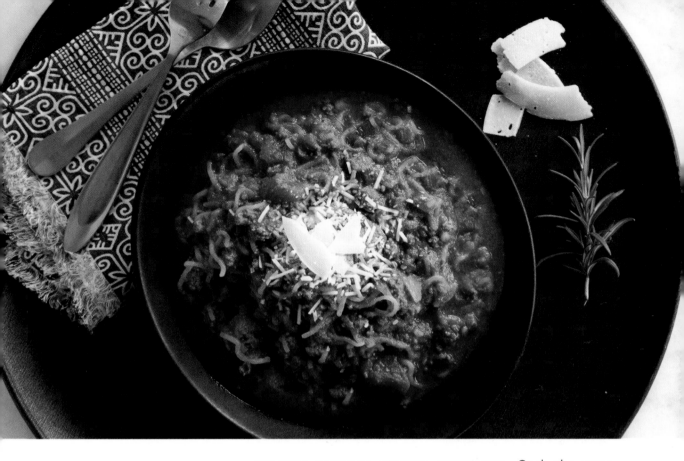

ELECTRIC PRESSURE COOKER DIRECTIONS: Cook the meat on sauté mode, then add the blended sauce and all the other ingredients (except the Parmesan and Troodles, if using) to the pot. Seal and cook at high pressure for 10 minutes. Use natural pressure release for at least 10 minutes followed by quick pressure release. If using Troodles, immediately add them after cooking so they can spend a few minutes softening in the piping hot sauce. Stir in the Parmesan cheese (if using).

MAKE A FAMILY MEAL: For the weight-loss plan, feel free to top your spaghetti with some extra Parmesan cheese or any grated cheese. Have a side salad with a vinaigrette dressing, and perhaps WWBB Garlic Bread (page 245). Growing children can enjoy a healthy carb such as whole-grain noodles in place of the noodle options here or they can have it with buttered sprouted-grain bread for a Crossover.

* FOR NSI: USE A GROCERY STORE ON-PLAN SWEETENER, OR LEAVE THE SWEETENER OUT. USE TROODLES (ZUCCHINI NOODLES) IN PLACE OF THE NOT NAUGHTY NOODLES OR TRIM HEALTHY NOODLES OR FIND KONJAC NOODLES AT YOUR GROCERY STORE (SEE PAGE 43).

* FOR DF: LEAVE OUT THE PARMESAN CHEESE.

totally dope chicken

S

FAMILY SERVE—FEEDS 6 TO 8 (HALVE IF YOUR FAMILY IS SMALLER, OR MAKE FULL AND FREEZE HALF)

8 slices bacon, diced (we use turkey, you can use any kind)

2½ pounds chicken tenderloins or boneless, skinless breasts or thighs, thawed if frozen

1½ (8-ounce) packages ⅓ less fat cream cheese

1 cup plain 0% Greek yogurt

1 tablespoon dried parsley flakes

2 teaspoons onion powder

2 teaspoons garlic powder, or 4 to 5 garlic cloves, minced

1½ teaspoons Mineral Salt

1 teaspoon black pepper

½ to 1 teaspoon Super Sweet Blend (optional)

½ to ¾ teaspoon red pepper flakes (optional)

PEARL CHATS: The title says it all, this stuff is addicting. What could be yummier than bacon- and ranch-flavored chicken? This dish usually goes by the name of Crack Chicken, but I thought that might offend some of you, so you can thank my sixteen-year-old son, Rocky, for its current name. I told him I thought "totally dope" may still be a tad offensive, so then he suggested calling it "Totally Dope Chicken on a Sunday" to appease our fellow churchgoing crowd. Hmmm . . . perhaps not. I'll let you rename this if the title is not to your liking—the chicken itself is sure to be!

Sadly, most crack chicken recipes call for packets of store-bought ranch seasoning. That stuff is usually laden with MSG, or if not, contains fillers, sugar, and other junk ingredients. No need to put that stuff in your body. It won't take you more than a few seconds to add the pure seasonings here that give all the ranch flavor you crave.

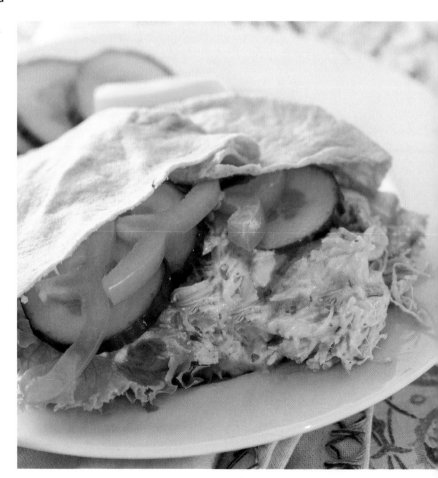

1. Cook the bacon until crisp in a skillet over medium heat.
2. Add the bacon and all the other ingredients to a crockpot and stir to combine. Cover and cook on low for 5 hours. Shred the chicken with 2 forks inside the crock and stir all well.

ELECTRIC PRESSURE COOKER DIRECTIONS: Cook the bacon on sauté mode until crispy. Add all the other ingredients (except the cream cheese and yogurt) to the pot along with 1 cup chicken broth. Seal and cook at high pressure for 8 minutes. Use natural pressure release for 5 minutes followed by quick pressure release. Stir in the cream cheese and yogurt.

MAKE A FAMILY MEAL: For the weight-loss plan, there are so many ways to eat this . . . stuff it into low-carb pitas or wraps (including lettuce wraps or Wonder Wraps 2, page 251); make a sandwich using Wonderful White Blender Bread (page 242) or Fifteen-Minute Focaccia Bread (page 247); put it over a salad or between slices of cucumber, or you can even put it in a nori wrap. Growing children can have a healthy carb on the side like a piece of fruit or a glass of whole milk, or they can enjoy their chicken in a whole-grain bread item for a Crossover.

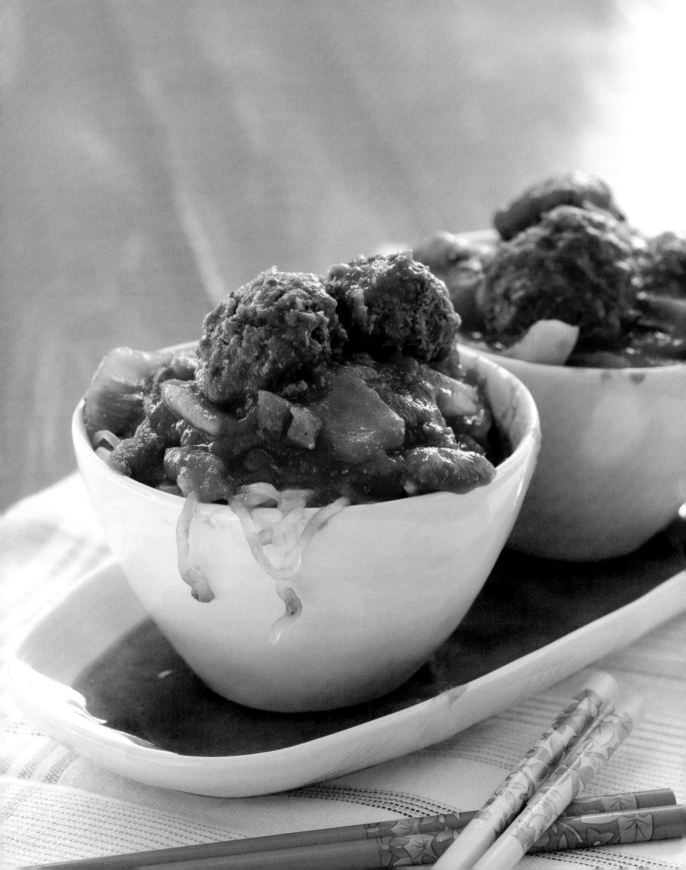

sweet and sour meatballs

FP WITH S AND E OPTIONS

FAMILY SERVE—FEEDS 6 TO 8 (HALVE IF YOUR FAMILY IS SMALLER, OR MAKE FULL AND FREEZE HALF)

2 (10- to 12-ounce) bags frozen large-cut seasoning blend (see page 35); if your kids don't like onions, you can leave the seasoning blend out and just use 2 red bell peppers or no veggies at all

35 Marvelous Make-Ahead Meatballs (page 208), mostly thawed from frozen

1 (6-ounce) can tomato paste

3 tablespoons rice vinegar or apple cider vinegar

¼ cup plus 1 tablespoon Gentle Sweet* (or more to taste)

¾ teaspoon Mineral Salt

½ teaspoon black pepper

½ teaspoon onion powder

¼ to ½ teaspoon red pepper flakes (stay with ¼ if you don't like a lot of heat, but we love even more)

2 cups water

1 teaspoon Gluccie*

Please make these . . . they are so yummy for an evening meal or as leftovers for lunch, and they're great to take to a party! If you stock your freezer with a bunch of Marvelous Make-Ahead Meatballs (page 208), then making this meal will be a breeze. Transfer a baggie of the meatballs from the freezer to the fridge the night before you make this meal and they'll be mostly thawed and ready enough for the crockpot. Or you can use fully frozen meatballs in an electric pressure cooker. (If you choose to use frozen meatballs in the crockpot, that's sorta against the rules. You'd be a rebel but we doubt it will kill ya.) If we can't twist your arm into making your own meatballs, you can buy store-bought frozen meatballs; however, you'll need to find some with 3 or less grams of carbs since any more carbs than that means too many fillers.

1. Put the seasoning blend in the bottom of a crockpot. Place the meatballs on top. Blend all the other ingredients in a blender for 1 minute, then pour over. Cover and cook on low for about 5 hours. (We have started with frozen meatballs before and cooked on high; we're still living to tell the tale, but don't sue us if you try the same and things don't work out.)

ELECTRIC PRESSURE COOKER DIRECTIONS: Spray a pressure cooker pot with coconut oil and add all the ingredients, including the blended sauce. Seal and cook at high pressure for 15 minutes. Use quick pressure release.

MAKE A FAMILY MEAL: For the weight-loss plan, you can eat these as an FP in a bowl over Cauli Rice (page 263) if you use the ultra-lean meat called for in the FP version of the meatballs. Throw down a side salad with a lean dressing and you're set. Or put them over brown rice for an E. If using regular beef in your meatballs, these will be an S (most store-bought meatballs will be an S also), so omit the brown rice and use sautéed Not Naughty Rice, Trim Healthy Rice, or riced cauliflower. Children can include a carb like whole-grain rice, plus a fat such as a creamy dressing on a salad, for a Crossover.

* FOR NSI: SUB XANTHAN GUM FOR THE GLUCCIE AND USE A GROCERY STORE ON-PLAN SWEETENER.

succulent barbacoa beef

S

FAMILY SERVE–FEEDS 6 TO 8 (HALVE IF YOUR FAMILY IS SMALLER, OR MAKE FULL AND FREEZE HALF)

2½ to 3 pounds beef chuck roast, cut into thirds

1 onion, cut into chunks

1 to 3 chipotle peppers in adobo sauce from a can (using 3 is lovely and spicy, but if you don't like a whole lot of spice, pull back to 1 or 2 and rinse the sauce off a little)

4 to 6 garlic cloves, minced

2 to 3 tablespoons lime juice (fresh or bottled)

3 tablespoons apple cider vinegar

¾ cup water or beef broth

1 tablespoon ground cumin

2 teaspoons dried oregano

1½ teaspoons Mineral Salt

1 teaspoon black pepper

We love Chipotle restaurants—so easy to stay on plan there using their bowl option. We love ordering their barbacoa beef or chicken, including the sautéed veggies, and putting it all over lettuce and salsa, then topping with lots of guac and a sprinkle of cheese for an S meal. Mmmm . . . amazing! Or sometimes we add some brown rice and beans for a healthy Crossover. You can also order an E meal there . . . grilled chicken breast, beans, brown rice, and all the veggies and fresh salsas. Just leave off the guac, and if you include cheese, make sure it is only a small garnish amount. You can make something similar to their succulent beef (our very favorite menu item there) at home. Here is our version.

1. Place the beef in the bottom of a crockpot. Put all the other ingredients in a blender and blend well. Pour the contents of the blender over the beef. Cover and cook on low for 7 to 8 hours. Break the beef apart once cooked . . . you don't have to completely shred, but pulling most of it apart allows it to drink up all the delicious juices.

ELECTRIC PRESSURE COOKER DIRECTIONS: Coat the pressure cooker pot with coconut oil spray and place all the ingredients in the pot, including the blended sauce. Seal and cook at high pressure for 50 minutes. Use natural pressure release.

MAKE A FAMILY MEAL: For the weight-loss plan, put this over lettuce and add salsa, cheese, guacamole, and optional sour cream for the "bowl" version. Or stuff it into Wonder Wraps 2 (page 251) or low-carb tortillas. Growing children can enjoy it with a healthy carb option like whole-grain rice or even baked corn chips.

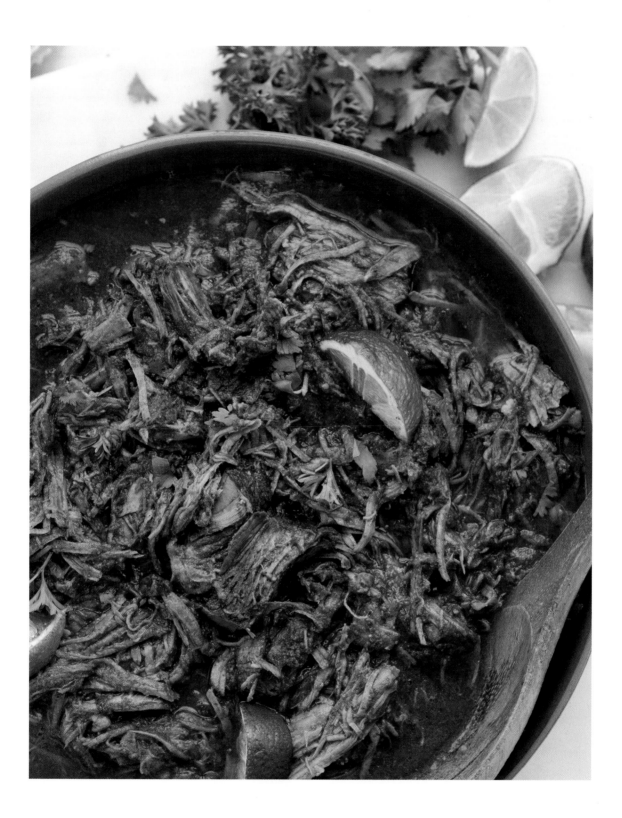

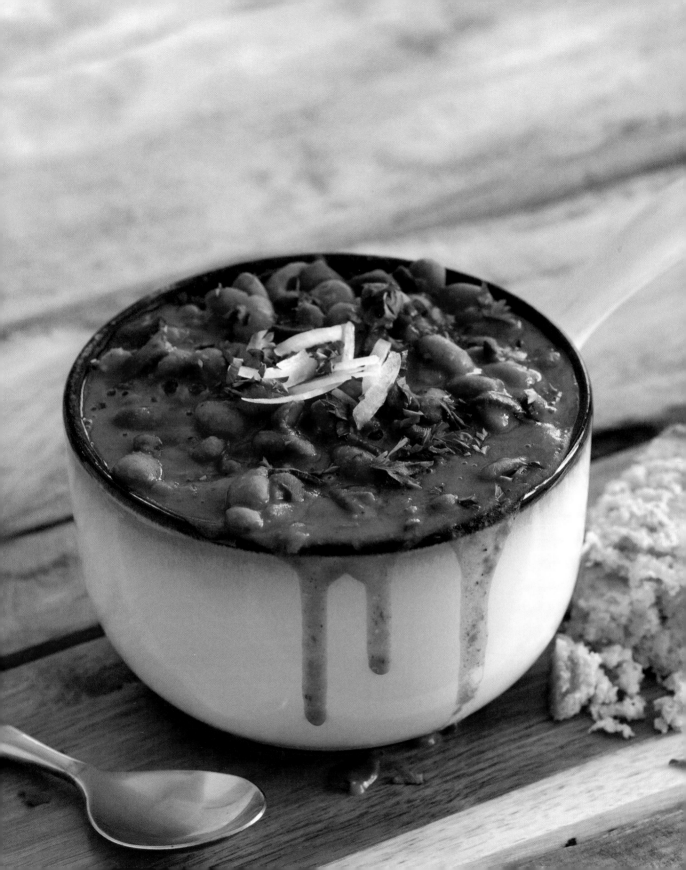

beans 'n' cornbread

Ⓔ

FAMILY SERVE—FEEDS 6 TO 8 (HALVE IF YOUR FAMILY IS SMALLER, OR MAKE FULL AND FREEZE HALF)

1½ pounds dried pinto beans

5 cups water (with an optional
  4 tablespoons Integral Collagen or
  Just Gelatin for added protein,
  see page 40)

2 to 3 ounces real turkey bacon bits
  or crumbles (using turkey here to
  keep within E fat guidelines)

1 tablespoon dried onion flakes

1½ teaspoons garlic powder

½ teaspoon black pepper

2½ to 3 teaspoons Mineral Salt

Nuke Queen's Cornbread
  (page 246)

This is an inexpensive but extremely tasty meatless meal. We love our beans 'n' cornbread nights!

1. Right before you go to bed the night before, put the beans in a large bowl and fill the bowl with water. Cover and allow the beans to soak for at least 7 hours. You can do this during the day if you'd rather cook the beans all night. Once soaked, drain the beans and place them in a crockpot.

2. Add the 5 cups water and collagen or gelatin (if using), the bacon bits, onion flakes, garlic powder, and pepper (don't add the salt yet, as it can stop the beans from softening). Stir, cover, and cook on high for 7 to 8 hours (if the beans absorb too much water and dry out, add a bit more). During the last hour, add the salt, starting with 2½ teaspoons and only adding the other ½ teaspoon if needed (we like the full amount, but some may find that too salty). Grab a potato masher and mash up some of the beans, leaving most whole (the mashed beans add a bit of texture).

3. While the beans are cooking, make the cornbread so it is ready once the beans are done.

ELECTRIC PRESSURE COOKER DIRECTIONS: Combine the soaked or nonsoaked (up to you) beans and all the seasonings except the salt in a pressure cooker. Seal and cook at high pressure for 30 minutes. Use natural pressure release. Follow the salt and mashing directions from the crockpot version.

MAKE A FAMILY MEAL: For the weight-loss plan, the beans and cornbread are perfect with a cucumber salad using a lean dressing. Don't forget your veggies, even with a meal like this. Chopped onions are fabulous sprinkled on the beans, too! Growing children can have butter on their cornbread for a Crossover, while you will use no more than 1 teaspoon of butter or just crumble your cornbread dry into your beans to keep this an E . . . yummy!

cream of spinach and chicken soup

FAMILY SERVE—FEEDS 6 TO 8 (HALVE IF YOUR FAMILY IS SMALLER, OR MAKE FULL AND FREEZE HALF)

2½ pounds boneless, skinless chicken breast, thawed if frozen

1 quart chicken broth (with an optional 3 to 4 tablespoons Just Gelatin or Integral Collagen, see page 40)

2 cups water

2 teaspoons Mineral Salt

1 teaspoon black pepper

1 teaspoon onion powder

2 teaspoons garlic powder, or 4 garlic cloves, minced

Shakes of cayenne pepper (optional, if you are a heat lover like us)

3 cups just off the boil water

1 (8-ounce) package ⅓ less fat cream cheese

2 cups frozen diced okra

1¼ teaspoons Gluccie*

1 cup powder-style Parmesan cheese (from the green can)

16 ounces fresh spinach (you can chop it a little if you want but you don't have to)

If you're a creamed spinach lover, you are going to love this flavorful soup.

1. Put the chicken in a crockpot along with the chicken broth with the collagen and gelatin (if using) and water. Add the salt, black pepper, onion powder, garlic powder, and cayenne (if using) and stir.

2. Put the 3 cups just-boiled water, cream cheese, and okra in a blender and blend well. Hold the lid down and blend like you're competing for the blending Gold Medal for smoothness. Vent hot air, then blend again until no tiny pieces of okra are left. Add to the crockpot. Cover and cook on low for 5 hours.

3. During the last hour, remove the chicken and cut it into pieces (don't shred). Don't return it yet. Scoop out 1½ cups broth and put it in the blender. Add the Gluccie and blend (holding the lid down tightly) for 30 seconds. Let hot air vent, then blend for another full minute or so until thickened. Return the puree to the pot, and add the Parmesan, chicken pieces, and spinach. Stir and cook for the last hour. Taste and adjust seasonings until you "own it."

ELECTRIC PRESSURE COOKER DIRECTIONS: Place the chicken, broth, 2 cups water, and seasonings in a pressure cooker. Seal and cook at high pressure for 12 minutes. Use natural pressure release. Meanwhile, blend the just-boiled water, okra, and cream cheese until smooth. Remove the chicken from the pressure cooker when done, but leave the cooker on the "keep warm" setting. Cut the chicken and set it aside. Stir the blended okra mixture into the pressure cooker. Then ladle out 1½ cups of the broth and blend with the Gluccie. Return to the pot and stir again. Add the Parm, chicken, and spinach to the pot. Cover and continue to use the "keep warm" setting for 5 to 10 minutes to allow the spinach to wilt.

MAKE A FAMILY MEAL: For the weight-loss plan, enjoy with a side salad and an optional S-friendly bread item from the Breads chapter (page 240) or half of a buttered Joseph's pita. Growing children can have buttered sprouted-grain bread for a Crossover.

* FOR NSI: SUB XANTHAN GUM FOR THE GLUCCIE.

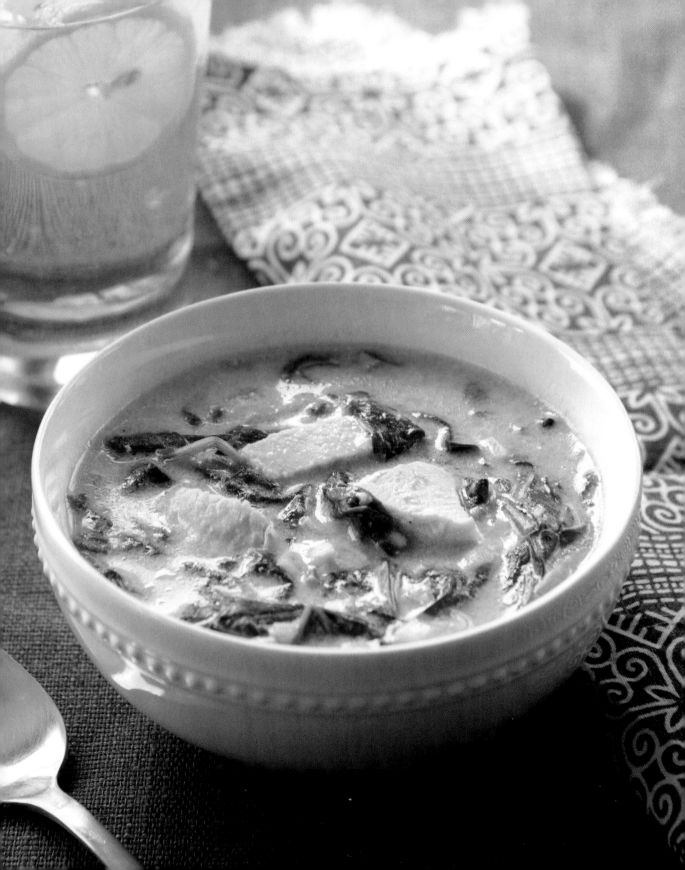

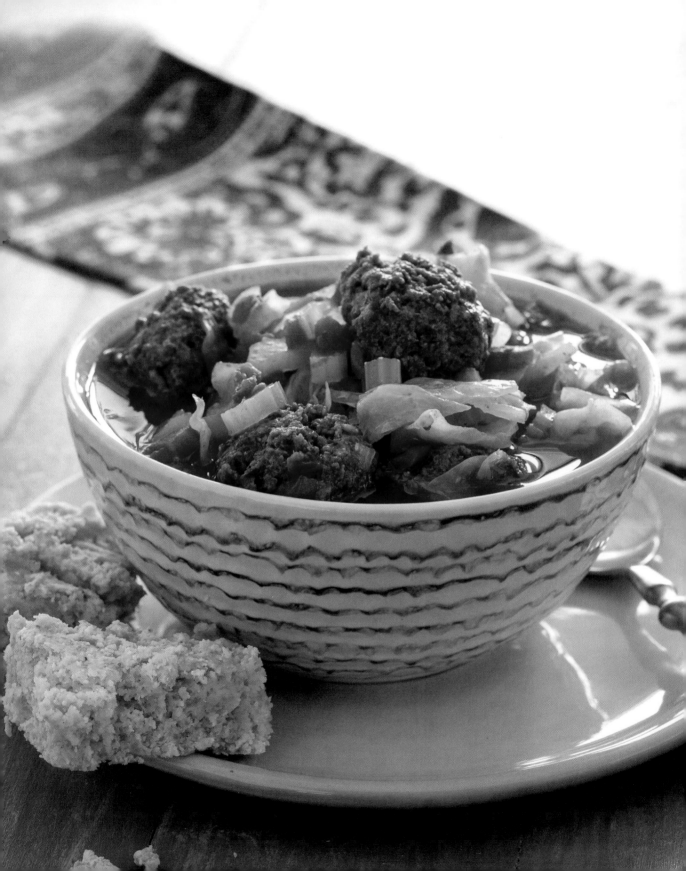

meatball soup

FAMILY SERVE—FEEDS 6 TO 8 (HALVE IF YOUR FAMILY IS SMALLER, OR MAKE FULL AND FREEZE HALF)

20 to 30 mostly thawed frozen Marvelous Make-Ahead Meatballs (page 208)

1 large cabbage, sliced into large bite-size pieces

1 onion, sliced

6 celery stalks, sliced

3 (14.5-ounce) cans diced tomatoes

1 quart beef broth

1½ teaspoons Mineral Salt

1 teaspoon black pepper

⅛ teaspoon cayenne pepper (optional)

½ cup brown rice or hulled barley (optional for E)

Slow-cooked cabbage with meatballs in a tomato and beef broth base . . . what's not to like? Stock your freezer with Marvelous Make-Ahead Meatballs (page 208) and prep is ridiculously easy. Transfer a family-size baggie of the meatballs from the freezer to the fridge the night before you make this meal and they'll be mostly thawed and ready enough for the crockpot, or you can use fully frozen with an electric pressure cooker. Guess we can't force you to make our meatballs, darn it, so if you prefer to buy store-bought meatballs, look for ones with 3 or less grams of carbs as any more than that means too many starchy fillers.

1. Put all the ingredients in a crockpot. Cover and cook on low for 5 to 6 hours (we have started with frozen meatballs before and cooked on high and are still alive, but we don't necessarily encourage it). The meatballs will come apart some once you gently stir at the end of cooking, but that makes the soup even better. But don't stir so that they become mincemeat.

ELECTRIC PRESSURE COOKER DIRECTIONS: Add all the ingredients to a pressure cooker. Seal and cook at high pressure for 30 minutes. Use quick pressure release.

MAKE A FAMILY MEAL: For the weight-loss plan, if using ultra-lean meat in your Marvelous Make-Ahead Meatballs, this soup will be an FP and can be eaten as is for an ultra-weight-loss meal. Or you can add the rice or barley to the pot during cooking for an E and still have room for a piece of sprouted-grain toast with a small smear of butter on the side. If you use regular beef for your meatballs (or store-bought meatballs), this soup will be an S, and you can have it with a piece of Fifteen-Minute Focaccia Bread (page 247) with butter. Growing children can have grated cheese on top and buttered sprouted-grain toast for a Crossover.

Comforting Casseroles & Bakes

Oven-baked casseroles and bakes are the meals that draw your family around the table and create lasting memories of the taste of home. Now they are Trimming and healthy, too!

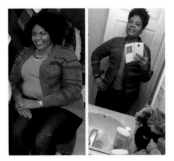

Here is the same outfit one year later (this time with a really tight belt—if not, the pants will fall off!). After nine months of trying to conceive, I was told I was insulin resistant and that I would need assistance to have a baby. My husband and I were both overweight. I had been on fad diets in the past but never stuck with them. We would both exercise, and I even dropped my caloric intake to 1,600 calories. I was still stuck at 268 pounds, eating 1,600 calories a day and exercising 3 times a week!

As a (self-proclaimed) sugar-holic, I found it difficult to consider reducing my sugar intake. However, on Easter morning in 2015, I was introduced to Trim Healthy Mama. A dear sister-in-Christ told me about a plan where people were kicking their sugar habits, having babies left and right, and losing weight. I went to Amazon, ordered the book, and signed up for every Facebook group. I dreamed about it and felt that God led me to this plan. I felt such an urge to do it and do it well. By the next day, I had done some grocery shopping and started separating fuels. I was so excited about every next meal and ready to wake up each day anticipating what I had prepared for the next day. This book had to have a special anointing for people like me!

After a few months, the pounds started coming off, and then people noticed. I love that there is forgiveness on this plan. If you mess up, start over again. And the best part is, I have messed up so many times but have not returned to sugar, white potatoes, or white flour. My habits have been solidified even when I want to indulge. Sugar is not my Master or Lord any-more! I feel great, my hormones are balanced, and although we have not yet conceived, I am confident that we will! **–JASMINE Y.**

drive-thru sue's chicken quiche S

FAMILY SERVE–FEEDS 6 TO 8 (HALVE IF YOUR FAMILY IS SMALLER, OR MAKE FULL AND FREEZE HALF)

Coconut oil cooking spray

10 eggs

2 cups egg whites (carton or fresh)

1½ teaspoons Creole seasoning
(we use MSG-free Tony Cachere's)

¾ teaspoon black pepper

Sprinkle of red pepper flakes
(optional, but recommended for a
little kick)

12 ounces shredded or grated
cheddar cheese

2 (12-ounce) cans chicken breast, or
3 cups diced cooked chicken (see
page 45 for cooking methods)

1 (10- to 12-ounce) bag frozen
small-cut seasoning blend
(see page 35)

PEARL CHATS: To all my fellow Drive-Thru Sue's—you can do it! This is fast . . . no frills . . . inexpensive . . . tasty . . . a cinch . . . come on . . . you have the skills! This is a crustless quiche but you won't miss it (or you can use the savory version of Beauty Blend Base Pie Crust, page 508).

1. Preheat the oven to 350°F. Spray a 9 × 13-inch baking dish with coconut oil.

2. Whisk together the whole eggs, egg whites, and seasonings in a large bowl. Add all the other ingredients and stir until combined.

3. Pour the mixture into the baking dish and bake for 45 minutes.

MAKE A FAMILY MEAL: For the weight-loss plan, serve with a giant salad or a smaller salad and another veggie like Killer Green Beans (page 261) or broccoli. Growing children or other family members at Crossover stage can have a healthy carb on the side, such as sprouted-grain bread and butter, a piece of fruit, a baked potato with butter, or brown rice.

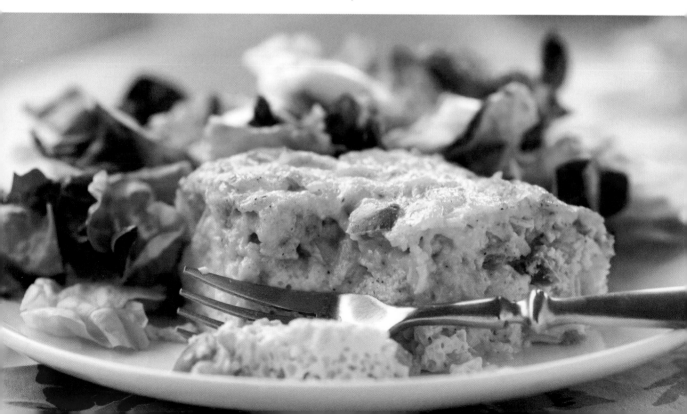

taco pie

S

2 to 2½ pounds ground beef, thawed if frozen

1½ cups sugar-free pizza sauce or the same amount Perfect Pizza Sauce (page 516)

2 to 3 teaspoons chili powder (depending upon your love of chili)

1½ teaspoons ground cumin

1 teaspoon onion powder

1 teaspoon garlic powder

Mineral Salt

12 ounces shredded cheddar or Mexican blend cheese

4 ounces ⅓ less fat cream cheese

3 large eggs

⅓ cup heavy cream

Black pepper

This is a twist on our famous cheeseburger pie. If you have any family members reluctant to jump on the Trim Train, they won't even realize they are doing it with this meal. Dish it up to picky husbands or children and watch them go back for seconds.

1. Preheat the oven to 350°F.

2. Brown the meat in a large skillet over high heat, then drain off any fat. Add the pizza sauce, chili powder, cumin, onion powder, garlic powder, and 1½ teaspoons salt. Spread the meat mixture in a 9 × 13-inch baking pan and mix in half of the shredded cheese.

3. Combine the cream cheese, eggs, cream, and a dash of both salt and pepper in a food processor and blend. Spread over the meat mixture, then top with the remaining shredded cheese. Bake for 35 minutes, or until bubbling.

MAKE A FAMILY MEAL: Pair with a big salad with a vinegar/oil dressing for a nice balance since this is a heavy S meal. You can add any nonstarchy veggie if you want something else on your plate. Growing children can have a healthy carb option on the side, such as buttered sprouted-grain bread or whole-grain rice or a baked potato with butter.

cheesy chicken spaghetti casserole ⓢ

FAMILY SERVE—FEEDS 6 TO 8 (HALVE IF YOUR FAMILY IS SMALLER, BUT DON'T FREEZE, AS KONJAC NOODLES DON'T FREEZE WELL)

4 single-serve bags Trim Healthy Noodles or Not Naughty Noodles,* well rinsed and drained

5 cups diced cooked chicken breast (see page 45 for cooking methods), or diced rotisserie chicken

1 (10-ounce can) Ro-tel-style diced tomatoes and green chilies, drained

1½ (8-ounce) packages ⅓ less fat cream cheese

½ cup chicken broth

1½ teaspoons Mineral Salt

½ teaspoon black pepper

1 teaspoon paprika

1 teaspoon chili powder

½ teaspoon onion powder

½ teaspoon garlic powder

3 cups (12 ounces) grated cheddar cheese

This is ooey-gooey, noodley, cheesy goodness. Regular white noodles when mixed with cheese are one of the most fattening and health-destroying foods on this planet. Konjac noodles such as our Trim Healthy or Not Naughty noodles allow you to enjoy that oh-so-magnificent combination of cheese and noodles without widening your waistline. On page 43, you can read more about them and find where to get them if you don't have our brand.

1. Preheat the oven to 375°F.
2. Snip the noodles a bit smaller with kitchen scissors so they are not too terribly long. Put the diced chicken, noodles, and diced tomatoes and chilies in a 9 × 13-inch baking dish.
3. Put the cream cheese, broth, salt, pepper, paprika, chili powder, onion powder, and garlic powder in a blender and blend until smooth. Scrape the mixture into the baking dish using a spatula. Mix in 2 cups of the cheddar. Top with the remaining cheddar and bake for 30 to 35 minutes. Broil for just a couple minutes at the end to make sure all the cheese is golden brown and bubbling, but watch it doesn't burn.

MAKE A FAMILY MEAL: Enjoy with a large side salad with vinaigrette and an optional nonstarchy veggie for a side, such as steamed asparagus with a little melted butter or coconut oil and salt. This is an ultracheesy main dish, so think moderation if you also want cheese or ranch on your salad or on your side veggies. If you feel like eating some dessert, try a baby-size shake or smoothie in the Shakes and Smoothies chapter (page 468) or perhaps an Incredible Peanut Butter Cookie Muffin (page 371). No need to tag on more cream cheese or cream in your dessert. We always want to respect the heavy S fats and not overdo them. Growing children and other Crossie peeps can include whole-grain garlic bread or another healthy starch.

* FOR NSI: USE GROCERY STORE KONJAC NOODLES (SEE PAGE 43).

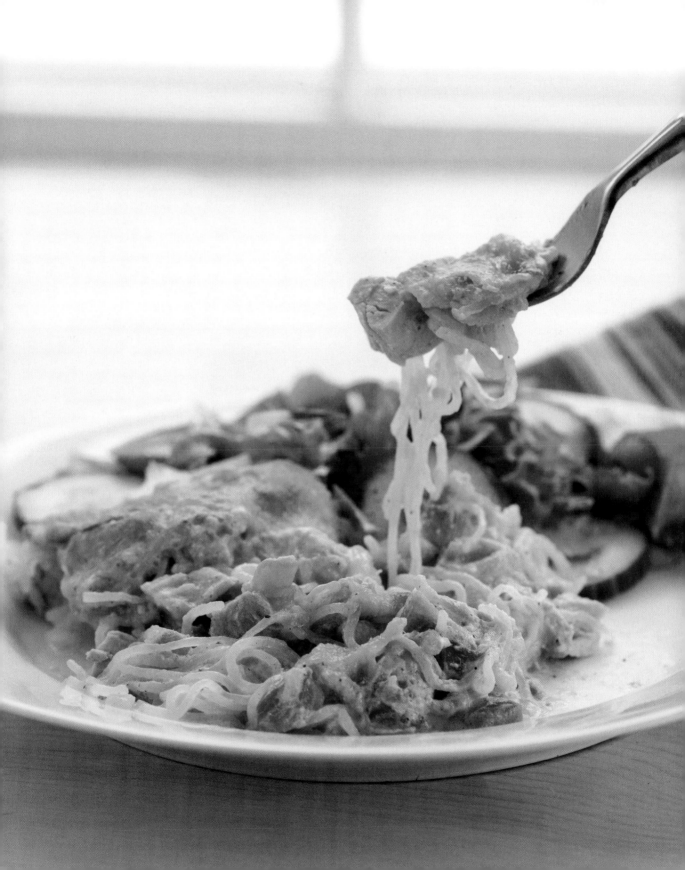

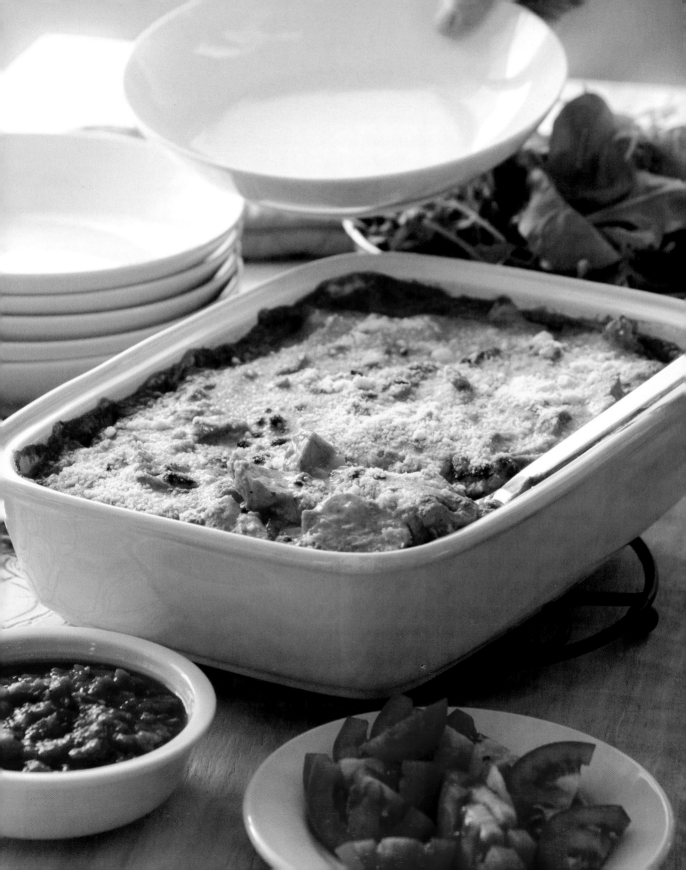

queso chicken bake   **E**

FAMILY SERVE–FEEDS 6 TO 8 (HALVE IF YOUR FAMILY IS SMALLER, OR MAKE FULL AND FREEZE HALF)

Coconut oil cooking spray

4 to 5 cups diced cooked chicken breast (see page 45 for cooking methods)

2 (15-ounce) cans black beans, drained

1 (15-ounce) can corn kernels, drained

1 cup cooked brown rice

1 (10-ounce) can Ro-tel-style diced tomatoes and green chilies (hot, medium, or mild), drained

1 (14.5-ounce) can diced tomatoes, drained

8 wedges Laughing Cow Light cheese* (see Note)

1¾ to 2 cups unsweetened cashew or almond milk (use the smaller amount if you prefer less cheese sauce)

1 cup frozen diced okra (optional, but great)

2 teaspoons chili powder

1½ teaspoons ground cumin

1¾ teaspoons Mineral Salt

1 teaspoon Gluccie*

¼ cup powder-style (from the green can) Parmesan cheese* (optional)

So extremely tasty . . . this E dinner is going to wow your family over to the Trim and Healthy side and keep them here!

1. Preheat the oven to 365°F (yes, that temperature is correct). Spray a 9 × 13-inch baking dish lightly with coconut oil.

2. Place the chicken, beans, corn, rice, Ro-tel, and tomatoes in the dish and mix together.

3. Put the cheese wedges, milk, okra (if using), chili powder, cumin, salt, and Gluccie in a blender and blend well until completely creamified . . . blend the very soul out of it so no bits of okra can be seen!

4. Pour the contents of the blender into the baking dish and stir it all in with the other ingredients. Sprinkle the Parmesan (if using) over the top and bake for 40 minutes. Let sit for a few minutes before serving.

MAKE A FAMILY MEAL: For the weight-loss plan, you can top with a little Greek yogurt and diced green onions if desired to stay in E mode. Pair with a side salad with an E-friendly dressing and you have a great meal. Growing children or others at Crossover stage can enjoy this topped with sour cream and plenty of grated cheese or sliced avocado as toppings.

NOTE: If you are a purist like Serene or are dairy-free and don't want to use Laughing Cow Light cheese, you can sub in her Hello Cheese recipe, which can be found free on our website or in *Trim Healthy Mama Cookbook*.

* FOR NSI: SUB XANTHAN GUM FOR THE GLUCCIE.

* FOR DF: OMIT THE LAUGHING COW AND PARMESAN CHEESES AND SUB HELLO CHEESE OR USE A STORE-BOUGHT DAIRY-FREE CHEESE (MAKING SURE IT HAS LESS THAN 5 GRAMS OF FAT PER SERVING).

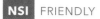

lazy chicken lasagna

S

FAMILY SERVE–FEEDS 6 TO 8 (HALVE IF YOUR FAMILY IS SMALLER, OR MAKE FULL AND FREEZE HALF)

4 tablespoons (½ stick) butter

1 onion, diced

2 celery stalks, diced

1 tablespoon dried basil

1 tablespoon dried parsley flakes

½ teaspoon dried oregano

1 to 2 teaspoons garlic powder, or 4 to 6 garlic cloves, minced

½ teaspoon Mineral Salt

¼ cup THM Baking Blend*

1 cup unsweetened cashew or almond milk

2 to 3 cups small-diced cooked chicken breast (see page 45 for cooking methods) or diced rotisserie chicken

1 (8-ounce) package ⅓ less fat cream cheese

1 (14-ounce) container 1% cottage cheese

2 large eggs

16 ounces frozen spinach, thawed, drained, and squeezed, or 16 ounces fresh spinach

8 ounces grated part-skim mozzarella cheese

¼ cup powder-style Parmesan cheese (from the green can)

One of the hits from *Trim Healthy Mama Cookbook* was Lazy Lasagna. Here is a creamy white version using chicken you are going to love.

1. Preheat the oven to 350°F.

2. Melt the butter in a skillet over medium-low heat. Add the onion and celery and cook for 5 minutes, or until soft. Add the herbs, garlic powder, and salt and cook for another couple minutes.

3. Add the Baking Blend, increase the heat to high, and cook for 90 seconds. Slowly add the nut milk, about 2 tablespoons at a time, whisking well and letting the sauce thicken after each addition. Add the chicken and simmer until heated through.

4. Put the cream cheese, cottage cheese, and eggs in a food processor and process until smooth.

5. Layer half the chicken sauce in the bottom of a 9 × 13-inch baking dish. Top with half the cream cheese mixture, then layer on half the spinach. Follow with half the grated mozzarella. Repeat the layers, ending with the mozzarella. Top with the Parmesan and bake for 40 minutes, or until bubbling.

* FOR NSI: SUB THE FRUGAL FLOUR OPTION (SEE PAGE 40) FOR THE BAKING BLEND.

cheesy tuna casserole

S

FAMILY SERVE—FEEDS 6 TO 8 (HALVE IF YOUR FAMILY IS SMALLER, OR MAKE FULL AND FREEZE HALF)

2 (16-ounce) bags frozen cauliflower florets, or 1 large head fresh cauliflower, cut into florets

3 (12-ounce) cans water-packed tuna, drained

1 tablespoon butter or coconut oil

1 onion, diced

8 ounces sliced mushrooms (optional)

2 (8-ounce) packets ⅓ less fat cream cheese

½ teaspoon Mineral Salt

½ teaspoon black pepper

¾ cup frozen peas

6 ounces grated or shredded cheese of any kind

Optional: 1 piece of plan-approved, S-friendly bread, such as Fifteen-Minute Focaccia Bread (page 247), Wonderful White Blender Bread (page 242), or 1 Joseph's pita or low-carb tortilla (ground into crumbs in a blender)

This is the sort of "regular food" casserole you can feed your family and know with a smile that this is an eating plan you can all enjoy for life!

1. Preheat the oven to 375°F.
2. Steam the cauliflower until nice and tender (you don't want it crunchy). Transfer to a 9 × 13-inch baking dish. Chop bigger cauli pieces smaller. Add the tuna, breaking up the flakes with a fork.
3. Melt the butter in a skillet over medium heat. Add the onion and mushrooms (if using) and sauté until the onions are translucent. Add the cream cheese, salt, and pepper and stir until melted. Add the peas and combine well. Pour over the cauliflower and tuna and stir. Top with the grated cheese and crumbs (if using).
4. Bake for 15 minutes, or until the cheese is bubbling. (Alternatively, broil for a few minutes, being careful not to burn the top.)

MAKE A FAMILY MEAL: For the weight-loss plan, serve with a giant salad or a smaller salad and another veggie like green beans or broccoli. Growing children and other Crossies can have sprouted-grain bread and butter, brown rice, or a baked potato with butter on the side for a Crossover.

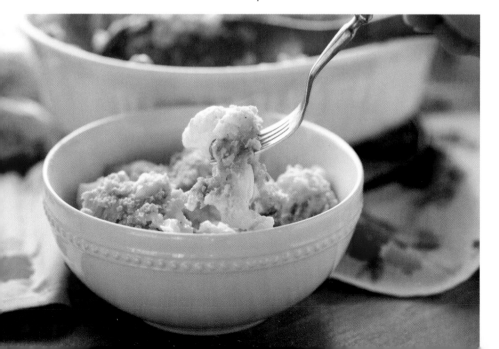

easy pizza casserole S

Coconut oil cooking spray

2 (10- to 12-ounce) bags frozen riced cauliflower

3 large eggs

1 cup egg whites (carton or fresh)

¾ teaspoon Mineral Salt

½ teaspoon garlic powder

2 cups grated part-skim mozzarella cheese

1 pound mild, medium, or hot Italian-style sausage meat (we use turkey, but you can use any kind), thawed if frozen

1 (10-ounce) bag frozen small-cut seasoning blend (see page 35)

5 ounces pepperoni, diced (we use turkey, but you can use any kind)

½ teaspoon dried oregano

Red pepper flakes to taste

1 (14-ounce) jar sugar-free pizza sauce, or 1 batch Perfect Pizza Sauce (page 516)

No special ingredients and just easy steps get this dish done.

1. Preheat the oven to 400°F. Spray a 9 × 13-inch baking dish with coconut oil.

2. Mix together the cauliflower rice, whole eggs, egg whites, salt, garlic powder, and 1 cup of the mozzarella in a large bowl. Scrape the mixture into the baking dish, then spread it evenly and smooth the top with a spatula. Cover and bake for 20 minutes. Uncover and bake for another 20 minutes (a total of 40 minutes).

3. While the base of the casserole is baking, make the topping. Set a skillet over medium-high heat and add the sausage, seasoning blend, and half of the diced pepperoni and brown the meat. Add the oregano and red pepper flakes. Cook the meat and seasoning blend until all the liquid has evaporated. Stir in the pizza sauce and remove from the heat.

4. Remove the casserole base and set the oven to high broil. Pour the meat sauce mixture over the casserole base, top with the remaining 1 cup mozzarella, then the remaining pepperoni. Return to the broiler and broil until the cheese is bubbling and the pepperoni gets slightly browned.

MAKE A FAMILY MEAL: For the weight-loss plan, all this dish really needs to be paired with is a large side salad, but if you feel like more on your plate, add a nonstarchy veggie or WWBB Garlic Bread (page 245). Crossover family members can enjoy this meal with a piece of fruit added as a healthy carb.

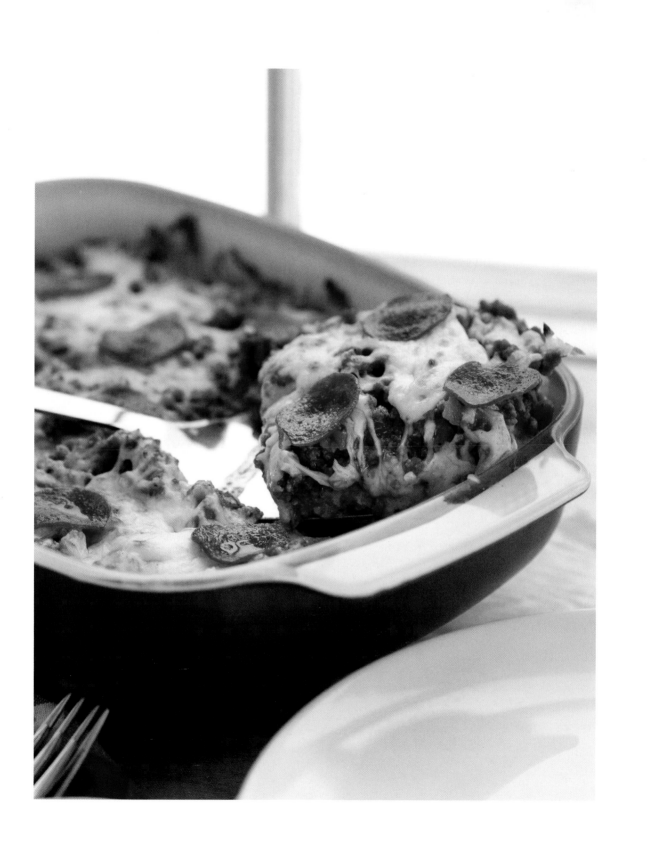

meatball casserole

S

FAMILY SERVE—FEEDS 6 TO 8 (HALVE IF YOUR FAMILY IS SMALLER, OR MAKE FULL AND FREEZE HALF)

35 frozen Marvelous Make-Ahead Meatballs (page 208), or freshly made One-Batch Meatballs* (recipe follows)

2 (14-ounce) jars sugar-free pizza sauce (we use Walmart Great Value brand), or 2 batches Perfect Pizza Sauce (page 516)

8 ounces shredded part-skim mozzarella cheese

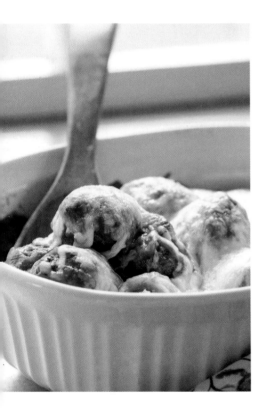

This is too easy! Simply pull out a family-size batch of our Marvelous Make-Ahead Meatballs from your freezer, top with sauce and cheese, add a side salad, and you've got supper! If you haven't made the meatballs ahead of time, never fear. They don't take long to whip up and can be made without special ingredients. Following this recipe is One-Batch Meatballs, which makes one meal's worth. Okay, okay . . . we can hear some of you muttering about not having time for all this homemade meatballs nonsense! You're a Prepackaged Pam and are not yet ready to change! Alright, you can use store-bought meatballs if you must, not quite as healthy, but hey, this is all about baby steps, so don't get down on yourself. You're doing your best at your own pace. Do try to find meatballs with 3 grams or less of carbs; any more than that means there are too many starchy fillers used.

1. If using frozen meatballs, preheat the oven to 400°F. If using freshly made, follow the baking instructions in the One-Batch Meatballs recipe (opposite) and when the meatballs are done, take them out of the oven and set the oven temperature to 400°F.

2. Arrange the frozen meatballs or the freshly cooked meatballs in a 9 × 13-inch baking dish. Top the meatballs with the sauce and then the mozzarella. Bake until the cheese is bubbling and the meatballs are heated through, 35 to 40 minutes for frozen meatballs, 15 minutes for the freshly cooked meatballs.

MAKE A FAMILY MEAL: For the weight-loss plan, pair with a large salad and/or a nonstarchy veggie or WWBB Garlic Bread (page 245). Growing children can enjoy a healthy carb on the side like whole milk, sprouted-grain bread, rice, or whole-grain noodles for a Crossover.

* FOR NSI: SEE SUBSTITUTIONS LISTED IN THE ONE-BATCH MEATBALLS RECIPE (OPPOSITE) OR USE STORE-BOUGHT MEATBALLS.

ONE-BATCH MEATBALLS

FP WITH S OPTION

MAKES ABOUT 35 MEATBALLS

1 cup frozen diced okra

2 tablespoons apple cider vinegar

2 tablespoons tomato paste

1 rounded teaspoon Mineral Salt

2 garlic cloves, minced, or
   ¾ teaspoon garlic powder

1½ teaspoons onion powder

½ to ¾ teaspoon black pepper

1¼ tablespoons Just Gelatin*

1¼ tablespoons THM Baking Blend
   or old-fashioned rolled oats

2 tablespoons grated Parmesan
   cheese (the green can kind is fine)

2 tablespoons Nutritional Yeast

⅓ teaspoon Italian seasoning (for
   Italian-style meatballs) or
   ⅓ teaspoon sage (for neutral
   meatballs)

2½ tablespoons egg whites (carton
   or fresh)

2 pounds ground meat (beef for S;
   venison, 96% lean grass-fed beef,
   or 96% lean turkey for FP), thawed
   if frozen

½ cup loosely packed finely diced
   fresh parsley (about ½ bunch with
   stems removed)

Coconut oil cooking spray

1 cup water mixed with a splash of
   soy sauce (for extra flavor),
   or chicken or beef broth, for
   cooking the meatballs

1. Preheat the oven to 400°F.

2. Put the okra in a food processor and process until completely broken down. Add all the other ingredients (except the meat, parsley, cooking oil, and water with soy sauce) and process until it becomes a paste.

3. Place the meat in a large bowl and add the paste and parsley. Mix well with your hands (or a fork), then form into small balls (a hair smaller than a golf ball).

4. Spray a large rimmed baking sheet with coconut oil. Put the meatballs on the baking sheet and bake for 10 minutes. Pour in the water or broth. Reduce the oven temperature to 350°F and continue baking for another 20 to 25 minutes.

* FOR NSI: USE A GROCERY STORE UNFLAVORED GELATIN.

loaves and fishes bake Ⓔ

FAMILY SERVE–FEEDS 6 TO 8 (HALVE IF YOUR FAMILY IS SMALLER, OR MAKE FULL AND FREEZE HALF)

Coconut oil cooking spray

1 pound tilapia or other white fish fillets, thawed if frozen

2 cups tightly packed fresh spinach, roughly chopped

2 tablespoons capers (optional)

4 garlic cloves, minced (6 for garlic lovers)

4 green onions, finely diced

1 tablespoon dried dill

1 (16-ounce) carton liquid egg whites

2 cups boiling water

2 tablespoons Just Gelatin*

1½ tablespoons (1 scoop) Integral Collagen* (optional)

¼ teaspoon Sunflower Lecithin* (optional)

1 tablespoon Mineral Salt

3 tablespoons Nutritional Yeast

½ teaspoon black pepper

2 tablespoons apple cider vinegar

1 tablespoon MCT oil (or extra-virgin olive oil in a pinch if you don't have MCT)

12 to 13 slices sprouted-grain bread (such as Ezekiel), cut into cubes

SERENE CHATS: *This hearty E meal, baked in a delicious white dill sauce, is a simple answer for what to make for dinner when there is perhaps only one loaf of bread hanging around, and a packet of fish at the bottom of your freezer. It will remind you of the wonderful miracle in the Bible of the loaves and fishes. Though of course not nearly as ultra-awesome as the Biblical event, it takes a loaf of bread and kind of multiplies it so that instead of a measly little portion of bread you can have a giant square on your plate. Although chock-full of protein, this bake satisfies the hankering for a carb fest without all the excess carbs. Those who want to use chicken breasts instead can just sub it out for the same amount of shredded cooked chicken or venison.*

1. Preheat the oven to 350°F. Spray a 9 × 13-inch baking dish with coconut oil.

2. Place the tilapia in a shallow saucepan with just enough water to start lapping up the sides of the fillets but not covering them. Bring to a boil, then reduce the heat and simmer for 2 minutes, or until opaque. Drain well.

3. Put the fish in a large bowl and flake it with a fork. Add the spinach, capers (if using), garlic, green onions, dried dill, and liquid egg whites and mix all together.

4. Put the boiling water, gelatin, collagen (if using), lecithin (if using), salt, nutritional yeast, pepper, vinegar, and MCT oil in a blender and blend well. Pour it into the bowl of fish and veggies and stir well.

5. Spread half of the fish mixture into the bottom of the baking dish. Add all of the cubed bread, then ladle the rest of the fish mix over the top. Spray the top lightly with coconut oil and bake for 55 minutes.

MAKE A FAMILY MEAL: For the weight-loss plan, a generous side of Cottage Citrus Dip (page 523) on the side of your plate sets this meal off perfectly. We also love to drizzle this bake with Fiery Fermented Hot Sauce (page 522) or Kickin' Dippin' Sauce (page 518). Pair with a large garden salad with an E-friendly vinaigrette or a small side of fruit to give you some more E-nergy. Growing children can have cheese or creamy dressing on their salad or whole milk with their meal to make it a Crossover.

* FOR NSI: USE A GROCERY STORE UNFLAVORED GELATIN. LEAVE OUT THE COLLAGEN AND LECITHIN AND SUB THE MCT OIL WITH OLIVE OIL EVEN THOUGH WE DON'T USUALLY ENDORSE COOKING WITH OLIVE OIL.

loaves and fishes bake—spicy tomato style Ⓔ

FAMILY SERVE–FEEDS 6 TO 8 (HALVE IF YOUR FAMILY IS SMALLER, OR MAKE FULL AND FREEZE HALF)

Coconut oil cooking spray

1 pound tilapia or other whitefish
fillets, thawed if frozen

1 (16-ounce) carton liquid egg
whites

2 (14.5-ounce) cans petite diced
tomatoes

4 garlic cloves, minced (6 for garlic
lovers)

1 small bunch fresh parsley, finely
diced (stems removed), or
2 tablespoons dried parsley flakes

2 tablespoons capers (optional)

3 tablespoons apple cider vinegar

1 tablespoon mesquite liquid
smoke

4 tablespoons Nutritional Yeast

1 tablespoon ground cumin

4 teaspoons onion powder

2½ to 3 teaspoons Mineral Salt
(use the larger amount for savory
heads)

½ teaspoon red pepper flakes

⅛ teaspoon cayenne pepper
(or ½ teaspoon black pepper for
those who prefer milder spices)

12 to 13 slices sprouted-grain bread
(such as Ezekiel), cut into cubes

FOR THE TOPPING

1 (6-ounce) can tomato paste

1 tablespoon apple cider vinegar

¼ teaspoon Mineral Salt

⅛ teaspoon black pepper

2 to 3 large tomatoes, sliced, for
decoration (optional)

Grated, garnish amount of Parmy
cheese or Pecorino Romano
sheep's cheese,* for sprinkling
(optional)

A twist on the original Loaves and Fishes Bake (opposite), this one uses no special ingredients and bursts with flavor . . . you're welcome!

1. Preheat the oven to 350°F. Spray a 9 × 13-inch baking dish with coconut oil.

2. Place the tilapia in a shallow saucepan with just enough water to start lapping up the sides of the fillets but not covering them. Bring to a boil, then reduce the heat and simmer for 2 minutes, or until opaque. Drain well.

3. Put the fish in a large bowl and flake it with a fork. Add all the other ingredients except the cubed bread and mix well.

4. Spread half of the fish mixture into the bottom of the baking dish. Add all of the cubed bread, then ladle the rest of the fish mix on top. Mix the can of tomato paste with the apple cider vinegar, salt, and pepper, and baste the top of the dish. If desired, decorate with sliced tomatoes and sprinkle with some cheese, keeping to E amounts. Bake for 55 minutes.

MAKE A FAMILY MEAL: For the weight-loss plan, once again this is fabulous with a side of Cottage Citrus Dip (page 523) and a side salad. Growing children can have cheese or creamy dressing on their salad or whole milk with their meal to make it a Crossover.

* FOR DF: LEAVE OFF THE CHEESE.

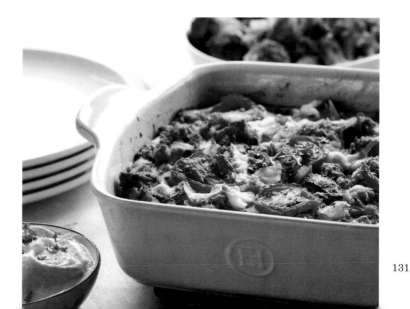

chicken enchilada stuffed spaghetti squash Ⓢ

FAMILY SERVE—FEEDS 6 TO 8 (HALVE IF YOUR FAMILY IS SMALLER, OR MAKE FULL AND FREEZE HALF)

2 large spaghetti squash

2 tablespoons butter

1 (10- to 12-ounce) bag frozen large-cut seasoning blend (see page 35)

3 tablespoons chili powder

2 teaspoons ground cumin

2 teaspoons garlic powder

1½ teaspoons Mineral Salt

½ teaspoon Super Sweet Blend (optional, but gives more of an enchilada-sauce taste as most contain sugar)

¼ cup THM Baking Blend or almond flour

1 (8-ounce) can tomato sauce

1 (15-ounce) can black beans, rinsed and drained

4 cups diced cooked chicken (see page 45 for cooking methods)

12 ounces cheddar cheese, grated

This dish makes use of our wonderful, nonstarchy friend spaghetti squash. God thought of everything when he made food . . . a vegetable containing noodles . . . oh yeah! You can present this two ways: baked in a regular baking dish or baked in the squash shells themselves.

1. Preheat the oven to 375°F.

2. Pierce the spaghetti squash in several places and place whole on a baking sheet. Bake for 1 hour 10 minutes. (Alternatively, halve the squash lengthwise, scoop out the seeds, and place cut side down on a baking sheet coated with coconut oil spray. Bake for 40 minutes.) We prefer to bake whole, because squash is easier to cut after baking and you can prebake squash any ol' time and keep it in the fridge. (If you are halving the recipe, you can cook 1 squash in your electric pressure cooker in 6 to 8 minutes.)

3. Halve the spaghetti squash lengthwise. Scrape out the seeds and discard. Using a fork, scrape all the flesh from 1½ of the squash into a 9 × 13-inch baking dish (or into a large bowl if baking in the squash shells). Divide the spaghetti strands from the remaining half squash into two baggies and freeze for 2 other single-serve meals to top with any sauce or one of our crockpot meals. If baking in the squash shells, set them on a baking sheet.

4. Melt the butter in a large skillet over medium-high heat. Add the seasoning blend and sauté for about 3 minutes. Stir in the chili powder, cumin, garlic powder, salt, and sweetener (if using). Add the Baking Blend, tomato sauce, and black beans and cook for a few more minutes. Add this to the spaghetti squash in the baking dish or bowl. Add the chicken pieces and half of the cheddar and mix all the ingredients well with a fork.

5. If baking in the baking dish, top with the remaining cheddar. If baking in the shells, divide the mixture among them and top with the cheddar. Raise the oven temp to 400°F and bake for 30 to 35 minutes.

MAKE A FAMILY MEAL: Enjoy with a side salad and another veggie such as green beans. Growing children can have a healthy carb side such as whole milk, sprouted-grain bread, or whole-grain rice.

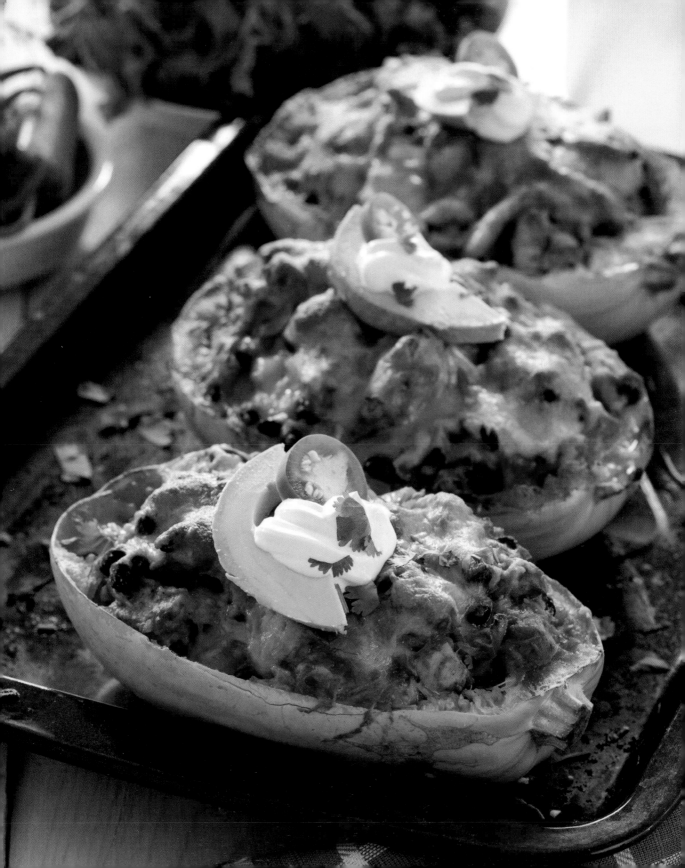

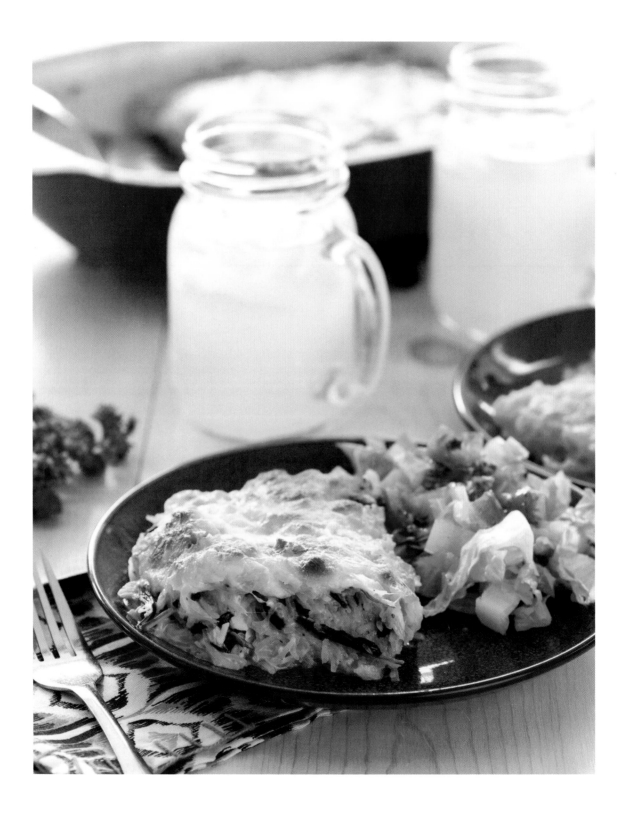

creamy garlic spinach spaghetti squash bake Ⓢ

FAMILY SERVE—FEEDS 6 TO 8 (HALVE IF YOUR FAMILY IS SMALLER, OR MAKE FULL AND FREEZE HALF)

2 medium spaghetti squash

2 tablespoons butter

8 garlic cloves, minced (or even more for garlic lovers)

16 ounces fresh spinach

4 ounces ⅓ less fat cream cheese

½ cup heavy cream

¾ cup grated Parmesan cheese (the green can kind is fine)

1 teaspoon Mineral Salt

1 teaspoon black pepper

A generous sprinkle of red pepper flakes (optional)

4 cups diced cooked chicken (see page 45 for cooking methods)

6 ounces part-skim mozzarella cheese, grated

Another dish that makes use of our wonderful, nonstarchy pal spaghetti squash. We predict this will become a go-to family favorite in your home, or take it to a potluck and watch it get devoured before you can blink an eye!

1. Preheat the oven to 375°F.

2. Pierce the spaghetti squash in several places and place whole on a baking sheet. Bake for 1 hour 10 minutes. (Alternatively, halve the squash lengthwise, scoop out the seeds, and place cut side down on a baking sheet coated with coconut oil spray. Bake for 40 minutes.) We prefer to bake whole, because squash is difficult to cut before baking but easy afterward and you can prebake squash any ol' time and keep it in the fridge until ready to make the casserole. (If you are halving the recipe, you can cook 1 squash in your electric pressure cooker in only 6 to 8 minutes.)

3. Halve the spaghetti squash lengthwise. Scrape out the seeds and discard. Using a fork, scrape all the flesh from 1½ of the squash into a 9 × 13-inch baking dish. Divide the spaghetti strands from the remaining squash into two baggies and freeze for 2 other single-serve meals to top with any sauce or one of our crockpot meals . . . you'll thank us for that later.

4. Melt the butter in a large skillet over medium-high heat. Add the garlic and toss in the butter for a minute. Add the spinach and toss until it is wilted down. Add the cream cheese, heavy cream, ½ cup of the Parmesan, the salt, black pepper, and red pepper flakes (if using). Stir, then add to the baking dish with the spaghetti squash. Add the diced chicken and stir together very well. Top with the grated mozzarella and the remaining ¼ cup Parmesan. Increase the oven temperature to 400°F and bake for 35 minutes.

MAKE A FAMILY MEAL: For the weight-loss plan, enjoy with a side salad with an S-friendly dressing and another cooked nonstarchy veggie if desired. Growing children can enjoy a healthy carb, such as whole milk, buttered sprouted-grain bread, or a baked potato with butter for a Crossover.

zippy zucchini rice bake

E

FAMILY SERVE—FEEDS 6 TO 8 (HALVE IF YOUR FAMILY IS SMALLER, OR MAKE FULL AND FREEZE HALF)

Coconut oil cooking spray

3 medium zucchini, chopped into a few large pieces for the processor or sliced into thin half-moons for the throw-together version

2 cups egg whites (carton or fresh)

2 cups 1% cottage cheese

1½ teaspoons Mineral Salt

¼ teaspoon black pepper

1 teaspoon onion powder

1½ teaspoons garlic powder

2 to 3 tablespoons turkey bacon bits or crumbles (optional)

1¼ cups "minute" (parboiled) brown rice (you can't use regular brown rice here)

¼ to ⅓ cup powder-style Parmesan cheese (from the green can)

Optional: 2 to 3 Wasa light rye crackers, 2 pieces sprouted-grain bread, or WWBB for One (page 244), crumbled, for topping

Got a feeling this quick and easy dish will be a regular on your table. It is a budget-friendly, meatless meal (if you don't use the bacon crumbles), yet still has adequate protein in the form of egg whites and cottage cheese. It is a great way to use up all that zucchini that is so abundant in the summer. But hopefully you'll love this casserole so much, you'll make it year-round. We love this recipe because the moisture from the zucchini helps quick-cook the rice! Brilliant! Choose from two easy ways to make this: if your family doesn't love zucchini, process it all up and they'll barely notice it; if you love zucchini, do the easy throw-together method.

1. Preheat the oven to 375°F. Spray a 9 × 13-inch baking dish with coconut oil.

2. **FOR THE PROCESSED VERSION:** Put the zucchini pieces in a processor and process until the size of rice. Add the egg whites, cottage cheese, salt, pepper, onion powder, and garlic powder and whiz until well combined. Scrape into the baking pan. Add the bacon bits (if using) and minute rice and mix well.

   FOR THE THROW-TOGETHER VERSION: Mix the zucchini, egg whites, cottage cheese, salt, pepper, onion powder, garlic powder, bacon bits (if using), and minute rice together in a bowl, then scrape into the prepared pan.

3. Sprinkle on the Parm. If you want a breading, crumble the crackers or bread over the top. Bake for 40 minutes. Allow to sit for 5 minutes before serving.

MAKE A FAMILY MEAL: Although this recipe includes some brown rice, there is room here to add in some more carbs for your E meal. Feel free to mix it into a salad with a lean dressing, have some fruit on the side, or pair with a baby-size E or FP shake from the Shakes and Smoothies chapter (page 468). Growing children can have this with extra fat, such as a full-fat dressing on their salad or sprouted-grain bread with butter, to make a Crossover.

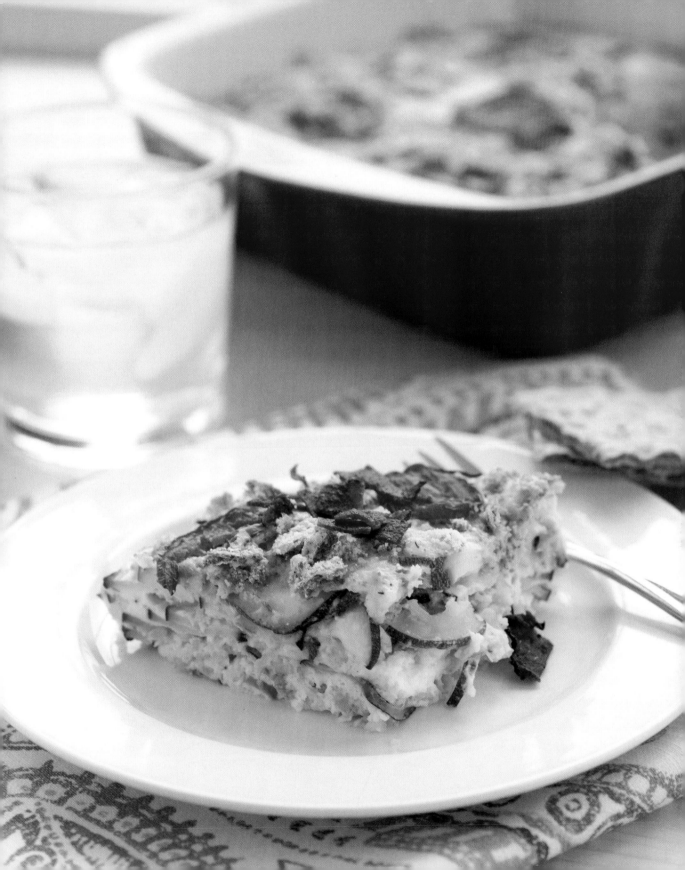

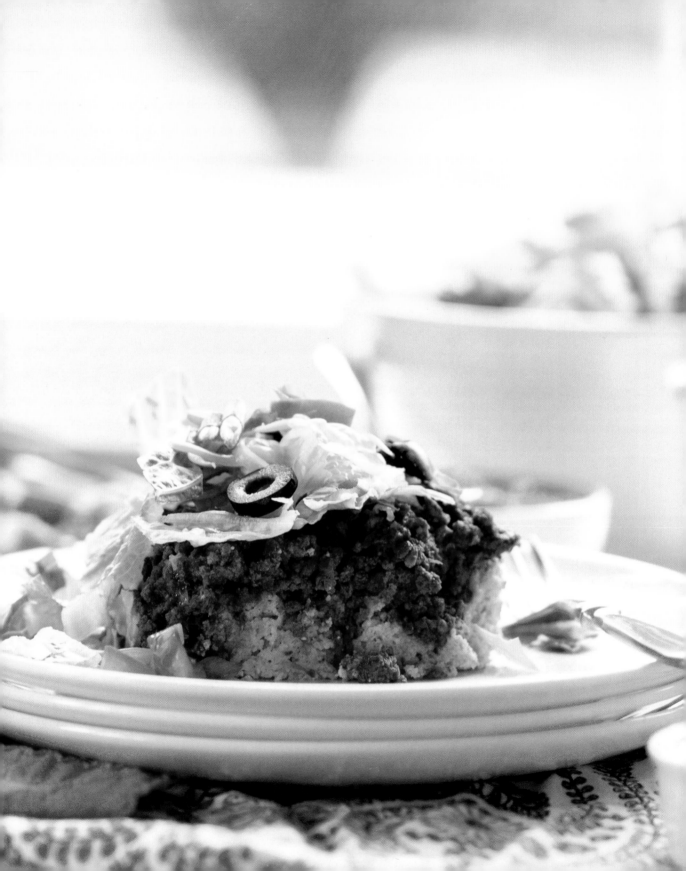

taco cornbread bake

Ⓢ

FAMILY SERVE—FEEDS 6 TO 8 (HALVE IF YOUR FAMILY IS SMALLER, OR MAKE FULL AND FREEZE HALF)

FOR THE MEAT SAUCE

2 pounds ground beef, venison, or turkey, thawed if frozen
1 teaspoon garlic powder
1 teaspoon onion powder
2 tablespoons chili powder
2½ teaspoons paprika
2 teaspoons ground cumin
1½ teaspoons Mineral Salt
1 (8-ounce) can tomato sauce
1 (12- to 15-ounce) jar salsa (hot, medium, or mild)

FOR THE CORNBREAD BASE

1½ cups THM Baking Blend*
1 tablespoon aluminum-free baking powder
1 teaspoon Super Sweet Blend*
½ teaspoon Mineral Salt
½ teaspoon paprika
¼ teaspoon ground turmeric
1 cup egg whites (carton or fresh)
1½ cups water
5 tablespoons coconut oil or butter

FOR THE TOPPINGS

4 to 5 generous cups chopped lettuce
2 large tomatoes, chopped
2 cups grated cheddar cheese*
½ cup sliced olives
Sliced green onions to taste
Dollops of sour cream* or sliced avocado (optional)

You can't go wrong with the match up of cornbread and hearty, well-seasoned taco meat, piled high with festive toppings. You have all the taste and texture of cornbread here in a hearty S recipe without any actual corn igniting your blood sugar and mixing with the fat, causing weight gain. We have a feeling this will become a Trimming family favorite in your home. (This is incredible heated as leftovers the next day. Place pieces with crust side down in a greased hot skillet and heat from the bottom up. Lettuce will stay mostly cool and still crunchy.)

1. Preheat the oven to 425°F.
2. Make the meat sauce. Brown the meat in a large skillet over medium to medium-high heat. Pour off any grease, then add the garlic powder, onion powder, chili powder, paprika, cumin, salt, tomato sauce, and salsa and let simmer on low.
3. While the sauce is simmering, make the cornbread base. Put the Baking Blend, baking powder, sweetener, salt, paprika, turmeric, egg whites, water, and 4 tablespoons coconut oil in a food processor and process well, scraping down the sides so that all the batter is mixed.
4. Melt the remaining 1 tablespoon oil in a 9 × 13-inch baking dish in the hot oven. Take the pan out and swish the oil around to fully cover the pan, then pour the batter into the pan.
5. Bake for 10 minutes, take out and pour the meat sauce over the top, return to the oven, and bake for another 15 to 17 minutes.
6. Allow the dish to cool for just a few minutes, then top with the lettuce and tomatoes, followed by the cheese, olives, green onions, and sour cream or avocado (if using).

MAKE A FAMILY MEAL: This is great in a bowl on its own with a baby-size S-friendly shake from the Shakes and Smoothies chapter (page 468) or Speedy Chocolate Milk (page 457). Growing children need a healthy carb side for a Crossover, so they can top theirs with black beans or have a side of refried beans or brown rice.

* FOR NSI: USE THE FRUGAL FLOUR OPTION (SEE PAGE 40) AND A GROCERY STORE ON-PLAN SWEETENER.

* FOR DF: LEAVE OFF THE CHEESE OR USE A NONDAIRY CHEESE.

chicken bacon rice casserole

FAMILY SERVE–FEEDS 6 TO 8 (HALVE IF YOUR FAMILY IS SMALLER, OR MAKE FULL AND FREEZE HALF)

5 cups diced cooked chicken or turkey (see page 45 for cooking methods), or diced rotisserie chicken

6 slices bacon, diced (we use turkey, but you can use any kind)

1 teaspoon butter (optional)

2 (10- to 12-ounce) bags frozen riced cauliflower (see page 36)

1 (10- to 12-ounce) bag frozen small-cut seasoning blend (optional; leave out if your kids don't like onions)

¼ cup chicken broth

¾ cup mayonnaise

1 cup 0% Greek yogurt

¼ cup water

1 teaspoon Mineral Salt

1 teaspoon black pepper

1½ teaspoons onion powder

1½ teaspoons garlic powder

2 teaspoons dried onion flakes

2 teaspoons dried parsley flakes

6 ounces cheddar cheese, grated or shredded

PEARL CHATS: My kids gobble this up, go back for seconds, and don't have a clue this uses cauliflower rice in place of regular rice. They say it tastes like Grandma's stuffing . . . Feel free to use leftover Thanksgiving turkey meat here.

1. Preheat the oven to 375°F. Place the diced chicken in a 9 × 13-inch baking dish.

2. Cook the bacon in a large skillet over medium-high heat. Transfer to a plate. If you used turkey bacon, add the butter to the skillet (otherwise you'll use the bacon fat in the pan). Add all the cauliflower rice and the seasoning blend (if using). Toss in the skillet for a couple minutes, allowing the veggies to soak up the bacon flavor. Stir in the broth, cover, and cook for 8 minutes, stirring every few minutes. Add to the baking dish with the chicken.

3. Place the mayonnaise, yogurt, water, and all the seasonings in a medium bowl and whisk well. Pour the mixture into the baking dish and stir all the ingredients well. Top with the cheddar and bake for 25 minutes.

MAKE A FAMILY MEAL: For the weight-loss plan, serve with a giant salad or a smaller salad and another veggie like green beans or broccoli. Children can have sprouted-grain bread and butter or brown rice on the side for a Crossover.

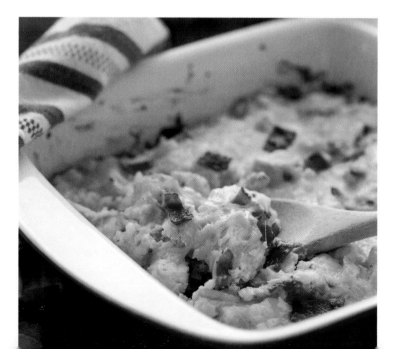

creamy mushroom chicken casserole   Ⓢ

FAMILY SERVE—FEEDS 6 TO 8 (HALVE IF YOUR FAMILY IS SMALLER, OR MAKE FULL AND FREEZE HALF)

2½ pounds chicken tenderloins or
  boneless, skinless chicken breasts
  or thighs, thawed if frozen
¾ cup THM Baking Blend*
½ teaspoon Mineral Salt
½ teaspoon black pepper
½ teaspoon onion powder
4 tablespoons butter or coconut oil
1 large onion, sliced
4 garlic cloves, minced
16 ounces mushrooms, sliced

FOR THE SAUCE
2 cups chicken broth
½ cup heavy cream
¾ teaspoon Gluccie*
½ teaspoon Mineral Salt
½ teaspoon black pepper

⅓ cup powder-style Parmesan
  cheese (from the green can)

1. Preheat the oven to 350°F.
2. Cut the chicken into 1-inch strips (easily done with kitchen scissors) and put in a bowl. Mix the Baking Blend with the salt, pepper, and onion powder. Pour the Baking Blend over the chicken pieces and toss to thoroughly coat.
3. Melt 3 tablespoons of the butter in a large skillet over medium-high heat. Add all the chicken pieces and cook, turning once, for 5 to 6 minutes. It doesn't matter if the chicken is not cooked all the way through, because you are just browning. Transfer the chicken to a 9 × 13-inch baking dish.
4. Add the remaining 1 tablespoon butter to the pan. Add the onion, garlic, and mushrooms and sauté for about 3 minutes, tossing the veggies several times. Pour the veggies over the chicken.
5. Make the sauce. Put the broth, cream, Gluccie, salt, and pepper in a blender and blend well for 10 to 20 seconds. Pour the cream mixture over the chicken and veggies. Sprinkle the Parmesan on top and bake for 45 minutes.

MAKE A FAMILY MEAL: For the weight-loss plan, serve with a giant salad or a smaller salad and another nonstarchy veggie of choice. Children can have a whole-grain pita and butter, a baked potato with butter, or brown rice on the side for a Crossover.

* FOR NSI: USE THE FRUGAL FLOUR OPTION (SEE PAGE 40) AND SUB XANTHAN GUM FOR THE GLUCCIE.

award-winning chili pie

FAMILY SERVE—FEEDS 6 TO 8 (HALVE IF YOUR FAMILY IS SMALLER, OR MAKE FULL AND FREEZE HALF)

2 pounds ground beef or venison, thawed if frozen

1 onion, diced

2 tablespoons chili powder

2 teaspoons Mineral Salt

1 teaspoon onion powder

Garlic powder to taste

1 to 2 squirts Bragg liquid aminos (optional)

1 (8-ounce) can tomato sauce

1 (14.5-ounce) can diced tomatoes

2 cups frozen diced okra

2 (10-ounce) cans Ro-tel-style diced tomatoes and green chilies, drained

1½ cups egg whites (carton or fresh)

1 (15-ounce) can pinto beans (see Note), rinsed and drained

8 ounces cheddar cheese, shredded or grated

PEARL CHATS: What could be better than chili itself? Chili you can eat with a fork! This has all the flavor of my original, award-winning chili (known as Pearl's Chili in the first two THM cookbooks), but there is no soup spoon required here.

My head is so big over my chili recipe winning multiple awards. People have entered it into chili cook-offs all over the country and it has won first prize several times. This is a fact I rub in to Serene as frequently as I can. I know pride doth come before a fall but hey, she invented Good Girl Moonshine and started the okra in brownies and smoothies craze so I'm always trying to play catchup. And okay, I admit it, I'm stealing from Serene's idea of including that secret, weight-loss ingredient here so she still beats me . . . drat! My family loves this pie, none of them knows about the secret okra ingredient, and they ask for it frequently, especially my oldest son, Bowen, who thinks okra is a demon (if you ever meet him don't show him this page).

1. Preheat the oven to 365°F (yes, 365°F—might be weird but it works).

2. Brown the meat in a large skillet over high heat. Drain off any excess fat, then add the onion, chili powder, salt, onion powder, garlic powder, and liquid aminos (if using) and cook for 2 to 3 minutes.

3. Put the tomato sauce, diced tomatoes, and okra in a blender and blend extremely well . . . totally blend the gajeebers out of it so no little green flecks of okra are left. Add this puree to the meat and simmer over medium heat for 10 minutes. Remove from the heat.

4. Put the tomatoes and chilies, egg whites, pinto beans, and half of the cheddar into the bottom of a 9 × 13-inch baking dish and stir very well until combined. Add the meat mixture, mix very well again, top with the remaining cheddar, and bake for 40 to 45 minutes.

MAKE A FAMILY MEAL: For the weight-loss plan, serve with a giant salad or a smaller salad and another veggie like green beans, asparagus, or broccoli. Children can have a whole-grain pita and butter or brown rice on the side for a Crossover.

NOTE: The one can of pinto beans here really doesn't add enough carbs to pull this meal out of S mode.

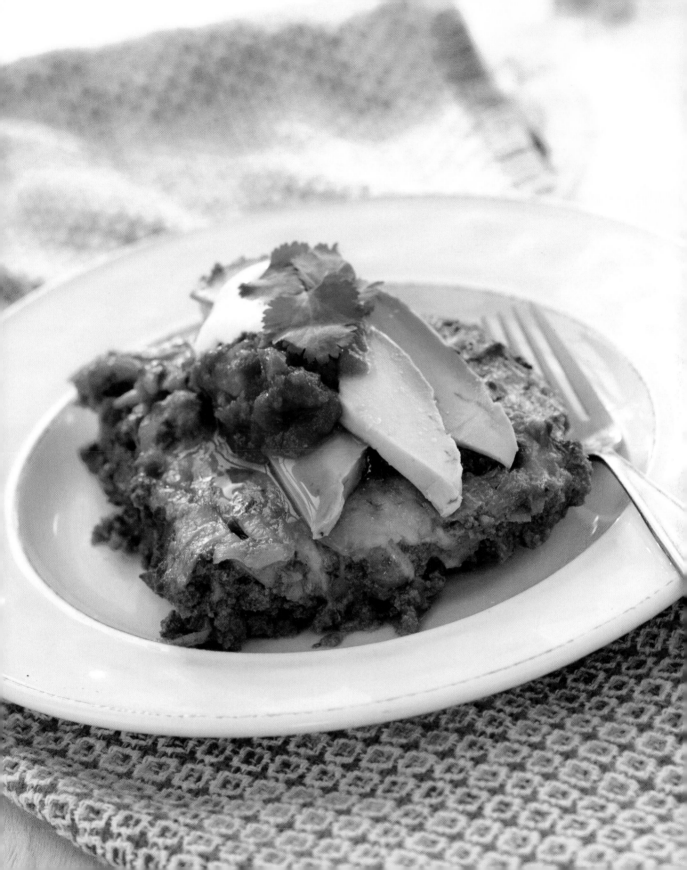

taste of home casserole

S

FAMILY SERVE—FEEDS 6 TO 8 (HALVE IF YOUR FAMILY IS SMALLER, OR MAKE FULL AND FREEZE HALF)

⅓ cup mayonnaise

1 cup 0% Greek yogurt or sour cream

2 tablespoons dried onion flakes

2 pounds ground beef, thawed if frozen

2 to 3 garlic cloves, minced

1 teaspoon Mineral Salt

1 teaspoon black pepper

½ teaspoon onion powder

1 to 2 tablespoons Nutritional Yeast (optional)

4 (15-ounce) cans green beans, drained

1 (8-ounce) can mushrooms, drained

12 ounces cheddar cheese, grated

This is comfort food to the max . . . the sort of dish that brings to mind good ol' American food (to our Canadians and other international folk . . . we still love you). You can even take this to Thanksgiving in place of regular green bean casserole and you won't miss out on any flavor or goodness.

1. Preheat the oven to 350°F.
2. Mix together the mayonnaise, yogurt, and onion flakes in a small bowl and set aside.
3. Brown the meat in a skillet over medium-high heat. Drain any fat. Add the garlic, salt, pepper, onion powder, and nutritional yeast (if using) and toss with the meat for 2 to 3 more minutes.
4. Transfer the mixture to a 9 × 13-inch baking dish. Add the green beans, mushrooms, mayo/Greek yogurt mixture, and cheddar and combine well. Bake for 45 minutes.

MAKE A FAMILY MEAL: For the weight-loss plan, serve with a giant salad or a smaller salad and another veggie like Mashed Fotatoes (page 264) or broccoli. Children can have whole-grain bread and butter, mashed potatoes, or brown rice on the side for a Crossover.

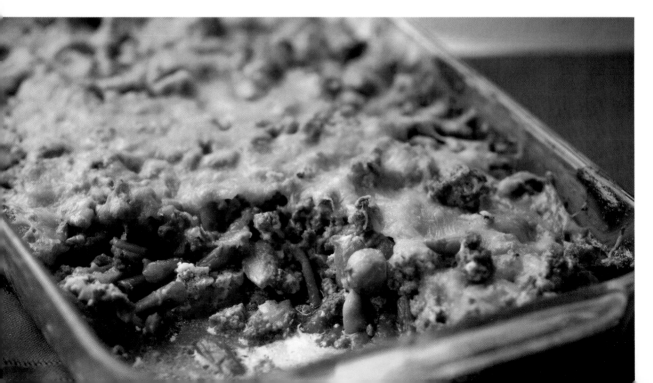

super salmon easy bake

Ⓢ

FAMILY SERVE—FEEDS 6 TO 8 (HALVE IF YOUR FAMILY IS SMALLER, OR MAKE FULL AND FREEZE HALF)

Coconut oil cooking spray

¼ cup warm water

2 tablespoons coconut oil

2 (15-ounce) cans salmon, drained

5 eggs

2 tablespoons apple cider vinegar

3 to 4 garlic cloves, minced, or
½ teaspoon garlic powder

2 to 3 teaspoons mesquite liquid
smoke

5 tablespoons THM Baking Blend*

1½ teaspoons aluminum-free
baking powder

2 tablespoons Nutritional Yeast

1½ tablespoons (1 scoop) Integral
Collagen* (optional)

2 tablespoons Baobab Boost
Powder* (optional)

1 teaspoon Mineral Salt

½ teaspoon black pepper

1 teaspoon red pepper flakes

2 tablespoons dried parsley flakes

2 teaspoons onion powder

FOR THE KETCHUP GLAZE

1 (6-ounce) can tomato paste

1 tablespoon apple cider vinegar

¼ teaspoon Mineral Salt

⅛ teaspoon black pepper

1 doonk Pure Stevia Extract Powder
(optional)

OPTIONAL TOPPINGS

3 large tomatoes, sliced, for
decoration

A little sprinkling of Pecorino
Romano sheep's cheese or
Parmesan cheese

This simple bake was born out of our love for the Super Salmon Patties from our first book but not super loving the longer process of frying them all up. This delivers the same yummy flavor with less hassle. Turn the oven on and dinner is solved. It's delicious served sliced and layered in romaine "taco shells" or cabbage leaves, topped with generous amounts of avocado and lively drizzles of hot sauce.

1. Preheat the oven to 350°F. Spray a 9 × 13-inch baking dish with coconut oil.

2. Mix the warm water and coconut oil in a mug to soften and stir well. Place the mixture in a bowl with the salmon, eggs, vinegar, garlic, and liquid smoke and mash with a fork. Combine the Baking Blend, baking powder, nutritional yeast, collagen (if using), baobab powder (if using), salt, black pepper, pepper flakes, parsley flakes, and onion powder. Get out all the lumps and bumps, then add it to your salmon. Stir together well, then transfer to the baking dish.

3. Make the ketchup glaze. Combine all the ingredients in a small bowl and mix well with a fork.

4. Brush the salmon bake with the ketchup glaze and then add toppings (if using). Bake for 40 minutes.

MAKE A FAMILY MEAL: For the weight-loss plan, serve with a giant salad, a smaller salad plus another veggie such as Mashed Fotatoes (page 264) or broccoli, or serve in lettuce wraps. Children can have whole-grain bread and butter, mashed potatoes. or brown rice on the side for a Crossover.

* FOR NSI: USE THE FRUGAL FLOUR OPTION (SEE PAGE 40). LEAVE OUT THE COLLAGEN. USE A GROCERY STORE BAOBAB POWDER (IF YOU CAN FIND IT), OR LEAVE IT OUT AND USE A GROCERY STORE ON-PLAN SWEETENER.

Big Eats Soups

You have arrived at the largest chapter in the book and that is no accident. It is LAAAAARGE for good reason. A study published in June 2005 in *Obesity Research* found that diets that include broth-based soup on a daily basis resulted in almost double the amount of weight loss of other diets. But we have a feeling that was very boring weight loss. The problem with typical diet soups is that yes, while they do make you lose weight at first, they also make you feel deprived and "hangry." They say insulting stuff like "a serving size is 1 cup" . . . who eats only 1 cup of soup? That sort of diet mentality leads only to more all-or-nothing, yo-yo dieting failure! You dream of pouring your insipid soup down the kitchen sink and filling up on a 12-inch sub followed by a Twinkie. So inevitably, you fall off your diet.

Our soups harness all the weight-loss and health-giving powers of broth-based soups, but smash their "diet" stereotype to smithereens. You get to eat big hearty bowlfuls. These soups are not starters or sides to your meal, they *are* your meal, and they leave you feeling nourished, nurtured, and full to the brim. Ladle a huge comforting bowlful, sit down to bliss, and say . . . "Aahh . . . now this I can do for life!" Then if you're not satisfied . . . have another smaller bowl.

You'll notice we've split up these stovetop soups into two sub chapters. We had to separate them because they couldn't play nice. We take two different approaches when it comes to soup. Pearl's soups come first because she uses shortcuts and is all about getting you started or keeping you on plan with yummy ease. Serene's soups are exotic, historic, adventurous, more "from scratchy," and have longer ingredient lists, but they do wonders for fat-loss and health. Both approaches are going to rock your world, so don't stay only in either Serene or Pearl land. You can start out with Pearl's simple soups since they use few if any special ingredients. Then, once you've found your Trim Healthy feet, branch out and try Serene's Trimmy Bisques. Reap the rewards from both sister cultures. (Be sure to read Serene's write-up on page 162 on why she wants you to make her Trimmy Bisques.)

creamy lemon chicken and quinoa soup Ⓔ

FAMILY SERVE—FEEDS 6 TO 8 (HALVE IF YOUR FAMILY IS SMALLER, OR MAKE FULL AND FREEZE HALF)

2 (16-ounce) bags frozen cauliflower florets, or 1 large head cauliflower, cut into florets

2 quarts chicken broth

3 cups water

3 ounces ⅓ less fat cream cheese

3 cups chopped carrots

3 cups chopped celery

1 large onion, diced

¾ cup uncooked quinoa

2 to 2½ teaspoons Mineral Salt

1¼ teaspoons dried thyme

1 teaspoon dried tarragon

1 teaspoon black pepper

4 to 5 cups diced cooked chicken breast (see page 45 for cooking methods)

⅓ to ½ cup lemon juice (fresh or bottled)

PEARL CHATS: This will comfort your body and soul. It is so creamy, it is hard to believe . . . but yes, it is an E!

1. Put the cauliflower, broth, and water in a soup pot and bring to a quick boil over high heat. Reduce the heat a little and simmer until the cauliflower is tender (it takes just a few minutes).

2. Scoop out the cauliflower with a slotted spoon and transfer it to a blender. Add 2 cups of the broth and the cream cheese, blend well, and set aside.

3. Add the carrots, celery, onion, and quinoa to the soup pot along with all the seasonings. Simmer for 20 to 30 minutes, until the veggies are tender. Add the contents of the blender to the soup pot and stir. Add the chicken and simmer for another 15 minutes or so. Add the lemon juice just before serving.

MAKE A FAMILY MEAL: For the weight-loss plan, enjoy a big bowl or two of soup alone or with a side salad with an E-friendly (lean) dressing. Growing children or others (like Skinny Jimmy husbands) will need an added fat for a Crossover, such as a swirl of cream in their soup or a full-fat dressing on their salad.

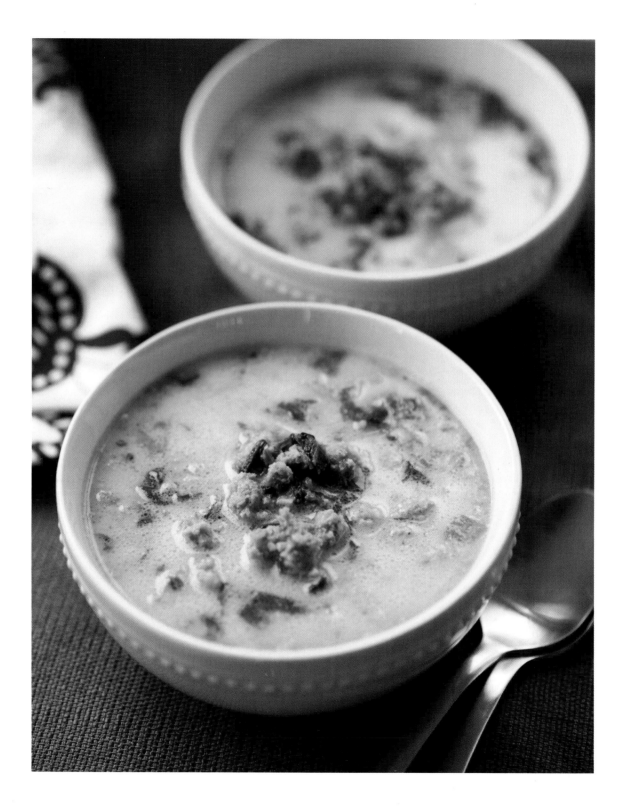

whoop whoop soup Ⓢ

FAMILY SERVE—FEEDS 6 TO 8 (HALVE IF YOUR FAMILY IS SMALLER, OR MAKE FULL AND FREEZE HALF)

2 pounds ground sausage meat (we use turkey or venison, but you can use pork if desired), thawed if frozen

2 quarts chicken broth or bone stock

1 cup water

¾ to 1 cup heavy cream

1 (10-ounce) box chopped spinach, thawed or still frozen

1 teaspoon Mineral Salt

1 teaspoon black pepper

1 teaspoon onion powder

1 teaspoon garlic powder

1 teaspoon red pepper flakes

1½ teaspoons Gluccie*

PEARL CHATS: Are you new to this Trim Healthy journey? Feeling overwhelmed and like you need some handholding? Allow this tasty, filling soup to kick-start you into success! It can be on your table in 15 minutes flat. It freezes well for other "no-think" meals and requires no special ingredients (if you sub out the Gluccie and sub in xanthan gum, easily found in your grocery store). That's enough to make you do a whoop whoop, fist pump, and happy dorky dance! Eventually you may want to purchase some Gluccie. One bag will last you about a year and it has so many weight-loss and health benefits. But no need to concern yourself with filling your cupboards with strange (to you) foods right now. Just start separating your fuels, fill up on delicious meals like this one, and you'll be making giant strides toward a trimmer and healthier you!

1. Brown the sausage in a large soup pot over medium-high heat. Add all the other ingredients (except for the Gluccie). Allow the soup to come to a low boil, then reduce the heat to medium. If you added frozen spinach, wait until it thaws in the hot soup before adding the Gluccie.

2. Once the spinach has thawed, stir it in well, then add the Gluccie a little at a time by tapping your teaspoon containing the Gluccie on the edge of your pot to add small amounts little by little. Use your other hand to whisk it in well while you are adding so it doesn't clump. Reduce the heat to medium-low and allow the soup to simmer for 5 to 15 more minutes, depending on how much time you have available.

MAKE A FAMILY MEAL: For the weight-loss plan, this is fantastic with a side salad (with vinaigrette or creamy dressing) and/or a bread like Wonderful White Blender Bread (page 242) or the Fifteen-Minute Focaccia Bread (page 247). Children or other Crossover family members can enjoy a healthy carb side such as buttered sprouted-grain toast.

* FOR NSI: SUB XANTHAN GUM FOR THE GLUCCIE.

pizzeria tomato soup

FAMILY SERVE—FEEDS 6 TO 8 (HALVE IF YOUR FAMILY IS SMALLER, OR MAKE FULL AND FREEZE HALF)

1 to 1½ pounds mild sausage meat (I use turkey, but you can use any kind), thawed if frozen

4 ounces pepperoni, diced (I use turkey, but you can use any kind)

1 (14-ounce) jar sugar-free pizza sauce or the same amount Perfect Pizza Sauce (page 516)

2 (8-ounce) cans tomato sauce

1½ cups frozen diced okra

1 quart chicken broth (with an optional 3 to 4 tablespoons Just Gelatin or Integral Collagen; see page 40)

2 cups water

½ teaspoon dried basil

½ teaspoon dried oregano

½ to ¾ teaspoon garlic powder

⅛ teaspoon cayenne pepper (adjust to your liking)

Mineral Salt and black pepper

½ cup heavy cream

ADDITIONS FOR LOADED VERSION

1 (10- to 12-ounce) bag frozen small-cut seasoning blend (see page 35)

8 ounces sliced mushrooms

2 to 3 ounces diced black or green olives

PEARL CHATS: This is a whole new way to eat tomato soup, and it will be devoured before your eyes! Not a soul will ever guess about the secret veggie; it just makes the soup creamier. This is a hit with every kid I have ever served it to, and even more exciting—it's done from start to finish within 15 minutes! There are two ways of making this . . . one is picky-kid friendly, the other is loaded up for appreciative adults. Both versions are delish!

1. Brown the sausage with the pepperoni in the bottom of a large soup pot over medium-high heat. (If making the loaded version, add in the seasoning blend, mushrooms, and olives at the same time and sauté along with the meats while they are browning.)

2. Put the pizza sauce, canned tomato sauce, and okra in a blender and blend. Blend like a champ until smooth as silk and no little green okra bits are there to tell the tale.

3. Pour the blender mixture into the pot along with the chicken broth with the optional gelatin and collagen (if using) and the water. Add the basil, oregano, garlic powder, cayenne, salt and pepper to taste (only ½ to ¾ teaspoon salt is needed), and the heavy cream. Bring to a quick boil, then reduce to a simmer and cook for another 5 to 10 minutes.

MAKE A FAMILY MEAL: For the weight-loss plan, this soup is perfect with WWBB Garlic Bread (page 245) or a grilled cheese sandwich using WWBB or store-bought Joseph's pita. Or simply have a big bowl of soup alone or with a side salad. Crossover-stage family members like growing children love it with lots of buttered sprouted-grain toast for dunking.

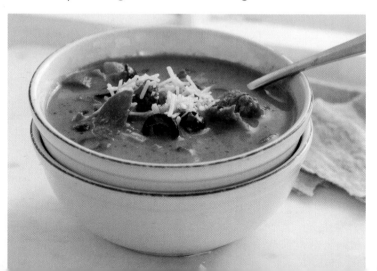

insanely simple chicken fiesta soup Ⓔ

FAMILY SERVE—FEEDS 6 TO 8 (HALVE IF YOUR FAMILY IS SMALLER, OR MAKE FULL AND FREEZE HALF)

2 quarts chicken broth (with an optional 3 to 4 tablespoons Just Gelatin or Integral Collagen; see page 40)

2 cups water

5 cups shredded cooked chicken breast (see page 45 for cooking methods)

2 (15-ounce) cans black beans, rinsed and drained

1 (10-ounce) can Ro-tel-style diced tomatoes and green chilies

1 (14.5-ounce) can fire-roasted tomatoes

1 (12-ounce) bag frozen corn kernels

1 rounded teaspoon paprika (smoked or regular)

1 rounded teaspoon ground cumin

1 rounded teaspoon Mineral Salt

¾ teaspoon black pepper

1 or 2 squirts Bragg liquid aminos (optional)

½ bunch fresh cilantro, stems removed, finely chopped, or 1 tablespoon dried parsley flakes

PEARL CHATS: Ever have those nights when nothing but an insanely simple dinner recipe will work otherwise you'll go insane? Yeah, that's me all too often. This is both insanely simple yet insanely tasty, and it's all hot and ready within 30 minutes! Sometimes you need a break from sneaky ingredients, too. We'll put plenty of sneaky stuff (like okra and other veggies) in other soups, but not here, so not even a blender is needed. Feel free to add the optional collagen or gelatin for a more balanced amino acid profile, but hey . . . you don't even have to do that if that's just one more thing to stress over! Don't stress! You're making great strides little by little and you don't have to be perfect.

1. Put all the ingredients except for half the cilantro into a large soup pot. Bring to a low boil, then cover and simmer over medium-low heat for 20 to 25 minutes. Own the flavors . . . add more seasonings after tasting if you like. Sprinkle with the remaining cilantro when serving.

MAKE A FAMILY MEAL: For the weight-loss plan, there is still room in your E quota of carbs for a few crumbled baked corn chips to top this soup. Delish! Or dollop with some 0% Greek yogurt. For a more filling factor, enjoy with a side salad with an E-friendly dressing. Growing children or other Crossie family members can enjoy with lots of grated cheese for a Crossover.

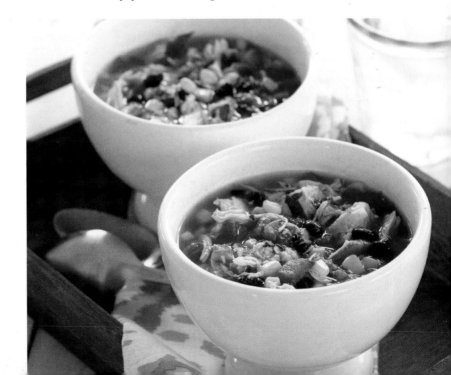

loaded broccoli and cheese soup Ⓢ

FAMILY SERVE–FEEDS 6 TO 8 (HALVE IF YOUR FAMILY IS SMALLER, OR MAKE FULL AND FREEZE HALF)

2 (14- to 16-ounce) bags frozen broccoli florets, or 1 large head fresh, cut into florets

10 cups water, or 2 quarts chicken broth plus 2 cups water (with an optional 3 to 4 tablespoons Just Gelatin or Integral Collagen*; see page 40)

2 level cups frozen diced okra

2 cups 1% cottage cheese

⅓ cup heavy cream

2 scoops (½ cup) unflavored Pristine Whey Protein Powder*

2 to 2½ teaspoons Mineral Salt (you'll need more salt or Bragg liquid aminos if you use water versus chicken broth, so start with less, then taste test at the end)

1 teaspoon black pepper

1 teaspoon onion powder

1 teaspoon garlic powder (or more if you love it)

¼ teaspoon cayenne pepper (really helps to bring out the flavor of the small amount of cheese, so if you are afraid of spice, don't leave it out but reduce to ⅛ teaspoon)

A couple squirts Bragg liquid aminos or coconut aminos (optional)

¼ teaspoon liquid smoke (optional)

1½ to 2 generous teaspoons Gluccie*

2 to 3 ounces real bacon bits (I use turkey, but you can use any kind)

1 cup grated cheddar cheese

PEARL CHATS: This may be one of the creamiest broccoli and cheese soups you have ever eaten, but there is very little cream and very little regular cheese. Only 1 cup of grated cheese for this big pot of soup! On the Trim Healthy Mama plan we don't shun foods like heavy cream and cheese, but we shouldn't abuse them, either. We need to respect their delight wisely and this soup demonstrates how. While this is almost a meatless meal (except for the bacon bits), it is chock-full of protein from the cottage cheese, whey protein, and collagen. Hey . . . please don't get frustrated if you don't want to use special ingredients. Just see the suggestions for substitutions (opposite). No worries!

Serene and I were both determined to put our versions of this soup in the book because we both believe our own are the best. You can find her Trimmy Bisque version on page 173. Yes, it is good, but put hers and mine side by side for a cook-off? I mean, I know pride cometh before a fall, but you're going down, Serene!

1. Put the broccoli and water or broth with the optional collagen and gelatin (if using) in a large soup pot and bring to a boil over high heat. Reduce to medium and simmer the broccoli until tender.

2. Put all the remaining ingredients except the Gluccie, bacon bits, and cheddar in a blender. Add about one-third of the cooked broccoli to the blender and just a small amount of the hot broth to help things blend. Add a generous 1½ teaspoons Gluccie, hold the lid down real tight, and blend for about 30 seconds. Let rest for a few seconds, then blend again until completely creamified. Don't let us find any little flecks of okra . . . blend, girl, blend! (If you're a guy, same goes.)

3. Pour the blended mixture back into the soup pot. Add the bacon bits. Break up the remaining broccoli pieces with a fork or potato masher so they are more bitsy but not smashed up completely. Stop worrying about the frothy white stuff on top of the soup . . . it will go away and become perfectly creamy. Cover, reduce to a low simmer, and go away while it cooks. Come back in 20 minutes, stir, and behold the miracle of creaminess. Add the cheddar, stir again, then taste and adjust the seasonings until you love it. If it is not thick enough for your preference, scoop some more broth into the blender, add that other ½ teaspoon Gluccie, and blend for a minute before returning it to the pot.

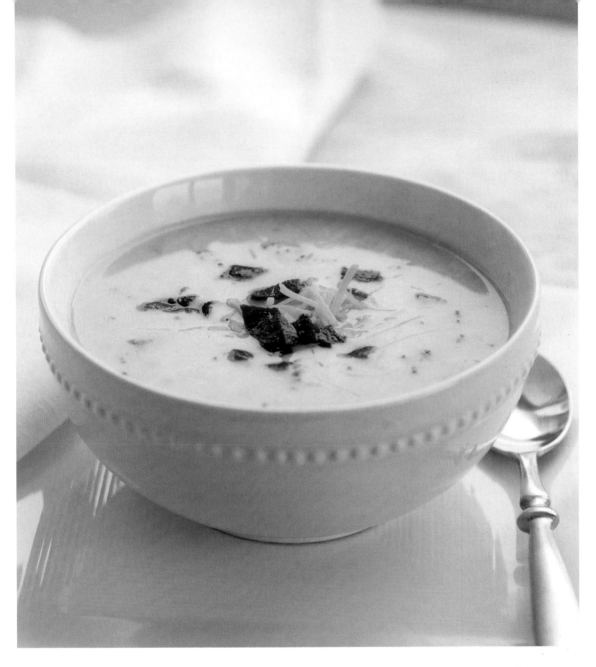

MAKE A FAMILY MEAL: For the weight-loss plan, this soup is perfect with buttered on-plan bread from the Breads chapter (page 240). Or simply pair with a side salad and have a couple big bowlfuls of soup. Crossover family members can enjoy buttered sprouted-grain toast on the side.

* FOR NSI: NIX THE WHEY PROTEIN AND USE AN UNFLAVORED GELATIN (FROM THE GROCERY STORE). FOR ADDED PROTEIN, USE 4 TO 6 TABLESPOONS INSTEAD OF THE 3 TO 4 CALLED FOR. AND YOU CAN ALWAYS SUB XANTHAN GUM FOR THE GLUCCIE.

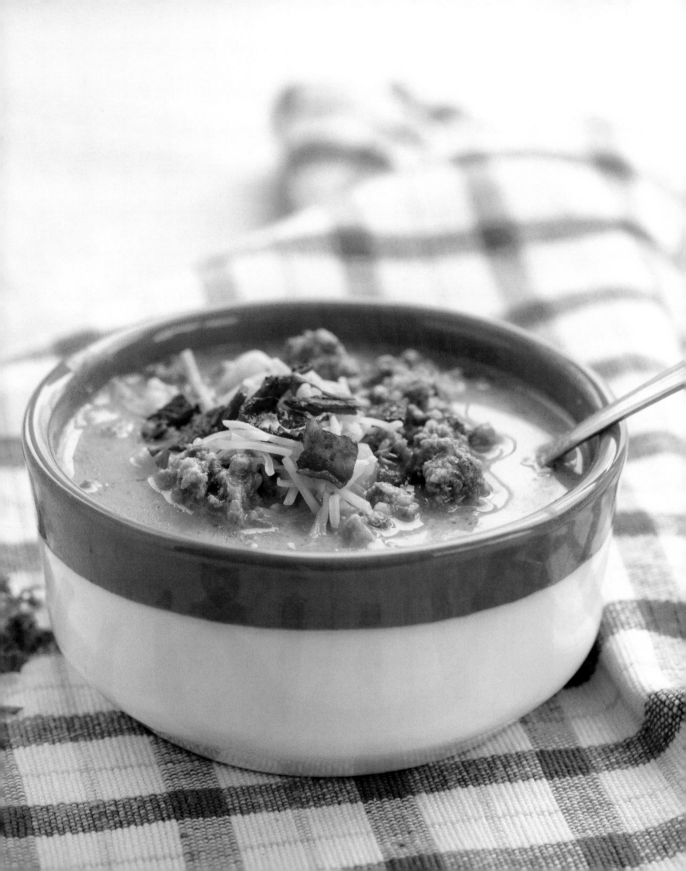

cheeseburger soup

S

FAMILY SERVE—FEEDS 6 TO 8 (HALVE IF YOUR FAMILY IS SMALLER, OR MAKE FULL AND FREEZE HALF)

1½ to 2 pounds ground beef, thawed if frozen

1 (10- to 12-ounce) bag frozen small-cut seasoning blend, or 1 large onion, diced

1 quart chicken broth (with an optional 3 to 4 tablespoons Just Gelatin or Integral Collagen; see page 40)

5 cups water

1 medium-large yellow squash, or 2 smaller squash, roughly chopped

2 (16-ounce) bags frozen cauliflower florets

2 to 2½ teaspoons Mineral Salt (start with 2, adding more at the end if needed)

1 teaspoon black pepper

1 teaspoon onion powder

1 to 2 teaspoons garlic powder

½ teaspoon paprika

¼ teaspoon ground turmeric (optional, but helps develop the cheesy color)

¼ teaspoon cayenne pepper (or more to taste . . . yummy)

1 teaspoon dried basil

2 tablespoons Nutritional Yeast

A squirt or two Bragg liquid aminos (optional)

2 teaspoons Gluccie*

1 teaspoon dried parsley flakes

⅓ cup heavy cream

2 cups grated cheddar cheese

PEARL CHATS: This filling soup is going to bless your socks off! It tastes super cheesy and creamy yet it doesn't go overboard abusing calories with multiple cups of cream or oodles and oodles of cheese like most cheeseburger soups do (then they add cornstarch or flour to thicken for a fat explosion . . . yikes!). This big ol' pot of soup feeds a large crowd, yet there are only a very sensible ⅓ cup of cream and 2 cups of grated cheese in it. The yellow squash gives the lovely golden, creamy, cheesy color and works in tandem with the cauliflower and Gluccie to thicken up and "creamify" things beautifully without the need for waist-exploding white flour or cornstarch.

1. Brown the meat in the bottom of a large soup pot over medium-high heat. Drain the meat (to remove the fat) and return the meat to the pot. Add the seasoning blend (or onion) and cook with the meat for a couple minutes.

2. Add the broth with the optional gelatin and collagen (if using), the water, yellow squash, cauliflower, the seasonings, nutritional yeast, and liquid aminos (if using). Bring to a boil over high heat. Reduce the heat to medium, cover, and allow to simmer for 5 minutes.

3. Scoop out roughly one-half to two-thirds of the cauliflower, along with all the squash pieces, and place in a blender (doesn't matter if a little seasoning blend goes in the blender or even if a few crumbles of meat sneak in, but try to avoid the rest). Add 1½ to 2 cups of the hot broth and the Gluccie. Blend on high for 30 seconds, holding the lid on tightly. Stop the blender, vent the hot air, then blend again, holding onto the lid for another full minute.

4. Stir the contents of the blender into the soup. Cover and simmer over medium-low heat for another 15 minutes or so. Add the parsley flakes, heavy cream, and cheddar, stirring until the cheese is melted. Taste and adjust the seasonings until it absolutely rocks your world, then serve.

MAKE A FAMILY MEAL: For the weight-loss plan, enjoy with an optional side salad and an S-friendly bread item from the Breads chapter (page 240). Growing children or others at Crossover stage can have buttered sprouted-grain toast on the side.

* FOR NSI: SUB XANTHAN GUM FOR THE GLUCCIE.

grandma's chicken noodle soup

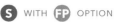 **S** WITH **FP** OPTION

FAMILY SERVE—FEEDS 6 TO 8 (HALVE IF YOUR FAMILY IS SMALLER, OR MAKE FULL WITHOUT NOODLES, AS THE NOODLES DON'T FREEZE WELL. SET HALF ASIDE TO FREEZE AND ADD JUST 1 TO 2 BAGS NOODLES TO TONIGHT'S AMOUNT, OR USE TROODLES)

1½ tablespoons butter or coconut oil

1 onion, diced

4 garlic cloves, minced

3 cups diced celery

1 cup finely diced carrots

2 quarts chicken broth (plus an optional 3 to 4 tablespoons Just Gelatin or Integral Collagen; see page 40)

2 to 3 cups water

1 (16-ounce) bag frozen cauliflower florets, or 1 large daikon radish, diced

2 teaspoons Mineral Salt

1 teaspoon black pepper

1 teaspoon onion powder

1 teaspoon dried sage

1 teaspoon dried thyme

3 to 4 cups diced cooked chicken (see page 45 for cooking methods)

2 to 3 single-serve bags Trim Healthy Noodles or Not Naughty Noodles,* well rinsed, drained, and snipped a bit smaller

½ cup heavy cream* (omit cream for FP; see Note)

Generous ½ teaspoon Gluccie (optional, but it gives a phenomenal result to soup texture)

PEARL CHATS: This is body and soul healing stuff! If your grandma or great-grandma made her soup from scratch and captured all the goodness out of chicken bones for her stock . . . that was healing elixir in a bowl! The only thing Grandma did wrong was to put white, starchy noodles in her soup. Those will fatten you up quick smart, so of course we are not going to do that! We are also not going to spend hours in the kitchen like Grandma . . . well, at least I am not, but Serene may want to. If you want to cook down bones for stock like Serene's always doing, more power to ya, but I'm happy simply spooning in gelatin or collagen for bone goodness. Speaking of Serene, be sure to try her Granny's Hug Trimmy Bisque (page 194). I give Serene a hard time about her extra steps and extra ingredients, but I have to admit that soup is incredible and, yes, not hard to make despite the "from scratchness."

I actually "borrowed" the amazing flavors in this soup from her Comfy Cozy Chicken Dumpling Soup from *Trim Healthy Mama Cookbook*. That recipe was way too much work for a lazy cook like me. So I present to you all the nurturing flavor with none of the fuss in this soup! Last thing . . . I'm not lying with the title for this soup—Serene may not look like a grandma, but she is one! Ha ha . . . love you, Grandma Serene. I'm ripping off your recipe, and I predict my much quicker version is destined to be a hit!!!

1. Melt the butter in a large soup pot over medium-high heat. Add the onion, garlic, celery, and carrots and sauté for about 3 minutes. Add all the remaining ingredients (except the cream and Gluccie). Bring to a quick boil, then reduce to a low simmer and cook for 20 to 30 minutes.

2. Transfer about 1½ cups of the broth to a blender. Add the cream and Gluccie (if using). Blend for about 30 seconds, holding on tightly to the lid. Vent the hot air, then blend again for another 20 seconds. This blending together of the cream and Gluccie is essential to the smooth, ever so slightly thickened texture of the soup . . . not slimy at all . . . promise! Return to the soup pot and simmer for a few more minutes. Taste to "own it" before serving.

MAKE A FAMILY MEAL: For the weight-loss plan, have a couple generous bowls alone or pair with an S-friendly side salad or bread from the Breads chapter (page 240). For an FP version,

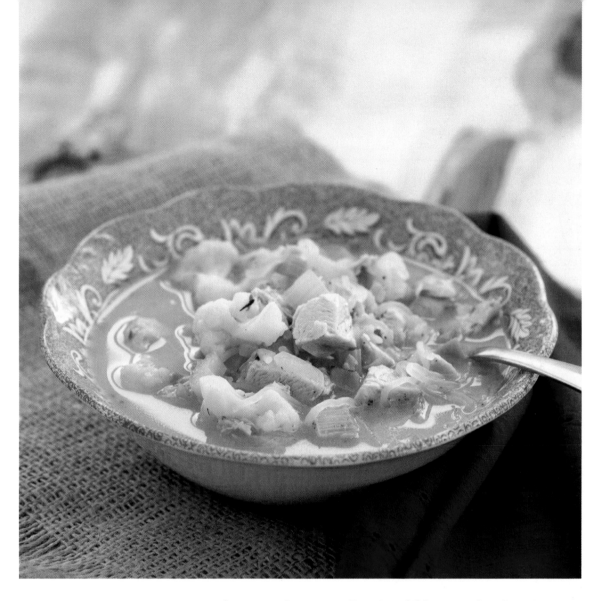

leave out the cream. Growing children or other Crossie peeps can enjoy buttered sprouted-grain toast for a Crossover with the S version of this soup.

NOTE: The FP version of this soup is fantastic when you are sick and need hot, healing, nutritious fare. If you have a stomach bug, leave out the noodles as they take a little more effort to digest.

* FOR NSI: FIND KONJAC NOODLES (SEE PAGE 43) AT YOUR GROCERY STORE. OR USE 2 CUPS TROODLES (ZUCCHINI NOODLES); IF USING TROODLES, DON'T ADD THEM UNTIL THE LAST FEW MINUTES OF COOKING. OR LEAVE OUT THE NOODLES ALTOGETHER.

* FOR DF: LEAVE OUT THE CREAM.

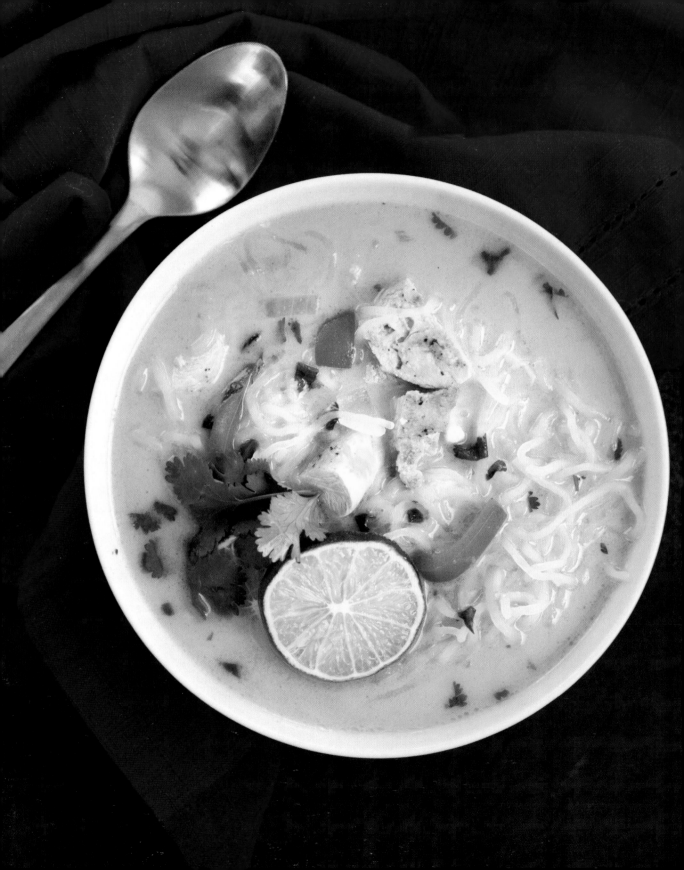

fat-burning chicken noodle soup Ⓢ

FAMILY SERVE—FEEDS 6 TO 8 (HALVE IF YOUR FAMILY IS SMALLER, OR MAKE FULL WITHOUT NOODLES, AS THE NOODLES DON'T FREEZE WELL. SET HALF ASIDE TO FREEZE AND ADD JUST 1 TO 2 BAGS NOODLES TO TONIGHT'S AMOUNT, OR USE TROODLES)

1 tablespoon coconut oil

4 to 6 garlic cloves, minced, or 2 teaspoons garlic powder

1 (10- to 12-ounce) bag frozen large-cut seasoning blend (see page 35)

1 (15-ounce) can full-fat coconut milk

¾ cup frozen diced okra

2 quarts chicken broth (with an optional 3 to 4 tablespoons Just Gelatin or Integral Collagen; see page 40)

4 to 5 cups diced cooked chicken (see page 45 for cooking methods)

2 tablespoons lime juice (optional)

¾ to 1 teaspoon red pepper flakes (adjust to your liking . . . I always prefer more!)

2 teaspoons Mineral Salt (or pull back on the salt a tad and add a couple good squirts fish sauce)

1 teaspoon black pepper

1 teaspoon ground ginger, or 1 to 2 teaspoons finely grated fresh ginger

1 teaspoon Super Sweet Blend, or 1 to 2 doonks Pure Stevia Extract Powder*

3 single-serve bags Trim Healthy Noodles or Not Naughty Noodles,* well rinsed, drained, and snipped a bit smaller

¼ bunch fresh cilantro, stems removed, chopped (optional)

PEARL CHATS: While my Grandma's Chicken Noodle Soup (page 156) uses traditional flavors, this soup is Asian inspired. Coconut-based meals like this one nourish your thyroid gland, which in turn helps rev your metabolism. The konjac-based noodles kick up the fat-burning even further, and the blended okra shoots it through the roof! This is a light S . . . you need these sometimes for dietary balance. It is also dairy-free, soul-warming, body-nourishing, and, of course, fat-burning!

1. Heat the coconut oil in a large soup pot over medium-high heat. Add the garlic and seasoning blend and toss around the bottom of the pot for about 3 minutes.

2. Put the coconut milk and okra in a blender and blend until smooth . . . really blend it to billio! Still see flecks of okra? Blend again! Pour it into the pot, add the broth with the optional gelatin and collagen (if using), and whisk together until smooth. Add the cooked chicken, lime juice (if using), pepper flakes, salt, black pepper, ginger, sweetener, and noodles. Bring to a quick boil, then reduce the heat to a low simmer and cook for 15 to 20 minutes. Add the cilantro (if using) in the last few minutes.

MAKE A FAMILY MEAL: For the weight-loss plan, enjoy a generous bowlful or two alone or pair with an S-friendly side salad and/or bread item from the Breads chapter (page 240). Growing children can enjoy a piece of fruit such as an orange after their soup for a Crossover.

* FOR NSI: USE A GROCERY STORE ON-PLAN SWEETENER. FIND KONJAC NOODLES AT YOUR GROCERY STORE (SEE PAGE 43 FOR WHAT TO LOOK FOR).

trim train italian soup

FP WITH S AND E OPTIONS

MAKES A HUGE AMOUNT (SEE NOTE)

2 pounds ground beef or venison, thawed if frozen

1 (10- to 12-ounce) bag frozen small-cut seasoning blend (see page 35)

6 to 8 garlic cloves, minced

1 quart fat-free chicken broth

2 tablespoons dried parsley flakes

1½ tablespoons dried basil

2 teaspoons dried oregano

2 to 3 teaspoons Mineral Salt (start with less and adjust at the end as needed)

1 teaspoon black pepper

2 (14.5-ounce) cans diced tomatoes

1 (6-ounce) can tomato paste

1 (8-ounce) can tomato sauce

1 (12-ounce) bag frozen cauliflower florets

7 cups just off the boil water

3 cups frozen diced okra

4 tablespoons Just Gelatin* or Integral Collagen (see page 40)

3 tablespoons extra-virgin coconut oil

Here is a delicious Italian version of the Trim Train Taco Soup we developed for *Woman's World* magazine, which they called Secret Ingredient Soup. They asked us to come up with an ultraslimming, ultratasty soup they could publish for those just starting our plan to help make the beginning of their Trim Healthy Mama journey easier. We developed the taco version and it was a hit! Trim Train not only helps beginners have a quick meal to fall back on when they are just starting and feeling overwhelmed, but it has also helped many of our seasoned Trim Healthy Mamas get through weight-loss stalls and simplify their weekly menus! You can find the original recipe on our website, www.trimhealthymama.com. Our head admin for the THM Facebook groups, Jessica Myers, came up with this Italian version.

1. Brown the meat in a large soup pot. If the meat you are using is not at least 96% lean, rinse it well under very hot water in a colander to release all the fat. Return the meat to the pot, add the seasoning blend and garlic, and sauté with the meat until the veggies thaw and begin to tenderize. Add the chicken broth, seasonings, diced tomatoes, tomato paste, and tomato sauce and let simmer.

2. While the soup is simmering, put the frozen cauliflower florets in a blender with 3 cups of the boiled water and puree until perfectly smooth (if you have a small blender this may require two batches). Add the creamed cauliflower to the soup pot.

3. Put the frozen okra in the blender with the remaining 4 cups boiling water, the gelatin, and coconut oil. Blend well until completely smooth and creamified. (Blend, baby, blend! There should be no little bits of okra left.) Add to the pot and simmer for another 15 to 20 minutes. The longer you simmer, the less you will notice any signs of okra at all. Taste test to "own it." You may want to go heavier with the seasonings, but it's up to you.

MAKE A FAMILY MEAL: For the weight-loss plan, enjoy a couple big bowlfuls as written for an FP. Top with grated cheese for an S or add a side salad with a creamy dressing. To make this an E, either add some cannellini beans to the soup or have sprouted-grain toast or 2 or 3 Wasa light rye crackers on the side with a

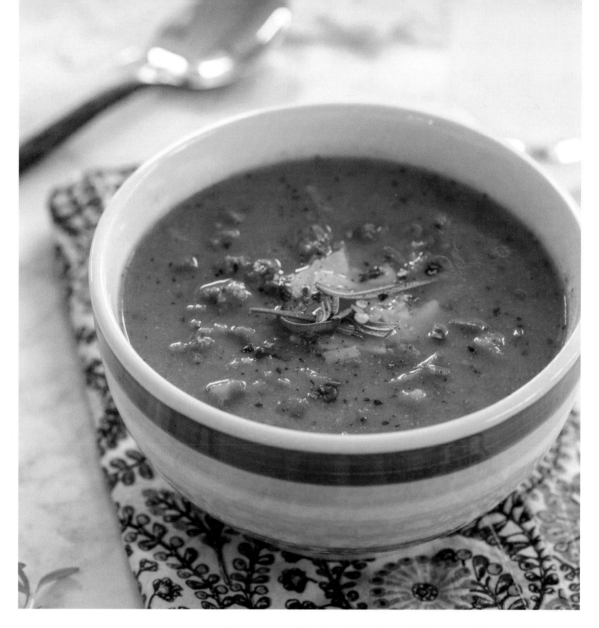

thin smear of butter. Growing children or others at Crossover stage can top this with grated cheese and include the beans, bread, or cracker items to merge carbs and fats.

NOTE: This makes 12 ginormous servings or 14 large servings. Dish up half of this soup as a hearty dinner to feed a family of 6, then set aside the rest for quick single-serve meals throughout the week. It will easily last 5 to 7 days in the fridge, but it also freezes well in individual portions.

* FOR NSI: USE AN UNFLAVORED GROCERY STORE GELATIN IF YOU WANT TO MAKE THIS SOUP AND DON'T HAVE THM JUST GELATIN.

TRIMMY BISQUES

SERENE CHATS: *A Trimmy Bisque is not your ordinary bowl of soup. Why can't Pearl get that? I had to create my own subchapter here to protect the value and preciousness of these soups as they were written (not as Pearl wants them to be written!). Can the words "comforting" and "superfoods" go together? If you're talking about a Trimmy Bisque, they can. What about "slimming" and "filling"? A thousand times yes!*

Now you know I love my big sister, but we have a problem. She has bossed me since we shared a room together growing up and that hasn't stopped. She's always going on about making our recipes as simple as possible, trying to force me to leave out what she calls "unnecessary" ingredients and suggesting shortcuts for everything. I sent over these recipes for her to place in the book and she called me saying, "Nobody will make these, Serene . . . everyone is too busy to use all those ingredients. You need to make your soups easier like mine." She wanted to chop this and change that and delete this and sprinkle these recipes throughout this soup chapter willy-nilly . . . to put them right next to her recipes that call for cream cheese and seasoning blend almost every single time! Then she said, "Why are you including ghee? I'll never put ghee in anything and neither will our readers . . . take it out! Miso . . . huh? Get rid of the miso, too!"

Enough is enough! She can be as Drive-Thru Sue or as Prepackaged Pam as she wants. Go ahead and enjoy Pearl's "normal" soups in the first half of this chapter, but believe me when I tell you I am going to change your world for the better with my Trimmy Bisques. Your health will thrive, your body will trim down, and you won't feel like the recipes are a burden to you, even though at first glance you may feel like there are more ingredients than in Pearl's recipes (most of them are seasonings, and sprinkling in seasonings takes two seconds). Open your mind to these Trimmy Bisques and your body will start to sing with vibrant health and shed fat as it hums its tune!

Now let me be really honest and transparent. Even though I love creating with food, more often than not, dinner in our house is a Trimmy Bisque. Why? Because they're the easiest for my big crowd! I'm not kidding. I make ginormous pots of them at all times (in much bigger batches than what I've listed here). I even have a fridge especially christened with space big enough for a couple of huge cauldrons of Trimmy Bisque to always have a home. Our lives here on our hilltop at the Allisons could be described as beautiful, joyful chaos, and I always have a huge houseful to feed. Our dinner is spent together, but we have grown and married children (with their little ones) popping in for lunch or an afternoon pick-me-up, and hordes of hungry cousins hanging around. Everyone knows that they are welcome to heat up a giant bowl of Trimmy Bisque and dunk a thick slice or two or three . . . (or eight if you are one of my teenage boys) of my homemade artisan sourdough bread into it (find that recipe in Trim Healthy Mama Cookbook*). My children who still live at home but go off to work for the day almost always take a "to go" Trimmy Bisque in a thermos or heat it up in the dreaded microwave (of course I give them a lecture).*

Huge pots of Trimmy Bisque are my survival mechanism for feeding us all healthy and hearty, even when I am not able to get home to make a meal. They are my parachute that saves the day, and they fill "hangry" mouths that would otherwise go out to Pizza Hut. If I am hangry I know there is always a batch of Trimmy Bisque that I can heat up in a jiffy and forgo the temptation to grab a spoon and dive into a giant jar of peanut butter. If you were to come over for dinner you would probably get a Trimmy Bisque shoved under your nose.

So, Pearl . . . let me be me. You can help our Mamas in your way, but I am going to help them in mine. They're better off with the balance from our different approaches. We have always done the plan uniquely and both our paths have been successful! Sorry, Pearl, but these Trimmy Bisques need my special list of ingredients, and believe me, I have already tamed them down a tad to appease you. Once our Mamas buy a tub of miso and ghee or a bag of Baobab Boost Powder, they will last them for a good while. Those things are easy to find too. I buy ghee at Costco for goodness' sake, I don't have to fly to India or South Asia to get it! It gives a much fuller flavor that's needed in some of these recipes and is a great option for dairy-free Mamas. Yes, we offer our brand of baobab powder online, but I have also spied it at regular grocery stores. Pearl, once our Mamas get used to these ingredients, they will become normal residents in their fridge, just like your precious cream cheese and store-bought almond milk. My suggested ingredients won't feel so weird after some time.

Getting fired up now, Pearl! I'm going to take our Mamas on trips back to ancient times with my bisques and on taste journeys from Europe to Asia . . . from simple to exotic . . . from creamy white to vivid green and every shade in between. Purists will be fist-pumping and high-fivin', and Drive-Thru Sue's will be catchin' on quick. If Mamas can't eat dairy? No probs! Many of my Trimmy Bisques are dairy-free, and if not I have easy-fix suggestions to make them fit for most.

THE SECRET TO TRIMMY BISQUES

So let's get down to the nitty-gritties of a Trimmy Bisque. If you are a THM vet, remember your creamy Trimmy (trimmaccino) hot drinks that you have grown to love? Well, I married this idea with savory dinnertime heartiness, and Trimmy Bisques were born.

A Trimmy Bisque needs four main things: hot liquid in a blender, a hygroscopic (attracts water) protein like gelatin, some superfood fat, and sunflower lecithin. To help you begin to recognize and understand your core Trimmy ingredients more, they are listed in a colored font. You whiz these four stars up in a blender and a creamed-up bisque base to your soup magically appears.

To ensure these soups are budget-friendly, I have made collagen optional—as gelatin is less expensive and the two serve a similar purpose—but I do use both. We list the option of using grocery store gelatin so you can go ahead and get started making soups without having to order online. But these are designed to be superfood soups, and we'd prefer you to use pure pasture-raised beef gelatin (like our Just Gelatin) rather than pork gelatin, about whose purity we have no clue. (Also note that grocery store gelatin is no less expensive ounce for ounce than the THM brand; in fact, it is usually more.) While Pearl is forcing me to also make sunflower lecithin optional in these recipes, it really helps make for a creamier texture and ensures the soup base doesn't separate after refrigeration. These bisques are simply better when you use it. Honestly, you use so little: one bag of that stuff will last you most of the year, so it is not much of an expense. But if you don't have sunflower lecithin, you should start on these bisques without it, then get it when you can.

Since we live in a world of boneless, skinless meat, collagen and gelatin provide missing amino acids from our modern diet. You can read more about their importance to the plan on page 40. These proteins are at the heart of a Trimmy, and are a quick and easy way to harmonize the need for the healing benefits of bone stocks with the necessity of a quick throw-it-together dinner for our fast-paced lives.

If you are a purist with the time to make your own low, slow, simmer stock, then by all means . . . you can use that in these bisque recipes (I often do). Clear broth becomes super creamy when whipped in a blender. If your broth is not skimmed, you won't have to add any fat. But since we don't know how much fat your stock contains, you should consider unskimmed stock an S.

Even if using homemade stock, you can still add a small amount of gelatin and/or collagen to your Trimmy to enhance the amount you have received from your own simmering pot of bone-in meat. Unless you add very collagen-rich parts of the chicken or beef bones (such as chicken feet), your Trimmy might need a little boost of these supplements to have an ultimate supply of their healing amino acids.

I do have one special bisque that uses homemade stock included here. It is designed to merge the two worlds of Purists and Drive-Thru Sue's even closer together than my regular Trimmy Bisques. This is a bone-in style made in the crockpot. Check out Granny's Hug Trimmy Bisque (page 194) to see how easy starting from scratch can be.

OTHER IMPORTANT INGREDIENTS

You'll notice there are a handful of other key ingredients chosen for their natural umami flavor and taste-bud tap-dancing that I often blend into the Trimmy . . . yellow miso, nutritional yeast, and apple cider vinegar (or the milder rice vinegar). Those are key in balancing and enhancing the perfect full and robust flavor profile to every mouthful. Beyond the joy of taste, these ingredients are powerful natural medicines. You have heard us rant about nutritional yeast and ACV (apple cider vinegar) before, but miso and a few others need their own explanation. Pearl especially needs to know why I have them in here and they ain't budging!

Miso: Miso is an enzyme-rich food that restores beneficial probiotics to your intestines. It is also a high-quality source of B vitamins, especially B12. And being high in antioxidants means it protects you against the free radicals that initiate aging and disease. It is a blood builder and lymph tonic. It protects the body from radiation and toxic overload and chelates heavy metals from the body. There is much more to this yummy little tub of fermented bean paste, but to cut a long story short, it also helps reduce the risk of colon, breast, prostate, and lung cancers and strengthens the immune system. Oh, and let me add that because it contains all essential amino acids, it is a complete protein. You can find it at many grocery stores in the international aisle or in natural foods stores. I use mellow yellow or white miso in these bisques.

Baobab: All my bisques are rich in veggies, specifically veggies that are high in vitamin C, which builds your immune system and beautifies your skin and hair. If you add Baobab Boost Powder to your bisque like some of my recipes suggest, you're injecting rich amounts of bioavailable vitamin C into every spoonful. Vitamin C is the crucial balance to a protein-rich diet, unlocking the benefits of gelatin and collagen, making these soups all the more powerful. Read about how it helps you shed weight on page 42.

Tea: Don't get weirded out if you see tea bags included in your ingredient list for some Trimmy Bisques. Tea is an amazing broth enhancer and helps impart deep, rounded base notes; light, fresh, and grassy high notes; or herby midtones to the flavor profile, depending on the tea of choice. Adding the teas I have chosen enriches your bisque with extra Trimmifying Trimminess from their metabolic revving and blood sugar stabilizing compounds. Your health, mood, and physical luster are all supported with these tea-brewed Trimmy Bisques.

sunny southwestern trimmy bisque

Ⓔ

FAMILY SERVE–FEEDS 6 TO 8 (HALVE IF YOUR FAMILY IS SMALLER, OR MAKE FULL AND FREEZE HALF)

2 to 3 pounds browned 96% lean ground turkey or venison or very lean grass-fed beef (thawed if frozen)

4 cups coarsely chopped carrots

1 onion, chopped

6 garlic cloves, minced

6 cups water

2 tablespoons ghee (clarified butter), MCT oil, or coconut oil

2 tablespoons Just Gelatin*

1 to 2 tablespoons Integral Collagen (optional)

¼ teaspoon Sunflower Lecithin (optional but preferred)

1½ teaspoons mesquite liquid smoke

2½ teaspoons ground cumin

3 tablespoons lemon or lime juice

¼ teaspoon Cajun seasoning

2 level doonks Pure Stevia Extract Powder*

3 to 3½ teaspoons Mineral Salt

¾ teaspoon chipotle powder

⅛ teaspoon cayenne pepper, or ½ teaspoon black pepper

3 tablespoons Nutritional Yeast (optional)

1 quart chicken broth

2 (15-ounce) cans black beans, rinsed and drained, or 3 cups home-cooked

1 (14.5-ounce) can petite diced tomatoes

½ teaspoon red pepper flakes

½ bunch fresh cilantro, chopped

SERENE CHATS: *The sunny golden hue of this soup and the hearty Southwestern flavors make you want to smile after a long, hard day. It features slow-burning, energizing carbs to put a bit of pep back into your evening, and it bursts with a happy sweetness that will bring a grin as it's gobbled up. My family loves it with Artisan Sourdough Bread (from* Trim Healthy Mama Cookbook*) or sprouted-grain bread toasted, cubed up, and thrown in. It's slimming, it's sunny, and super-duper yummy. . . . Yeehaaaaw!*

1. Brown the ground meat in a large skillet over medium-high heat. If the meat is not at least 96% lean, rinse it thoroughly under very hot water to get all the extra fat out of it. Set the meat aside.

2. Place the carrots, onion, and garlic in a soup pot with 5 cups of the water. Cover and bring to a boil. Reduce to a simmer and cook until the veggies are tender.

3. Ladle 2 cups of the hot broth into a blender and add the Trimmy ingredients: ghee, gelatin, collagen (if using), and lecithin (if using). Add the liquid smoke, cumin, lemon juice, Cajun seasoning, stevia powder, salt, chipotle powder, cayenne, and nutritional yeast (if using). Blend until smooth and creamy and return the puree to the soup pot.

4. Now put three-fourths of the tender veggies into the blender along with the remaining 1 cup water. Blend until nice and smooth and return the puree to the pot. Add the chicken broth, black beans, tomatoes, meat, pepper flakes, and cilantro and bring to a perfect serving temperature. Taste and adjust the flavors to "own it."

MAKE A FAMILY MEAL: For the weight-loss plan, there is still E carb room here to add a piece of sprouted-grain toast for dunking or a couple of Wasa light rye crackers. Or finish the meal with a piece of fresh fruit or with an add-on E-friendly shake from the Shakes and Smoothies chapter (page 468). Children can have a Crossover with butter on their bread and cheese on their soup if desired.

* FOR NSI: USE A GROCERY STORE UNFLAVORED GELATIN AND GROCERY STORE ON-PLAN SWEETENER.

cream of mushroom trimmy bisque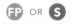

FAMILY SERVE—FEEDS 6 TO 8 (HALVE IF YOUR FAMILY IS SMALLER, OR MAKE FULL AND FREEZE HALF)

2 quarts water

1 large onion, diced

8 garlic cloves, minced

16 ounces baby bellas (cremini)
   or button mushrooms, sliced

1 teaspoon dried thyme, or leaves
   from 2 sprigs fresh thyme,
   finely diced

2 bay leaves

1½ teaspoons Mineral Salt

1 teaspoon black pepper

2 tablespoons rice vinegar

1 to 2 tablespoons red wine
   (optional)

2 tablespoons Nutritional Yeast,
   or 1 tablespoon yellow miso for
   umami burst

2 tablespoons ghee (clarified
   butter)

2 tablespoons Just Gelatin*

1 scoop Integral Collagen (optional)

½ teaspoon Sunflower Lecithin
   (optional but preferred)

¼ to ½ teaspoon Gluccie*
   (depending on thickness desired)

¼ cup heavy cream* (for a lovely
   and luscious S, leave out for FP
   version)

Protein options: ½ cup unflavored
   Pristine Whey Protein Powder or
   4 cups diced cooked chicken
   breast (see page 45 for cooking
   methods)

½ bunch fresh flat-leaf parsley,
   stems removed and finely diced

SERENE CHATS: *If you love cream of mushroom soup but don't love the pounds that creep up on you due to the added starches and other junk usually added to that soup, then dig in to this angel of a Trimmy Bisque. This bisque is delicate and lovely and can be enjoyed without meat by using the whey protein option instead of the chicken breast if preferred.*

1. Put the water, onion, garlic, sliced mushrooms, herbs, salt, pepper, vinegar, wine (if using), and nutritional yeast in a soup pot. Cover and bring to a boil. As soon as it boils, reduce to a simmer and let the veggies become tender and the herbs release their fragrance.

2. Ladle all the mushrooms, some onions (leave out the bay leaves), and some broth into a blender until it reaches the 4-cup mark. Add the core Trimmy ingredients: ghee, gelatin, collagen (if using), and lecithin (if using) plus the Gluccie and blend to Trimmy it up until smooth and yumzers. Pour this back into the pot, using a spatula to get every flavorful bit out.

3. Stir everything well. Add the cream (for an S; or drizzle cream on each individual bowl). Add your protein of choice. If using whey protein, remove ½ cup of the broth, add a couple ice cubes to cool the broth down, then stir in the whey with a fork until there are no lumps (if you don't cool it down it will clump). While stirring constantly, slowly add the whey mix to your soup. Bring the soup back up to the perfect serving temp and stir in the parsley. Taste and adjust the flavors to "own it." Remove the bay leaves before serving.

MAKE A FAMILY MEAL: For the weight-loss plan, enjoy a generous bowlful or two alone, or add in a side salad and/or a bread item from the Breads chapter (page 240). Children can enjoy buttered sprouted-grain bread on the side or a piece of fruit for a Crossover.

* FOR NSI: USE A GROCERY STORE UNFLAVORED GELATIN AND XANTHAN GUM FOR THE GLUCCIE.

* FOR DF: LEAVE OUT THE CREAM.

Sunny Southwestern Trimmy Bisque (page 165)

Cream of Mushroom Trimmy Bisque (opposite)

Red Russian Borscht Trimmy Bisque (page 168)

Irish King Trimmy Bisque (page 169)

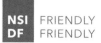
red russian borscht trimmy bisque ⓢ

FAMILY SERVE—FEEDS 6 TO 8 (HALVE IF YOUR FAMILY IS SMALLER, OR MAKE FULL AND FREEZE HALF)

2 large beets

Greens from the 2 beets, coarsely diced

2 quarts water

1 tablespoon Mineral Salt

2 teaspoons dried dill

2 bay leaves

½ head red cabbage, chopped

1 large red onion, chopped

About 15 red radishes, chopped

2 large celery stalks, diced

8 garlic cloves, minced

2 tablespoons MCT oil, flavorless coconut oil, or butter

2 tablespoons Just Gelatin*

1½ tablespoons Integral Collagen (optional)

¼ teaspoon Sunflower Lecithin (optional but preferred)

5 tablespoons apple cider vinegar

2 tablespoons mellow white or yellow miso

1 to 2 teaspoons mesquite liquid smoke (use the smaller amount if your sausages are smoked)

1 teaspoon black pepper

4 doonks cayenne pepper

½ tablespoon Gentle Sweet*

1½ to 2 pounds cooked smoked sausage links (use turkey sausage with no more than 3 net carbs per serving), finely sliced

FOR THE TANGY BORSCHT TOPPER*

1 cup 0% Greek yogurt

Juice of 1 lemon

½ tablespoon MCT oil or flavorless coconut oil

½ tablespoon dried dill

¼ teaspoon Mineral Salt

Thin slices lemon, for garnish

SERENE CHATS: *This brilliant, beautiful red bisque is a delicious zinger for the tongue and a potent health-builder for your body. You can literally see God's goodness gleaming. Red and purple veggies contain a long list of amazing nutrients, including substances called anthocyanins. These "anthy" things lower your risk of colon cancer, help treat stomach ulcers, and fight obesity and diabetes. They help preserve better balance, short-term memory, and vision as we age. The superstar of this bisque is the beet, which not only does all that but helps boost your immune system and purifies and builds your blood. This bisque of beauty makes us feel as strong as a homegrown Russian.*

1. Remove the beet greens. Wash the beets and cut them into large chunks without peeling. Put the beets in a food processor and process until they look like bright red, small-curd cottage cheese. Don't process the beet greens; place them in a large soup pot with the water, salt, dill, bay leaves, cabbage, onion, radishes, celery, garlic, and the processed beets. Cover and bring to a boil, then reduce to a gentle simmer.

2. Ladle out about 4 cups of the soup broth (trying not to get veggies with it) into a blender. Add your core Trimmy ingredients: **MCT oil, gelatin, collagen** (if using), and **lecithin** (if using). Add all the remaining ingredients (except the sausage). Hold the blender lid down tightly and Trimmy it up nice and smooth. Scrape it back into the soup pot.

3. Add the sausage to the pot and let everything simmer together for a while so the flavors meld. It should start to lose any pink froth, and a deep red hue will be revealed.

4. Make your tangy borscht topper. Whisk all the ingredients in a bowl until smooth. Remove the bay leaves from the bisque.

5. Drizzle a tablespoon of the borscht topper onto your bowl of bisque broth, and lay a lemon slice (if using) on top.

MAKE A FAMILY MEAL: For the weight-loss plan, enjoy a bowlful or two alone or pair with a side salad and/or an S-friendly bread from the Breads chapter (page 240). Children can finish the meal with a side of fruit or have whole-grain rice or sprouted-grain bread on the side.

* FOR NSI: USE A GROCERY STORE UNFLAVORED GELATIN AND AN ON-PLAN SWEETENER.

* FOR DF: LEAVE OFF THE BORSCHT TOPPER.

irish king trimmy bisque

E

FAMILY SERVE—FEEDS 6 TO 8 (HALVE IF YOUR FAMILY IS SMALLER, OR MAKE FULL AND FREEZE HALF)

2 quarts chicken broth

6 garlic cloves, minced

2 large leeks, washed well and thinly sliced

4 large carrots (see Note), finely diced*

2 celery stalks, finely diced

2 bay leaves (optional)

½ teaspoon dried thyme

1 cup old-fashioned rolled oats

4 to 6 chamomile tea bags (optional)

1 cup just off the boil water

2 tablespoons butter, MCT oil, or flavorless coconut oil

2 tablespoons Just Gelatin*

1½ tablespoons Integral Collagen (optional)

¼ teaspoon Sunflower Lecithin (optional but preferred)

2 tablespoons apple cider vinegar

1½ to 2 teaspoons Mineral Salt (the larger amount for savory heads; add the extra after final tasting)

¼ teaspoon black pepper

2 teaspoons onion powder

4 to 5 cups diced cooked chicken breasts (see page 45 for cooking methods)

½ bunch fresh parsley, stems removed and finely diced, for garnish

SERENE CHATS: *Archaeologists have discovered ancient Irish archives that describe a dish called* brotchan roy. *Made with the traditional Irish staples of yore—oats, leeks, butter, and milk—many historians believe this recipe dates all the way back to the ancient Druids. "Brotchan" means broth and "roy" can be translated as king. It was a simple dish beloved by royalty and peasants alike. Of course I've gone and Trim Healthy Mammafied it so it can help make you both feel and look your "Queenliest" . . . or "Kingliest" if you are a dude. With a few simple tweaks and a whiz of your Trimmy blender, the timeworn taste of brotchan roy can be yours (the Trimming way). Bring your family the experience . . . the flavors . . . and the history of the harvest fields of ancient Ireland.*

1. Put the broth, garlic, leeks, carrots, celery, bay leaves (if using), and thyme in a large soup pot. Cover and bring to a boil, then reduce the heat, add the oats, and gently simmer.

2. If using chamomile tea, brew it in the 1 cup of boiled water for a few minutes. Now assemble your Trimmy: Place the brewed tea or 1 cup boiled water into a blender. Add the core Trimmy ingredients: butter, gelatin, collagen (if using), and lecithin (if using). Add the vinegar, salt, pepper, and onion powder. Hold the lid down tightly on the blender and whip until smooth and creamy. Stir the puree back into the soup pot. Add the chicken. Taste and adjust the flavors to "own it." Remove the bay leaves. Garnish with the parsley, and serve up hearty bowls of Irish heritage.

MAKE A FAMILY MEAL: For the weight-loss plan, this bisque is a light E, so you have carb room to dunk ripped-up pieces of sprouted-grain toast in your bowl, or serve a refreshing fruit salad for dessert. Growing children or others not on the weight-loss track can have a Crossover with butter on their bread.

NOTE: Parsnip lovers can use 3 medium parsnips instead of carrots. Parsnips are as sweet as yams and will make your bisque very sweet, so be prepared.

FOR NSI: USE A GROCERY STORE UNFLAVORED GELATIN.

rustic andouille sausage trimmy bisque   S WITH FP OPTION

FAMILY SERVE–FEEDS 6 TO 8 (HALVE IF YOUR FAMILY IS SMALLER, OR MAKE FULL AND FREEZE HALF)

1 quart cold water

1 (10-ounce) box frozen spinach

1 (12-ounce) bag frozen cauliflower florets

1 (12-ounce) bag frozen broccoli florets

1 large onion, diced

2 red or orange sweet bell peppers, coarsely chopped

6 garlic cloves, minced

2 teaspoons dried basil

1 (14.5-ounce) can petite diced tomatoes

2 cups frozen diced okra

4½ cups just off the boil water

2 tablespoons mellow yellow or white miso

1 tablespoon balsamic vinegar

1 tablespoon rice vinegar or apple cider vinegar

1 (6-ounce) can tomato paste

1 tablespoon oil-packed sun-dried tomatoes, rinsed (optional, but it gives amazing tomato flavor burst)

1 tablespoon ghee (clarified butter)

1 tablespoon MCT oil, flavorless coconut oil, or butter

2 tablespoons Just Gelatin*

1½ tablespoons (1 scoop) Integral Collagen (optional)

¼ teaspoon Sunflower Lecithin (optional but preferred)

2 tablespoons Nutritional Yeast

1 tablespoon Mineral Salt

¼ to ½ teaspoon black pepper

¼ teaspoon cayenne pepper

2 teaspoons onion powder

1 teaspoon ground cumin

2 teaspoons mesquite liquid smoke

2 doonks Pure Stevia Extract Powder*

SERENE CHATS: *This is a favorite on my table when flavorful food and contented tummies are in order. This creamy bisque has sweet balsamic undercurrents, but it is conquered by smoky sausage heartiness. French immigrants and Acadian exiles birthed the beloved andouille sausage into Louisiana Cajun culture. Now the town of LaPlace, Louisiana, nestled at the edge of the Mississippi River, is nicknamed the Andouille Capital of the World. Andouille sausage is traditionally made with garlic, onions, peppers, and pork, then smoked—sometimes even double smoked—into andouille perfection. I use smoked chicken sausage and add an extra punch of mesquite liquid smoke for good measure (but you can use pork if desired).*

1. Put the cold water in a large soup pot, then add the spinach, cauliflower, broccoli, onion, bell peppers, garlic, and basil. Cover and bring to a boil, then reduce the heat to a simmer and cook until the veggies are tender. Add the diced tomatoes.

2. The first blend: Put the okra, 3 cups of the boiled water, the miso, both vinegars, the tomato paste, and sun-dried tomatoes (if using) in a blender and blend well. Add this to the gently simmering veggies and stir well.

3. Now let's make the Trimmy blend: In the same dirty blender, combine the remaining 1½ cups boiled water and our core Trimmy ingredients: **ghee, MCT oil, gelatin, collagen** (if using), and **lecithin** (if using). Add the nutritional yeast, seasonings, liquid smoke, and stevia powder. Hold the lid down and whiz whiz, then pour this creamy yumminess into your pot.

4. Add the diced sausage links and heat through. (If using whey protein to beef up the protein amounts, ladle out some soup broth into a cup, trying not to get any fixin's in there, and drop a couple of ice cubes in to cool it down. Now add the whey and stir well until all the clumps are gone. Return the whey mixture slowly to the pot, stirring constantly as you add it back.)

5. Taste and adjust the flavors to "own it" and dig in, baby!

MAKE A FAMILY MEAL: For the weight-loss plan, feel free to top the soup with a little grated cheese if you want. Have a big bowl or two of this soup alone or add a side salad and/or an S-friendly bread item. If you would like to make this soup an

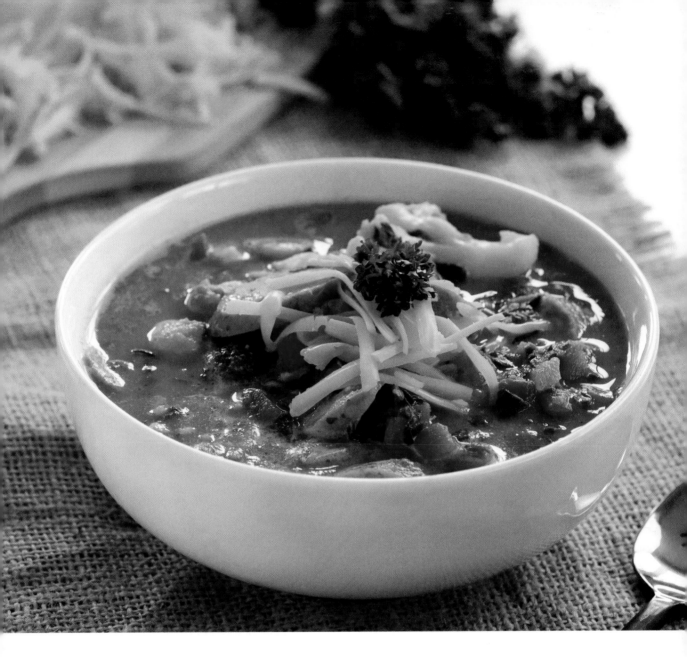

2 to 3 packages smoked chicken sausage links, sliced (enough so each person gets 1½ to 2 links, or use just 1 pack to save dollars and follow the whey protein addition option)

¼ to ½ cup Pristine Whey Protein (optional; use if you don't have enough sausage links)

FP, you can use 4 to 5 cups of precooked diced chicken breast in place of the sausage links and add another 1 to 2 teaspoons liquid smoke. Growing children or others needing Crossovers can finish their meal with some fruit or have rice or sprouted-grain toast on the side.

* FOR NSI: USE A GROCERY STORE UNFLAVORED GELATIN AND GROCERY STORE ON-PLAN SWEETENER.

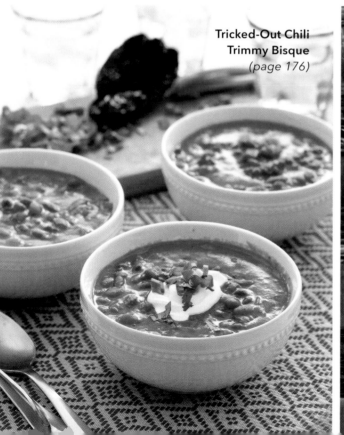

Better Than Pearl's Broc and
Cheese Trimmy Bisque
(opposite)

Peasant's Garden
Trimmy Bisque
(page 174)

Tricked-Out Chili
Trimmy Bisque
(page 176)

Peanut Satay
Trimmy Bisque
(page 175)

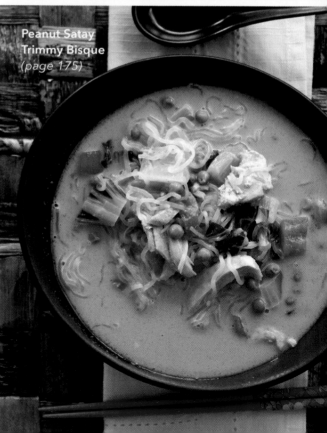

better than pearl's broc and cheese trimmy bisque ⓢ

FAMILY SERVE–FEEDS 6 TO 8 (HALVE IF YOUR FAMILY IS SMALLER, OR MAKE FULL AND FREEZE HALF)

3 (12-ounce) bags frozen broccoli florets

6 cups water

6 garlic cloves, minced

3 cups just off the boil water

1 to 2 tablespoons ghee (clarified butter)

2 tablespoons Just Gelatin*

1½ tablespoons (1 scoop) Integral Collagen (optional)

¼ teaspoon Sunflower Lecithin (optional but preferred)

1 tablespoon toasted sesame oil

2 tablespoons yellow miso

¾ cup powder-style Parmesan cheese (from the green can) or freshly grated Pecorino Romano cheese (grated on the finest holes for better measuring)

⅓ cup Nutritional Yeast

1 tablespoon onion powder

1 to 2 tablespoons Baobab Boost Powder (optional), the smaller amount for budgeting Mamas

1 tablespoon Mineral Salt

¼ teaspoon cayenne pepper

¼ teaspoon black pepper

1 teaspoon mesquite liquid smoke

1 teaspoon soy sauce

1 teaspoon Gluccie*

2 cups frozen diced okra

¼ large red bell pepper

2 tablespoons apple cider vinegar

Protein options: ½ cup unflavored Pristine Whey Protein Powder, or 4 to 5 cups diced cooked chicken (see page 45 for cooking methods) or pulled rotisserie chicken

SERENE CHATS: *Big Sis Pearl dared to say her Loaded Broccoli and Cheese Soup (page 152) was superior to mine! I hope she knows this does mean war! My precious version is not just a soup, it's a Trimmy Bisque for goodness' sake. . . . You did read my Trimmy Bisque sermon starting on page 162, right? There is no competing with Trimmy Bisque level! Of course, I am tooting my own horn in full awareness that I am being a total bad egg here. I am sure Pearlie's is wonderful, but I've never tasted it because I'm too busy enjoying mine. Maybe we can tie. If you like hers better, just keep it to yourself . . . Okay?*

1. Place the broccoli in a soup pot with the 6 cups water and the garlic. Bring to a boil and then reduce the heat and simmer. Using a potato masher (not a blending device), mash the broccoli in the water until the florets are broken up.

2. Now make your Trimmy: Put 2 cups of the boiled water in a blender with the core Trimmy ingredients: **ghee, gelatin, collagen** (if using), and **lecithin** (if using). Add the sesame oil, miso, Parmesan, nutritional yeast, onion powder, baobab powder (if using), salt, cayenne, black pepper, liquid smoke, soy sauce, and Gluccie. Trimmy it all up in the blender until creamy and add it to your pot of broccoli.

3. Using the same blender (don't wash), blend the remaining 1 cup boiled water with the okra, bell pepper, and vinegar until smooth. Blend like you're a blending champ and there are no green okra bits left. Stir into the pot.

4. Add your protein of choice. If using whey protein, remove ½ cup of the broth, add a couple ice cubes to cool the broth down, then stir in the whey with a fork until there are no lumps (if you don't cool it down it will clump). While stirring constantly, slowly add the whey mix to your soup. Simmer a little longer, taste, and adjust the flavors to "own it!"

MAKE A FAMILY MEAL: For the weight-loss plan, enjoy a big bowlful or two alone or add a side salad and/or a bread item from the Breads chapter (page 240). Growing children or other Crossie-lovers can end their meal with a piece of fruit or enjoy buttered sprouted-grain toast on the side.

* FOR NSI: USE A GROCERY STORE UNFLAVORED GELATIN AND SUB XANTHAN GUM FOR THE GLUCCIE.

peasant's garden trimmy bisque

(FP)

FAMILY SERVE—FEEDS 6 TO 8 (HALVE IF YOUR FAMILY IS SMALLER, OR MAKE FULL AND FREEZE HALF)

1 large head cabbage, or
   1½ smaller heads, chopped
10 garlic cloves, minced
1 onion, chopped
1 quart plus 2½ cups water
1 tablespoon Mineral Salt
6 chamomile tea bags (optional)
3 tablespoons Nutritional Yeast
4 tablespoons grated Parmesan
   cheese (the green can kind is fine)
2 tablespoons apple cider vinegar
2 teaspoons dried rosemary
1½ teaspoons black pepper
2 teaspoons Gluccie*
2 tablespoons ghee (clarified
   butter)
2 tablespoons Just Gelatin*
2 scoops (3 tablespoons) Integral
   Collagen (optional)
¼ teaspoon Sunflower Lecithin
   (optional but preferred)

PROTEIN OPTIONS
2 cups 1% cottage cheese plus
   ½ cup water
½ cup unflavored Pristine Whey
   Protein Powder plus 1 cup
   lukewarm water
3 cups pulled rotisserie chicken or
   small-diced cooked chicken breast
   (see page 45 for cooking
   methods)

SERENE CHATS: *Thick and wonderful, this Trimmy Bisque will catapult you back to a little thatched-roof cottage where all meals are richly filled with humble veggies. Of course they are freshly pulled from the rich loamy black soil in the backyard garden. The optional chamomile tea in this soup is like a health shot! Chamomile goes way beyond a digestive aid, reducing cancerous cells, fighting off dangerous microbes, and leveling blood sugar.*

1. Place the cabbage, garlic, and onion in a large soup pot. Add all the water and the salt, cover, and bring to a boil. Reduce the heat and simmer until the veggies are tender. If using chamomile tea bags, take out 1 cup of the hot broth (avoid getting the veggies) and simmer the tea in it for a few minutes while your veggies are simmering.

2. Now blend all your veggies. You'll need to do this in a couple batches. Ladle some soup broth into your blender. If using tea, remove the bags and add the tea to the blender along with half of the veggies. Add the nutritional yeast, Parmesan, vinegar, rosemary, pepper, and 1 teaspoon of the Gluccie. Blend well. Pour that mixture into a bowl. Ladle more soup water into the blender, add the rest of your veggies along with the remaining 1 teaspoon Gluccie and your core Trimmy ingredients: ghee, gelatin, collagen (if using), and lecithin (if using). Blend well, then return to the pot along with the blended mix from the bowl. Stir.

3. Add your protein of choice. If using cottage cheese, put it in the same dirty blender with the water and blend until smooth, then add it to the soup. If using whey powder, mix it with the lukewarm water until there are no clumps, then add it slowly to the pot while whisking. Bring the soup to the perfect serving temp. Taste and adjust the flavors to "own it."

MAKE A FAMILY MEAL: Enjoy a big bowlful or two of soup alone or pair it with a side salad (with a lean dressing to stay FP) and/or a slice or two of Fifteen-Minute Focaccia Bread (page 247) or Wonderful White Blender Bread (page 242). Growing children or others in the Crossie club can top it with cheese and add fruit on the side or sprouted-grain bread for a Crossover.

* FOR NSI: USE A GROCERY STORE UNFLAVORED GELATIN AND SUB XANTHAN GUM FOR THE GLUCCIE.

* FOR DF: USE A CHICKEN PROTEIN OPTION.

peanut satay trimmy bisque

(S)

FAMILY SERVE–FEEDS 6 TO 8 (HALVE IF YOUR FAMILY IS SMALLER, OR MAKE FULL AND FREEZE HALF, BUT LEAVE OUT THE NOODLES IF FREEZING)

2 quarts chicken broth

4 garlic cloves, minced

1 bunch green onions, diced

1 head bok choy, sliced

2 cups frozen peas

2 large red bell peppers, diced

1 (15-ounce) can full-fat coconut milk

1 cup just off the boil water

1 tablespoon toasted sesame oil

2 tablespoons Just Gelatin*

1 scoop Integral Collagen (optional)

¼ teaspoon Sunflower Lecithin (optional but preferred)

½ cup Pressed Peanut Flour*

2 tablespoons sugar-free natural-style peanut butter

1 teaspoon Gluccie*

2 tablespoons soy sauce, or a couple good squirts Bragg liquid aminos or coconut aminos

2 tablespoons fish sauce

4 doonks Pure Stevia Extract Powder plus 1 tablespoon Gentle Sweet*

4 to 8 tablespoons Thai red curry paste (you can start with 4 and add more at the end if you want; I use 8)

Juice of 2 limes or lemons

3 tablespoons Baobab Boost Powder (optional)

½ teaspoon red pepper flakes (more for hotheads)

3 to 4 single-serve bags Trim Healthy Noodles or Not Naughty Noodles,* well rinsed, drained, and snipped a bit smaller

4 to 5 cups diced cooked chicken breast or thighs (see cooking methods on page 45), or pulled rotisserie chicken

A handful of sliced fresh basil (optional)

SERENE CHATS: *This Trimmy Bisque boasts a smooth and rich mouthfeel drenched with the exotic flavors of Thai cuisine. Bold peanut lingers long on the tongue while bright refreshing bursts of lime and Thai ginger from the curry paste tease the taste buds. A much-beloved Thai dish served up with a Trimmy twist so it can please your waistline as well as your palate.*

1. Place the chicken broth in a large soup pot and add the garlic, green onions, bok choy, peas, and three-fourths of the diced bell pepper. Cover, bring to a boil, then reduce the heat and gently simmer until tender.

2. Put the coconut milk in a blender, add the boiled water and the core Trimmy ingredients—sesame oil, gelatin, collagen (if using), and lecithin (if using)—the peanut flour, peanut butter, Gluccie, soy sauce, fish sauce, stevia powder, Gentle Sweet, red curry paste, lemon juice, baobab powder (if using), and the remaining bell pepper. Hold the lid on tightly and blend well. Pour your Trimmy into the pot, stir well, then add the pepper flakes. Add the noodles and chicken. Taste and adjust the flavors to "own it." Heat to the perfect serving temperature. Garnish with basil (if using) and visit Thailand for the evening.

MAKE A FAMILY MEAL: For the weight-loss plan, it is perfect on its own, or you can add a side salad such as the Thai-Kissed Cucumber Salad (page 268). A pot of steamed brown jasmine rice is extra filling for Crossover family members who can add it to their soup. If you are at S Helper stage, a ¼ cup of this rice adds a nice dimension of texture.

* FOR NSI: SUB XANTHAN GUM FOR THE GLUCCIE. USE A GROCERY STORE UNFLAVORED GELATIN, ON-PLAN SWEETENER, AND SUGAR-FREE DEFATTED PEANUT FLOUR. WHILE YOU'RE THERE, FIND KONJAC NOODLES IF YOU DON'T WANT TO USE THM BRAND.

tricked-out chili trimmy bisque

(E)

FEEDS A HUGE CROWD (TALKING A BIG FAMILY MEAL HERE WITH LOTSA HANDY LEFTOVERS THAT YOU CAN WARM UP FROM THE FRIDGE OR FREEZE)

1½ pounds dried pinto beans

5 tablespoons apple cider vinegar

8 garlic cloves, minced, or
  1½ teaspoons garlic powder

2½ to 3 pounds lean ground beef
  (we'll magically get it even leaner
  soon), venison, or turkey (if ya
  want), thawed if frozen

2 (14.5-ounce) cans petite diced
  tomatoes

3 whole dried ancho chilies
  (easy to find at grocery stores;
  I use San Miguel brand)

3 cups boiling water

2 tablespoons tahini (sesame paste)
  or almond butter

1 tablespoon toasted sesame oil

2 tablespoons Just Gelatin*

1½ tablespoons (1 scoop) Integral
  Collagen (optional)

½ teaspoon Sunflower Lecithin
  (optional but preferred)

1 (6-ounce) can tomato paste

1½ tablespoons onion powder

2 tablespoons plus 1 teaspoon
  Mineral Salt (see Note)

4 teaspoons mesquite liquid smoke

1 tablespoon ground cumin

3 tablespoons Nutritional Yeast

SERENE CHATS: *Tricked-Out Chili Trimmy Bisque is made to "bring it!" It satisfies hard-to-fill, starving, scarfing, and scrounging mouths. Men or teenage boys with huge appetites . . . or a Mama who feels like she could eat a bear . . . Tricked-Out Chili Trimmy Bisque to the rescue! It's an E. Not just E for E-nergy but E for E-normous! You get to have seconds of this bisquey boy and the firsts don't need to be dainty, neither! Part of the trick here is being able to use beef in an E chili (thanks to our rinsing method described in the directions), so there is nothing diety tasting or feeling about it. I'm not saying you can't use turkey, but I prefer grass-fed beef or venison for the heartiness factor.*

This makes more than my usual Trimmy Bisques, 'cause this one is for big eaters and big potlucks and big backyard barbies and big leftovers for quickie lunches. It's thick 'n' hearty like that good ol' canned Hormel Chili that hardworkin' men with big ol' farm boots swear by. After supper tonight, you can close the kitchen and turn off the light 'cause all the bellies will be good and stuffed.

I'm not apologizing that you'll be making beans from scratch here. It is another part of the "trick" for the hearty texture of the soup. Don't be put off by that because this is a cinch. If you want a chili using beans from a can, Pearl has a couple in the crockpot chapter (page 76), but if you skip mine, scared of one little extra step, you'll be missing out. Game's on, and it is finally time for me to win the chili competition. I'll admit her chili from our first book beat mine (she rubs that in my face a lot), but "Tricked-Out" ain't going down!

1. Soak the beans. You can do this either before you go to bed the night before or in the morning the day you're making your chili. To soak, rinse the beans, then put them in your BIG soup pot. Add 2 tablespoons of the vinegar and enough cold water to amply cover. Soak overnight (or for about 7 hours).

2. Drain the beans in a colander, rinse, and put them back in the pot. Add enough water to cover by a good inch and add the garlic. If this is the morning and you're rinsing after an overnight soak, just leave the beans sitting there in the new water until midafternoon when you can start cooking them. If you're soaking during the day and you're out of the house, rinse and add more water back in as soon as you get home . . . like ASAP. Cover the pot, bring to a boil, then reduce the heat to low and simmer until the beans are very tender, almost mushy. (If you are rushing home from work, simmer at

a higher temp such as medium-low as it will take a good hour to cook them.)

3. While the beans are simmering, brown your meat. Once it's done, rinse it extremely well under very hot (better yet, boiling) water in a colander, rinsing then re-rinsing to get every bit of fat out to make it E-friendly. Add the meat and canned tomatoes to the pot with the simmering beans.

4. While the meat is browning, prepare your ancho chilies. You can choose to wear gloves, but I just wash my hands really well afterward and don't put my fingers near my eyes or my babies before I wash up. Slice along the sides of each ancho to open it up completely and cut away the stem. Scrape out all of the seeds and veins if you don't want a fiery chili, but if you want a bit of a kick, leave in about 15 or so seeds (this is what I do). If you are a hot maniac, then leave a bunch more. Lightly rinse the chilies under water, then put them in a bowl with 1 cup of the boiling water to soften them. Set them aside for 15 minutes to soak.

5. Scoop out 1 cup of the broth from the cooked beans (do your best to avoid getting any beans with it) and put it in a blender. Add the softened chilies and their soaking water, the core Trimmy ingredients—tahini, sesame oil, gelatin, collagen (if using), and lecithin (if using)—the tomato paste, the remaining 3 tablespoons vinegar, the onion powder, salt, liquid smoke, cumin, and nutritional yeast. Hold the lid down tightly and whiz until smooth, then add it to the soup pot along with the remaining 2 cups boiled water. Stir together, taste, and adjust the flavors to "own it." Bring it to the perfect serving temperature, then start filling up your hungry crowd.

MAKE A FAMILY MEAL: For the weight-loss plan, eat a big ol' bowl or two as is—or there is a little bit of room in your E quota of carbs to sprinkle on a few baked corn chips or to top with a dollop of Greek yogurt. Side salads are always welcome, just keep your dressing lean. Growing children or others in Crossover mode can top their chili with grated cheese and/or sour cream and enjoy those baked corn chips.

NOTE: Don't freak out. This amount of salt is perfect for this huge batch of chili, and Mineral Salt is good for ya!

* FOR NSI: USE A GROCERY STORE UNFLAVORED GELATIN.

vibey cream of cilantro trimmy bisque · S

FAMILY SERVE–FEEDS 6 TO 8 (HALVE IF YOUR FAMILY IS SMALLER, OR MAKE FULL AND FREEZE HALF)

3 large rainbow bell peppers
  (red, orange, and yellow), cut into
  medium dice

1 large onion, diced

6 garlic cloves, minced

3 cups cold water

6 ITO EN green tea bags

7½ cups just off the boil water (or
  cold water for reducing caffeine)

1 bunch fresh cilantro

2 tablespoons ghee (clarified
  butter)

2 tablespoons Just Gelatin*

1½ tablespoons (1 scoop) Integral
  Collagen (optional)

¼ teaspoon Sunflower Lecithin
  (optional but preferred)

½ cup powder-style Parmesan
  cheese (from the green can)

2 tablespoons Nutritional Yeast

¼ teaspoon black pepper

2½ teaspoons Mineral Salt

2 teaspoons onion powder

3 to 4 tablespoons Baobab Boost
  Powder (optional but preferred)

2 cups frozen diced okra

1 to 2 loose tablespoons grated
  fresh ginger (grated on the finest
  option on your grater)

½ teaspoon red pepper flakes

Juice of 1 lemon

2 doonks Pure Stevia Extract
  Powder*

½ to 1 teaspoon matcha powder
  (optional; only use if serving at
  lunch as the matcha adds more
  caffeine)

4 cups diced cooked chicken breast
  (see page 45 for cooking
  methods)

SERENE CHATS: *There is ugly green food (like my Ugly Duckling Trimmy Bisque on page 182, which tastes awesome so don't let Pearl scare you away from it) and beautiful green food and then there is a green that brings loveliness to a new level. That's where this vibey soup fits . . . somewhere at the loveliest of all levels. Bright, popping orange, yellow, and red bell peppers add to the alluring artistry, but the flavor merriment of this Trimmy Bisque might be the best part of all. It will be the topic of conversation at hip luncheons or potluck parties, and it brings a fresh new taste sensation to the family table.*

You'll notice this soup calls for ITO EN green tea (a blend of sencha and matcha). Don't freak out at the strange name. I buy this tea at Costco and have even spied it at Walmart. And if you can't find it in a store, it is very easily found online. The flavor of this tea is divine, very bright tasting without a lot of bitter tannin taste, and it brews up into a vibrant, almost lime green color. While it does have a little caffeine (you can do my cold brew method if you don't want caffeine), I do a regular hot brew for this and my kids still sleep well at bedtime. But the choice is yours.

1. Place the bell peppers, onion, and garlic in a soup pot with the 3 cups cold water. Cover, bring to a boil, reduce the heat, and simmer until tender.

2. While the veggies are simmering, place the tea bags in 4½ cups of the boiled water and let steep for a few minutes before squeezing the tea bags and removing them from the water. (Alternatively, brew the tea in the same amount of cold water to avoid caffeine.)

3. Divide the cilantro bunch in half. Remove the stems from one half, finely chop the leaves, and set aside. From the other half, remove only the large, tough stems and coarsely chop (this gets used next, in the Trimmy blend).

4. Make your Trimmy: Place the brewed tea (if using cold-brewed, heat the tea after the bags are removed so your fat and hygroscopic protein Trimmy up just right) in a blender. Add the coarsely chopped cilantro and the core Trimmy ingredients—**ghee, gelatin, collagen** (if using), and **lecithin** (if using)—the Parmesan, nutritional yeast, pepper, salt, onion powder, and baobab powder (if using). Hold the lid down and whiz, then pour into the veggie pot.

5. In the same dirty blender, place the okra and the remaining 3 cups boiled water and blend until perrrrfectly smooth. Add

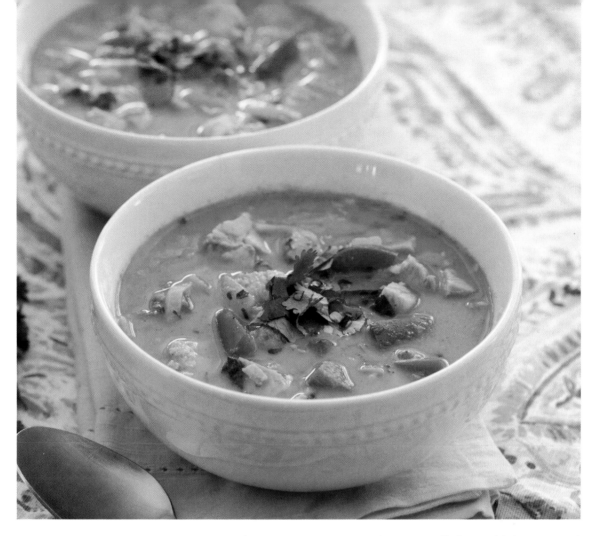

the puree to your pot, stir super well, then add the reserved cilantro, grated ginger, pepper flakes, lemon juice, stevia powder, matcha (if using), and chicken and bring to a perfect serving temperature. Taste and adjust the flavors to "own it."

6. Serve your Trimmy Bisque in gorgeous "vibey" bowls and experience unorthodox flavor winsomeness. You might like to float a few ripped-up pieces of toasted and lightly salted seaweed on top like Asian lily pads, but if that doesn't float your boat, then pretend you didn't read this.

MAKE A FAMILY MEAL: This is delicious served with Cheesy Flower Biscuits (page 248) and a lacy spring mix side salad with a sesame vinaigrette. Or just eat a big bowlful or two and be done. Steamed brown jasmine rice is the perfect addition for Crossover family members.

* FOR NSI: USE A GROCERY STORE UNFLAVORED GELATIN AND AN ON-PLAN SWEETENER.

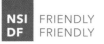
chicken paprikash trimmy bisque   Ⓢ

FAMILY SERVE–FEEDS 6 TO 8 (HALVE IF YOUR FAMILY IS SMALLER, OR MAKE FULL AND FREEZE HALF, BUT DON'T USE NOODLES IF FREEZING)

3 tablespoons ghee (clarified butter)

1 large onion, diced

6 to 7 garlic cloves, minced

Protein options: 1 whole uncooked chicken, jointed (for traditional method); or meat from 1 whole rotisserie chicken, pulled apart and off the bone; or 4 to 5 cups diced or sliced cooked chicken breasts or thighs (see page 45 for cooking methods)

¼ cup Hungarian paprika (see Note)

2 red bell peppers, diced

1 (14.5-ounce) can petite diced tomatoes

2 quarts chicken broth

3 single-serve bags Trim Healthy Noodles or Not Naughty Noodles,* well rinsed, drained, and snipped a bit smaller (optional; this soup doesn't need them to be great but Hungarians like their noodles, so include if you want)

1 cup boiling water

2 tablespoons Just Gelatin*

1½ tablespoons (1 scoop) Integral Collagen (optional)

¼ teaspoon Sunflower Lecithin (optional but preferred)

2 teaspoons fish sauce

¼ teaspoon black pepper

3 doonks cayenne pepper (add more for spice heads)

1 to 1½ teaspoons Mineral Salt (the chicken broth provides most of the salt; add more at the end if needed)

SERENE CHATS: *Fragrant with spice, sailing you across the seas, this bisque is kissed with the terra-cotta earthiness of dried red sweet peppers. Its deep, slightly smoky flavor undertones sing the Hungarian national anthem on your tongue. No . . . ¼ cup of Hungarian paprika is not a misprint. Tonight we celebrate this Hungarian favorite the Trimming way! Whether this is a comfort food from your childhood and you'd prefer to make this the traditional way with bone-in chicken, or it's a new exotic food adventure that you want to keep simple with pre-cooked diced chicken . . . Chicken Paprikash Trimmy Bisque is what's for dinner.*

1. Melt 2 tablespoons of the ghee in a large soup pot over medium heat. Add the onion and garlic and sauté until translucent.

2. If you are a purist, traditionalist Mama who wants to use bone-in chicken pieces here, rub them with salt and pepper and sear them in the ghee, garlic, and onions, then transfer them to a plate. (You'll have to do a couple of searing batches.) If you're not using bone-in chicken, simply cook the garlic and onions with the ghee alone.

3. Reduce the heat to low, add the paprika to the veggies, and stir for a couple minutes (make sure not to scorch this lovely spice as it will ruin the flavor). Add the bell peppers and tomatoes, increase the heat to medium, and simmer for a couple/few minutes. It's now time to add the broth, noodles (if using), and chicken (including the seared bone-in chicken). Cover and simmer while you make your Trimmy. (If using bone-in chicken, be sure to simmer until the chicken is cooked.)

4. Make the Trimmy: In a blender, place the boiling water and core Trimmy ingredients—remaining 1 tablespoon **ghee,** the **gelatin, collagen** (if using), and **lecithin** (if using)—the fish sauce, black pepper, cayenne, salt, nutritional yeast, lemon juice, liquid smoke (if using), and Gluccie. Hold the lid down tightly, press blend, and Trimmy it up, baby! Add it to your bisque and simmer for a few more minutes. Remove the pot from the heat and slowly stir in the yogurt. Taste and adjust the flavors to "own it." Purists running the extra mile with this bisque can serve each bowl with bone-in chicken or choose to fish the pieces out and de-bone. Whichever way you create this delish dish . . . dig in and enjoy.

2 tablespoons Nutritional Yeast

2 tablespoons lemon juice (fresh or bottled)

1 teaspoon mesquite liquid smoke (optional)

¾ teaspoon Gluccie*

1½ cups plain 0% Greek yogurt*

MAKE A FAMILY MEAL: For the weight-loss plan, enjoy a big bowlful or two alone—or pair it with a side salad and/or a bread item from the Breads chapter (page 240). Growing children can have a piece of fruit or buttered sprouted-grain toast on the side.

NOTE: Just look for "product of Hungary" on the label and make sure the paprika hasn't been sitting in your cupboard for years . . . stale paprika can ruin this recipe.

* FOR NSI: USE A GROCERY STORE UNFLAVORED GELATIN AND SUB XANTHAN GUM FOR THE GLUCCIE. LEAVE OUT THE NOODLES OR FIND GROCERY STORE KONJAC NOODLES.

* FOR DF: SUB 1 CAN COCONUT MILK PLUS 1 ADDITIONAL TABLESPOON LEMON JUICE FOR THE GREEK YOGURT.

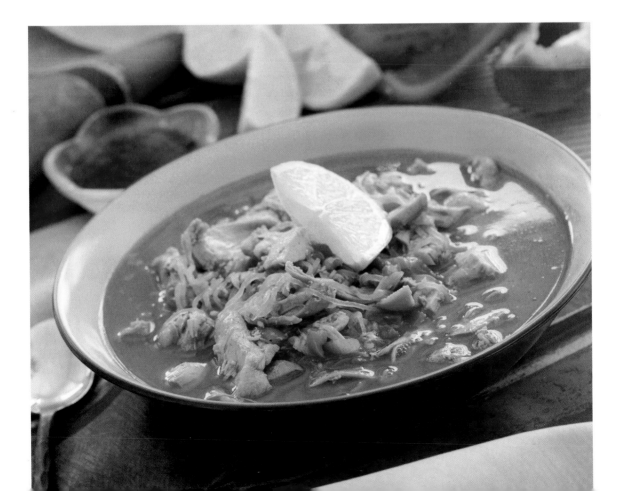

ugly duckling trimmy bisque

FP WITH S AND E OPTIONS

FAMILY SERVE–FEEDS 6 TO 8 (HALVE IF YOUR FAMILY IS SMALLER, OR MAKE FULL AND FREEZE HALF)

2½ to 3 pounds ground beef or venison (thawed if frozen)

1 onion, diced

6 to 7 garlic cloves, minced

1 (12-ounce) bag fresh kale

2 quarts water

4 rooibos tea bags, or ½ teaspoon chaga extract (I use Vitajing Herbs brand)

2 tablespoons ghee (clarified butter)

2 tablespoons Just Gelatin*

1 tablespoon Integral Collagen (optional)

Generous ¼ teaspoon Sunflower Lecithin (optional but preferred)

½ dried habanero (or black pepper to taste if you don't like heat)

2 tablespoons Nutritional Yeast

2 tablespoons apple cider vinegar

2½ teaspoons Mineral Salt

2 teaspoons mesquite liquid smoke

1 teaspoon onion powder

½ teaspoon chipotle powder

1 pound red radishes, or 1 large daikon radish, finely chopped

Greens from the radishes, or 4 to 6 ounces additional kale

SERENE CHATS: *What's with the crazy name? I had to fight to keep this bisque in the book as Pearl thought it was too ugly to go in. She didn't win because, while I admit it may not be beautiful, I love the taste and you can't possibly find a healthier more detoxifying soup. Pearl shouldn't judge a bisque by its cover! You might find this soup turns from an overlooked ugly duckling to a flying swan of taste and nutrition, becoming a welcomed, ultraslimming favorite in your life. So there, Pearl!*

1. Brown the meat with the onion and garlic in a skillet over medium-high heat and set aside.

2. Place the kale in a soup pot with the water and bring to a boil. Cover, reduce to a simmer, and cook until tender.

3. Ladle out 2 cups of this veggie water (not caring if you get a few kale floaters in there), and if using tea, brew the tea in this water for 5 minutes, then remove the tea bags. Pour the water or brewed tea into a blender with the core Trimmy ingredients: ghee, gelatin, collagen (if using), and lecithin (if using). Add the dried habanero, nutritional yeast, vinegar, salt, liquid smoke, onion powder, and chipotle powder and blend well. Really Trimmy it up perfectly creamy and smooth.

4. Pour this Trimmy bisque cream into your pot. With a slotted spoon, fish out all of the greens and place it in the same blender, adding enough of the broth to blend until perfectly silky smooth, before returning to the pot. Add the chopped radishes and radish greens or extra kale. Bring back to a quick boil, then turn down to a simmer. Add the meat and cook until the radishes are tender. Taste and adjust the flavors to "own it."

MAKE A FAMILY MEAL: For the weight-loss plan, enjoy this alone or have it with a side salad and an FP- or S-friendly bread option from the Breads chapter (page 240). To make this an S, top it with grated cheese or to have as an E, enjoy a piece or two of sprouted-grain bread on the side with a thin smear of butter. Growing children can have both grated cheese and sprouted-grain toast for a Crossover.

* FOR NSI: USE A GROCERY STORE UNFLAVORED GELATIN.

cheesy no cheese trimmy bisque

FP

FAMILY SERVE–FEEDS 6 TO 8 (HALVE IF YOUR FAMILY IS SMALLER, OR MAKE FULL AND FREEZE HALF)

2 quarts plus 1 cup water

2 large celery stalks, cut into chunks

2 red bell peppers, cut into chunks

1 large onion, cut into chunks

2 (12-ounce) bags frozen cauliflower florets

6 garlic cloves, minced

2 tablespoons Baobab Boost Powder (optional)

Juice of ½ to 1 lemon (use the smaller amount if using baobab)

6 tablespoons Nutritional Yeast

½ teaspoon mesquite liquid smoke

1 tablespoon Mineral Salt

½ teaspoon chili powder (optional, for a lil' kick)

2 teaspoons onion powder

¼ to ½ teaspoon black pepper

2 doonks cayenne (this is not spicy and brings a sharper cheese flavor)

1½ tablespoons toasted sesame oil

½ tablespoon ghee (clarified butter)*

2 tablespoons Just Gelatin*

1½ tablespoons (1 scoop) Integral Collagen* (optional)

¼ teaspoon Sunflower Lecithin (optional but preferred)

¾ teaspoon Gluccie*

Protein options: ½ cup unflavored Pristine Whey Protein Powder, or 4 to 5 cups diced cooked chicken breast (see page 45 for cooking methods)

¼ cup packed fresh parsley, stems removed, finely chopped

SERENE CHATS: *Who said those with dairy allergies have to have a cheeseless life? Don't say pooh-pooh to the delicious taste of moo moo. This dairy-free cheese soup will make you celebrate the taste of cheese once again. And if you are not someone who has to be dairy-free? Neither am I, but still give this soup a whirl. Including pasteurized dairy in every single meal can cause stalls, so change it up and give dairy a break! (I do list whey powder as one of the protein options, but many dairy-sensitive people can use our Pristine Whey, as the lactose has been removed. However, you can use chicken breast instead.)*

1. Put the water, vegetables, garlic, baobab powder (if using), lemon juice, nutritional yeast, liquid smoke, and seasonings in a soup pot. Cover and bring to a boil, then reduce the heat and let it gently simmer until tender.

2. Ladle 2 to 3 cups of the hot broth into a blender. Add half of the veggies and your core Trimmy ingredients: sesame oil, ghee, gelatin, collagen (if using), and lecithin (if using). Hold the blender lid tightly down and whiz until creamy (venting hot air once), then pour into a bowl. Now fill the blender with the rest of the veggies, a couple more cups broth, and the Gluccie. Holding the lid down tightly, whiz until smooth. Scrape the mixture into the soup pot, then pour the contents of the bowl back into the pot, too.

3. Add your protein of choice to the pot. If using whey protein, remove ½ cup of the broth, transfer it to a bowl, add a couple ice cubes to cool the broth down, then stir in the whey with a fork until there are no lumps (if you don't cool it down it will clump). While stirring constantly, slowly add the whey mix to your soup. Bring the soup back to the desired temperature and add the parsley. Taste test to "own it," then serve.

MAKE A FAMILY MEAL: For the weight-loss plan, have a big bowlful or two alone or pair with a side salad with lean dressing to stay in FP mode. If you add sprouted-grain toast on the side, you'll be having an E, which is perfectly fine. Crossover-stage family members can have generous butter on their toast.

* FOR NSI: USE A GROCERY STORE UNFLAVORED GELATIN AND SUB XANTHAN GUM FOR THE GLUCCIE.

* FOR DF: IF YOU ARE DAIRY-FREE TO THE POINT OF NOT ALLOWING GHEE, THEN USE EITHER ANOTHER ½ TABLESPOON SESAME OIL OR TAHINI.

indian madras trimmy bisque

S

FAMILY SERVE—FEEDS 6 TO 8 (HALVE IF YOUR FAMILY IS SMALLER, OR MAKE FULL AND FREEZE HALF)

2 quarts water

1 large onion, diced

6 garlic cloves, minced

1 (16-ounce) bag frozen spinach

2 cups frozen peas

1 (16-ounce) bag frozen cauliflower florets

2 tablespoons ghee (clarified butter)

2 tablespoons Just Gelatin*

1½ tablespoons Integral Collagen (optional)

¼ teaspoon Sunflower Lecithin (optional but preferred)

1 (15-ounce) can full-fat coconut milk

1 (6-ounce) can tomato paste

1 tablespoon apple cider vinegar

3½ tablespoons mild Madras curry powder (I use Sadaf brand; use another mild curry powder if you can't find it, or order it online)

½ teaspoon ground cumin

3½ to 4 teaspoons Mineral Salt (use the larger amount for salt lovers)

3 tablespoons Nutritional Yeast

1 teaspoon onion powder

¼ teaspoon cayenne pepper

½ teaspoon black pepper

2 cups frozen diced okra

Protein options: diced cooked chicken breasts or thighs (see page 45 for cooking methods); or pulled rotisserie chicken; or 2½ pounds browned ground beef or venison

SERENE CHATS: *Thick and fragrant with the alluring aroma of a spice market in a bustling town in India, this Trimmy Bisque fills your belly with warm, exotic flavors. It is super easy (take that, Pearl!)—just boil and blend and it really satisfies without the need for the usual huge mound of white rice that comes with many Indian dishes. This is not too spicy as written, so increase the cayenne if you like a spicier curry, or take it back to just ⅛ teaspoon if you're not a spice head.*

1. Put the water in a soup pot with the onion, garlic, spinach, peas, and cauliflower. Cover, bring to a boil, then reduce the heat and simmer until the veggies are tender.

2. Put about 2 cups of the hot broth in a blender. Try to avoid the veggies, but don't stress over it. Add your core Trimmy ingredients—**ghee, gelatin, collagen** (if using), and **lecithin** (if using)—the coconut milk, tomato paste, vinegar, curry powder, cumin, salt, nutritional yeast, onion powder, cayenne, black pepper, and okra. Holding the lid down tightly, blend with Super Mama powers so no bits of okra are left floating around. Scrape the whipped sauce into the pot and stir very well to combine all the flavors.

3. Add your protein choice and bring to a perfect serving temperature. Taste and adjust the flavors to "own it."

MAKE A FAMILY MEAL: For the weight-loss plan, enjoy a large bowlful or two alone, or add on a side salad or an S-friendly bread item from the Breads chapter (page 240). Hard-to-fill growing children, Skinny Jimmy hubbies, or even those who are pregnant or nursing babies can have a large scoop of steaming brown basmati rice added to their soup for a Crossover.

* FOR NSI: USE A GROCERY STORE UNFLAVORED GELATIN.

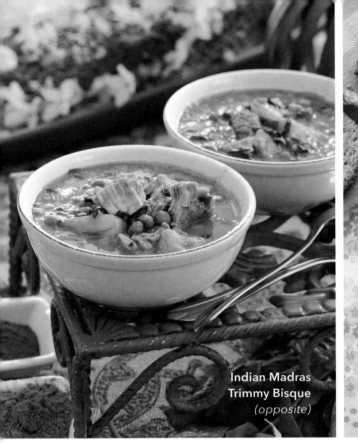

Indian Madras Trimmy Bisque
(opposite)

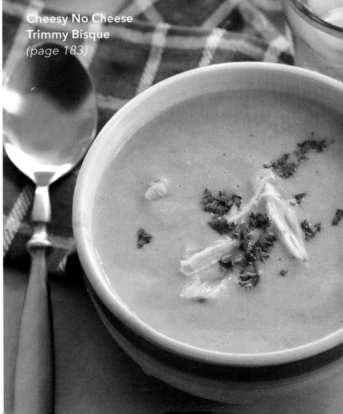

Mother England's Trimmy Bisque
(page 190)

Ugly Duckling Trimmy Bisque
(page 182)

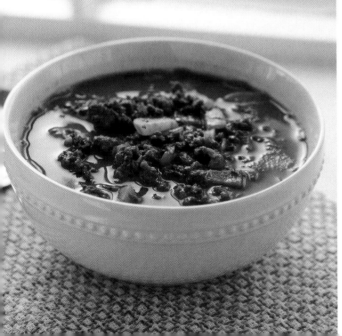

Cheesy No Cheese Trimmy Bisque
(page 183)

thai lullaby trimmy bisque

S

FAMILY SERVE—FEEDS 6 TO 8 (HALVE IF YOUR FAMILY IS SMALLER, OR MAKE FULL AND FREEZE HALF, BUT LEAVE OUT NOODLES IF FREEZING)

1 quart cold water

3½- to 4-ounce knob fresh ginger, coarsely diced (you should end up with just shy of ½ cup loosely packed ginger pieces)

1 (12-ounce) bag frozen broccoli florets

1 (12-ounce) bag frozen cauliflower florets

2 cups frozen peas

3 large rainbow bell peppers (red, orange, and yellow)

1 large onion, diced

6 garlic cloves, minced

1 cup snow peas (optional)

1 cup sliced mushrooms

½ teaspoon red pepper flakes (pull back a tad if you are not a heat lover)

4 to 6 ITO EN green tea bags (sencha/matcha blend; see page 178 for where to get this)

1 quart boiling water (or 1 quart cold water for reduced-caffeine cold-brewing)

2 tablespoons extra-virgin coconut oil

2 tablespoons Just Gelatin*

1½ tablespoons (1 scoop) Integral Collagen (optional)

¼ teaspoon Sunflower Lecithin (optional but preferred)

1 (15-ounce) can full-fat coconut milk

3 tablespoons Baobab Boost Powder (optional)

1 tablespoon mellow miso (yellow or white)

1 tablespoon fish sauce

2 tablespoons soy sauce

4 doonks Pure Stevia Extract Powder*

2 teaspoons Mineral Salt

Juice of 1 lemon

1 tablespoon rice vinegar (optional)

½ tablespoon onion powder

4 to 5 cups diced cooked chicken breasts or thighs (see page 45 for cooking methods), or pulled rotisserie chicken

3 to 4 single-serve bags Trim Healthy Noodles or Not Naughty Noodles*

A handful of fresh basil leaves, coarsely cut and bruised between your hands (optional but delicious)

> **SERENE CHATS:** *Soothing, comforting, and creamy dreamy, this Trimmy Bisque sings a Thai lullaby over you as it goes down like warm, liquid velvet. You might think it's contradictory to use the word "lullaby" in a dinner brewed with green tea, but this delicately Thai-kissed dinner tastes and feels like a bowl of consoling restfulness. Taste and experience it for yourself.*

1. Place the cold water in a blender with the ginger pieces and blend on low for a minute. Pour it through a fine-mesh sieve into a bowl and press the ginger to get all the ginger juice out. Place this juice in a soup pot along with the broccoli, cauliflower, peas, bell peppers, onion, garlic, snow peas (if using), mushrooms, and red pepper flakes.

2. Brew your tea hot in the boiling water (or cold in 1 quart cold water) and let it steep for 3 to 5 minutes. Squeeze out the tea bags and pour the tea into your soup pot. Cover, bring to a boil, then reduce the heat and simmer until the veggies are tender.

3. Time for your Trimmy blend: Ladle out 1 cup of the veggie water (trying not to catch any veggies) and add it to a blender. Add the core Trimmy ingredients—oil, gelatin, collagen (if using), and lecithin (if using)—the coconut milk, baobab powder (if using), miso, fish sauce, soy sauce, stevia powder, salt, lemon juice, rice vinegar (if using), and

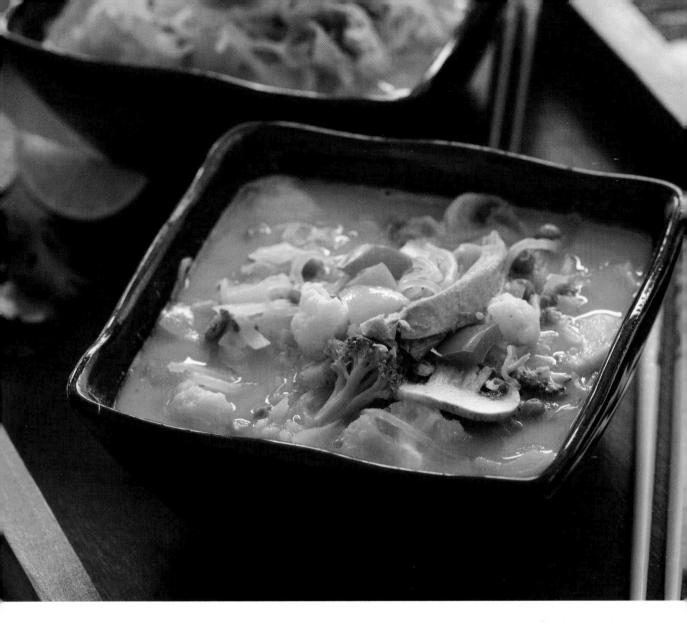

onion powder. Hold the lid down tightly while you whiz until smooth. Pour it into the pot. Add the diced chicken breast, noodles, and fresh basil (if using). Taste and adjust the flavors to "own it."

MAKE A FAMILY MEAL: For the weight-loss plan, this is perfect with a side of Thai-Kissed Cucumber Salad (page 268). Steamed jasmine brown rice is a lovely accompaniment for those members in the family needing to have a Crossover meal.

* FOR NSI: USE A GROCERY STORE UNFLAVORED GELATIN AND AN ON-PLAN SWEETENER. WHILE YOU ARE THERE, FIND KONJAC NOODLES (SEE PAGE 43).

sopa de quinoa trimmy bisque

Ⓔ

FAMILY SERVE—FEEDS 6 TO 8 (HALVE IF YOUR FAMILY IS SMALLER, OR MAKE FULL AND FREEZE)

35 frozen Marvelous Make-Ahead
  Meatballs, FP style (page 208), or
  freshly made One-Batch Meatballs
  (page 129)

2 quarts plus 2 cups water

1 cup uncooked quinoa, rinsed

1 cup frozen peas

1 (12-ounce) bag fresh kale, or 2 to
  3 medium zucchinis, coarsely
  chopped

1 onion, diced

6 garlic cloves, minced

4 carrots, sliced

3 celery stalks, diced

1½ teaspoons dried oregano

2 cups just off the boil water

2 tablespoons MCT oil

2 tablespoons Just Gelatin*

1½ tablespoons (1 scoop) Integral
  Collagen (optional)

¼ teaspoon Sunflower Lecithin
  (optional but preferred)

1 tablespoon Mineral Salt

4 tablespoons Nutritional Yeast

2 teaspoons onion powder

½ teaspoon black pepper

FOR THE SUNSHINE SAUCE

2 large yellow or orange bell
  peppers, coarsely chopped
  (see Note)

½ dried habanero (if you can't take
  the heat, add a doonk or two of
  cayenne pepper instead)

Juice of 2 limes or 1 large lemon

2 tablespoons Baobab Boost
  Powder (optional but preferred)

¼ teaspoon Mineral Salt

1 doonk Pure Stevia Extract
  Powder* (see Note)

3 to 4 tablespoons 1% cottage
  cheese*

SERENE CHATS: *Have an adventurous spirit? Travel with me tonight to the majestic Andean mountains of Peru. In an entrancing world where the clouds make their nest on earth, a pale yellow broth swimming with quinoa, native oregano, and vibrant colored vegetables is ladled into rustic bowls. Quinoa is not technically a grain but an edible seed that boasts a long list of vitamins and minerals, contains more fiber than most whole grains, and has a large amount of flavonoids. It is anti-inflammatory, antiviral, anticancer and also fights depression.*

Sopa de quinoa is traditionally served with meatballs and a vibrant orange sauce made from a local chili pepper called ají amarillo. Just in case you were thinking of skipping this condiment, in Peru ají amarillo is considered part of the national condiment trio, along with onions and garlic. To make this dinner a true Peruvian experience, you owe it to yourself and your family to take the 2 extra minutes to whiz up its golden gloriousness. This is a bit of a "faker" recipe because it is not easy to get your hands on ají amarillo peppers unless you live in the countries where they grow natively. This vibrant orange chili pepper is very fruity, with a citrus burst and a spicy afterglow. I chose sunshiny orange bell peppers to match the color and provide a base of sweet peppery goodness.

1. Preheat the oven to 400°F. Reheat the frozen meatballs until warm (about 15 minutes) or bake fresh meatballs.

2. Meanwhile, bring 2 cups of the water to a boil in a medium saucepan. Add the quinoa and return to a boil. Reduce the heat to a simmer, cover, and cook for 15 to 20 minutes.

3. While the quinoa is cooking, place the remaining 2 quarts water in a soup pot and add the peas, kale (or zucchini), onion, garlic, carrots, celery, and oregano and bring to a boil. Cover, reduce the heat, and simmer until tender.

4. Make your Trimmy: Place the 2 cups boiled water in a blender and add your core Trimmy ingredients—MCT oil, gelatin, collagen (if using), and lecithin (if using)—the salt, nutritional yeast, onion powder, and black pepper. Hold the lid down tightly, blend, then pour it into the soup pot. Add the quinoa and stir everything well, tasting to adjust the flavors to "own it." Bring it to a perfect serving temperature, then add your oven-heated meatballs. Don't do too much agitating and stirring after the meatballs are added or they will fall apart.

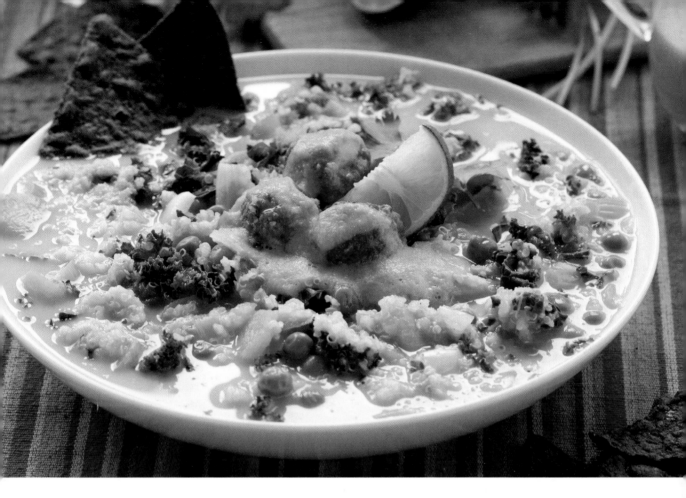

FOR SERVING
Fresh cilantro
Lime wedges (optional)
Baked blue corn chips

5. Make the sunshine sauce. Throw all the sauce ingredients into a blender and blend until creamy.

6. To serve, ladle the soup into bowls and garnish with the cilantro and lime wedges (if using). Serve the sauce and baked blue corn chips on the side.

MAKE A FAMILY MEAL: For the weight-loss plan, have a big bowlful or two alone, or pair it with a side salad with lean dressing to stay in E mode. Crossover-stage family members can have a generous helping of butter on a toasted whole-grain pita or sprouted bread.

NOTE: If you are only using this sauce for E purposes, you can leave out the stevia, sub in ¼ to ½ mango, and take ¼ to ½ bell pepper away.

* FOR NSI: USE A GROCERY STORE UNFLAVORED GELATIN FOR THE SOUP AND AN ON-PLAN SWEETENER FOR THE SAUCE.

* FOR DF: LEAVE THE COTTAGE CHEESE OUT OF THE SAUCE—IT'S STILL GOOD.

mother england's trimmy bisque

(E)

FAMILY SERVE—FEEDS 6 TO 8 (HALVE IF YOUR FAMILY IS SMALLER, OR MAKE FULL AND FREEZE HALF)

1 pound dried green split peas

2 quarts plus 1 cup water

1 onion, diced

4 green onions, diced

6 large celery stalks diced

6 garlic cloves, minced

1½ teaspoons rubbed sage

2 bay leaves

1 tablespoon dried parsley flakes

2 tablespoons MCT oil or butter

2 tablespoons Just Gelatin*

1½ tablespoons (1 scoop) Integral
   Collagen (optional)

¼ teaspoon Sunflower Lecithin
   (optional but preferred)

1 tablespoon apple cider vinegar

4 teaspoons Mineral Salt

½ to 1 teaspoon black pepper

2 doonks cayenne pepper

¼ to ½ teaspoon garlic powder

1 tablespoon mesquite liquid
   smoke

4 tablespoons Nutritional Yeast

1½ cups frozen diced okra

1 cup frozen green peas

2 cups finely diced cooked chicken
   breast (see page 45 for cooking
   methods)

SERENE CHATS: *Our mother loved reading us nursery rhymes when we were growing up Down Under in New Zealand and Australia. One of our favorites to learn was:*

> *Pease porridge hot, pease porridge cold,*
> *Pease porridge in the pot nine days old,*
> *Some like it hot, some like it cold,*
> *Some like it in a pot nine days old.*

It was not until we reached adulthood that we realized this was about split pea soup! "Pease," the Middle English plural form of "pea," was traditionally made into a protein-rich, inexpensive, staple pottage beloved by eighteenth-century England. But the history of this soup goes back even further. Around 500 to 400 BC the Greeks and Romans cultivated the precious pea, and the streets of Athens bustled with vendors selling steaming hot pea soup.

I'm excited to bring this historically nourishing food to the limelight again, but with a Trim Healthy twist. Peas are one of the highest protein legumes so I have included a smaller amount of chicken breast.

1. Place the split peas and the water in a large soup pot. Cover the pot, bring to a boil, then reduce the heat and simmer. While the peas are simmering, add the onion, green onions, celery, garlic, sage, bay leaves, and dried parsley. Simmer until the split peas have lost their form and are mushy.

2. Now make your Trimmy: Discard your bay leaves first, then ladle 4 cups pea and vegetable soup into a blender. Add your core Trimmy ingredients—MCT oil, gelatin, collagen (if using), and lecithin (if using)—the vinegar, salt, black pepper, cayenne, garlic powder, liquid smoke, nutritional yeast, and okra. Hold the lid down tightly and blend to creamy perfection, then pour it back into the pot.

3. Add the frozen peas and chicken and let simmer for several minutes more until everything is beautifully cooked through and the flavors have melded. Taste and adjust the flavors to "own it." Keep history alive on your table!

MAKE A FAMILY MEAL: For the weight-loss plan, this is delicious with crumbled toasted sourdough or sprouted-grain bread. Add a side salad with lean dressing if you want. Crossover-stage family members can use heavy slabs of butter on the bread.

* FOR NSI: USE A GROCERY STORE UNFLAVORED GELATIN.

moroccan trade winds trimmy bisque   Ⓔ

FAMILY SERVE—FEEDS 6 TO 8 (HALVE IF YOUR FAMILY IS SMALLER, OR MAKE FULL AND FREEZE HALF)

1 pound dried red lentils (no other kind will sub), rinsed and drained

2 quarts water

2 large carrots, diced

2 large celery stalks diced

1 large onion diced

6 garlic cloves, minced

⅓ cup tightly packed chopped fresh parsley (stems and leaves), or 3 tablespoons dried parsley flakes

2 (14.5-ounce) cans petite diced tomatoes

½- to 1-inch piece fresh ginger, grated on the finest setting, or 1 teaspoon dried ground ginger

1 teaspoon ground cinnamon

1 teaspoon ground coriander

1 teaspoon ground turmeric

1 teaspoon ground cumin

2 teaspoons Hungarian paprika

2 teaspoons onion powder

¼ to ½ teaspoon garlic powder (optional; for garlic lovers)

2 tablespoons ghee (clarified butter)

2 tablespoons Just Gelatin*

1½ tablespoons (1 scoop) Integral Collagen (optional)

¼ teaspoon Sunflower Lecithin (optional)

Juice of 1 lemon

1 tablespoon mellow white or yellow miso

2 tablespoons Nutritional Yeast

½ teaspoon black pepper

½ dried habanero, or ½ teaspoon red pepper flakes

2 cups 1% cottage cheese,* 0% Greek yogurt, and/or diced cooked chicken breast* (see Note)

1 tablespoon Mineral Salt

SERENE CHATS: *In the days of Christopher Columbus, Morocco became a celebrated stopping point on the spice trade route between Europe and the Far East. In Moroccan cuisine, spices are tossed in with generous abandon, celebrated and mixed one upon the other to create deep and complex flavors. Like an artist with a colorful palette for one single picture, a Moroccan dish does not proclaim "less is more" when it comes to spices. Ras el hanout, the most celebrated Moroccan spice mixture, combines 27 spices to create its iconic flavor. Spices are actually delicious medicines that help protect your DNA, brain, liver, heart, pancreas, kidneys, and skin and promote overall vitality. This Trimmy Bisque is blown in on the gusty trade winds of Moroccan spice ports. It is tangy and gorgeous, and warms your soul as well as your body with its many healing spices.*

1. Place the lentils, water, carrots, celery, onion, garlic, parsley, tomatoes, ginger, spices, onion powder, and garlic powder (if using) in a soup pot. Cover, bring to a boil, reduce the heat, and simmer for about 40 minutes, or until the red lentils are super soft and mushy. You may need to stir occasionally to make sure nothing catches on the bottom. Remove from the heat.

2. Now make the Trimmy: Ladle 1 cup of the hot lentil soup base into a blender. Add the core Trimmy ingredients—ghee, gelatin, collagen (if using), and lecithin (if using)—the lemon juice, miso, nutritional yeast, black pepper, habanero, and cottage cheese. Hold the lid down and Trimmy it up, smooth as silk, then scrape every drip back into your lentil pot. Now add the salt and chicken (if using) and stir super-duper well. Turn the heat back on and bring it to a perfect serving temperature. Taste and adjust the flavors to "own it."

MAKE A FAMILY MEAL: For the weight-loss plan, this is delicious with crumbled toasted sourdough or spouted-grain bread. Add a side salad with lean dressing if you want. Crossover-stage family members can use heavy slabs of buttAH on the bread.

NOTE: You can choose to eat this as a vegetarian dish or add some cooked chicken breast. If using both cottage cheese and chicken, use only 2 cups diced chicken.

* FOR NSI: USE A GROCERY STORE UNFLAVORED GELATIN.

* FOR DF: OMIT THE COTTAGE CHEESE AND USE 4 TO 5 CUPS DICED COOKED CHICKEN BREAST (SEE PAGE 45 FOR COOKING METHODS).

Moroccan
Trade Winds
Trimmy Bisque
(page 191)

Top and Tail
Trimmy Bisque
(opposite)

top and tail trimmy bisque

S

FAMILY SERVE—FEEDS 6 TO 8 (HALVE IF YOUR FAMILY IS SMALLER, OR MAKE FULL AND FREEZE HALF)

2 to 3 pounds ground beef, venison, or turkey (thawed if frozen)

2 quarts plus 1 cup water

1 to 2 pounds red radishes, quartered, or 1 large daikon radish, coarsely chopped

4 to 6 garlic cloves, minced

1 large onion, coarsely chopped

1 (12-ounce) bag fresh kale, coarsely chopped, or a similar amount of the daikon or red radish greens

1 (15-ounce) can full-fat coconut milk

2 tablespoons extra-virgin coconut oil

2 tablespoons Just Gelatin*

1½ tablespoons (1 scoop) Integral Collagen (optional)

¼ teaspoon Sunflower Lecithin (optional but preferred)

½ dried habanero

½ teaspoon garlic powder

1 teaspoon dried oregano

1 teaspoon ground cumin

2 teaspoons onion powder

2 tablespoons apple cider vinegar

2 tablespoons yellow miso

½ teaspoon chaga extract (optional, but gives a beefy flavor)

1 teaspoon fish sauce

1 tablespoon Mineral Salt

SERENE CHATS: *No waste here. We use the tops and the tails of our starring veggie, the radish! This soup was inspired by my wonderful backyard garden put in by my nephew Zadok Johnson, a master organic gardener. (I had no time to do it myself this year due to this book.) His gardens are pure art—things of beauty and vibrant brilliance. In season I harvested giant daikon radishes and their huge bouquet of gorgeous greens every night and threw them in this yummy Trimmy Bisque. I realize that many folks may not have a Zadok living next door on a hilltop like us, or time or space for their own garden, so I have tweaked this recipe so everyone can enjoy it.*

1. Start by browning the ground meat in a skillet over medium-high heat. While the meat is browning, place the water, radishes, garlic, onion, and kale (or daikon or radish greens) in a large soup pot. Cover and bring to a boil. Reduce the heat and simmer until the veggies are tender.

2. Meanwhile, ladle 1 cup of the soup broth into a blender. Add the coconut milk and the core Trimmy ingredients—1 tablespoon of the **coconut oil**, the **gelatin**, **collagen** (if using), and **lecithin** (if using)—the habanero, garlic powder, oregano, cumin, onion powder, vinegar, miso, chaga extract (if using), fish sauce, and salt. Hold the lid down tightly and whip, then add this to the pot. Add the browned meat and remaining 1 tablespoon coconut oil. (I add the oil last so that it forms little yummy beadlets on top of the bisque.) Stir everything together well, take your bisque off the heat, and taste to adjust the flavors and "own it."

MAKE A FAMILY MEAL: For the weight-loss plan, enjoy a big bowlful or two and perhaps add a little grated cheese on top if you desire. Always feel free to pair this with a side salad. The Crossover peeps in the family can have sprouted-grain bread with butter or a piece of fruit to end their meal.

* FOR NSI: USE A GROCERY STORE UNFLAVORED GELATIN.

granny's hug trimmy bisque

(S)

FAMILY SERVE—FEEDS 6 TO 8 (HALVE IF YOUR FAMILY IS SMALLER, OR MAKE FULL AND FREEZE HALF)

1 whole chicken, thawed if frozen

6 cups water

2 tablespoons apple cider vinegar

2 bay leaves

1 teaspoon rubbed sage (optional)

2 large onions, halved

4 to 6 garlic cloves, minced

1 large turnip or daikon radish, halved, or 1 pound red radishes (don't cut 'em)

½ bunch fresh parsley, stems and leaves separated (tie the stems together with twine or a tea bag string and chop the leaves)

6 celery stalks, diced

1 bunch green onions, diced

2 cups frozen peas

1 to 2 tablespoons Just Gelatin*

1½ tablespoons (1 scoop) Integral Collagen (optional)

¼ teaspoon Sunflower Lecithin (optional but preferred)

1 tablespoon Mineral Salt

½ teaspoon black peppercorns

1 to 2 tablespoons Nutritional Yeast (optional)

3 cups boiling water

SERENE CHATS: *This is chicken soup made from scratch just like Granny would make, but it is not too time consuming, even for a Drive-Thru Sue. Easier than it looks, this Trimmy Bisque merges time-honored home-cooked wholesomeness with an "I can actually do this" possibility. Each healing mouthful brings Grannified comfort big time. It cuddles you all up in its warmth and simple goodness. It is rich in the wonders of folk medicine. Chicken soup from scratch is Jewish penicillin and is thought to fix practically anything you've got bothering you.*

You'll notice in the ingredients list that the oil, ghee, or butter is missing from the core Trimmy ingredients. That is because the natural fat in the broth from slow-cooking a whole chicken takes its place. This broth also naturally contains gelatin, but the small added amount helps complete this recipe.

PREP TIP: This recipe should be started in the morning, so if you have to rush off to work or elsewhere, prep the veggies the night before and separate them as described in the directions.

1. Rinse the chicken well, remove any giblets, and cut off any large globs of fat from the opening of the cavity. Put it in a crockpot. Add the water, vinegar, bay leaves, sage (if using), onions, garlic, turnip or radishes, and tied parsley stems. Just pack all these veggies in wherever you can, pinning them around the chicken.

2. Place the celery and green onions in a zippy bag with the peas and diced parsley leaves. Refrigerate until they get added later, in the final 30 minutes of cooking time.

3. Cover the crockpot, set to low, and forget all about it for 7½ to 8 hours. Uncover, locate the parsley stems, and throw them away. Now, with an oven mitt in each hand, pour the contents of the crockpot through a colander set over a large soup pot. Once all the crock juices have drained through, place the colander over a plate so your counter doesn't get messy. Ladle 4 cups of the crock juice into a blender and set aside.

4. Using tongs or any kitchen utensil that works, fish out the onions and turnip (or radishes) from the colander, cut their tender yumminess into soup-size morsels, and add them to the soup pot. Next, using a couple of forks, break open your delicious slow-cooked chicken and remove all the bones (a

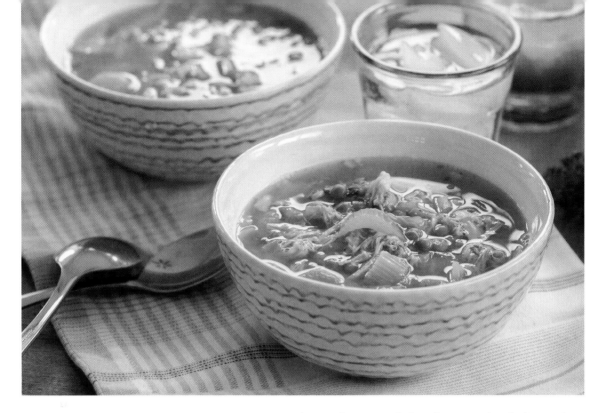

surprisingly quick process). Put the meat (and skin, unless there are huge pieces that gross you out) into the soup pot. Discard the bay leaves.

5. To the blender with the crock juice, add the core Trimmy ingredients—**gelatin, collagen** (if using), and **lecithin** (if using)—the salt, pepper, and nutritional yeast (if using). Hold the lid down tightly and blend to Trimmy it up. Pour your Trimmy back into the soup pot along with the 3 cups boiled water. Add the veggies from the refrigerated zippy bag and allow all to simmer for another 30 minutes or so in the pot, or until the veggies are tender. Stir, taste, and adjust the flavors to "own it." Maybe you need a little more salt and pepper . . . maybe a hint more sage, or you might want to add a little more boiling water to increase the broth. Since this is an S, if you would like it even more rich tasting, you can ladle out a cup or two of the broth and put it back in the blender with a tablespoon or two of MCT oil, coconut oil, or ghee and whip up an even creamier Trimmy.

MAKE A FAMILY MEAL: For the weight-loss plan, enjoy a big bowlful as is or have a side salad and/or an S-friendly bread item. Family members at Crossover stage can enjoy fruit to end the meal or have it with buttered sprouted-grain toast.

* FOR NSI: USE A GROCERY STORE UNFLAVORED GELATIN.

Supper Salads

Most people think of salads as sides when it comes to supper-time, but these salads stand proudly alone, big enough for the whole family to enjoy as a hearty meal. They have ample protein, and you can really go whole hog with hefty portions. Full salad supper meals are a great way for you and your kids to get more leafy greens in your life without feeling like you are eating light, diety rabbit food.

NOTE: Don't forget about Salad Bar Night (page 284) in the Family Theme Nights chapter (page 273), and please check out our Trim Mac Salad in our *Trim Healthy Mama Cookbook*—it rocks!

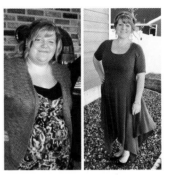

I was at least 350 at my biggest. I stopped weighing myself because I had given up. I had accepted the fact that I was broken beyond repair—I had broken myself—and there was no diet, no plan of action that would ever help me, because I was too far gone physically and mentally. I was miserable. I spent a few months in India and accidentally lost some weight—that's what happens when you live on lentils and veggies for months. But then I got back to the States and gained much of it back. I did, however, see a glimmer of hope. Maybe I wasn't broken after all. I began learning about nutrition and tried more diets unsuccessfully.

So when my aunt suggested this new thing called Trim Healthy Mama, I saw it as just another fad. But then my sister started doing it for her whole family, and they started losing. I sat on the sidelines and watched her for a while. It seemed like too much information—too much to know/memorize/relearn. Then I decided, what the heck. I had spent my entire life learning how to eat crap—I could spend a few months learning how to eat right. And I did.

I'm now 110 pounds down and counting; 75 of that with THM. Everything has changed, as cliché as it sounds. My skin is glowy, my nails are growing like crazy, I'm no longer on blood pressure meds, I no longer feel like I'm trying to just stay afloat for the whole day. I feel like I radiate a different air. I've started running recently, and I like it! I know I've added years to my life.

I'm single, so my THM lifestyle is very different from that of my sister (who has a husband and two kids). THM really is something you make your own. For me, if it's not fast and easy, it's not my cup of tea (#DriveThruSue), but there's a way to do THM that works even for me. I keep my menu simple, with ready quick proteins like precooked chicken, eggs, and canned tuna for wraps, salads, stir-fries, etc. I memorized two quick on-plan desserts. I can make them so fast, it would take me longer to go to the store to buy cookies. My biggest tip would be to encourage others not to have an all-or-nothing mentality. You will screw up. A lot. Start over again in three hours. Not tomorrow.

—BRITTANY C.

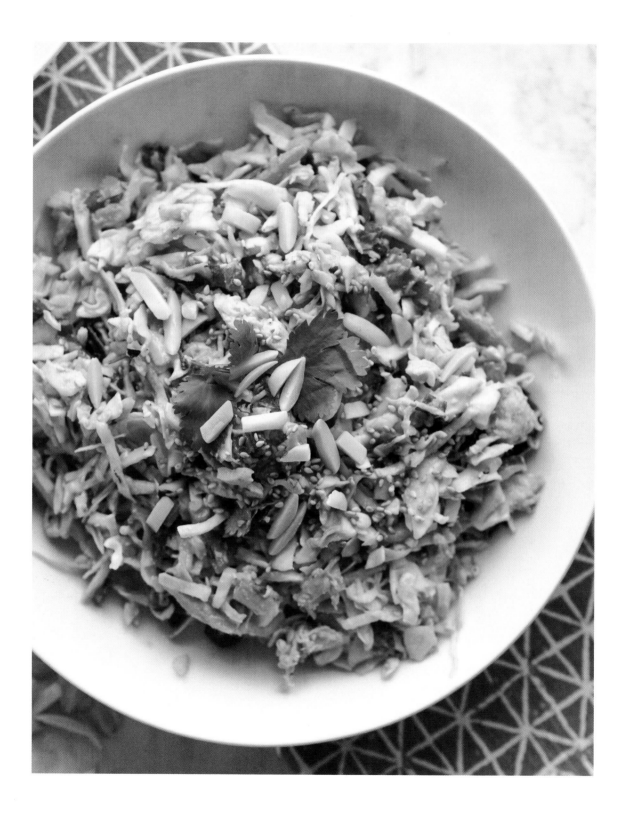

ten-minute chinese chicken salad ⓢ

FAMILY SERVE—FEEDS 6 TO 8 (HALVE IF YOUR FAMILY IS SMALLER)

2 to 3 (12- to 16-ounce) bags coleslaw

½ bunch fresh cilantro, stems removed, chopped

3 to 4 green onions, diced

4 cups diced cooked chicken (see page 45 for cooking methods), or pulled rotisserie chicken

Mineral Salt and black pepper

FOR THE DRESSING

¼ cup sugar-free natural-style peanut butter, tahini, or almond butter

¼ cup Pressed Peanut Flour*

2 to 3 tablespoons toasted sesame oil

⅓ cup unsweetened cashew or almond milk

2 tablespoons rice vinegar

2 tablespoons apple cider vinegar

3 tablespoons soy sauce, or a couple generous squirts Bragg liquid aminos

½ teaspoon Mineral Salt

¾ to 1 teaspoon ground ginger

⅛ teaspoon cayenne pepper (optional)

2 to 3 tablespoons Gentle Sweet* (or more to taste)

FOR THE TOPPINGS

½ cup slivered almonds

2 tablespoons sesame seeds

1 to 2 avocados, sliced (optional)

Here's a way to get your entire family enjoying salad. The bagged coleslaw makes it a speedy-to-put-together meal, full of sweet and savory Asian flavor, perhaps not precisely Chinese cuisine, but definitely inspired by the Orient. We say 10 minutes, but if you are a slow chopper of green onions and cilantro, it might take you 15 minutes max. Depending on how big the eaters are in your home, you will choose to use either 2 or 3 bags of the coleslaw. If you have leftovers, all the better; this makes for a great leftover lunch. If you prefer, you can use a large head of cabbage, finely sliced, and 2 shredded carrots in place of the bagged coleslaw.

1. Toss the bagged coleslaw with the cilantro and green onions in a very large salad bowl. If not already seasoned, sprinkle the cooked chicken with Mineral Salt and pepper, then add to the salad and toss.

2. Make the dressing. Whisk together all the ingredients in a small bowl.

3. Add the dressing to the salad bowl and toss well so the dressing drenches through all the veggies and chicken. Allow it to sit for 2 to 3 minutes, then toss again. Taste and adjust if needed. Perhaps you need more soy sauce or salt or sweetener or ginger? Top with the almonds, sesame seeds, and avocado (if using).

MAKE A FAMILY MEAL: For the weight-loss plan, just a big ol' bowl or two of this salad is filling and all you may need. Or pair with a baby-size shake from the Shakes and Smoothies chapter (page 468) if desired. To fill up more, feel free to have a buttered slice of Wonderful White Blender Bread (page 242) on the side. Crossover family members can have brown rice added to their salad as a healthy carb or enjoy a side of fruit.

* FOR NSI: USE A GROCERY STORE ON-PLAN SWEETENER AND SUGAR-FREE DEFATTED PEANUT FLOUR.

ranch hand taco salad

Ⓔ

FAMILY SERVE–FEEDS 6 TO 8 (HALVE IF YOUR FAMILY IS SMALLER)

2 pounds ground turkey, venison, or beef, thawed if frozen

1½ tablespoons chili powder

2 teaspoons ground cumin

2 teaspoons paprika (smoked or regular)

1 teaspoon garlic powder

1 teaspoon onion powder

1 teaspoon Mineral Salt

¾ cup water

3 to 4 large heads romaine lettuce, chopped (use the larger amount if you have big eaters)

1 pint cherry tomatoes, halved

2 (15-ounce) cans pinto beans, rinsed and drained, or 3 cups home-cooked beans

1 (15-ounce) can black beans, rinsed and drained, or 1½ cups home-cooked beans

1 (15-ounce) can corn kernels, rinsed and drained

FOR THE EASY RANCH DRESSING*

Rounded ½ cup plain 0% Greek yogurt

1 rounded teaspoon garlic powder

1 rounded teaspoon onion powder

Rounded ½ teaspoon Mineral Salt

1 rounded teaspoon black pepper

2 teaspoons dried parsley flakes

OPTIONAL TOPPINGS

Crumbled baked corn chips

Salsa

Greek yogurt

This salad is hearty enough to fill up the hungriest ranch hand after working all day! There's no way you're going to think you are eating an E meal. Dig in!

1. Brown the meat in a large skillet over medium-high heat. If the meat is not at least 96% lean, once cooked, rinse it very well under hot (better yet, boiling) water to release all the fat. Return the meat to the skillet and add the chili powder, cumin, paprika, garlic powder, onion powder, salt, and water. Simmer for 2 to 3 minutes, then remove from the heat.

2. Put the chopped lettuce, tomatoes, beans, and corn in a large salad bowl.

3. Make the ranch dressing. Combine the yogurt, seasonings, and parsley flakes in a small bowl.

4. Dump the dressing into the large bowl with the salad and mix well to coat. Add the seasoned meat. Toss all the ingredients well. Add the toppings if desired.

MAKE A FAMILY MEAL: For the weight-loss plan, have a big bowl or two just as written. Or you can pair this with a baby-size FP shake or smoothie from the Shakes and Smoothies chapter (page 468) for more a filling factor. Or have Speedy Chocolate Milk (page 457) on the side. Growing children can enjoy fats like grated cheese and avocado on their salad for a Crossover.

* FOR DF: OMIT THE YOGURT-BASED DRESSING AND USE ANY LEAN (LESS THAN 5 GRAMS OF FAT) HOMEMADE OR STORE-BOUGHT DRESSING WITHOUT DAIRY.

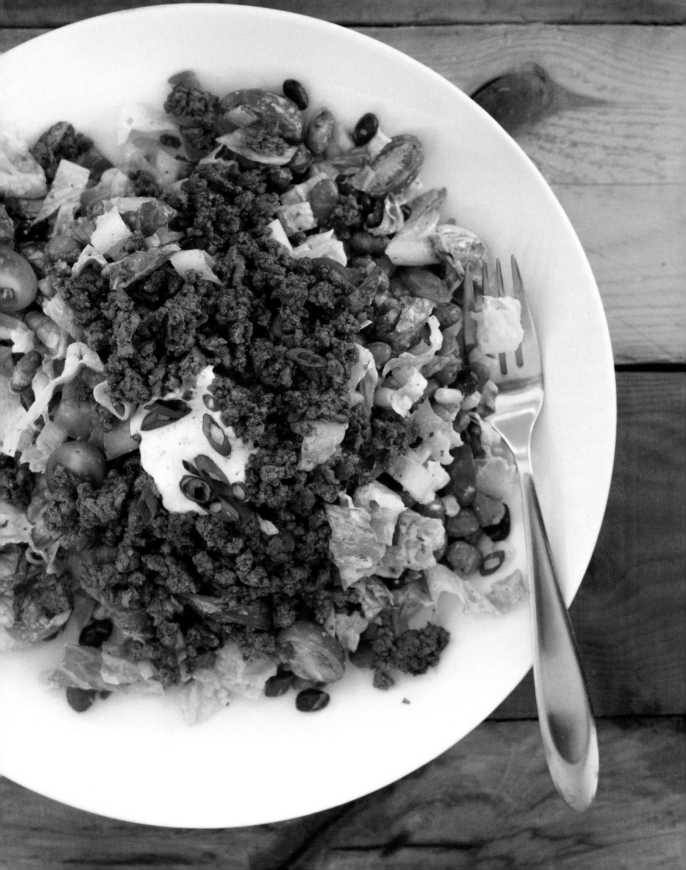

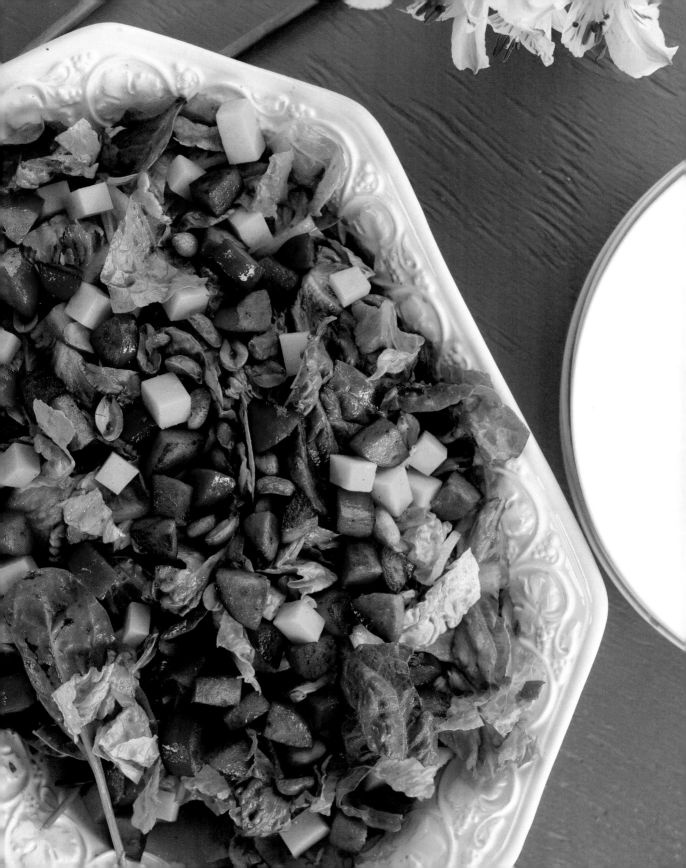

smoked sausage salad (S)

FAMILY SERVE–FEEDS 6 TO 8 (HALVE IF YOUR FAMILY IS SMALLER)

3 large heads romaine lettuce, sliced

Several large handfuls of fresh spinach or kale (really pile it in as it will wilt down)

¼ cup extra-virgin olive oil

2 tablespoons balsamic vinegar (find one with no more than 2 grams carbs)

2 tablespoons apple cider vinegar

2 to 3 teaspoons Gentle Sweet, or a doonk or 2 of pure stevia extract*

Couple generous squirts Bragg liquid aminos, or ¼ teaspoon Mineral Salt

1 tablespoon butter

13 to 16 ounces smoked sausage, diced or sliced (we use turkey, but you can use any kind)

Coconut oil cooking spray

½ to ¾ cup peanuts or other chopped nuts

Cayenne pepper or Bragg liquid aminos or soy sauce, for seasoning the peanuts

4 ounces sharp cheddar cheese,* diced small

PEARL CHATS: This is a hearty, extremely tasty, family-pleasing salad, and it takes me only 10 to 15 minutes to get it on the dinner table. As you can see, this chapter is small with only three recipes. That is because I find it challenging to make full meals of salad for my teen boys. They think salad doesn't fill them enough, but they never complain about this one (nor the other two in this chapter). Male-friendly salad . . . is that such a thing? It is now. This has a beautiful combination of savory hot meat, tangy wilted greens, scrumptious cheese, and spicy nuts . . . how could they not love it?

1. Put the lettuce and spinach in a huge bowl. You want lots and lots of greens to start with, as they wilt down a lot. Pour the oil, vinegars, sweetener, and liquid aminos over the leaves and toss well. Set aside.

2. Melt the butter in a skillet over medium-high heat. Add the diced sausage pieces and toss well for a few minutes until they get nicely browned and a bit crispy.

3. Preheat the oven to a high broil. Spray a baking pan with coconut oil and add the nuts. Sprinkle them with the cayenne pepper (use just a little if you don't like things too spicy, or coat them well if you are a spice freak like us) and pour on a squirt or two of liquid aminos and toss. Broil for just a couple minutes, or until the peanuts start to brown . . . don't let them burn.

4. Toss the greens once again. Add the cheddar and mix it in a little. Top with the sausage and peanuts.

MAKE A FAMILY MEAL: This salad really needs only a bread and butter side. You can use Wonderful White Blender Bread (page 242) or Fifteen-Minute Focaccia Bread (page 247). If you're still hungry, end with a baby-size shake from the Shakes and Smoothies chapter (page 468). Growing children or others in Crossover stage can enjoy a buttered pita or sprouted-grain bread or fruit as a side.

* FOR NSI: USE A GROCERY STORE ON-PLAN SWEETENER.

* FOR DF: LEAVE OFF THE CHEDDAR OR USE A NONDAIRY CHEESE IN ITS PLACE.

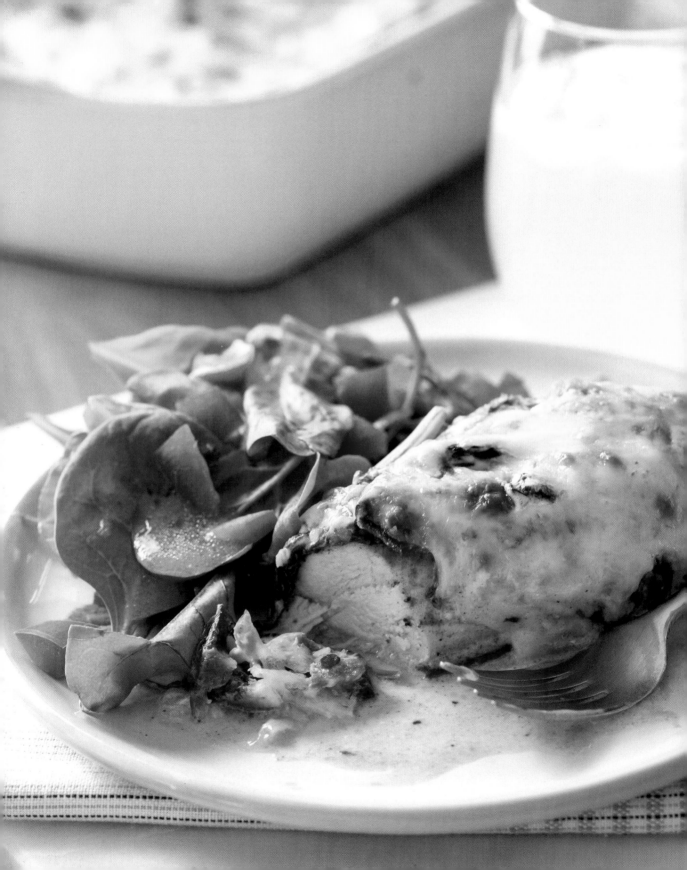

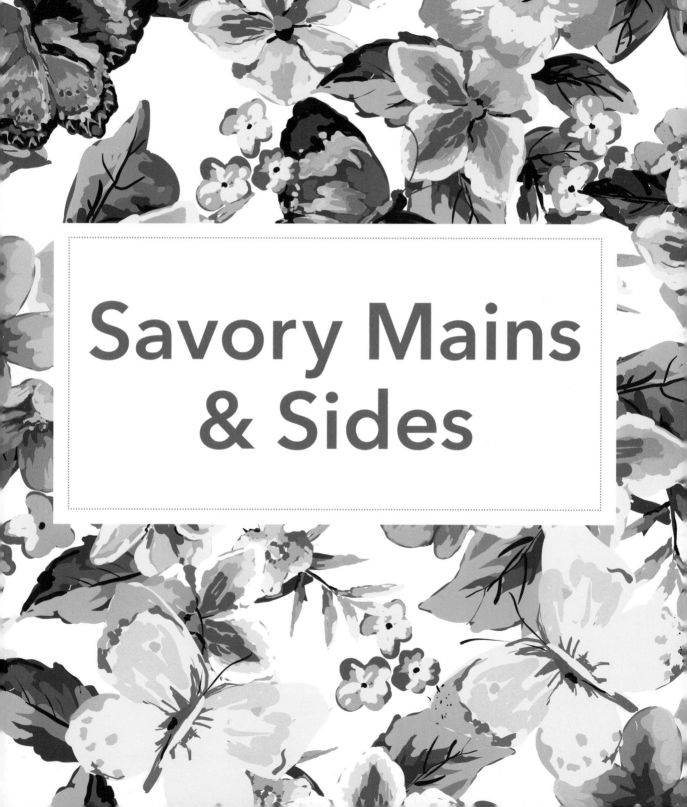

Savory Mains & Sides

Oven-Baked
Meats
&
Fish

Meatloaf, meatballs, baked chicken, and fish . . . all your regular family staple meals are now Trimmified!

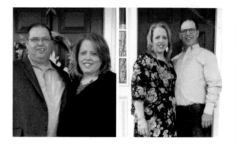

A year ago today, my husband and I started fully on plan. Over twenty-two years of marriage and having four children, we had both been overweight or obese for most of that time. With a parent who died too young from heart disease and another parent suffering through health issues directly related to obesity (high blood pressure, heart disease, type 2 diabetes, kidney failure), we were ready to be healthy for ourselves, our marriage, and our kids . . . and we were in it together.

My handsome, funny, hard-working husband has lost 100 pounds this year with ZERO exercise. Whoop! He hopes to start working out this year. He tells people he just eats what I tell him to eat. He struggles with the E meals and still isn't crazy about veggies and fruit, but we have made it work. Truthfully, he has expanded his palate, learned the plan, and can even cook a few things on his own now!

As of this morning, I am down eighty pounds! I have been overweight most of my life. My kids have never known me this trim. I have forty pounds to go to get to my goal, which by the scale and BMI charts will still be overweight. I don't care, and my husband is VERY OKAY with where I am now! This body is what I have lived in for forty-five years, and it is a testimony of the four amazing kids it birthed and the choices I have made. It is a redeemed body that can bring God glory with its story and imperfections.

I love how my view/relationship with food as a THM has changed over the last year. The food of my past wasn't the friend I thought it was. It hurt me. The food I choose now is delicious fuel that feeds my health. When I choose wisely, it heals. If I choose poorly, it compromises my health. I don't feel controlled by cravings. I have a new perspective about treating myself. I look at taking the time to chop and sauté beautiful veggies for an omelet as a treat. Spending a little extra money and time on food that feeds my health is a treat (like avocados and dark chocolate!). I find joy in eating beautiful healthy food.

I value myself (and our family) enough to rearrange priorities (budget and time) to make this work. Sometimes we want off-plan stuff, but then we get back on board three hours later. I am a bit of a Drive-Thru Sue sometimes. With four kids, home-schooling, and working part-time, I utilize some personal choice items to make this sustainable for us. It has taken time and mistakes and grace to make this lifestyle second nature, but it really IS easy now. It wasn't in the beginning. So hold on if you are frustrated or confused.
—TAMMY M.

marvelous make-ahead meatballs

FP OR **S**

MAKES 140 MEATBALLS (IF YOU DON'T HAVE THE FREEZER ROOM FOR THIS MANY MEATBALLS, HALVE OR QUARTER THE RECIPE)

Coconut oil cooking spray

4 level cups frozen diced okra

½ cup apple cider vinegar

1 (6-ounce) can tomato paste

1 rounded tablespoon plus
1 teaspoon Mineral Salt

6 to 8 garlic cloves, minced, or 3 to
3½ teaspoons garlic powder

1 tablespoon plus 2 teaspoons
onion powder

1 tablespoon black pepper

1 tablespoon plus 2 teaspoons Just
Gelatin*

⅓ cup THM Baking Blend* or
old-fashioned rolled oats

½ cup grated Parmesan cheese*
(the green can kind is fine)

½ cup Nutritional Yeast

1 rounded teaspoon sage (for
neutral meatballs), or 1 to
2 rounded teaspoons Italian
seasoning (for Italian-style
meatballs)

¾ cup egg whites (carton or fresh)

8 pounds ground meat (beef for S;
venison, 96% lean grass-fed beef,
or 96% lean turkey for FP), thawed
if frozen

1 bunch fresh parsley, stems
removed, finely diced

Water with a splash of soy sauce
(for extra flavor), or chicken or
beef broth, for simmering
meatballs

Stock your freezer with these babies and you'll save yourself time in the future and, more important, save yourself from going off plan! Just a couple hours of your time per month will make quick meatball meals a cinch! Check out the Meatballs, Rice, and Gravy recipe (page 211), or try them in Meatball Casserole (page 128), in crockpot meals (see pages 107 and 115), or in a Trimmy Bisque (see page 188). Frozen meatballs can be heated up for a quick breakfast, popped into your mouth for snacks (dipped into ketchup or sugar-free pizza sauce), and they can top a salad or fill a sandwich. This recipe makes 140 meatballs, which is enough for four meals that feed 6 to 8 people (about 35 meatballs per meal). You can store the meatballs in single-serve baggies for lots of quick meals or snacks.

These can be a succulent S made with beef, but they absolutely rock as Fuel Pulls. They stay marvelously moist due to the secret ingredient (okra) and cooking method. Just make sure to keep the secret veggie at the heart of this recipe hush-hush while your picky fam gobbles them down. Making them as FP enables them to work with any meal, whether an S or an E. Yes, you get to eat meatballs with your E meals! Usually when you think about protein choices for E meals you think whitefish and chicken breasts, right? Meatballs open up a whole new exciting world for E meals! Enjoy them over quinoa or brown rice . . . perfect meal partners!

1. Preheat the oven to 400°F. Spray 4 large rimmed baking sheets with coconut oil (or just use 2 pans if that is all you have, as you may have to cook a couple batches anyway if that is all your oven can hold).

2. Place the okra in a food processor and process until it forms a powdered snow (or appears as broken down as possible). Stop the processor and push the okra back down into the blades with a spatula a couple times, then run it again to make sure to get it all processed. Add the vinegar, tomato paste, salt, garlic, onion powder, pepper, gelatin, Baking Blend (or oats), Parmesan, nutritional yeast, herb of your choice, and egg whites. Process well until it forms a paste.

3. Put the ground meat in a large bowl and add the processed paste and parsley. Mix with your hands until well combined. Form the mixture into balls (just a tad smaller than golf balls)

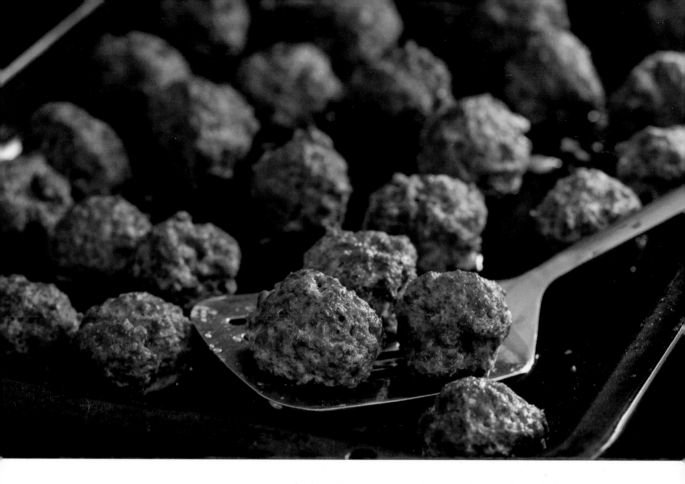

and place them on your baking sheets about ½ inch apart. Spray the tops of the balls with coconut oil spray.

4. Bake for 10 minutes (doing this causes a faux sear), then pour about 1 cup of seasoned water or broth into each pan to cover about ⅓ inch of the pan depth—this keeps the meatballs moist for the rest of the cooking time. Reduce the oven temperature to 350°F and finish baking them for another 20 to 25 minutes. You may have to do a couple batches of meatballs to get them all cooked.

5. Once cooled, leave out how many meatballs you want to use for your week and place the rest into baggies and freeze. If making meatballs to use in any of the family-serve recipes in this book, portion them into 35 meatballs per gallon-size baggies.

* FOR NSI: USE A GROCERY STORE UNFLAVORED GELATIN AND OATS INSTEAD OF THE BAKING BLEND.

* FOR DF: OMIT THE PARMESAN AND USE 2 TO 3 ADDITIONAL TABLESPOONS NUTRITIONAL YEAST.

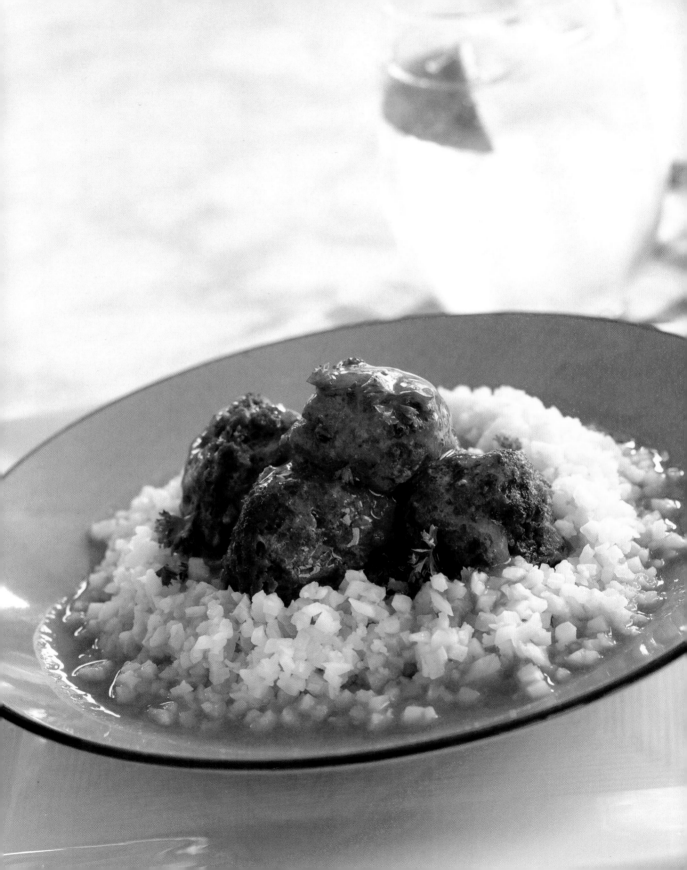

meatballs, rice, and gravy

E OR **S**

FAMILY SERVE—FEEDS 6 TO 8 (HALVE IF YOUR FAMILY IS SMALLER, OR MAKE FULL AND FREEZE HALF)

Coconut oil cooking spray

35 frozen Marvelous Make-Ahead Meatballs* (page 208) or freshly made One-Batch Meatballs* (page 129)

2½ cups water or chicken/beef broth

½ teaspoon Mineral Salt

½ teaspoon onion powder

1 tablespoon Nutritional Yeast

Few shakes of cayenne pepper

Generous squirt or 2 of Bragg liquid aminos or coconut aminos

1½ to 2 teaspoons Gluccie*

Cooked brown or wild rice (for E) or sautéed cauli rice (for S), for serving

1. **FOR FROZEN MEATBALLS:** Preheat the oven to 400°F. Spray a large baking sheet with coconut oil and heat the meatballs for 15 to 20 minutes, or until heated through.

   FOR FRESH MEATBALLS: Bake as directed. When the meatballs are done, pour any leftover cooking juices into a 4-cup measuring cup and add enough water or chicken/beef broth to come to 2½ cups.

2. To make the gravy, add the 2½ cups water (or the water plus cooking juices if you made fresh meatballs), the salt, onion powder, nutritional yeast, cayenne, and liquid aminos to a small saucepan. Bring it to a boil, then reduce the heat to medium-low. Add the Gluccie a little at a time by tapping the spoon on the side of the saucepan and letting it sprinkle in, while whisking with your other hand so it doesn't clump. Let the gravy simmer for a few minutes, and add more liquid if it gets too thick or a little more Gluccie if it's not thick enough. Taste and adjust the seasonings to your liking.

MAKE A FAMILY MEAL: For the weight-loss plan, put the FP meatballs over ¾ cup brown or wild rice for an E option. Then top it with gravy. Enjoy it with a side salad and/or another nonstarchy veggie like green beans. For an S, put FP or S meatballs over sautéed cauli rice, Not Naughty Rice, or Trim Healthy Rice. You can sauté the cauli or konjac-based rice in more oil for an S. Crossover family members can enjoy brown rice mixed with melted butter with their meatballs and gravy.

* FOR NSI: IN THE GRAVY, USE XANTHAN GUM IN PLACE OF THE GLUCCIE. IN THE MEATBALLS, USE A GROCERY STORE UNFLAVORED GELATIN AND USE GROUND OATS IN PLACE OF THE BAKING BLEND.

* FOR DF: OMIT PARMESAN IN THE MEATBALLS AND USE 3 TABLESPOONS NUTRITIONAL YEAST.

burger bombs

S

FAMILY SERVE—FEEDS 6 TO 8 (HALVE IF YOUR FAMILY IS SMALLER, OR MAKE FULL AND FREEZE HALF)

3 pounds ground beef, thawed
if frozen
3 large eggs
1 onion, quartered
3 garlic cloves, peeled but whole
2 rounded teaspoons Mineral Salt
1 teaspoon black pepper
¼ cup THM Baking Blend* or
ground up oats (oat flour)

FOR THE TOPPING
1 (6-ounce) can tomato paste
1 tablespoon apple cider vinegar
1 tablespoon water
1½ to 2 teaspoons Super Sweet
Blend, or 4 teaspoons Gentle
Sweet*
¾ teaspoon Mineral Salt
¼ teaspoon onion powder
Prepared mustard

In reality, these are mini meatloaves (not trying to pretend they're not . . . well, actually we sort of are to our kids). The ketchup and mustard topping brings to mind a juicy burger. One of our Trim Healthy Mamas posted on our main Facebook group that she calls her mini meatloaves Burger Bombs and that they go over much better with her kids with that title. We've adopted the name with her consent, and, yes, it works . . . our kids scarf these up! These are also incredibly kid-friendly, since the blending of the onion and garlic with the eggs introduces lots of flavor but doesn't leave suspicious onion chunks in the view of picky eaters. We enjoy Burger Bombs by putting lettuce down on plates, smearing on some mayo, then placing the bomb on top. Feel free to sprinkle on some cheese and optional chopped tomato.

1. Preheat the oven to 350°F.

2. Put the meat in a large bowl and set aside.

3. Place the eggs, onion, garlic, salt, pepper, and Baking Blend (or oats) in a blender or food processor and blend or process well. Add the blended mixture to the beef and combine well. Fill 16 to 18 cups of muffin tins with the meat mixture.

4. Make the topping. Mix together the tomato paste, vinegar, water, sweetener, salt, and onion powder in a small bowl.

5. Smear the topping mixture generously over the top and exposed sides of the meat mounds (use it all up, as this is what adds great flavor to the bombs). Top each bomb with a little swirl of mustard. Place the muffin tins on baking trays to capture any juice that oozes out of the muffin cups. Bake for 35 to 40 minutes.

MAKE A FAMILY MEAL: For the weight-loss plan, WWBB Garlic Bread (page 245) is awesome with this meal. Growing children or others needing Crossovers can have the garlic bread, but made with sprouted grains.

* FOR NSI: USE OATS IN THE MEATLOAF MIXTURE AND A GROCERY STORE ON-PLAN SWEETENER FOR THE SAUCE.

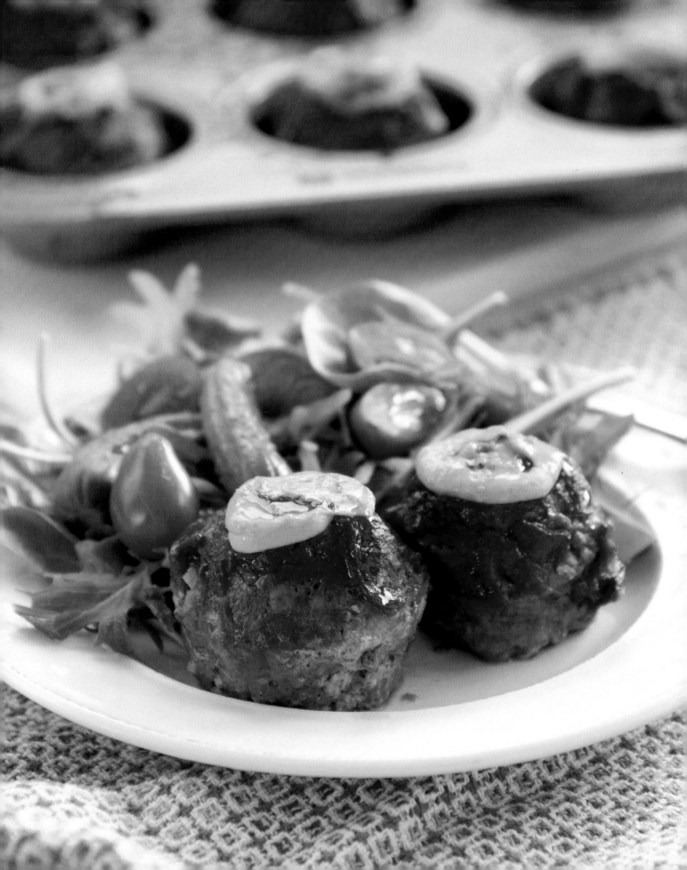

mama mia meatloaf

S

FAMILY SERVE–FEEDS 6 TO 8 (HALVE IF YOUR FAMILY IS SMALLER, OR MAKE FULL AND FREEZE HALF)

2 large eggs

1 onion, quartered

3 garlic cloves, peeled but whole

1 tablespoon Worcestershire sauce

1 tablespoon dried parsley flakes

1¾ teaspoons Mineral Salt

1 teaspoon black pepper

¼ cup powder-style Parmesan cheese (from the green can)

¼ cup THM Baking Blend* or old-fashioned rolled oats

2 pounds ground beef, thawed if frozen

1 pound Italian sausage meat (any kind, we use turkey), thawed if frozen

FOR THE SAUCE

1 (14.5-ounce) can diced tomatoes

1 (8-ounce) can tomato sauce

2½ teaspoons dried oregano

1½ teaspoons dried basil

2 teaspoons Super Sweet Blend, or 2 doonks Pure Stevia Extract Powder*

1½ teaspoons onion powder

1 teaspoon garlic powder

8 ounces shredded part-skim mozzarella cheese

This Italian-style meatloaf is a crowd-pleaser. It is moist and flavorful with a marinara sauce harmonizing superbly with mozzarella cheese. Picky onion-despising children won't know it is in here because the onion is processed into the sauce.

1. Preheat the oven to 350°F.

2. Put the eggs, onion, garlic, Worcestershire sauce, parsley, salt, pepper, Parmesan, and Baking Blend (or oats) in a food processor and process well for a minute or two until smooth.

3. Add the contents of the food processor to the meat in a 9 × 13-inch baking dish and mix all thoroughly together.

4. Make the sauce. Don't bother washing the food processor. Add the canned tomatoes, tomato sauce, oregano, basil, sweetener, onion powder, and garlic powder and process until smooth.

5. Pour half of the sauce into the baking dish and mix well with the meat. Smooth the meat into a flat loaf inside the dish. Pour the remaining tomato sauce on top, then cover with the mozzarella cheese. Bake for 50 minutes. The loaf releases a lot of fluid. Pour half of it out once cooked, but keep some in, surrounding the loaf as it helps keep it moist and flavorful.

MAKE A FAMILY MEAL: For the weight-loss plan, WWBB Garlic Bread (page 245) and a side salad are beautiful accompaniments to this meal. Growing children or others needing Crossovers can have the garlic bread, but made with sprouted-grain bread in place of the WWBB bread.

* FOR NSI: USE OATS IN THE MEATLOAF MIXTURE AND A GROCERY STORE ON-PLAN SWEETENER FOR THE SAUCE.

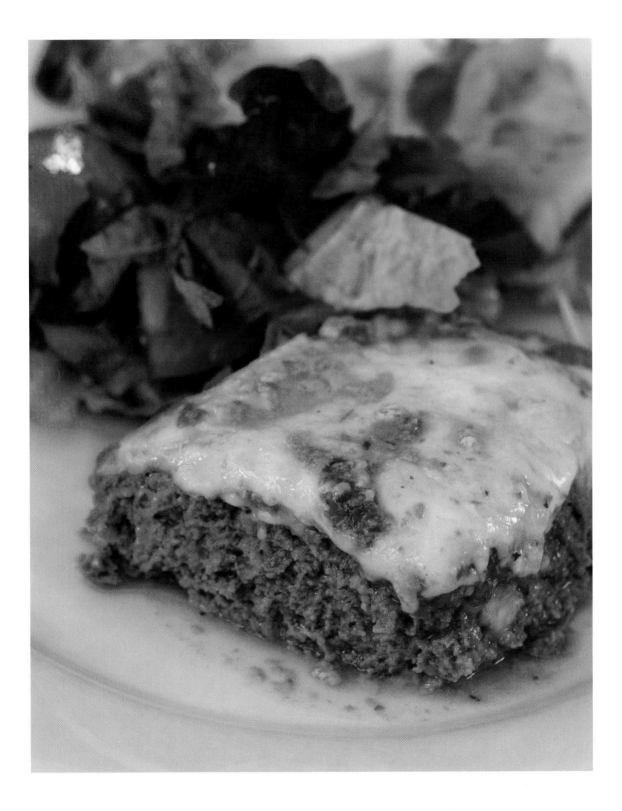

loaded philly cheese meatloaf

S

FAMILY SERVE–FEEDS 6 TO 8 (HALVE IF YOUR FAMILY IS SMALLER, OR MAKE FULL AND FREEZE HALF)

1 tablespoon butter or coconut oil

1 (16-ounce) bag frozen large-cut seasoning blend (see page 35)

8 ounces sliced mushrooms

3 pounds ground beef, turkey, or venison, thawed if frozen

3 large eggs

2½ teaspoons Mineral Salt

¾ teaspoon black pepper

2 teaspoons onion powder

2 teaspoons garlic powder

3 tablespoons Worcestershire sauce

2 tablespoons hot sauce

½ cup THM Baking Blend*

8 ounces provolone or cheddar cheese, grated

1. Preheat the oven to 365°F.

2. Melt the butter in a saucepan over high heat. Add the seasoning blend and mushrooms and sauté for 5 to 10 minutes, until wilted.

3. While the veggies are cooking, put the ground meat, eggs, salt, pepper, onion powder, garlic powder, Worcestershire sauce, hot sauce, Baking Blend, and half of the grated cheese in a bowl and combine very well.

4. Scrape the meat mixture into a 9 × 13-inch baking dish and spread out. Top with the sautéed veggies, then top with the remaining grated cheese. Bake for 45 minutes.

MAKE A FAMILY MEAL: For the weight-loss plan, pair this with any yummy nonstarchy veggie (such as Mashed Fotatoes on page 264) and an S-friendly side salad. Family members at Crossover stage can add a healthy carb such as buttered sprouted-grain bread, a baked potato with butter, or even a piece of fruit to end their meal.

* FOR NSI: USE THE FRUGAL FLOUR OPTION (SEE PAGE 40).

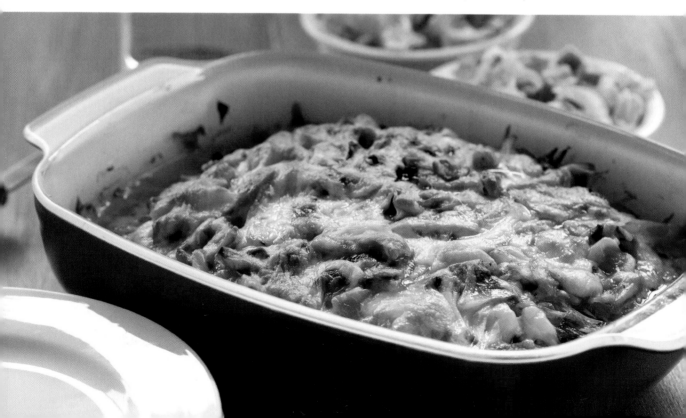

make it again chicken

S WITH FP OPTION

FAMILY SERVE—FEEDS 6 TO 8 (HALVE IF YOUR FAMILY IS SMALLER, OR MAKE FULL AND FREEZE HALF)

2½ to 3 pounds boneless, skinless chicken breasts or thighs, or
4 to 6 pounds bone-in chicken
Coconut oil cooking spray (if using boneless chicken)
3 tablespoons prepared yellow mustard
3 tablespoons mayonnaise, homemade (see page 517) or store-bought
⅓ cup plain 0% Greek yogurt*
1 tablespoon apple cider vinegar
¼ cup Gentle Sweet*
2 tablespoons butter (for searing boneless chicken)
Mineral Salt and black pepper

OPTIONAL TOPPINGS
Natural bacon bits (we use turkey)
Diced green onion
Fresh rosemary sprigs

If you love honey-mustard flavors, you'll love this chicken recipe, which works great for either boneless or bone-in chicken. It is so crazy easy that you might find yourself falling back on it again and again when you don't know what on earth to drum up for dinner. It tickles your taste buds with its sweet yet savory flavors and has an option for an awesome FP change-up, too. Don't be afraid of having the odd FP dinner to lighten things up sometimes.

1. Preheat the oven to 425°F for boneless chicken or 375°F for bone-in chicken. If cooking boneless chicken, spray a 9 × 13-inch baking dish with coconut oil.

2. Mix together the mustard, mayo, yogurt, vinegar, and Gentle Sweet in a bowl and set aside.

3. **FOR BONELESS CHICKEN:** Pound the breasts for a few seconds each to flatten them out a bit. Heat the butter in a large skillet over high heat. Add all the chicken and brown for 1 minute on each side to get a little seared here and there (it does not have to cook through). Transfer the chicken to the prepared baking dish, sprinkle lightly with salt and pepper, then pour the mustard mix over the top, followed by any optional toppings. Bake for 20 minutes, or until cooked through.

   FOR BONE-IN CHICKEN: Place the chicken pieces on the baking dish, sprinkle lightly with salt and pepper, then coat with the mustard sauce, using your hands to make sure each piece is coated well. Sprinkle with any optional toppings, and bake for 50 minutes (you can broil at the end for extra crispiness if desired).

MAKE A FAMILY MEAL: For the weight-loss plan, pair this with Cauli Rice (page 263) or Troodles (page 264) and a side salad with an S-friendly dressing. To make this an FP, use the boneless, skinless breasts option and sear in just 1½ tablespoons butter rather than 2, omit the mayonnaise, and add 3 more tablespoons of Greek yogurt. Growing children and others needing Crossovers can enjoy the S version with brown rice to soak up all the tasty sauce from the chicken.

* FOR NSI: USE A GROCERY STORE ON-PLAN SWEETENER.

* FOR DF: OMIT THE YOGURT AND USE AN ADDITIONAL ⅓ CUP MAYONNAISE (EITHER STORE-BOUGHT OR USING RECIPE FROM PAGE 517).

hubby lovin' chicken

S

FAMILY SERVE—FEEDS 6 TO 8 (HALVE IF YOUR FAMILY IS SMALLER, OR MAKE FULL AND FREEZE HALF)

Coconut oil cooking spray

4 to 6 pounds drumsticks, wings, thighs, or any other bone-in chicken pieces, thawed if frozen

6 tablespoons (¾ stick) butter,* melted

¾ cup grated Parmesan cheese* (we use powder-style from the green can)

¼ cup Nutritional Yeast (if you're out of this, use 1 full cup Parmy)

2½ tablespoons dried parsley flakes

2 teaspoons paprika

2 teaspoons garlic powder

1 teaspoon dried oregano

1 rounded teaspoon Mineral Salt

1 rounded teaspoon black pepper

¼ teaspoon cayenne pepper

This chicken is man-pleasing stuff, but we of the fairer sex devour our fair share, too.

1. Preheat the oven to 375°F. Spray 2 large shallow pans with coconut oil.

2. Put the chicken in a large bowl, pour the melted butter over it, and mix thoroughly with your hands so each piece is coated well.

3. On a dinner plate, mix together the Parmesan, nutritional yeast, parsley flakes, paprika, garlic powder, oregano, salt, black pepper, and cayenne. Roll each piece of butter-glazed chicken in the seasonings.

4. Place the chicken on the prepared pans and bake for 50 minutes, then broil on high for just a few minutes, until the tops are nice and brown (keep a watch so it doesn't burn).

MAKE A FAMILY MEAL: For the weight-loss plan, enjoy the chicken with any yummy S-style nonstarchy veggie, and don't forget your side salad. For veggies, try Killer Green Beans (page 261), or Green Fries (page 262), or simply steam up some broccoli and toss it with butter, salt, and pepper. Growing children can have a healthy carb side such as whole milk, sprouted-grain bread and butter, or a baked potato with butter.

* FOR DF: USE ALL OF THE NUTRITIONAL YEAST IN PLACE OF THE PARMESAN, AND USE FLAVORLESS COCONUT OIL IN PLACE OF THE BUTTER.

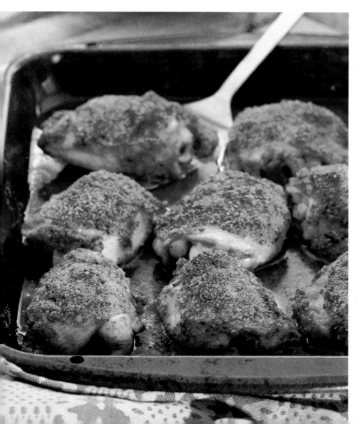

creamed spinach and bacon-smothered chicken ⓢ

FAMILY SERVE—FEEDS 6 TO 8 (HALVE IF YOUR FAMILY IS SMALLER, OR MAKE FULL AND FREEZE HALF)

Coconut oil cooking spray

6 to 8 slices bacon, diced (we use turkey; you can use any kind of bacon)

1 teaspoon butter (optional; for cooking the turkey bacon)

8 ounces fresh spinach

4 to 5 garlic cloves, minced

¾ teaspoon red pepper flakes (optional)

1 (8-ounce) package ⅓ less fat cream cheese

¼ cup water or chicken broth

2½ to 3 pounds boneless, skinless chicken breasts (cut large breasts in half), thawed if frozen

Mineral Salt, black pepper, and paprika, for sprinkling

4 to 6 ounces grated pepper jack cheese or part-skim mozzarella cheese

PEARL CHATS: Longing for moist, flavorful chicken topped with creamed spinach and bacon? Ain't nothing to it. Here's how.

1. Preheat the oven to 425°F. Spray a large rimmed baking sheet with coconut oil.

2. Meanwhile, cook the bacon in a large skillet over medium heat until crisp (if using turkey bacon, cook it in the butter so it doesn't stick to the skillet). Add the spinach, garlic, and pepper flakes (if using) and stir with the bacon for a minute or two until the spinach is wilted. Add the cream cheese and water and stir all the ingredients until the cream cheese melts.

3. Pound the chicken breasts for just a few seconds to flatten a little bit. Place them on the prepared baking sheet and sprinkle them generously with salt, pepper, and paprika. Spoon the creamed spinach mixture over the top of each breast, then top with the grated cheese.

4. Bake for about 25 minutes, or until cooked through.

MAKE A FAMILY MEAL: For the weight-loss plan, pair this with Troodles (page 264) and a side salad with an S-friendly dressing. Or make some Wonderful White Blender Bread (page 242) to have on the side. Growing children and others needing Crossovers can enjoy this with brown rice or WWBB Garlic Bread (page 245) made with sprouted-grain bread.

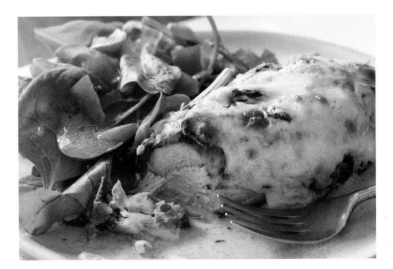

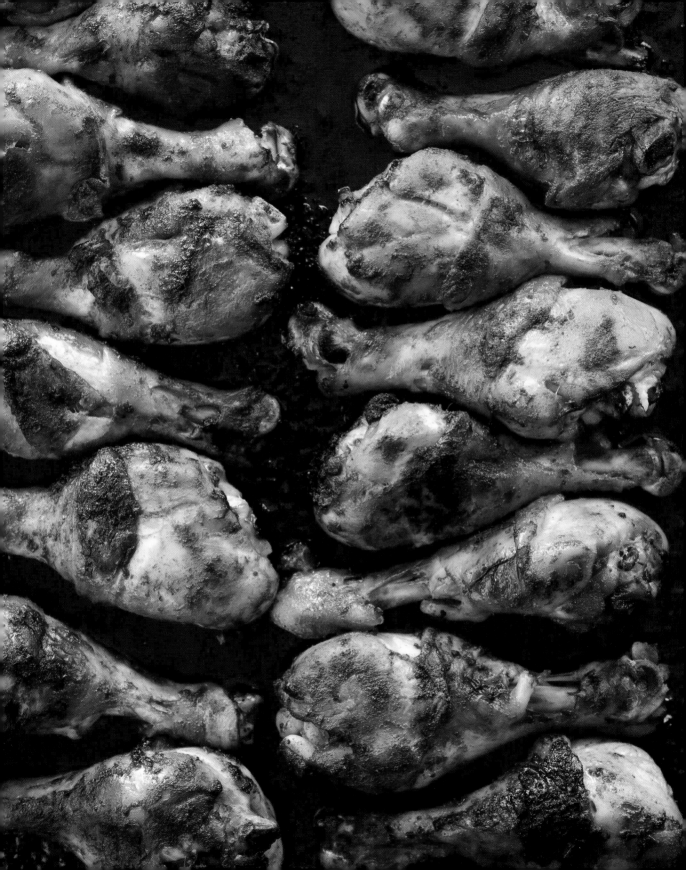

little sweet little spicy drumsticks

S

FAMILY SERVE–FEEDS 6 TO 8 (HALVE IF YOUR FAMILY IS SMALLER, OR MAKE FULL AND FREEZE HALF)

4 to 6 pounds chicken drumsticks

4 tablespoons (½ stick) butter, melted

2 teaspoons Super Sweet Blend, or 3 to 4 tablespoons Gentle Sweet*

1½ tablespoons garlic powder

1½ tablespoons paprika

1 tablespoon ground cumin

1 tablespoon chili powder

1 tablespoon chipotle powder, or 2 tablespoons chili powder

1½ teaspoons Mineral Salt

¼ to ½ teaspoon cayenne pepper (optional, for heat freaks)

We love chicken legs because they are one of the most inexpensive cuts of meat! Perfect for budget-minded Mamas feeding hungry mouths. And don't worry, we do mean only a little spicy here. These are kid friendly; they have just enough spice to let your mouth know it's flavor time! If your family is as heat loving as ours are, add the optional cayenne for more of a kick.

1. Preheat the oven to 375°F.
2. Pierce each chicken leg several times with a sharp knife, pulling downward to create holes in the chicken skin and meat so the flavors can creep in.
3. Mix together the melted butter, sweetener, and all the seasonings in a bowl. (It will become a paste.) Dip each drumstick into the paste, then use your hands to smear it all over the chicken, making sure each piece is well coated with the spice mixture. It will be clumpy; no worries, it will melt in the hot oven. Place the chicken pieces on 2 shallow baking pans or 1 extra-large pan.
4. Bake for 45 to 50 minutes, turning the pieces a couple times. At the end of cooking, turn the oven to high broil and crisp the top of the drummies even more for a few minutes. (They should be very browned, but not burned, so keep an eye on them while you broil.)

MAKE A FAMILY MEAL: For the weight-loss plan, pair this with a side salad and an S-friendly dressing. Add a steamed or roasted nonstarchy veggie if you like, seasoned up well and tossed with a little butter. Growing children or others at Crossover stage can enjoy a healthy carb on the side such as brown rice or quinoa noodles, or end the meal with a piece of fruit.

* FOR NSI: USE A GROCERY STORE ON-PLAN SWEETENER.

lemon cream chicken

S

FAMILY SERVE—FEEDS 6 TO 8 (HALVE IF YOUR FAMILY IS SMALLER, OR MAKE FULL AND FREEZE HALF)

2½ pounds chicken tenderloins or boneless, skinless chicken breasts (cut large breasts in half), thawed if frozen

Seasonings: Mineral Salt, black pepper, dried parsley flakes, and paprika

½ teaspoon dried thyme

4 tablespoons (½ stick) butter, melted

Juice of 1 big, juicy lemon or 2 small lemons

⅓ to ½ cup heavy cream

4 to 6 garlic cloves, minced

¼ to ⅓ cup grated Parmesan cheese (the green can kind is fine)

PEARL CHATS: Here's another way to make plain ol' chicken breasts or tenders amazingly good! My husband declared this tastes like something from a good restaurant . . . and he can be picky, so I took that as a win! If you have big eaters in your fam, use 3 pounds of chicken, but make sure to up the cream and butter amounts by a couple tablespoons each to compensate.

1. Preheat the oven to 425°F.
2. Put the tenderloins or breasts in a 9 × 13-inch or oval baking dish. Sprinkle liberally with the seasonings and thyme.
3. Combine the melted butter and lemon juice in a small bowl. Add the cream and garlic and whisk well. Spoon over the top of the chicken and spread out the mixture so the tops of all the chicken are well covered. Sprinkle on the Parmesan. Bake for 20 minutes for tenderloins or 25 to 30 minutes for breasts.

MAKE A FAMILY MEAL: For the weight-loss plan, pair with Cauli Rice (page 263) and a side salad with an S-friendly dressing. Growing children and others needing Crossovers can enjoy this with brown rice or quinoa to soak up all the tasty sauce from the chicken.

idiot's chicken

S

2½ to 3 pounds boneless, skinless chicken breasts (cut large ones in half) or thighs, thawed if frozen

2 tablespoons coconut oil or butter, melted

Mineral Salt and black pepper, for sprinkling

2 (14.5-ounce) cans fire-roasted, diced tomatoes, one can drained

4 to 6 garlic cloves, minced

1½ teaspoons dried oregano

1½ teaspoons Italian seasoning

1 tablespoon dried parsley flakes

Red pepper flakes (optional; we love using about ¾ teaspoon)

8 ounces of your favorite grated cheese

Hold on . . . before you think we're meany pants name-callers, hear us out. This recipe started out with the name "Idiot's Guide to Mouth-Watering Italian Chicken." We thought that was a fitting title because this recipe is just so easy, it begs to be made. But after making it a few times, tweaking it, and chatting about the recipe between ourselves, it got naturally shortened to Idiot's Chicken. That stuck. We're sorry 'bout that, but not about the easy, delicious meal.

1. Preheat the oven to 425°F.
2. Place the chicken in a 9 × 13-inch or oval baking dish. Pour the melted oil over the top, then sprinkle liberally with salt and pepper.
3. Mix together the canned tomatoes, garlic, ¾ teaspoon salt, oregano, Italian seasoning, parsley flakes, and pepper flakes to taste (if using). Pour over the chicken. Sprinkle the cheese over the top and bake for 25 minutes, or until the cheese is golden and bubbling and the chicken is cooked through.

MAKE A FAMILY MEAL: For the weight-loss plan, pair this with a nonstarchy veggie side and a side salad. WWBB Garlic Bread (page 245) goes great with this, too. Crossover family members can have the garlic bread made with sprouted-grain bread in place of the WWBB bread.

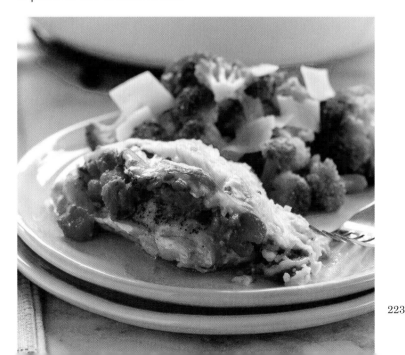

addictive greek chicken ⓢ

FAMILY SERVE—FEEDS 6 TO 8 (HALVE IF YOUR FAMILY IS SMALLER, OR MAKE FULL AND FREEZE HALF)

Coconut oil cooking spray

1 tablespoon butter or coconut oil

4 to 5 garlic cloves, minced

10 ounces fresh spinach

Mineral Salt and black pepper

2½ to 3 pounds boneless, skinless chicken breasts or thighs (enough for 1 piece each for every adult or big-eating child, perhaps 2 for a big guy in your life), thawed if frozen

5 ounces crumbled feta cheese

2 ounces diced or sliced olives (optional)

4 ounces grated part-skim mozzarella cheese

Paprika, for sprinkling

Yummy garlicky spinach and feta cheese stuffed into chicken . . . mmmm. It pairs well with Tzatziki Cucumber Salad (page 266).

1. Preheat the oven to 425°F. Spray a large rimmed baking sheet with coconut oil.

2. Melt the butter in a large skillet over medium-high heat. Add the garlic and sauté for about a minute. Add the spinach, ½ teaspoon salt, and ½ teaspoon pepper and toss for another couple minutes until wilted. Set aside.

3. Pound the chicken breasts or thighs just a little bit to flatten them somewhat. Butterfly each breast or thigh by slicing horizontally through the center (as if you are opening a book), but do not cut all the way through (keep the spine of the book intact—got it?). Lay the breasts or thighs flat and open (like an open book, just to keep being annoying with this analogy) on the prepared baking sheet. Spoon the spinach onto one side of each piece of chicken, add some feta, olives (if using), and mozzarella, then close over with the other side (like you're closing a— nah . . . done with that book spiel now).

4. Spray the tops of the chicken with coconut oil and sprinkle very well with salt, pepper, and paprika. Bake, uncovered, for 25 to 30 minutes, or until cooked through.

MAKE A FAMILY MEAL: For the weight-loss plan, pair with Tzatziki Cucumber Salad (page 266) or any other cucumber salad that you like and a nonstarchy veggie of your choice. Those eating Crossovers can include some buttered sprouted-grain pita bread.

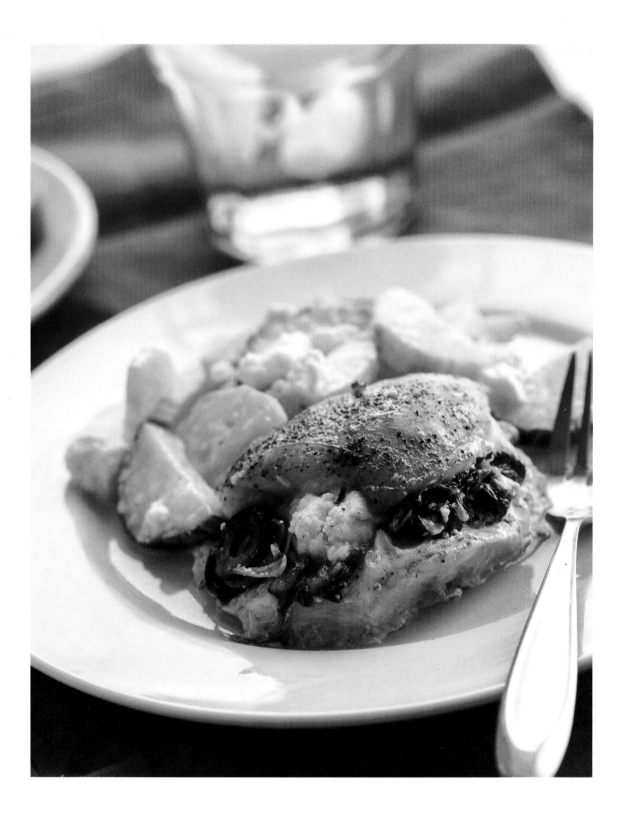

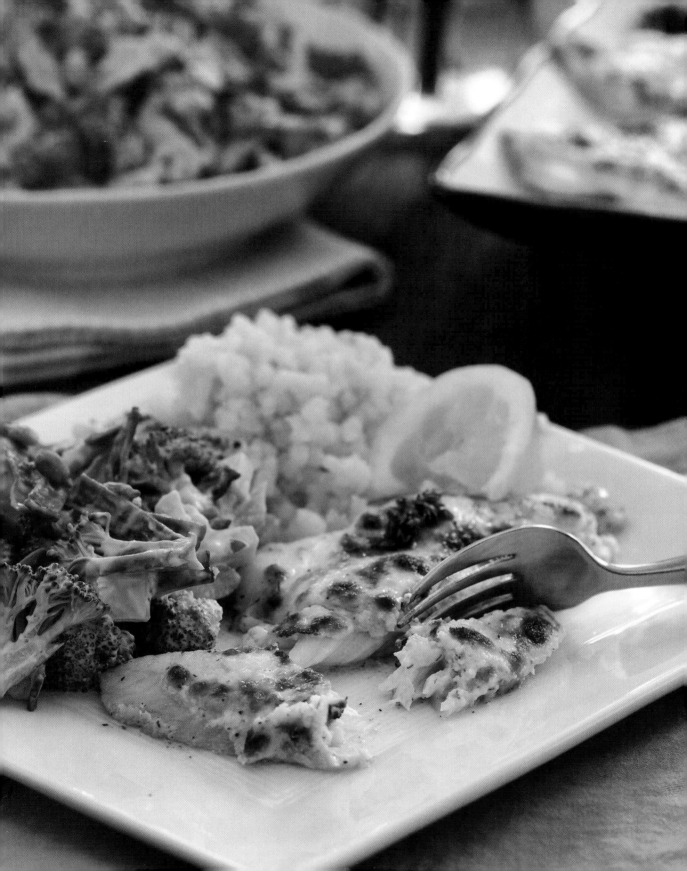

flaky parmesan tilapia

S

FAMILY SERVE—FEEDS 6 TO 8 (HALVE IF YOUR FAMILY IS SMALLER)

2 pounds tilapia or other thin whitefish fillets, thawed if frozen

4 tablespoons (½ stick) butter, melted

Black pepper

Red pepper flakes (optional)

¾ cup grated Parmesan cheese (we use powder-style from the green can)

¼ cup mayonnaise

2 heaping tablespoons Greek yogurt

¾ teaspoon dried dill

This is a quick and easy way to include more fish in your life. There is only so much chicken and red meat you can eat, so please make room for fish! It is a wonderful, slimming part of the balanced-protein approach in THM. This recipe is incredibly flaky and full of flavor, and it's a great way to get your children to start liking fish. It need not be expensive, either. You can buy 2 pounds of frozen tilapia fillets from any landlocked grocery store inexpensively and thaw them before cooking. If you don't like the idea of using tilapia, use any other thin whitefish of your liking.

1. Preheat the oven to a high broil.
2. Rinse the fish and pat it dry. Place it in a single layer (no overlap) in an extra-large baking dish or 2 medium baking dishes. Pour the melted butter over the top and turn each fillet in the butter to coat well on both sides. Sprinkle lightly with black pepper and pepper flakes (if using).
3. Combine the Parmesan, mayo, yogurt, and dill in a bowl and stir until a paste forms. Set aside.
4. Put the fish on the second rack from the top of the oven and broil for 3 minutes.
5. Remove from the oven, turn each piece over, and smear with some Parmesan paste to cover the top of the fish (easily done with a fork). Broil for another 4 to 5 minutes, until it's bubbling and golden brown on the top and flaky in the middle.

MAKE A FAMILY MEAL: For the weight-loss plan, enjoy it with a side salad and/or a veggie like broccoli tossed in butter and Mineral Salt or Cauli Rice (page 263). Growing children and others at Crossover stage can enjoy it with brown rice or buttered sprouted-grain bread.

garlic and herb butter tilapia

FAMILY SERVE—FEEDS 6 TO 8 (HALVE IF YOUR FAMILY IS SMALLER, OR MAKE FULL AND FREEZE HALF)

Coconut oil cooking spray

2 pounds tilapia or any thin white fish fillets, thawed if frozen

Mineral Salt and black pepper

8 tablespoons (1 stick) softened butter*

1 rounded teaspoon garlic powder, or 4 to 6 garlic cloves, minced

¾ teaspoon Italian seasoning

½ teaspoon dried dill (optional)

Dinner is on your table within 15 minutes tonight with this yumminess.

1. Preheat the oven to 400°F. Spray an extra-large baking dish or 2 medium baking dishes with coconut oil.

2. Lay the fillets in a single layer in the prepared dish and sprinkle with salt and pepper.

3. Mix the butter in a bowl with the garlic powder, Italian seasoning, and dill (if using). Spread the buttery mix over the tops of the fish. Bake for 10 to 12 minutes, until flaky.

MAKE A FAMILY MEAL: This fish is lovely paired with Mashed Fotatoes (page 264) or Cauli Rice (page 263) and an S-friendly salad. Brown rice is the perfect accompaniment for those in Crossover stage.

* FOR DF: SUB COCONUT OIL FOR THE BUTTER, OR PERHAPS USE GHEE IF YOU LIKE IT AND TOLERATE IT WELL. IF USING COCONUT OIL, IT WON'T SPREAD AS EASILY OVER THE FISH, BUT JUST DO YOUR BEST; IT TASTES JUST AS GOOD AT THE END. YOU CAN ADD A LITTLE EXTRA MINERAL SALT TO MAKE UP FOR THE BUTTERY TASTE.

cilantro-lime salmon

S

FAMILY SERVE—FEEDS 6 TO 8 (HALVE IF YOUR FAMILY IS SMALLER, OR MAKE FULL AND FREEZE HALF)

Butter or coconut oil cooking spray

2 pounds salmon fillets, skin on or not, either is fine (or 1 fillet for each adult or big eating child), thawed if frozen

Mineral Salt and black pepper

1 large bunch fresh cilantro (most of the stems removed)

4 garlic cloves, minced

Juice of 3 limes

¼ cup coconut oil

½ jalapeño (seeds and all, baby) for heat freaks (optional)

2 to 3 teaspoons Gentle Sweet (optional, for a sweeter sauce)

FOR THE AVOCADO CRÈME

2 avocados

Juice of 1 lime (or add more if you love it)

½ to 1 teaspoon garlic powder

½ teaspoon Mineral Salt

¼ teaspoon black pepper

2 tablespoons MCT oil or extra-virgin olive oil

¼ jalapeño (optional)

¼ to ½ cup water

Get an incredibly tasty and healthy dinner on the table in 15 minutes tonight. Time to stop thinking "yuck" when you think of salmon. To our salmon haters, here's a challenge for you: Make this (perhaps just halve or quarter the recipe to start if you and salmon are not best friends yet), then taste it with an open mind. We think your mind will be blown . . . or at least changed.

Salmon is highly anti-inflammatory and soooo good for your heart, your brain, and your skin. It is a balanced part of the protein intake of this plan. Don't beef and chicken your every meal. Salmon needs its turn! This recipe can help you baby-step your way into salmon loving. The avocado crème is optional but really takes it over the top. Oh, and salmon need not be expensive. We buy our wild-caught salmon at Aldi and get a packet of four frozen fillets for about five bucks. Pretty sweet!

1. Preheat the oven to 400°F or the broiler to high. Grease an extra-large baking dish or 2 medium baking dishes with butter or coconut oil.

2. Arrange the fish in the baking dishes and sprinkle liberally with salt and pepper.

3. Put the cilantro, garlic, lime juice, coconut oil, jalapeño (if using), and Gentle Sweet (if using) in a food processor and puree (see Note). You will likely have to stop the processor, scrape down the sides with a spatula, and stir a little every now and then to get it all processed. Once processed, take out the blade and stir the mixture. Using a spoon, smear some of the mixture over each fillet until the puree is all used up. Bake for 15 minutes or broil on the second rack from the top until just cooked through.

4. While the salmon is cooking, make the avocado crème. Put all the ingredients (except the water) in a blender and blend until smooth. Add the water a little at a time and keep blending until it thins to your liking.

MAKE A FAMILY MEAL: For the weight-loss plan, pair with a fresh salad and an optional nonstarchy veggie. Crossover family members can enjoy this with brown rice.

NOTE: You can replace the cilantro-lime mixture with Karate Chop Kale Pesto (page 524) or store-bought pesto for a change-up.

FRIENDLY

firecracker salmon

S

FAMILY SERVE–FEEDS 6 TO 8 (HALVE IF YOUR FAMILY IS SMALLER, OR MAKE FULL AND FREEZE HALF)

Coconut oil cooking spray

2 pounds salmon fillets, skin on or not is fine (or 1 fillet for each adult or big-eating child)

⅓ cup soy sauce

4 to 6 garlic cloves, minced

1½ teaspoons finely grated or minced fresh ginger

1½ to 2 teaspoons Super Sweet Blend, or 1 to 2 tablespoons Gentle Sweet*

1 to 2 tablespoons Sriracha sauce (Huy Fong brand . . . find it in the international foods aisle at your grocery store)

½ to 1½ rounded teaspoons red pepper flakes (all depends on your heat preference)

Coconut oil (1 rounded teaspoon for each piece of fish)

3 green onions, finely diced

1. Spray 1 extra-large baking dish or 2 medium baking dishes with coconut oil. Place the fillets in a single layer in the baking dish(es).

2. Mix together the soy sauce, garlic, ginger, sweetener, Sriracha, and pepper flakes in a bowl. Pour it over the salmon, making sure each piece is coated well on both sides.

3. Cover the dish(es) with plastic wrap, put them in the fridge, and allow the salmon to marinate for at least 1 hour. It's best for several hours or even overnight. (You can also bake or broil right away if you'd like.)

4. Preheat the oven to 400°F or the broiler to high.

5. Uncover the fish and put 1 teaspoon of coconut oil on each piece of fish. Bake for 15 minutes or broil on the second rack from the top until it's just done. Top with the green onions once they're cooked.

MAKE A FAMILY MEAL: For the weight-loss plan, Thai-Kissed Cucumber Salad (page 268) is wonderful with this salmon, or any S-friendly salad works. Pair it with Cauli Rice (page 263) or sautéed Trim Healthy Noodles or Troodles (page 264), or fill up with another nonstarchy veggie. Brown rice is always perfect with fish for Crossover members of your household.

* FOR NSI: USE A GROCERY STORE ON-PLAN SWEETENER.

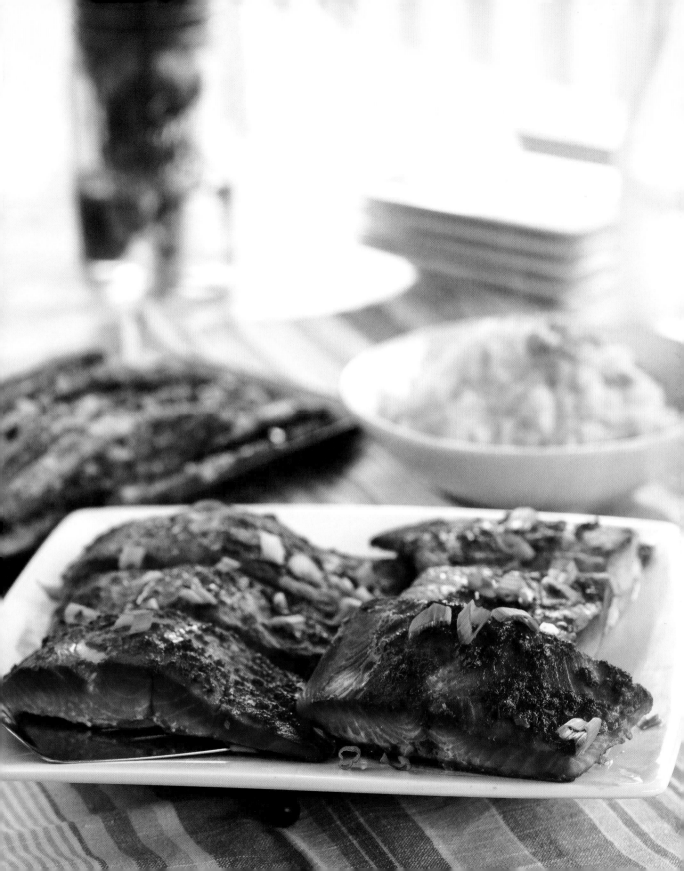

Patties,
Tenders
&
Fritters

Get your skillet ready for the tasty recipes in this chapter. Your kids will snatch these up, especially the chicken tenders! While not a recipe in this chapter, the Marvelous Make-Ahead Meatballs (page 208) also make great patties. You can also make up the One-Batch Meatballs (page 129) and brown patty-size amounts in butter and coconut oil as described for the recipes in this chapter.

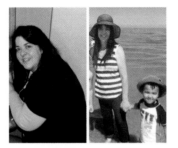

A hundred and five pounds gone at fifty-one and the nonscale victories keep coming! As a mom (and a grandma) who battled weight all my life, I never thought I would say it was easy, but THM is—but only if you lose the sugar and white carbs and learn to separate fuels. I got the original book in 2013 and thought it sounded too hard . . . but had a tiny seed of thought: "What if I start and have a testimony in a year's time?" Once you understand the principles (and the whys), then it all clicks and you see how easy this plan can be. Sure, there is a learning curve, and one's diet mentality is certainly challenged, but it's so, so worth it—and there is no suffering or starvation. Sixty pounds disappeared in that first year, and then another forty-five. My blood-test results are fantastic, and I have energy and stamina! I live in Australia, so I have done the plan without using a lot of special ingredients. I keep it simple, which is what makes this sustainable for me.

My husband also has lost forty pounds and has never read the book. He colors outside the lines a bit but loves eggs and bacon, meat and veggies, along with salads and the other simple foods I cook for him. It took a while to leave the garlic bread and chips, etc., but we have found enough alternatives to appease any cravings now. I can only wish you the life-changing energy and joy this can bring you, because it is up to you! I love shopping, I love cooking, I love food in its right place, I love all the good health benefits! I'm forever grateful for THM and for deciding to Just Do It! —JAN G.

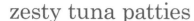

zesty tuna patties

S

FAMILY SERVE—MAKES ABOUT 14 PATTIES (HALVE IF YOUR FAMILY IS SMALLER)

3 (12-ounce) cans water-packed tuna, drained and mashed

3 large eggs

1 onion, finely diced

½ cup THM Baking Blend,* any crumbled S or FP bread from the Breads chapter (page 240), or ground up Joseph's pitas

3 tablespoons mayonnaise* or Greek yogurt

1 generous tablespoon diced pickled jalapeños

1 bunch fresh parsley or cilantro, stems removed, leaves finely chopped

Juice of 1 large lemon (or 2½ tablespoons bottled lemon juice), or juice of 2 limes (or 2½ tablespoons bottled lime juice)

½ teaspoon Mineral Salt

½ teaspoon black pepper

Flavorless coconut oil and/or butter,* for frying

Children love these patties and we Mamas love them because tuna is such a budget-friendly protein. If you have picky onion haters in your family, simply leave that ingredient out. You have a choice of making these two ways, with either lime and cilantro for a fresh bold taste or with lemon and parsley for a more traditional approach. Both are wonderful, but our favorite is the traditional lemon and parsley.

1. Place the tuna, eggs, onion, Baking Blend, mayo, and jalapeños in a bowl. Add the parsley and lemon juice for the parsley-lemon version; add the cilantro and lime juice for the cilantro-lime version. Add the salt and pepper.

2. Working in batches of 4 to 5 cakes, heat 1 tablespoon coconut oil and 1 tablespoon butter in a large skillet over medium to medium-high heat. Drop rounded ¼-cup amounts of the mix into the pan. Spread the patties out a little and sauté them until they're heated through and well browned on both sides. Repeat for more batches, each time using 1 tablespoon butter and 1 tablespoon coconut oil for frying.

MAKE A FAMILY MEAL: For the weight-loss plan, these patties are fabulous with some Cottage Citrus Dip or the herby variation (page 523) on the side of your plate. A side salad completes the meal, or enjoy Killer Green Beans (page 261). Growing children can enjoy brown rice or sprouted-grain bread on the side.

* FOR NSI: USE THE FRUGAL FLOUR OPTION (SEE PAGE 40) OR GROUND UP JOSEPH'S PITAS.

* FOR DF: USE ONLY THE COCONUT OIL, NOT THE BUTTER, TO FRY AND YOUR FAVORITE DAIRY-FREE MAYONNAISE.

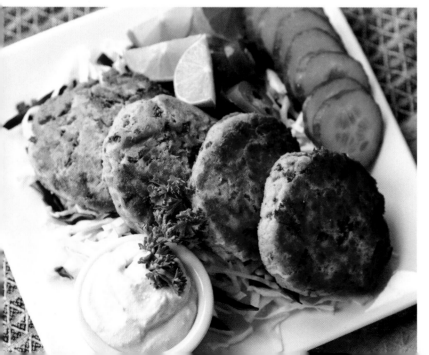

zucchini fritters

S

FAMILY SERVE–MAKES 16 TO 18 FRITTERS (HALVE IF YOUR FAMILY IS SMALLER)

4 medium to large zucchinis, grated
or shredded in a food processor
(6 to 7 cups)

1 teaspoon Mineral Salt

3 large eggs

⅓ cup THM Baking Blend*

¼ cup powder-style Parmesan
cheese* (from the green can)

4 to 6 garlic cloves

¾ teaspoon black pepper

Generous sprinkle Nutritional Yeast

¼ onion, very finely diced (optional)

Butter* and/or flavorless coconut
oil, for frying

Looking for a meatless meal that is tasty and filling? You just found it . . . and it's a fabulous way to use up bountiful zucchini in the summer months. Since these fritters don't have a lot of protein, be sure to have either Speedy Chocolate Milk (page 457) or one of the baby-size shakes (see pages 469 to 490) with or after your meal to amp up the protein, or end your meal with a hot drink with added collagen. Or pair them with Kickin' Dippin' Sauce (page 518), which is another tasty way to get more protein.

1. Place the grated zucchini in a colander over the sink. Toss with the salt and allow to sit for 5 to 10 minutes. After that time, squeeze down the zucchini using a clean cloth to drain out as much of the liquid as you can, but no big deal if some remains.

2. Transfer the zucchini to a large bowl and combine with eggs, Baking Blend, Parmesan, garlic, pepper, nutritional yeast, and onion (if using).

3. Working in batches, heat 1 tablespoon butter and 1 tablespoon coconut oil in a large skillet over medium to medium-high heat. Drop generous tablespoon-size mounds of the mixture into the skillet. Flatten them out with a spatula so the zucchini gets cooked through. Brown on both sides. Continue to cook more batches, each time using 2 tablespoons of the fat.

MAKE A FAMILY MEAL: For the weight-loss plan, pair this with Kickin' Dippin' Sauce (page 518) if desired and/or have it with Mashed Fotatoes (page 264). Children can enjoy this with brown rice or with fruit on the side.

* FOR NSI: USE THE FRUGAL FLOUR OPTION (SEE PAGE 40).

* FOR DF: REPLACE THE PARMESAN WITH THE SAME AMOUNT OF NUTRITIONAL YEAST. USE ONLY THE COCONUT OIL, NOT THE BUTTER, TO FRY.

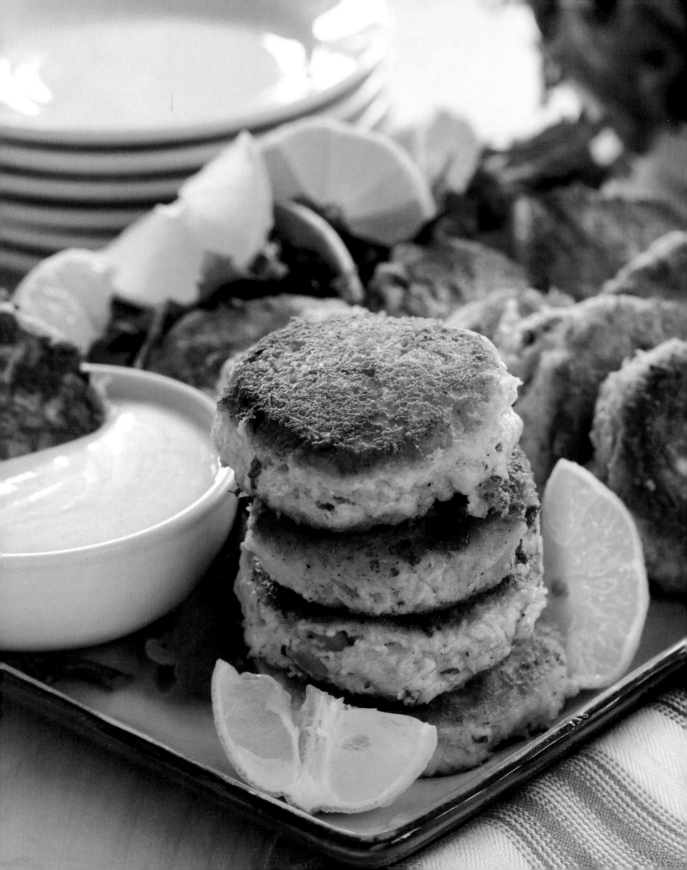

chicken cakes

S

FAMILY SERVE–MAKES 14 CAKES (HALVE IF YOUR FAMILY IS SMALLER)

2 teaspoons butter or coconut oil

4 garlic cloves, minced

½ (10- to 12-ounce) bag frozen small-cut seasoning blend (see page 35)

3 (12-ounce) cans chicken, drained

3 large eggs

¼ cup THM Baking Blend, ground-up oats, or ground-up Joseph's pitas

2 tablespoons mayonnaise

1 tablespoon prepared mustard

1¼ teaspoons Creole seasoning (we use MSG-free Tony Cachere's)

¾ teaspoon black pepper

¼ cup finely minced fresh parsley, or 1 tablespoon dried parsley flakes

Flavorless coconut oil and/or butter,* for frying

FOR THE RÉMOULADE SAUCE* (OPTIONAL)

¼ cup mayonnaise

¼ cup Greek yogurt

Juice of ½ lemon

1 to 1½ teaspoons Sriracha sauce (Huy Fong brand)

¼ teaspoon Creole seasoning

If you love crab cakes, you'll love these chicken cakes. They're great on their own but the rémoulade sauce kicks them up to extreme food-star stage. Chicken is a much easier find than crab (and we're not big crab fans), so these can be an easy staple in your home. If you have leftovers (we never do, sadly), they'll make a great lunch to reheat or even eat cold, crumbled over a salad.

1. Heat a large skillet over high heat. Add the butter and garlic and toss in the hot butter for half a minute. Add the seasoning blend and toss for another few minutes, until the seasoning blend is thawed and starting to cook through. Remove from the heat and transfer the veggie mix to a large bowl. Add the chicken, eggs, Baking Blend, mayo, mustard, Creole seasoning, pepper, and parsley. Mash the chicken with a fork while stirring well.

2. Working in batches of 4 or 5 cakes, heat 1 tablespoon coconut oil and 1 tablespoon butter in the same skillet over medium-high heat. Drop rounded ¼-cup amounts of the mix into the pan. Spread the cakes out a little and sauté them until heated through and well browned on both sides. Continue to cook more batches, each time using 1 tablespoon butter and 1 tablespoon coconut oil for frying.

3. Make the rémoulade sauce (if using). Mix together all the ingredients in a bowl. Serve alongside the cakes for dipping.

MAKE A FAMILY MEAL: For the weight-loss plan, have this with a large salad and an optional nonstarchy veggie cooked in your favorite S style. Growing children or others in Crossover mode can have a healthy carb side such as a piece of fruit, sprouted-grain bread, or brown rice.

* FOR DF: USE ONLY THE COCONUT OIL TO FRY. OMIT THE RÉMOULADE SAUCE OR USE ½ CUP DAIRY-FREE MAYO IN PLACE OF THE YOGURT AND MAYO.

snatch 'em up chicken tenders   **S**

FAMILY SERVE—FEEDS 6 TO 8 (HALVE IF YOUR FAMILY IS SMALLER, OR MAKE FULL AND FREEZE HALF)

2 large eggs

½ cup egg whites (carton or fresh)

2½ to 3 pounds chicken tenderloins or boneless, skinless chicken breasts (if using breasts, cut into tender-size pieces with kitchen scissors), thawed if frozen

1½ cups THM Baking Blend*

1 cup powder-style Parmesan cheese (from the green can)

1 teaspoon Mineral Salt

1½ teaspoons black pepper

1½ teaspoons onion powder

1½ to 2 teaspoons garlic powder (depending on your love for it)

⅛ teaspoon cayenne pepper (use either more or less depending on your love of spicy)

Flavorless coconut oil (if skillet-frying) or coconut oil cooking spray (if oven-frying)

Our children are gobbling machines when it comes to these tenders! They snatch them up so quickly that if we don't hide a couple somewhere for ourselves, we'll be out of luck. If you have children or teens (or perhaps husbands) who turn their noses up at the idea of eating healthy, just serve these up and don't mention anything about THM or healthy foods! They'll have no idea. Choose from the skillet-fry (our reliable favorite method), air-fry, or oven-fry methods. By the way, if you're penny-pinching, the frugal flour option (page 40) works great for this recipe, so no need to use up your Baking Blend.

1. Whisk together the whole eggs and egg whites in a large bowl. Put the chicken pieces in the egg mix and turn to coat well.

2. Mix together the Baking Blend, Parmesan, salt, black pepper, onion powder, garlic powder, and cayenne on a large dinner plate. Dip the egg-coated chicken pieces into the breading. Coat well, then put them on another plate waiting to fry.

3. **TO SKILLET-FRY:** Working in batches, heat 2 generous tablespoons (or a little more) of the coconut oil in a large skillet over medium heat. Brown the tenders on both sides and cook until "done" in the middle. Cook more batches, using 2 generous tablespoons of oil per batch. You should be able to get 3 pounds fried in 3 batches if your skillet is large enough.

   TO AIR-FRY: Set an air-fryer to 400°F. Fry the chicken for 15 to 20 minutes, according to the manufacturer's directions.

   TO OVEN-FRY: Preheat the oven to 425°F. Put 2 tablespoons butter or coconut oil on a large rimmed baking sheet, place it in the oven and allow the oil to melt while the oven preheats. Once it's melted and bubbling, take the baking sheet out and spread the fat around the sheet evenly. Place the chicken tenders on the baking sheet, spray the tops generously with coconut oil, and bake for 18 to 20 minutes.

MAKE A FAMILY MEAL: For the weight-loss plan, dip these tenders in ketchup (preferably sugar-free) or honey-mustard sauce (such as the sauce from Make It Again Chicken on page 217). Enjoy with buttered, steamed broccoli or cauliflower on the side and a fresh side salad. Children can get their carbs for a Crossover with a piece of fruit.

* FOR NSI: USE THE FRUGAL FLOUR OPTION (SEE PAGE 40).

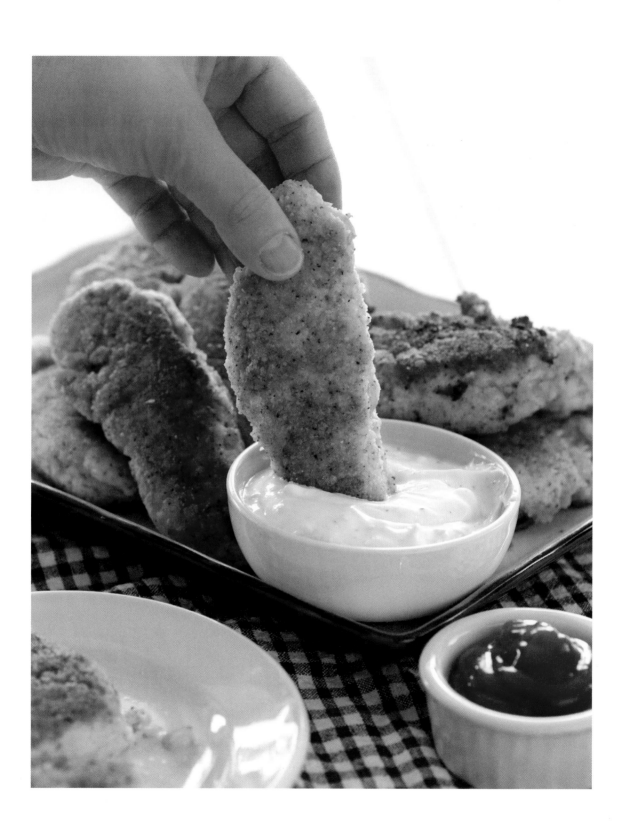

Breads, Wraps, Biscuits & Loaves

We think life without bread isn't life at all, so let's not deprive ourselves, okay? On THM you can enjoy sprouted whole-grain breads, artisan sourdough, or whole rye breads for E meals. But sometimes you want butter on your bread and that collision of fat and grain is a Crossover, which eaten too often can cause weight gain for most people. The following breads are either an FP or an S and allow you to have that blessed combination of bread and butter or bread and cheese. They are also all gluten-free.

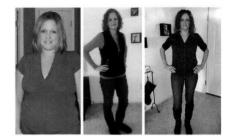

I am overjoyed to write this post. I am forever thankful to God for leading me to THM. I never dieted but did count calories. I would lose weight, only to gain it back and then some. I started Trim Healthy Mama feeling very defeated in April 2013. Amazingly, by November 2013 (middle picture), I had reached goal weight. I was so superexcited, because I honestly had come to believe that I would never lose the weight. And here I was, just months later, feeling better and at goal.

But what is almost as exciting (and maybe even more so) is that I have now maintained and have been eating this way for four years now! That's huge, ladies! Losing the weight is one thing, but being able to keep it off is a whole 'nother deal. Now I get to add in yummy occasional Crossovers instead of stressing about how I'm going to keep the weight off. So, if you're wondering if this is sustainable long-term—it is! This truly is a way of life rather than a diet. No more counting calories, no more being hungry, no more disliking the food I'm eating. I spent so many years of my life trying to lose the weight all the wrong ways. I never knew it could be so easy, fun, AND delicious! Let me encourage you to keep going. It really is worth it. You'll look back and be so happy you did! I am a THM for life! **–TAMMY S.**

wonderful white blender bread

FP

MAKES 1 LOAF

Coconut oil cooking spray

1½ cups egg whites (carton or fresh)

½ teaspoon xanthan gum

¾ cup unflavored Pristine Whey Protein Powder*

1 cup THM Baking Blend*

1 cup plain 0% Greek yogurt or 1% cottage cheese

2½ teaspoons aluminum-free baking powder

1 teaspoon Super Sweet Blend*

½ teaspoon Mineral Salt

Just blend and bake! Couldn't be easier. You don't know how excited we are to give you this white, fluffy bread, which we affectionately abbreviate to WWBB. It is going to change your world. After months of tweaking and trying for the ultimate low-carb, low-fat white bread, we have it! It makes perfect slices for sandwiches, grilled cheese, French toast, garlic bread; or just spread a piece with butter and sugar-free jelly and say "Mmm." Best of all, it is a Fuel Pull . . . and the crowd goes wild! There are plenty of low-carb bread options out there online, but most are loaded with almond flour and tons of whole eggs. You don't want to eat calorie-laden bread like that on a daily basis. We don't have to count calories, but piling butter or mayonnaise on top of bread that already has a bunch of fat can turn into calorie abuse; it is not the balanced Trim Healthy way. There's just no need to do that. Fuel Pull bread makes more sense for your daily bread. Now you can put some butter on your bread and really enjoy it!

1. Preheat the oven to 350°F. Spray a 9 × 5-inch (standard) glass loaf pan with coconut oil. You want your pan to be as straight-sided as possible. Slanted pans can cause the bread to fall over the pan as it rises. If your bread rises a bit lopsided, though, never fear, it will still taste great.

2. Put the egg whites and xanthan gum in a blender and blend on high for 1 minute, until thickened and frothy. Add all the other ingredients and blend well for another minute or so.

3. Using a spatula, scrape the batter into the loaf pan and bake for 40 minutes. If after 20 minutes the top of the bread looks like it's browning too much, place a folded piece of parchment paper over the top. Once the bread is out of the oven, allow it to sit for a couple minutes, then remove it from the pan (you may need to use a knife around the sides of the pan to help it come out). Let it cool at least another 10 to 15 minutes before carefully slicing your first piece or two with a serrated knife. Cover the rest of the loaf with a paper towel and put it in a gallon baggie. You can store it on the counter for the first day, if desired, but after that it is best kept in the refrigerator.

* FOR NSI: USE A GROCERY STORE ON-PLAN SWEETENER AND WHEY PROTEIN (SEE PAGE 43). USE THE FRUGAL FLOUR OPTION (SEE PAGE 40), BUT NOTE THAT THIS WILL TAKE THIS BREAD FROM AN FP TO AN S AND IT WON'T LOOK AS WHITE.

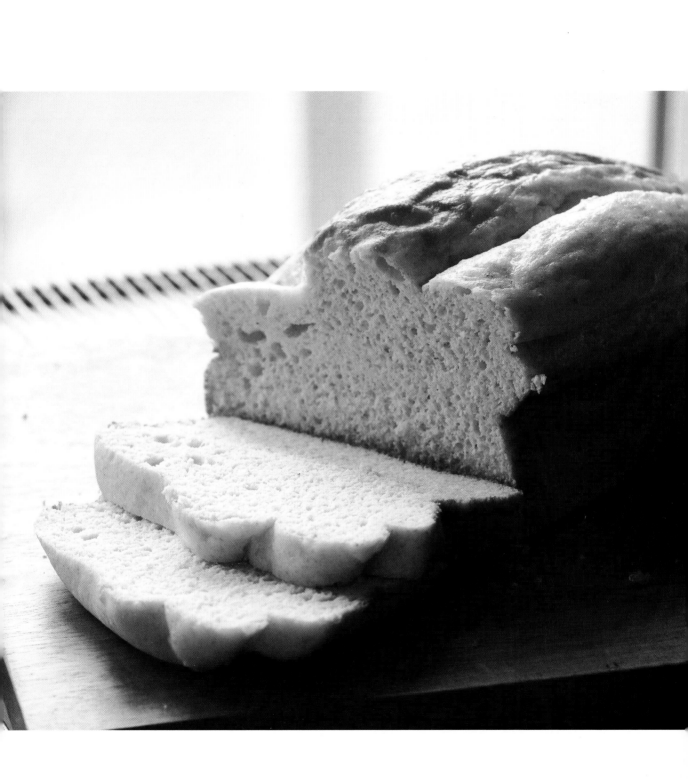

wwbb for one

FP

SINGLE SERVE

¼ cup egg whites (carton or fresh)

⅛ teaspoon xanthan gum

1½ tablespoons unflavored Pristine Whey Protein Powder*

2 tablespoons THM Baking Blend*

2 tablespoons plain 0% Greek yogurt or 1% cottage cheese

½ teaspoon aluminum-free baking powder

3 pinches Mineral Salt

⅛ teaspoon Super Sweet Blend*

Coconut oil cooking spray

PEARL CHATS: We had a feeling you'd love the loaf version of WWBB (page 242) enough that you'd ask us for a single serve. Here it is. Yes, it is microwaved so it doesn't quite have all the splendor of the full baked loaf, but it is still reasonably wonderful for a quick fix. Serene's sitting here grumbling about all this microwave "bidness," but she'll just have to get over it. If you feel the same way as she does, check out the awesome Personal Pan Pizza (page 310) made in a skillet with this single-serve recipe.

1. Put the egg whites and xanthan gum in a small bowl and blend for about 1 minute with a stick blender or put in a mini blender. Add the whey protein, Baking Blend, yogurt, baking powder, salt, and sweetener and stir in with a fork, or blend until well combined.

2. Spray a small slice of bread-size Pyrex (round or square) dish with coconut oil (don't use a mug . . . it doesn't work for this recipe). Scrape the batter into the dish and microwave it for 1 minute 50 seconds. Remove and slice it into 2 thin pieces of bread.

* FOR NSI: USE A GROCERY STORE ON-PLAN SWEETENER AND WHEY PROTEIN (SEE PAGE 43). USE FRUGAL FLOUR OPTION (SEE PAGE 40), BUT NOTE THAT THIS WILL TAKE THIS BREAD FROM AN FP TO AN S AND IT WON'T LOOK AS WHITE.

wwbb garlic bread (S)

MULTIPLE SERVE

Coconut oil cooking spray
Slices of Wonderful White Blender
  Bread* (page 242)
Butter or coconut oil
Garlic powder, parsley flakes, and
  Parmesan cheese, for sprinkling

Perfect with Pizzeria Tomato Soup (page 150) or any soup or stew—in fact, any S-friendly meal you wish to pair it with.

1. Preheat the oven to 450°F. Spray a rimmed baking sheet with coconut oil.

2. Smear the bread slices with butter or coconut oil and place them on the sheet. Sprinkle on garlic powder, parsley, and Parmesan and bake for about 5 minutes.

* FOR NSI: USE A GROCERY STORE ON-PLAN SWEETENER AND WHEY PROTEIN (SEE PAGE 43). USE THE FRUGAL FLOUR OPTION (SEE PAGE 40).

NSI DF FRIENDLY

nuke queen's awesome bread (FP)

MAKES 1 LOAF

1½ cups THM Baking Blend*
6 tablespoons water
2 cups egg whites (carton or fresh)
Scant ¼ teaspoon Mineral Salt
½ teaspoon Super Sweet Blend*
1 tablespoon aluminum-free baking
  powder

PEARL CHATS: If you are dairy-free and can't make WWBB (page 242), this can be a great alternative. Or if you are in a big hurry and don't have the time for baking in the oven—this bread is microwaved! (As you can imagine, Serene despises the microwave part so we do include a baking option.) This was my first attempt at a white FP bread and it went viral. You can watch the video on our website of us making it (I tie Serene up so she can't stop my nuking efforts). I have to admit that our WWBB has surpassed this as my favorite bread now, but Nuke Queen's can still serve a great purpose for some people who can't tolerate cottage cheese or whey protein.

1. Mix together all the ingredients in a large bowl. Transfer it to an 8½ × 4½-inch Pyrex loaf pan. Microwave it for about 10 minutes. (You can also bake it at 350°F for 45 minutes if preferred.)

* FOR NSI: USE A GROCERY STORE ON-PLAN SWEETENER AND USE THE FRUGAL FLOUR OPTION (SEE PAGE 40), BUT NOTE THAT THIS WILL TAKE THIS BREAD FROM AN FP TO AN S.

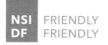
nuke queen's cornbread

FP

MULTIPLE SERVE

Coconut oil cooking spray

⅓ cup canned baby corn (put the leftovers in a baggie and freeze for the next time)

1⅓ cups THM Baking Blend*

⅓ cup powder-style Parmesan cheese* (from the green can)

1½ cups egg whites (carton or fresh)

½ cup unsweetened cashew or almond milk

½ teaspoon Mineral Salt

1 tablespoon aluminum-free baking powder

1 tablespoon butter, coconut oil, or ghee, melted

1 to 1½ teaspoons Super Sweet Blend,* or more to taste if you like sweeter cornbread (optional)

PEARL CHATS: You don't nuke this, you bake it, but since I am the Nuke Queen who invented the original FP Nuke Queen bread and this recipe was adapted from that . . . the name stuck. In *Trim Healthy Mama Cookbook*, we included an S-style cornbread, but we realized we needed a cornbread that could be a side to E or FP meals. Cornmeal is hard on your blood sugar, so that was out. And we could have used oat flour, but we didn't want to pile more carbs into your E meals. At last we found a remedy . . . the "corniness" in this recipe comes from baby corn, which is a nonstarchy veggie you can find in a can in the Asian section of any grocery store . . . so fun! Pair this with the crockpot pinto beans on page 111 for a lovely meal. Or put this on the side of any soup or stew.

1. Preheat the oven to 425°F. Spray a 9 × 13-inch baking dish thoroughly with coconut oil.

2. Put the baby corn in a food processor and process until fully broken down into tiny pieces. Put all the other ingredients in a bowl, add the processed corn, and stir together.

3. Pour the batter into the baking dish and bake for 25 to 30 minutes.

* FOR NSI: USE A GROCERY STORE ON-PLAN SWEETENER. USE THE FRUGAL FLOUR OPTION (SEE PAGE 40), BUT NOTE THAT THIS WILL TAKE THIS BREAD FROM AN FP TO AN S, SO WHILE IT WILL WORK IN S MEALS, IF YOU PAIR IT WITH E DISHES, YOU'LL HAVE A CROSSOVER.

* FOR DF: SUB NUTRITIONAL YEAST FOR THE PARMESAN.

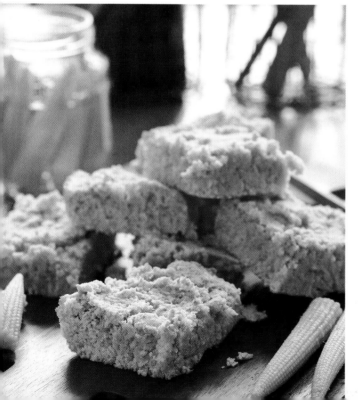

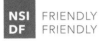
fifteen-minute focaccia bread

MULTIPLE SERVE

S

4 tablespoons butter or coconut oil, melted

4 large eggs

½ cup egg whites (carton or fresh)

⅓ cup water

1½ cups THM Baking Blend*

¼ cup powder-style Parmesan cheese* (from the green can)

⅓ cup unflavored Pristine Whey Protein Powder*

2 teaspoons aluminum-free baking powder

2 pinches Mineral Salt

Topping ideas: Parmesan cheese,* dried basil and rosemary (or chopped fresh herbs), onion powder, garlic powder (or minced fresh garlic), Mineral Salt

This savory, peasant-style bread is great for dipping or makes a lovely side to S or FP soups and stews. It can be used as a cornbread-style side for S recipes. It can even make a nice sandwich if you cut a piece, split it down the middle, and use the two sides, or butter them up and just enjoy!

1. Preheat the oven to 425°F. Line the bottom of a 9 × 13-inch baking dish with parchment paper.
2. Mix together all the ingredients (except the toppings) in a large bowl. Spread the mixture in the baking dish, patting down the top with your hands to smooth it. Sprinkle on the toppings of your choice and bake for 15 minutes.

* FOR NSI: USE THE FRUGAL FLOUR OPTION (SEE PAGE 40) AND LOOK FOR A GROCERY STORE WHEY PROTEIN ISOLATE (SEE PAGE 43).

* FOR DF: SUB THE NUTRITIONAL YEAST FOR THE PARMESAN AND USE COLLAGEN IN PLACE OF THE WHEY PROTEIN.

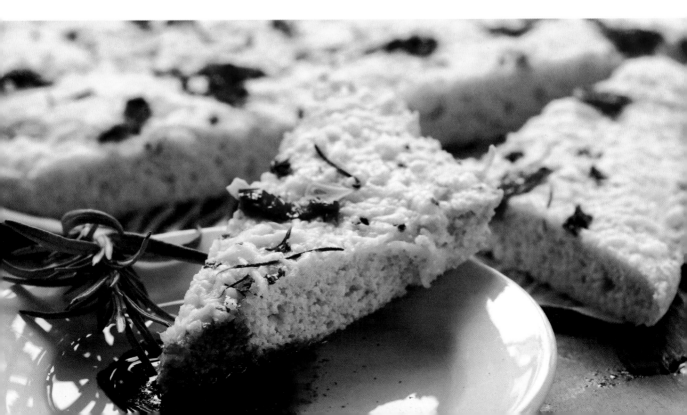

cheesy flower biscuits

S

MAKES 16 BISCUITS

Coconut oil cooking spray

1 (16-ounce) bag frozen cauliflower florets

1 cup THM Baking Blend

1 cup egg whites (carton or fresh)

4½ tablespoons (3 scoops) Integral Collagen

2 tablespoons Whole Husk Psyllium Flakes

2 teaspoons aluminum-free baking powder

½ to 1 teaspoon red pepper flakes (optional)

1 tablespoon onion powder

1 teaspoon garlic powder

½ teaspoon Mineral Salt

½ teaspoon Sunflower Lecithin (optional, but helps dough consistency)

6 tablespoons (¾ stick) butter, melted

1 cup freshly grated cheese (see Note) or ¾ cup powder-style cheese (such as Parmesan from the green can)

SERENE CHATS: *These are the perfect combination of crispy on the outside with a moist crumb structure in their yummy centers. Smeared with a little butter . . . ahhh . . . so amazing! The flour used here is from cauliflower, but don't let that deter you. They taste light and "naughty" like the white flour kind, not at all like the heavy bricks that many healthy substitutions for biscuits end up being. These babies boast more fiber than the whole-grain "sink ship" types and are way more Trimmifying. Packed with protein, they can be eaten alone for a snack or as a wonderful accompaniment to a main meal. Split in two and toast if you want to crisp them up again after refrigeration, or put in a hot oven for just 5 minutes. The first version here is perfectly cheesy, but please check out the variations because we don't want you to miss out on any of the yumminess! The plain version is used in Scones, Jam, and Cream Night (page 287) and you can find a yummy breakfast version called Sausage and Cheese Breakfast Biscuits (page 360).*

1. Position a rack in the top third of the oven and preheat to 350°F. Spray 2 large baking sheets with cooking oil (or use 1 very large pizza stone).

2. Make the "cauli snow." Put the frozen cauliflower in a blender (not a food processor) and pulse until it is broken down. Then blend it on a low setting until it turns into a powdery white snow (don't add any water, just keep blending until it is complete powder snow . . . no rice-size pieces left). Measure out 1 cup for this recipe. (Put the leftover cauli snow in a baggie in the fridge for the next time, or back into the freezer if you think it will be a while before you bake with cauli snow again.)

3. Put the snow in a bowl. Add all the other ingredients (except the melted butter and cheese) and use a stick blender to mix it into a dough. Add the melted butter and blend again. Stir in the cheese. (If you don't have a stick blender, whisk the dry ingredients first, then add the cauli snow and whisk well. Then add the melted butter and whisk whisk whisk, then stir in the cheese.)

4. With a large spoon, plop 16 mounds onto the greased baking sheets. Don't flatten them out. Bake for 35 minutes.

NOTE: Since these already use ¾ stick of butter, I use a lighter cheese such as Pecorino Romano (I get it from Costco and it

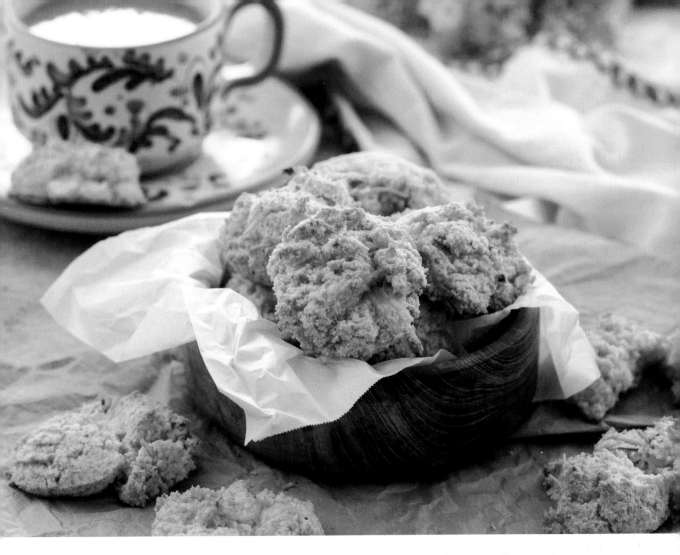

has an ultra-sharp flavor, so a little goes a long way) so as not to abuse calories—however, I'm not forcing you to do that. Rohnda (our photographer) really enjoyed these made with cheddar, but she also tried the Parmesan version and declared them super-yummy. I make these for special times, and the plain version more often since it doesn't require cheese.

VARIATIONS

(DF) PLAIN FLOWER BISCUITS OR SCONES: Leave out the cheese, garlic powder, onion powder, and pepper flakes. Reduce the salt to ¼ teaspoon. Bake as directed. Use for Scones, Jam, and Cream Night (page 287)—so yummy!

GARLIC AND CHEESE FLOWER BISCUITS: Leave out the pepper flakes, press close to a full bulb of garlic (not just a clove, but a large bulb), and add 2 tablespoons dried parsley.

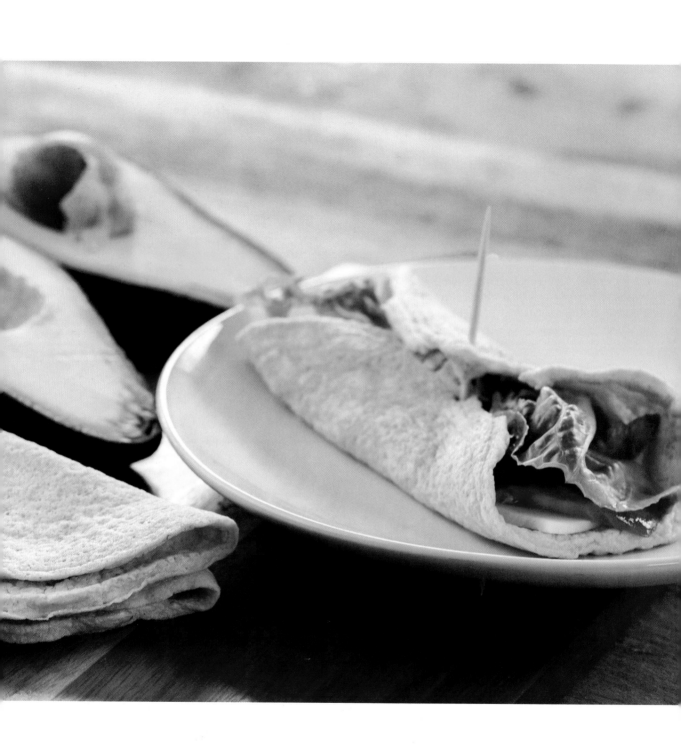

wonder wraps 2

FP

SINGLE SERVE (3 WRAPS) OR BIG BATCH (SEE THE VARIATION)

⅓ cup egg whites (carton or fresh)

1 tablespoon Whole Husk Psyllium Flakes

1 tablespoon THM Baking Blend

2 pinches Mineral Salt

Splash of hot sauce

1 rounded teaspoon powder-style Parmesan cheese (from the green can) or Nutritional Yeast (optional)

2 tablespoons water

Coconut oil cooking spray

If the iPhone can have upgrades, so can a couple of our standard recipes. This is version 2 of these wraps. If you love the first version, we won't hold it against you for being loyal to it (as it has fewer ingredients), but these have a lovely neutral flavor with no hint of rubbery egginess (we never found the original rubbery, but we got the odd bit of feedback about it . . . sniff).

For newbies . . . these wraps can revolutionize your world. They are gluten-free, low in carbs, low in fat, and low in calories, but high in wonderfulness. They make fast, no-think wraps for lunches for home or work, and they are sturdy enough to hold up well when stuffed with meats and veggies. Stuff them with chicken, avocado, and tomato, or make burritos and wrap them around seasoned beef, sour cream, salsa, and onion. Any way you would use a tortilla, you can use a Wonder Wrap in the same manner. We love stuffing them with a little cooked chicken and grated cheese, rolling them up, then putting them right back on the griddle with a little melted butter and crisping and melting them right up. Rocking snack or lunch! It is a great idea to make up a big batch (see the variation that follows) to have in the fridge for quick meals. You can watch the free video on our website on how to make them on the griddle.

1. Whisk together the egg whites, psyllium flakes, Baking Blend, salt, hot sauce, Parmesan (if using), and water in a small bowl. Let it set up for about 3 minutes while you heat the griddle.

2. Heat a nonstick electric griddle (you can find nontoxic ones these days) to about 300°F or a good nonstick pan to medium heat and lightly spray with coconut oil.

3. Put 2 rounded tablespoons of batter on the griddle and spread it out using the back of a spoon. Keep spreading until it reaches the size of a regular 4- to 6-inch tortilla. Flip after the first side is golden and brown the second side for about a minute or so. Repeat making wraps, spraying the griddle with oil each time.

VARIATION

BIG BATCH WONDER WRAPS 2: For a big batch that makes 18 wraps, use 2 cups egg whites, ⅓ cup psyllium flakes, ⅓ cup Baking Blend, ⅛ teaspoon salt, several splashes of hot sauce, 2 tablespoons Parmesan or nutritional yeast (if using), and ⅔ cup water. The cooking method is the same.

cheesy bread sticks or pizza crust

S

MAKES 2 TRAYS OF BREAD STICKS OR 2 PIZZA CRUSTS

1 large head fresh cauliflower or 1½ (16-ounce) bags frozen cauliflower florets

3 cups grated part-skim mozzarella cheese

1 cup egg whites (carton or fresh)

½ cup powder-style Parmesan cheese (from the green can)

½ teaspoon Mineral Salt

½ teaspoon dried oregano

½ to ¾ teaspoon garlic powder (depending on your love for garlic)

1 teaspoon dried parsley flakes

Toppings: Mineral Salt, red pepper flakes, minced garlic, Italian seasoning, etc.

PEARL CHATS: Dip these bread sticks into warmed-up sugar-free pizza sauce; kids love them! My husband loves to eat them while watching football, which usually means his poor Lions are losing! Good food eases the pain a little.

There are quite a few recipes for cauliflower cheese bread on the Internet, but they usually require you to cook the cauliflower first. I'm too lazy for all that. Serene and I have been doing a lot of experimenting with "cauli snow" (blended or processed cauliflower), so I thought I'd try that easy method with no precooking required. I was so shocked and happy when it worked. For these bread sticks I prefer fresh cauliflower processed into snow in the food processor, but if you have only frozen cauli snow, you can use your blender (frozen won't work in the food processor).

This basic recipe also makes fabulous pizza crusts, similar to our Fooled Ya Pizza Crusts in *Trim Healthy Mama Cookbook* but without the extra step of cooking the cauliflower. So much less effort! For pizzas, cook as directed, top with pizza sauce, cheese, and toppings, then put back in the oven and broil until the cheese is bubbling.

1. Preheat the oven to 425°F. Line 2 large 12 × 18-inch baking sheets with parchment paper.

2. **FOR FRESH CAULI SNOW:** Chop the fresh cauliflower into florets and place in a processor. Process completely, past rice size, all the way into snow (which is as fine as it can go . . . sort of like flour). You'll need to process in 2 batches to get the job done.

   FOR FROZEN CAULI SNOW: Put the frozen cauliflower into a blender and blend into a snowy powder. You'll need to process in 2 batches to get the job done.

3. Put all the cauli snow in a large bowl. Add 1 cup of the mozzarella, the egg whites, Parmesan, salt, oregano, garlic powder, and dried parsley. Mix well and divide onto the 2 prepared sheets.

4. Using a spatula or your hands, spread the dough out into large rectangles taking up most of the space on the baking sheets but not fully reaching the ends or sides. Don't let the edges get wispy. Push them in or they'll burn.

5. Bake for 25 minutes. Remove from the oven and top each with 1 cup mozzarella. Add toppings to your liking, return to the oven, and bake for another 5 minutes. Cut into small bread sticks ready for dipping.

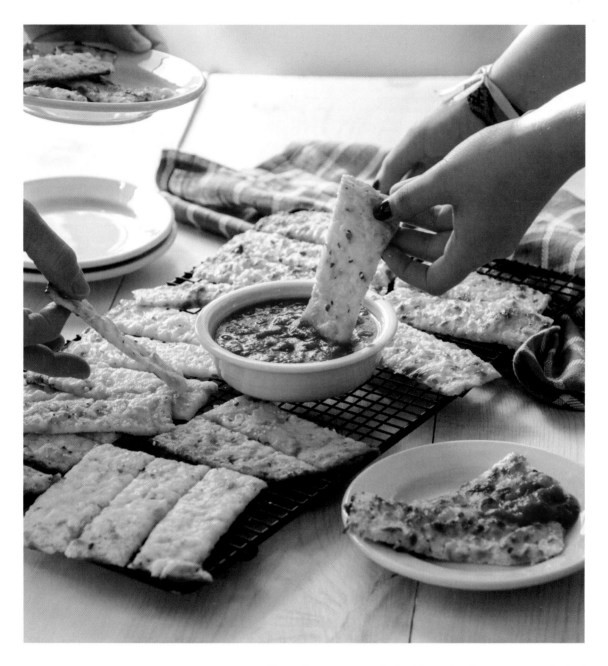

NOTE: There is some protein in this recipe but not a ton. I tried putting whey protein in the batter but didn't like the result. Then I tried collagen . . . nope, didn't work in this recipe. Best idea is to pair your bread sticks with Speedy Chocolate Milk (page 457), Speedy Strawberry Milk (page 457), a Trimmy, or any of our drinks that contains protein.

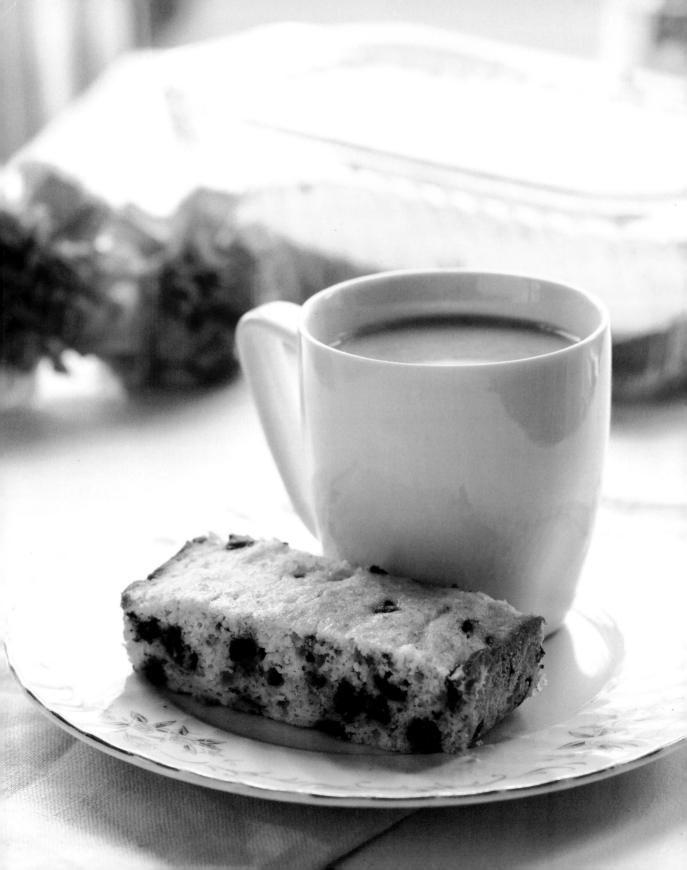

SWEET LOAVES

sweet flower bread ⓢ

MAKES 2 LOAVES

Coconut oil cooking spray

1 (16-ounce) bag frozen cauliflower florets

1 cup THM Baking Blend

1 cup egg whites (carton or fresh)

4 pinches Mineral Salt

4 tablespoons (½ stick) butter, melted

3 tablespoons (2 scoops) Integral Collagen

½ cup Gentle Sweet (plus ⅛ teaspoon Pure Stevia Extract Powder if you like a sweeter bread)

2 teaspoons aluminum-free baking powder

½ teaspoon Sunflower Lecithin (optional, but somehow gives a creamier result)

⅓ to ½ cup Trim Healthy Chocolate Chips, or ½ cup chopped walnuts (optional)

SERENE CHATS: *Perfect with a cuppa coffee. These cute loaves taste like something Sara Lee might bake up—sugar sweet, very moist, and white! How in the world can treats like this not only be super healthy but also help hack off some pounds? Well, the flour used is flower . . . as in cauliflower. You'd never know. FYI: these loaves are not supposed to rise high in your pans; they are more the size of brownies in a loaf pan. The batter is very moist, so it's much better to use two loaf pans rather than one.*

1. Preheat the oven to 350°F. Spray two 9 × 5-inch loaf pans with coconut oil.

2. Make the "cauli snow." Put the frozen cauliflower in a blender (not a food processor) and pulse until it is broken down. Then blend on a low setting until it turns into a powdery white snow (don't add any water, just keep blending until it is complete powder snow . . . no rice-size pieces left). Measure out 1 cup for this recipe. (Put the leftover cauli snow in a baggie in the fridge for the next time or back into the freezer if you think it will be a while before you bake with cauli snow again.)

3. Put the cauli snow in a bowl. Add all the other ingredients and mix well. Divide the batter between the loaf pans and bake for 40 to 45 minutes, until just done on top. Allow to cool in the pans, then carefully remove.

cinnamon swirl wwbb

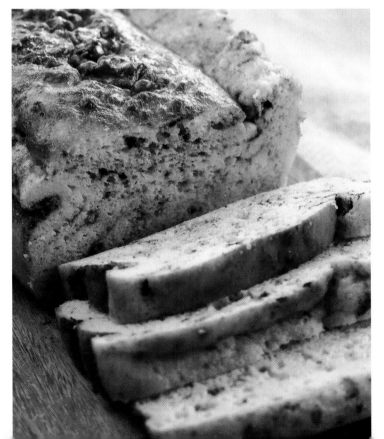

Coconut oil cooking spray
Batter from Wonderful White Blender Bread* (page 242), but reduce the salt to ¼ teaspoon and increase the sweetener to ½ cup Gentle Sweet*

FOR THE CINNAMON SWIRL
Cinnamon, for liberal sprinkling
3 tablespoons Gentle Sweet*

1. Preheat the oven to 350°F. Spray a 9 × 5-inch (standard) glass loaf pan with coconut oil. You want your pan to be as straight-sided as possible.

2. Make the bread batter with the changes indicated.

3. Make the cinnamon swirl. Put one-fourth of the batter into the loaf pan. Sprinkle extremely liberally with cinnamon (meaning keep sprinkling cinnamon until you get a good, well-covered, dark layer), then sprinkle on 1 tablespoon of the Gentle Sweet. Spoon in another one-fourth of the batter and sprinkle once more very generously with cinnamon and another 1 tablespoon of Gentle Sweet. Repeat one more time. Then add the final one-quarter of the batter to the loaf pan. Bake as directed in the WWBB recipe (page 242).

* FOR NSI: USE A GROCERY STORE ON-PLAN SWEETENER. FOR THE BREAD BATTER, USE A GROCERY STORE ON-PLAN WHEY PROTEIN (SEE PAGE 43) AND SUB THE FRUGAL FLOUR OPTION (SEE PAGE 40) FOR THE BAKING BLEND. BUT NOTE THAT THE FRUGAL FLOUR OPTION WILL TAKE THIS BREAD FROM AN FP TO AN S AND IT WON'T LOOK AS WHITE.

pumpkin chocolate chip wwbb

S

MAKES 1 LOAF

Coconut oil cooking spray

1½ cups egg whites (carton or fresh)

½ teaspoon xanthan gum

¾ cup unflavored Pristine Whey Protein Powder*

1 cup THM Baking Blend*

1 cup pure pumpkin puree

1 teaspoon pumpkin pie spice

2½ teaspoons aluminum-free baking powder

½ cup Gentle Sweet* (plus ⅛ to ¼ teaspoon Pure Stevia Extract Powder* for a sweeter loaf)

¼ teaspoon Mineral Salt

½ cup Trim Healthy Chocolate Chips*

1. Preheat the oven to 350°F. Spray a 9 × 5-inch (standard) glass loaf pan with coconut oil.

2. Put the egg whites and xanthan gum in a blender and blend on high for 1 minute, until thickened and frothy. Add all the other ingredients (except the chocolate chips) and blend well for another minute or so.

3. Using a spatula, scrape the batter into the loaf pan and bake for 40 minutes. Cover the top of the bread with a folded piece of parchment paper if it looks like it's browning too much. Once out of the oven, remove the loaf from the pan and allow it to cool at least 15 minutes before slicing.

* FOR NSI: USE A GROCERY STORE ON-PLAN SWEETENER AND WHEY PROTEIN (SEE PAGE 43). SUB THE FRUGAL FLOUR OPTION (SEE PAGE 40) FOR THE BAKING BLEND, BUT NOTE THAT THIS WILL TAKE THIS BREAD FROM AN FP TO A LIGHT S AND IT WON'T LOOK AS WHITE. SUB ½ CUP CHOPPED 85% CHOCOLATE FOR THE CHOCOLATE CHIPS.

Veggies
&
Salad Sides

We have some staple veggie side recipes here for you, including some from *Trim Healthy Mama Cookbook* that you'll probably find yourself constantly relying on. But just know that you don't really need a specific recipe when it comes to putting a veggie side on your dinner plate. Roast or steam any veggie (such as broccoli or cauliflower), add butter or coconut oil if using for an S or spritz with coconut oil for an E or FP, and generously season. The same goes for salads. We have some fun side salads here, but all you really have to do is rip or slice a generous amount of leafy greens, put them under your main dish or on the side of your plate, and add dressing.

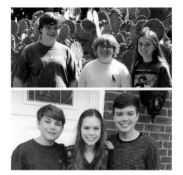

After eight months on Trim Healthy Mama, more than one hundred pounds have dropped off my triplets and me. I am a single mother who works a full-time job and prepares every meal. This plan is very workable, and it can be as easy or as difficult as the person makes it. We rarely eat out mainly because we love the good healthy food!

Our THM journey began after two ladies from church told me about this plan. I ordered the books online and decided to give it a try. I was a little concerned how my children would accept the new way of eating, so I began slowly with what we normally ate by separating our fuels, cooking with approved oils and sweeteners, and eliminating all sugar completely. To my surprise, my family loved it! The weight began to fall off. By the time school started again, I had lost forty-three pounds and both boys had lost well over thirty pounds each! People were blown away at their transformations! Prior to THM, both boys were on prescription medication for acid reflux, but today they are drug-free! My daughter's complexion has improved and she has lost all her "sugar" swell. We all are so thankful for being introduced to THM. It has changed our health and all of our lives forever. We simply cannot think of eating any other way. —STACEY N.

garlic parmesan asparagus

FAMILY SERVE—FEEDS 6 TO 8 (HALVE IF YOUR FAMILY IS SMALLER)

1 pound fresh asparagus
3 tablespoons butter or coconut oil, melted
Mineral Salt and black pepper
6 garlic cloves, minced
⅓ cup grated Parmesan cheese (the green can kind is fine)

1. Preheat the oven to 425°F.
2. Rinse the asparagus and trim off the end pieces. Spread out in a single layer on a large rimmed baking sheet.
3. Drizzle the melted butter or oil over the asparagus. Season with salt and pepper and sprinkle on the garlic and Parmesan. Using your hands, mix the asparagus with the butter and the rest of the ingredients, then lay them out in a single layer again. Bake for 9 to 10 minutes.

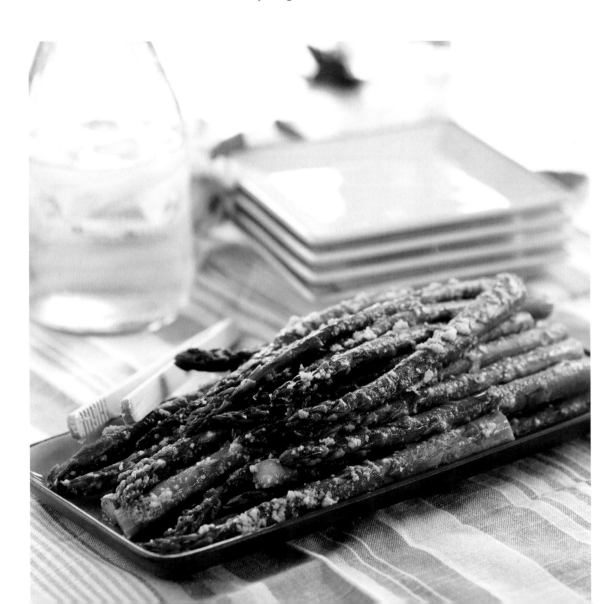

smashed radishes (S)

FAMILY SERVE—FEEDS 6 TO 8 (HALVE IF YOUR FAMILY IS SMALLER)

2 pounds radishes

4 tablespoons (½ stick) butter or coconut oil, melted

4 garlic cloves, minced

½ teaspoon Mineral Salt

Black pepper to taste

Sprinkling of thyme, rosemary, or another of your favorite herbs

Generous sprinkling of Parmesan cheese* or Nutritional Yeast

1. Preheat the oven to 425°F.

2. In a pot of boiling water, cook the radishes for 15 minutes. Drain and toss with the melted butter, garlic, salt, pepper, and herbs.

3. Transfer the radishes to a large baking sheet and smash with the bottom of a mug or mason jar. Pour any leftover butter mixture from the bowl over the radishes and top with the Parmesan. Bake for 20 minutes.

* FOR DF: LEAVE OFF THE PARMESAN CHEESE.

killer green beans (S)

FAMILY SERVE—FEEDS 6 TO 8 (REDUCE TO 1 TO 2 CANS IF YOUR FAMILY IS SMALLER)

2 to 3 (15-ounce) cans green beans, rinsed and drained

2 tablespoons butter or coconut oil

Seasonings: Mineral Salt, black pepper, and garlic powder

Calling all Drive-Thru Sue's . . . this is right down your alley! Green beans are impossibly good this way, and they take only a few minutes until done.

1. Put the green beans in a large skillet. Add the butter and sprinkle with the seasonings to taste. Let the beans cook over medium-high heat until they are a bit crispy and shrivel-y . . . amazing!

green fries

S

FAMILY SERVE—FEEDS 6 TO 8 (HALVE IF YOUR FAMILY IS SMALLER)

2 (16-ounce) bags frozen extra-fine green beans, thawed or still frozen

Seasonings: Mineral Salt, black pepper, Nutritional Yeast, cayenne pepper

Parmesan cheese (optional), for sprinkling

3 to 4 tablespoons butter or coconut oil

We couldn't leave these out of this book just in case you don't have *Trim Healthy Mama Cookbook*. These ugly-looking things are so yummy, and the uglier they get, the better they taste!

1. Preheat the oven to 375°F.
2. Empty the bags of green beans onto 2 rimmed baking sheets. Sprinkle with the seasonings to taste. Sprinkle with Parmesan (if using). Add the butter or coconut oil. Bake for 30 to 45 minutes, stirring once the butter or coconut oil has melted and then turning a couple times more during cooking, until the beans are shriveled and ugly.

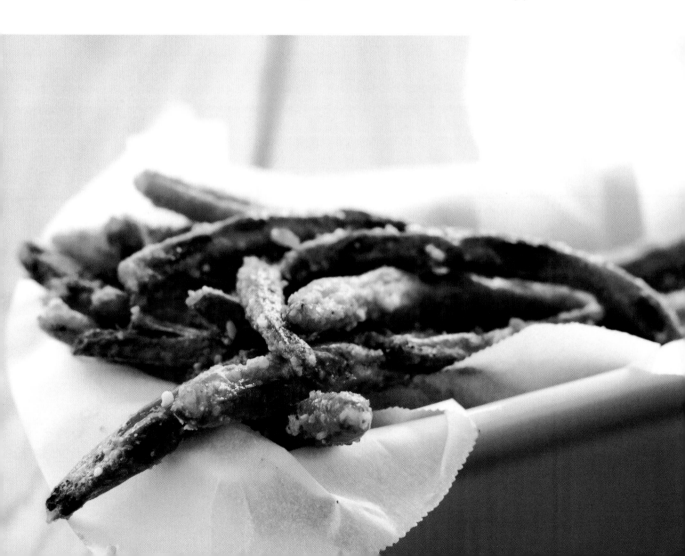

crispy, crunchy okra

S OR **FP** DONE IN AN AIR-FRYER

MULTIPLE SERVE

1 to 2 (12- to 16-ounce) bags frozen diced okra

2 tablespoons melted coconut oil or butter (for S), or coconut oil cooking spray (for FP)

Seasonings: Mineral Salt, black pepper, garlic powder, cayenne pepper, Nutritional Yeast, and Parmesan cheese (optional)

You don't have to think of okra as slimy. It is delicious, addictive stuff roasted in the oven or crisped in an air-fryer. Take your pick of how to make it.

1. **TO BAKE:** Preheat the oven to 400°F. Place the okra on 1 or 2 large rimmed baking sheets, toss with the oil and seasonings, and bake for 30 to 45 minutes, until browned and crispy in parts.

2. **TO AIR-FRY:** Spray the okra with coconut oil, then sprinkle on the seasonings and toss well. Fry at 400°F for 20 minutes (you may need another 5 minutes, depending on your fryer).

cauli rice

FP WITH **S** OPTION

FAMILY SERVE—MAKES ABOUT 6 SERVINGS (BUT IF YOU ARE THE ONLY ONE EATING IT, MAKE THE FULL BATCH, THEN FREEZE OTHER PORTIONS IN BAGGIES)

Coconut oil cooking spray, or 1 tablespoon chicken broth (for FP) or 1 tablespoons coconut oil or butter (for S)

2 (10- to 12-ounce) bags frozen riced cauliflower, or 1 large head cauliflower pulsed into rice-size pieces in a food processor

Mineral Salt and black pepper

Perfect under so many main dishes. You can keep it an FP with just a spritz of coconut oil, or sauté it in more generous amounts of coconut oil or butter for an S.

1. Spray a large skillet with coconut oil (for an FP), or heat the coconut oil or butter (for an S). Add the riced cauliflower, season with salt and pepper to taste, and sauté until tender.

mashed fotatoes

S

FAMILY SERVE–FEEDS 6 TO 8 (HALVE IF YOUR FAMILY IS SMALLER)

3 (16-ounce) bags frozen
   cauliflower florets, or use
   1 to 2 large heads fresh
¾ teaspoon Mineral Salt
¼ teaspoon black pepper
3 tablespoons butter
3 tablespoons heavy cream
½ to ¾ teaspoon garlic powder
   (optional)
3 tablespoons grated Parmesan
   cheese (optional; the green can
   kind is fine)
Turkey (or pork) bacon bits and
   diced green onions (optional)

This goes well with just about any S dinner where you would normally use mashed potatoes.

1. Steam the cauliflower until tender. Put it in a colander and squeeze out all the excess water.
2. Place it in a food processor, add the salt, pepper, butter, cream, garlic powder (if using), and Parmesan (if using) and process well. (You may need to stop the processor to scrape down the sides every now and then.)
3. If desired, serve topped with bacon bits and green onions.

troodles

FP WITH **S** OPTION

SINGLE SERVE (DOUBLE OR TRIPLE AMOUNTS IF MAKING FOR MORE THAN JUST YOU)

Coconut oil cooking spray (for FP)
   or a pat of butter or coconut oil
   (for S)
1 zucchini (spiralized into noodles)
Mineral Salt and black pepper

Trim noodles equal "Troodles"! These zucchini noodles are a fantastic, healthy, and slimming noodle replacement for the starchy, white, fattening kind. You can use the Troodle maker tool available on our website or find your own favorite spiralizing gadget for making these.

1. Spray a small skillet with coconut oil (for an FP) or smear with butter or coconut oil (for an S).
2. Set the skillet over medium-high heat, add the Troodles, season with salt and pepper, and cook for just 2 to 3 minutes, or until tender.

freshy bowl

S WITH **E** AND **FP** OPTIONS

FAMILY SERVE–FEEDS 6 TO 8 (HALVE IF YOUR FAMILY IS SMALLER)

9 large rainbow bell peppers

Juice of 3 lemons

6-inch finger fresh ginger, finely grated

1 large jalapeño, very finely diced (seeded if you can't take the heat)

3 garlic cloves, minced

2 teaspoons ground cumin

¼ cup MCT oil (see Note)

3 tablespoons apple cider vinegar

1½ teaspoons Mineral Salt

1 large bunch fresh cilantro, stems removed, finely diced

SERENE CHATS: *Unlike salads that use leafy greens, this stays fresh all week in the fridge. My children endearingly call this our "Freshy Bowl" since it is a staple on our table. I make up this lively, incredibly flavorful salad about once a week so I can always have an instant fresh side salad. It is the perfect side to any protein dish, but I love it as a bed for any meal. I put a layer of this onto my dinner plate, then simply put my main course over the top of it. What a delicious way to get in my high–vitamin C veggies!*

As written, this is a delightful S, perfect with any S protein dish like roasted chicken or even a steak. As an S, it is also beautifully complemented by sliced avocado. But it can easily be made FP- and E-friendly by reducing the oil to 2 tablespoons for an FP, then tossing with a couple cups quinoa or brown rice inside the bowl for an E. Enjoy this with a lean protein like grilled tilapia or chicken breast and you have a flavorful E meal!

1. Cut the peppers into ½- to 1-inch pieces and place them in a large salad bowl. Add all the other ingredients and toss well.

NOTE: If you do not have the MCT oil, then sub with olive or avocado oil . . . but the MCT oil is silkier and carries less flavor overtones, so it helps promote the true fresh flavors of this dish.

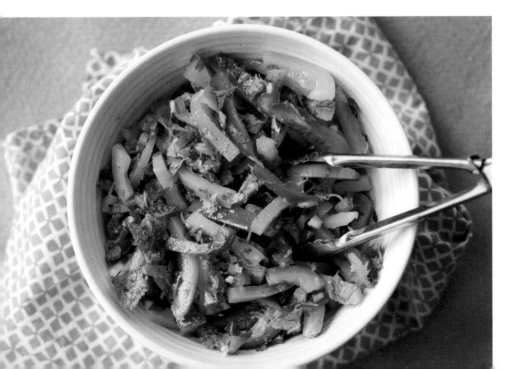

slender slaw

S

FAMILY SERVE—FEEDS 6 TO 8 (HALVE IF YOUR FAMILY IS SMALLER)

1 large cabbage, finely sliced or finely shredded in a food processor

¼ cup MCT oil (see Note)

1 large tomato, finely diced

⅓ cup plus 2 tablespoons apple cider vinegar

1½ teaspoons Mineral Salt

1¼ teaspoons Super Sweet Blend*

½ teaspoon black pepper

3 tablespoons dried parsley flakes

½ cup crumbled feta cheese (pack it down to measure)

6 hard-boiled eggs, crumbled (you don't want big egg white chunks, so break 'em up)

This only keeps getting better as it sits in the fridge. It is a perfect side to any S meal, but it also makes a great 2-minute single-serve Hangry Meal. Just scoop out a big bowlful. You already have protein with the egg, so just add a couple pieces of buttered Wonderful White Blender Bread (page 242) on the side, or put protein-rich Kickin' Dippin' Sauce (page 518) on the side. There are so many ways to enjoy this salad.

1. Put all the ingredients (except the feta and eggs) in a large bowl. Stir super well to combine all the flavors. Add the crumbled feta and crumbled hard-boiled eggs and stir well again. Who knew cabbage salad was this good!

NOTE: You can use 2 tablespoons of MCT plus 2 tablespoons of extra-virgin olive oil instead. Or if you don't have MCT oil, use avocado oil.

* FOR NSI: USE A GROCERY STORE ON-PLAN SWEETENER.

NSI

tzatziki cucumber salad

FP

FAMILY SERVE—FEEDS 6 TO 8 (HALVE IF YOUR FAMILY IS SMALLER)

1½ cups plain 0% Greek yogurt

2 medium to large cucumbers (peeled if not organic), finely diced or sliced

1 to 2 garlic cloves, minced

½ onion, finely sliced (optional)

½ to 1 teaspoon dried dill

Juice of 1 to 2 lemons, or 2 to 4 tablespoons bottled lemon juice

½ teaspoon Mineral Salt

¼ teaspoon black pepper

If you are a fan of Greek food you are probably already very familiar with tzatziki, which is a creamy, zesty dip made with Greek yogurt, cucumbers, garlic, lemon juice, and dill. We added more cucumber to make this an actual side salad and it is delish! This is the perfect side to Addictive Greek Chicken (page 224), or use it with any meal.

1. Combine all the ingredients in a bowl.

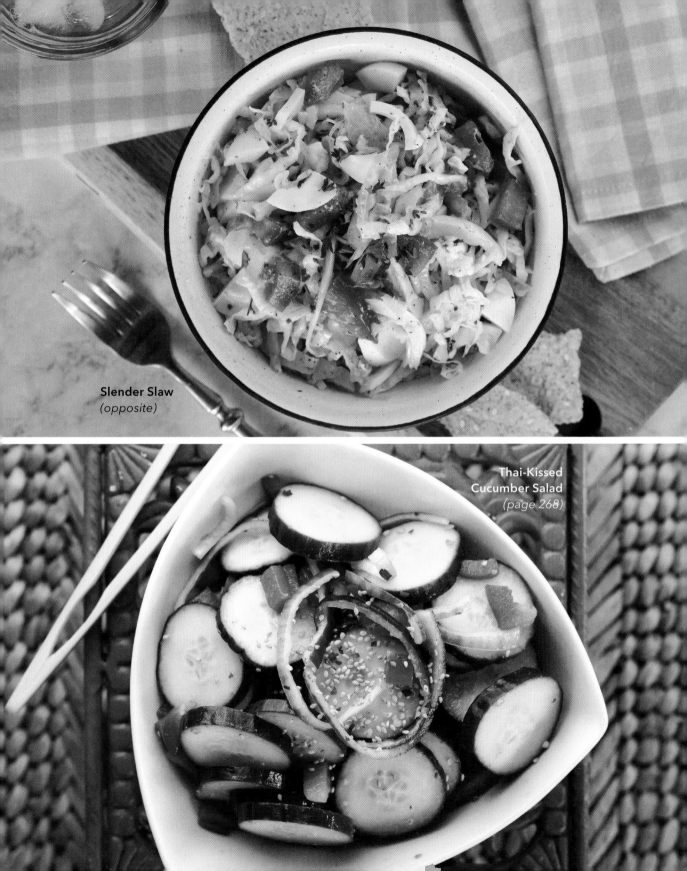

Slender Slaw
(opposite)

**Thai-Kissed
Cucumber Salad**
(page 268)

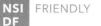
thai-kissed cucumber salad FP

FAMILY SERVE—FEEDS 6 TO 8 (HALVE IF YOUR FAMILY IS SMALLER)

3 to 4 cucumbers

1 large red bell pepper, finely diced

½ red onion, sliced into thin rings

⅓ cup rice vinegar

2 tablespoons Gentle Sweet*

2 to 3 teaspoons toasted sesame oil

4 teaspoons toasted sesame seeds

1 teaspoon ground ginger, or 1 to
   2 inches fresh ginger, finely grated
   or minced

¼ teaspoon garlic powder

¼ teaspoon red pepper flakes
   (optional, for extra heat)

1 to 2 teaspoons Mineral Salt

Dash of soy sauce (optional; if
   needed at the end after taste
   testing)

Refreshing and exotic, this side salad kisses the palate with the flavors of Southeast Asia. This stays fresh in the fridge and doesn't wilt or get slimy as the days go by. It is delicious served fresh and even better as it keeps. As an FP, it harmonizes with all Trim Healthy fuel categories. Imagine it nestled fresh and fragrant alongside a steaming serving of brown jasmine rice and a succulent braised chicken breast for an E. Or pair it with Peanut Satay Trimmy Bisque (page 175) or any other meal where crisp Asian marinated cucumbers make your taste buds come alive.

1. If the cucumbers are nonorganic, peel them. If they're organic, take a fork and scrape down the sides of your cucumber to make a pretty pattern. Slice them crosswise ⅛ inch thick (thinner makes them soggy after a day or two in the fridge). Lay the cucumber slices in a single layer on paper towels and cover them with a layer of paper towels. Leave them for 20 minutes so the towels can soak up the extra water.

2. Meanwhile, put the bell pepper and onion slices in a large bowl and toss them with the rice vinegar, Gentle Sweet, sesame oil, sesame seeds, ginger, garlic powder, and pepper flakes (if using).

3. After the cucumbers have drained for 20 minutes, add them to the bowl and toss well to coat with the dressing. Add 1 teaspoon of the salt. Taste and add more if needed or splash in a little soy sauce (if using). Delicious to serve fresh and even better as it keeps.

* FOR NSI: USE A GROCERY STORE ON-PLAN SWEETENER.

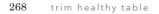

smokin' chipotle tuna salad

FP

FAMILY SERVE—FEEDS 6 TO 8 (HALVE IF YOUR FAMILY IS SMALLER)

5 large carrots, grated (dice them if you prefer a crunchy salad)

1 pound bag of mini rainbow bell peppers, sliced into thin rounds, or 1 of each (red, yellow, and green large bell peppers), diced

6 (4- to 5-ounce) cans water-packed tuna, drained

2 tablespoons MCT oil (or avocado or extra-virgin olive oil)

¼ cup rice vinegar

3 tablespoons apple cider vinegar

2 tablespoons grated Parmesan cheese* (the green can kind is fine)

2 tablespoons Nutritional Yeast

2 teaspoons mesquite liquid smoke

2 teaspoons Mineral Salt

1 teaspoon chipotle powder

1 teaspoon ground cumin

½ teaspoon garlic powder

Handful of finely diced fresh cilantro, for garnish (optional)

Lime quarters, for squeezing (optional)

This is a mouthful of flavor and fresh crunch and is packed full with protein goodness. All you need is an E side like baked sweet potatoes or brown rice and you have dinner! If you don't have a large family and would prefer to use this for single-serve meals, halve the recipe and you will get three protein-rich meals out of it. A quick idea is to spread it on toasted sprouted-grain or artisan sourdough for an E. If you'd rather eat it in a bowl alone or pair it with Wonderful White Blender Bread (page 242) to stay in an FP mode, have at it. This salad keeps well and the flavors just keep getting better.

1. Combine all the ingredients (except the lime quarters) in a large bowl and toss well. If desired, serve the limes for squeezing over individual servings.

* FOR DF: LEAVE OUT THE PARMESAN CHEESE.

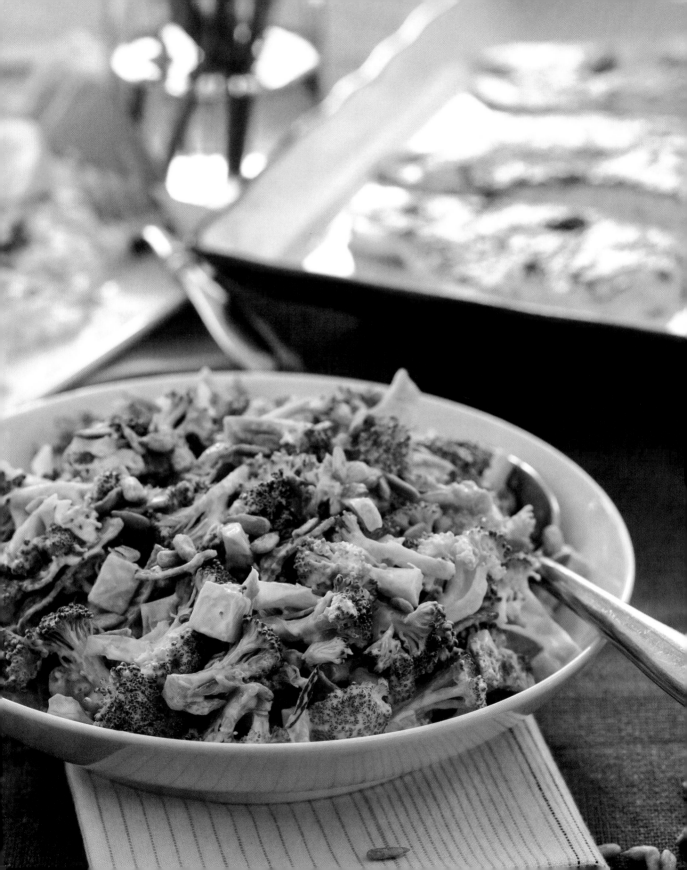

melissa's amish broccoli salad (S)

FAMILY SERVE–FEEDS A VERY BIG FAMILY OR LARGE GATHERING (HALVE FOR FEWER PEOPLE)

2 heads broccoli, chopped (keep the pieces small)

½ pound turkey (or other) bacon, crisped in a skillet and crumbled

4 to 6 ounces cheddar cheese, finely diced

½ red onion, finely chopped (optional)

¾ cup mayonnaise

¾ cup plain 0% Greek yogurt

2 to 3 tablespoons Gentle Sweet* (or more to taste . . . sweetness is up to you)

½ teaspoon Mineral Salt

Sprinkle of sunflower seeds (optional)

PEARL CHATS: Our cousin Melissa and her husband bought land right next to where Serene and I (and our sister Vange) all live on this hilltop in the middle of these Tennessee woods. She's the one to thank for the inspiration for this recipe. Although not Amish, Melissa and Cal moved here from Amish country with their eleven children, so Cal could help our husbands manage our fast-growing THM company. They are building a cob home with a living green roof! As you can envision, all our children have a blessed life running barefoot through the woods with all their cousins. Melissa is all the things my Drive-Thru Self has never attained but admires. She is an incredible pioneer woman, grows a fantastic garden, makes artisan sourdough bread, gathers fresh eggs every morning, and makes natural soaps, water kefir, and all kinds of fermented healthy concoctions. She brings this Amish salad (double the amounts you see here) to our big family gatherings, and we all scarf it up in record time. This is perfect to take to a church potluck, a picnic, or just to make for home use.

1. Put the broccoli in a big bowl and add the bacon, cheddar, and onion (if using). Mix together the mayonnaise, yogurt, Gentle Sweet, and salt in another bowl. Pour the dressing over the broccoli and toss to coat well. Sprinkle sunflower seeds (if using) on top.

NOTE: If you have some of this in the fridge and want a quick meal, simply add diced chicken breast to it and you have lunch!

* FOR NSI: USE A GROCERY STORE ON-PLAN SWEETENER.

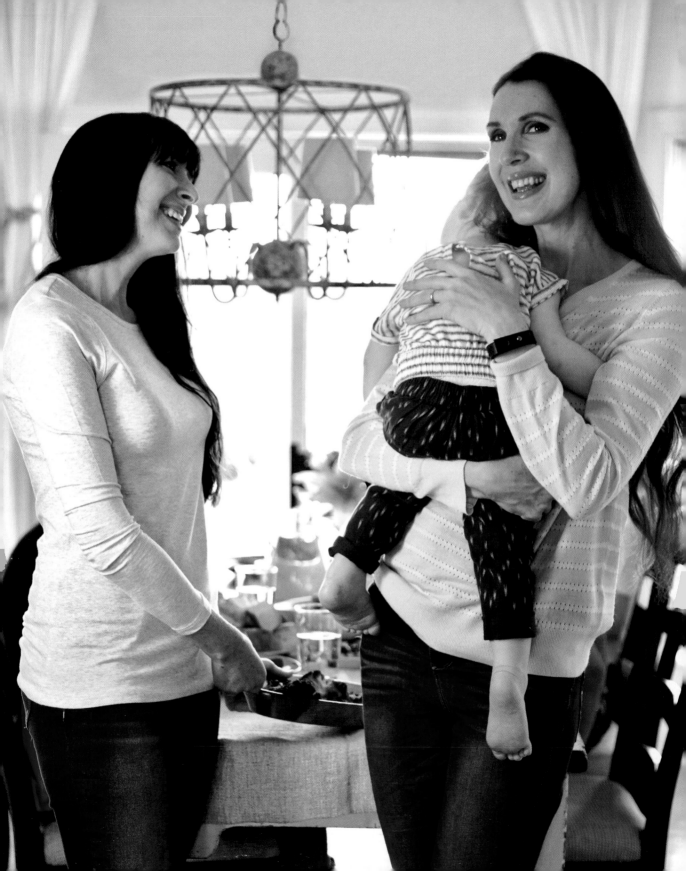

Family
Theme Nights

Make memories centered around good food and family
using these ideas for special nights.

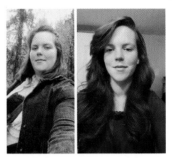

I had always been heavy all my life. I do not remember a time when I was skinny. I never had any of the issues associated with being overweight, though. Thank God for that. I was just a "healthy obese person" in my eyes. My sister-in-law shared Trim Healthy Mama with me. She came across it by accident on the Internet. I was actually excited to start. I wanted a change; something had to be done. After getting a few basic recipes from her, I went head-first into the plan. I hadn't fully read the book yet (I didn't have my own copy at the time) and with her calling me almost every day (we talk a lot), I just got the basics down and changed my whole family's way of eating. I was determined not to make two different meals.

Fast-forward to three years later. It has been three years and two months since I have been on plan. I have had two pregnancies in that time (one on earth, one in heaven) and am currently pregnant with another baby. I went from a size 22/24, 1t-3t, to a size 8 skirt and a size small/medium top. As a mom of three with one on the way, I am determined to teach my kids healthy eating habits now so that they don't have to struggle like I did for twenty-six years (my current age).

My biggest nonscale victory is playing the flute. Might seem a little odd that it isn't a clothing NSV, but in high school I was never able to play the thing. I got so mad at it. I just thought it wasn't for me. Looking back at it, it was my asthma and my weight around my upper body that held me back. Now I can play it with ease (sometimes a little out of breath on a long song), but it is amazing to me that I can now play this instrument.

My hubby has lost 90-plus pounds on THM. He was reluctant at first to start, as he loved (still does occasionally) white potatoes, pasta, and bread. But once he started seeing progress from me, he happily joined in. He didn't have a goal to reach, he just wanted to be at 200 pounds. When he finally got there, he wanted to see how far he could go (within healthy weight limits). He now stays at 175 pounds and is on maintenance mode for every meal (red sealed journeyman carpenter) and is very active all day long. He loves THM and would never go back to the old way of eating. Thank you, Pearl, Priscilla, and Serene. You have changed his life and he is so happy.

If I had any tips for anyone: Keep it simple. I did THM with No Special Ingredients for two and a half years. It wasn't until recently that I added in some different items from the THM store. You can do this, ladies. It isn't a race. Keep it going. **–KRYSTINE W.**

nacho night

FAMILY SERVE—FEEDS 6 TO 8 (HALVE IF YOUR FAMILY IS SMALLER)

2 large heads fresh cauliflower, cut into small florets, or
3 to 4 (16-ounce) bags frozen cauliflower florets

4 tablespoons (½ stick) butter or coconut oil, melted

Seasonings: Mineral Salt, black pepper, powder-style Parmesan cheese (from the green can), or Nutritional Yeast

2 pounds ground beef, venison, or turkey, thawed if frozen

Chili powder (optional)

Cumin (optional)

Paprika (optional)

16 ounces grated cheese

Toppings: Diced jalapeños, sliced olives, diced tomatoes, chopped green onions, and any other nacho toppings you love . . . use 'em!

PEARL CHATS: *No need to miss out on the good stuff in life like nachos. Simply use roasted, crispy cauliflower as the first nacho layer and you'll have no worries about your waistline exploding. "What the heck, Pearl . . . cauliflower . . . really?!" you say. Don't knock it till ya try it! Roasting cauliflower makes it the perfect vehicle to top with all the goodies you love, like seasoned meat, cheese, jalapeños, and olives.*

1. Preheat the oven to 425°F.

2. Divide the cauliflower between 2 large rimmed baking sheets. Toss with the butter and all the seasonings. Bake until browned and crispy, 30 minutes for fresh cauliflower, 35 to 45 minutes for frozen.

3. While the cauliflower is roasting, brown the meat in a large skillet on medium-high heat, seasoning as desired with chili powder, cumin, paprika, salt, and pepper. Drain off any excess fat if needed.

4. Remove the cauliflower from the oven and top it with the grated cheese. Sprinkle with the browned, seasoned meat and the rest of the toppings. Return it to the oven and bake for another few minutes. (Or broil until the cheese is melted. Watch it doesn't burn.)

MAKE A FAMILY MEAL: This is the perfect meal to pair with an add-on S-friendly shake from the Shakes and Smoothies chapter (page 468) or Speedy Chocolate Milk (page 457). Growing children can have a healthy carb side, such as whole milk or some beans and brown rice.

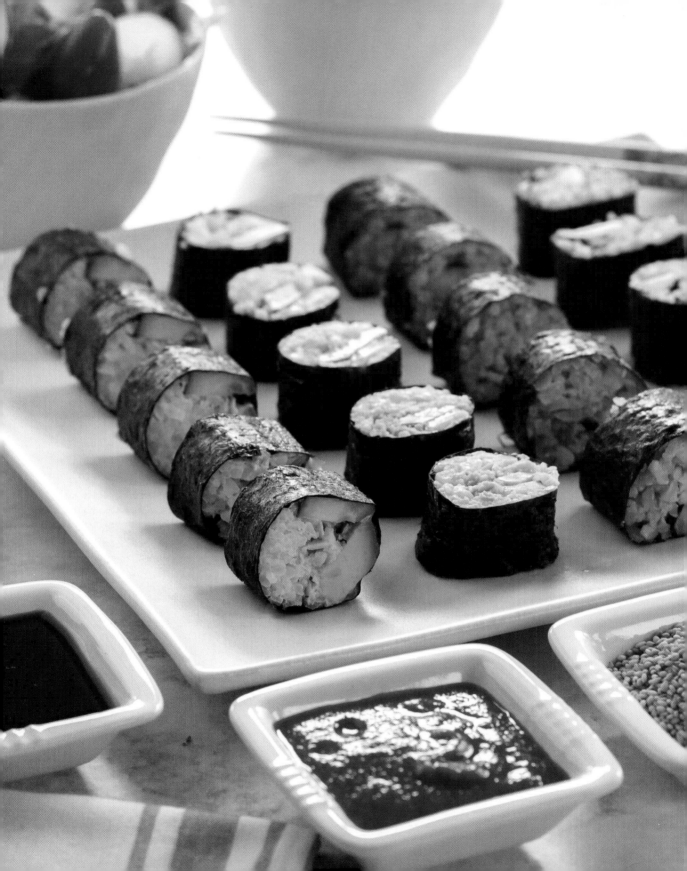

sushi night

E OR S

FAMILY SERVE—FEEDS 6 TO 8 (HALVE IF YOUR FAMILY IS SMALLER)

FOR E-STYLE SUSHI

3 cups freshly cooked brown rice
  (using 1 more cup water than
  normal when you cook it),
  still warm

3 tablespoons rice vinegar

2 to 4 teaspoons Gentle Sweet*
  (depending on your preference for
  a hint of sweetness)

½ teaspoon Mineral Salt

10 to 12 sheets nori

1 to 2 cucumbers, peeled, seeded,
  and cut into lengthwise strips, or
  any other veggie you desire

Protein options: 10 to 12 ounces
  smoked salmon; water-packed
  canned salmon; or sliced chicken;
  or 2 cups scrambled egg whites

FOR S-STYLE SUSHI

2 (10- to 12-ounce) bags frozen
  riced cauliflower

2 teaspoons toasted sesame oil

3 to 4 ounces ⅓ less fat cream
  cheese* or the same amount of No
  Moo Cream Cheese (page 441) or
  other dairy-free cream cheese

¼ to ½ teaspoon Mineral Salt

3 tablespoons rice vinegar

2 to 4 teaspoons Gentle Sweet*
  (depending on your preference for
  a hint of sweetness)

10 to 12 sheets nori

Toasted sesame seeds (optional)

2 avocados, cut into lengthwise
  slices

1 to 2 cucumbers, peeled, seeded
  and cut into lengthwise strips, or
  any other veggie you desire

Protein options: 10 to 12 ounces
  smoked salmon, water-packed
  canned salmon, or sliced chicken;
  or 2 cups scrambled eggs

OPTIONAL DIPPING SAUCES AND
CONDIMENTS

Soy sauce or Bragg liquid aminos

Sriracha sauce (Huy Fong brand)

Spicy mayo

Wasabi

Pickled ginger

Homemade sushi might sound intimidating, but it doesn't have to be. First, we need to apologize to the ancient art of traditional sushi-making. Our sushi is all shortcut, hodgepodge, and probably breaks all the rules, but it is delicious, healthy, and easy. You can have an amazing sushi dinner on your table within half an hour.

It takes the intimidation out of it if you think of sushi as a type of burrito. Just fill and roll! These days you can buy nori sheets at almost any grocery store, so there's really nothing scary about this meal. Choose if you want to make an E or S sushi or perhaps even both kinds if you have the time and have family members who Crossover. For an E sushi, you need sticky brown rice. That happens easily when you use one more cup of water than normal when you cook it. For protein you can use salmon (being sure it is lean for E guidelines), but you don't have to. Sliced chicken breast works, too; you can even use cooked egg whites. For an S sushi you can make a sticky rice out of cauli rice mixed with cream cheese. With an S you can use salmon or chicken but you can also go meatless and just use avocado (if doing so be sure to get your protein in a drink with or after your meal). You can stuff both an S and E sushi with any sliced veggies from your fridge, such as cucumber or shredded carrot, or even use leafy greens like spinach.

If the idea of rolling your own sushi still makes you feel a little overwhelmed, try this simple shortcut. Buy the smaller, seasoned snack-size nori (seaweed) squares. Lay out all your filling options on your table and let everyone make their own as they go. Just pile in the fillings you like, fold over, and eat

with your hands. Kids can make Crossovers and you can stick with your S or E fillings.

FOR E-STYLE SUSHI

1. Mix the warm rice with the vinegar, Gentle Sweet, and salt. Lay out your first nori sheet on a flat work surface and spread the rice in a thin layer, leaving a ¼-inch border at the edges that is free of rice. Pile your veggies and protein of choice at the very front of your nori strip, making sure they take up no more than one-quarter of the space on the nori sheet.

2. Roll the sushi firmly rather than loosely, but not so tight that you tear the nori sheet. Seal the edge by dipping your finger in water and running it across the open edge of the nori. This will make it sticky enough so it doesn't unravel. Slice into sushi-size pieces with a sharp knife.

3. Serve the sushi with the optional dipping sauces (nixing spicy mayo for an E) and pickled ginger.

FOR S-STYLE SUSHI

1. Put the cauliflower rice in a large skillet over high heat. Toss with the sesame oil for 3 to 4 minutes, until it thaws and starts to cook. Add the cream cheese, ¼ teaspoon salt, the vinegar, and Gentle Sweet and allow to cook for a couple more minutes, or until tender, stirring well. Taste and add another ¼ teaspoon salt if you feel you need it. Remove from the heat and cool just slightly.

2. Spread the cauli rice over a sheet of nori and sprinkle with the sesame seeds (if using). Fill and roll and in the same way as for the E sushi.

3. Serve with the optional dipping sauces and pickled ginger.

* FOR NSI: USE GROCERY STORE ON-PLAN SWEETENER.

* FOR DF: FOR THE S-STYLE SUSHI, USE NO MOO CREAM CHEESE (PAGE 441) OR ANOTHER DAIRY-FREE CREAM CHEESE INSTEAD OF THE DAIRY CREAM CHEESE.

brinner night

S

FAMILY SERVE–FEEDS 6 TO 8 (HALVE IF YOUR FAMILY IS SMALLER)

Blender Freezer Waffles*
(page 336), either made fresh or
thawed if frozen

Basic Pancake Syrup* (from the
waffle recipe, page 516), or
grocery store sugar-free syrup

Bacon (enough for 3 to 4 slices per
person, or more for guys or other
hungrier family members)

1 to 2 tablespoons butter

12 eggs

1 cup egg whites (carton or fresh)

Mineral Salt and black pepper

2 tablespoons water

3 to 4 ounces cheese, grated

Nutritional Yeast

You know what Brinner is, right? Breakfast for dinner. Nothing brings more family fun than waffles with bacon and eggs for your evening meal. We use turkey bacon, but you can use any kind you enjoy most.

1. It helps save time to have the waffles made ahead and frozen, then all you have to do is thaw them—but if not, make them fresh. Make the pancake syrup (or find a store-bought sugar-free pancake syrup without maltitol). Set aside.

2. Cook the bacon on a large griddle until crisp.

3. Melt the butter in a large skillet over medium heat. Add the whole eggs and egg whites, sprinkling with salt and pepper to taste, and whisk in the skillet. Cook, whisking frequently, until the eggs start to set and thicken. Once they are very close to done, remove the skillet from the heat, add the water, and whisk well into the eggs, until the soft heat from the still-hot pan finishes them. Finally stir in the grated cheese and nutritional yeast.

* FOR NSI: USE THE FRUGAL FLOUR OPTION (SEE PAGE 40), USE A GROCERY STORE ON-PLAN SWEETENER, AND FIND AN ON-PLAN, GENTLY PROCESSED WHEY PROTEIN ISOLATE (SEE PAGE 43) FOR THE WAFFLES. FOR THE PANCAKE SYRUP, USE A GROCERY STORE ON-PLAN SWEETENER AND XANTHAN GUM FOR THE GLUCCIE.

The following two pizza crust recipes satiate all your pizza cravings with binge-busting protein power. We tweaked and tweaked until they tasted so close to the real fattening, white, starchy kind. (You know, the kind that ignites overeating, cravings, and an exploding waistline.) You are now free from all that! Try both crusts to find your personal favorite. (First is Pearl's, second is Serene's.) Top these angelic crusts with your favorite toppings that you already enjoy on "bad for ya bod" pizza crusts. Hold nothing back and wow your taste buds!

Both of these crusts are Fuel Pulls. There are some awesome S pizza crust recipes out there that you may come across on Pinterest and, yes, we do sanction them. They are great for a now and then, but too often they are made with oodles of almond flour, plus cheese plus other fats. That means the crusts are filled with as many calories as all the pizza toppings themselves. Remember, while we don't count calories, there's no need to abuse them. Eating those pizza crusts may not be something you can pull off regularly if you are a turtle at losing weight. But even if you can eat those regularly and still lose weight, give our FP crusts a chance; we think they're going to wow you! (Also, for NSI friendly crusts, feel free to use any of these as a pizza crust: the batter from Wonder White Blender Bread on page 242, the Beauty Blend Thin and Crispy Pizza Crust on page 506, or the Cheesy Bread Sticks on page 252. And don't forget about the Personal Pan Pizza option on page 310.)

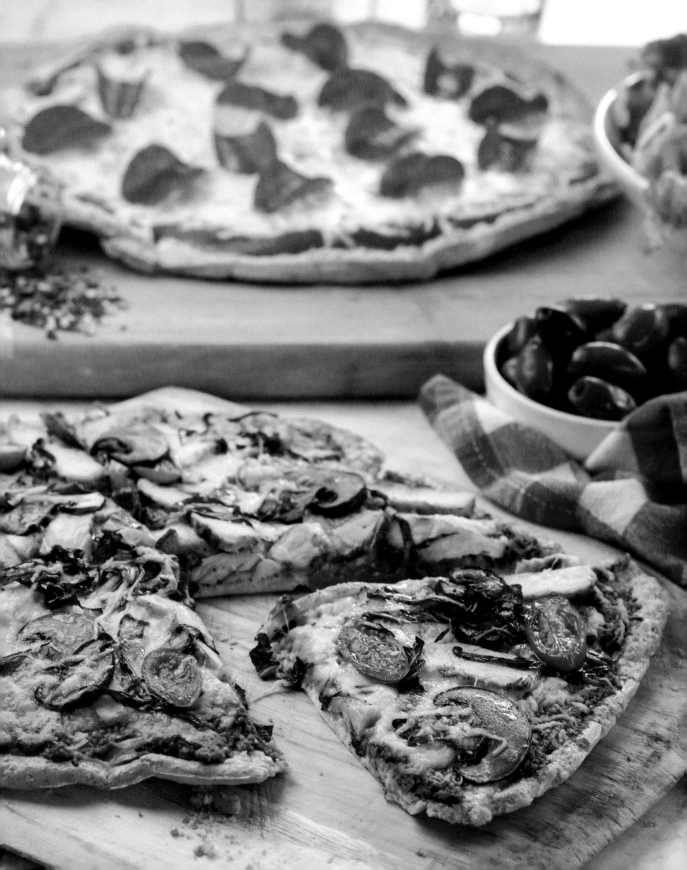

butterfly pizza

BUT **S** ONCE IT HAS CHEESE AND TOPPINGS

FAMILY SERVE—MAKES 2 MEDIUM TO LARGE PIZZA CRUSTS

FOR THE CRUSTS

Coconut oil cooking spray

⅓ cup unflavored Pristine Whey Protein Powder

¼ cup Whole Husk Psyllium Flakes

⅓ cup powder-style Parmesan cheese (from the green can)

¼ teaspoon Mineral Salt

½ teaspoon onion powder or garlic powder

½ teaspoon Italian seasoning

1 teaspoon parsley flakes (optional)

12 egg whites

½ teaspoon xanthan gum, or 1 teaspoon cream of tartar (we get best results with xanthan)

1 to 2 tablespoons melted butter or coconut oil, for brushing crusts

No-added-sugar pizza sauce, grated cheese, and pizza toppings of your choice

PEARL CHATS: This crust is crispy on the bottom and light and airy through the middle. . . . What more could you ask for? One of the very smart women on our THM Facebook groups had the idea to take the Butterfly Wings Cake from *Trim Healthy Mama Cookbook* and turn it into a pizza crust. We ran with it, tweaked the seasonings, amounts of ingredients, and baking methods and it is fabulous! The butterfly in the title represents your Trim Healthy metamorphosis into a healthier and more vibrant you! So whenever you bite into this pizza, envision yourself spreading your wings and rising above the chains of extra weight and health problems that once held you down.

Unlike Beat the Cheat Pizza (page 283), which works with carton egg whites, this crust works best with fresh. That means you need a full carton of eggs. Don't buy expensive eggs for this recipe, as you are using only the whites and not worrying about the yolks. If you can get a dozen eggs for about a buck fifty, this is really about the same price (or less) as a carton of liquid egg whites, so not too bad. If you do want to use up the yolks, put them in your children's egg scrambles.

1. Make the crusts. Preheat the oven to 400°F. Line 2 large baking sheets with parchment paper. Spray the paper well with coconut oil.

2. Whisk together the whey protein, psyllium flakes, Parmesan, salt, onion powder, Italian seasoning, and parsley flakes (if using) in a medium bowl. In a separate large bowl, beat the egg whites and xanthan (or cream of tartar) until soft peaks form. A little at a time, gently stir the dry mixture into the egg whites until fully incorporated.

3. Pour the batter into the prepared baking sheets, spreading it out into any shape you desire, either round, square, or rectangular. Bake for 15 minutes. Remove the crusts from the oven. Leave the oven on and increase the oven temperature to 425°F.

4. Flip the crusts over and brush the bottoms with 1 tablespoon of melted coconut oil or butter. Turn the crust again, right side up. Top them with the pizza sauce, cheese, and toppings of your choice, then carefully return them to the oven, this time sliding the crusts straight from the sheets onto the oven rack. Be careful as you transfer so they don't fall apart. Bake for another 10 minutes, or until the cheese is bubbling.

282   trim healthy table

beat the cheat pizza

FP BUT **S** ONCE IT HAS CHEESE AND TOPPINGS

FAMILY SERVE—MAKES 2 MEDIUM PIZZAS OR 1 EXTRA-LARGE

FOR THE DRY MIX (SEE NOTE)
1 cup THM Baking Blend

1 tablespoon Just Gelatin

1½ tablespoons (1 scoop) Integral collagen

1 tablespoon aluminum-free baking powder

½ teaspoon baking soda

4 tablespoons Whole Husk Psyllium Flakes

¼ teaspoon Mineral Salt

FOR THE WET MIX
1 cup 1% cottage cheese

2 cups egg whites (from a carton)

1 teaspoon xanthan gum

1 teaspoon cream of tartar

No-added-sugar pizza sauce, grated cheese, and pizza toppings of your choice

SERENE CHATS: *You have two options for making this crust. Option A takes a little longer and gives the ultimate result. But if you don't have a few spare minutes to beat your egg whites, try Option B. It is still yum but skips a few steps.*

1. Position a rack in the bottom third of the oven and preheat to 350°F. Line 2 baking sheets with parchment paper or grease a very large pizza stone.

OPTION A

2. Make the dry mix. Combine all the ingredients in a bowl and flatten any bumps (even tiny ones) with the back of a spoon, pressing against the sides and bottom of the bowl. Set aside.

3. Make the wet mix. Put the cottage cheese in a blender or food processor and blend until smooth. Set aside. With a handheld electric mixer, beat the egg whites with the xanthan gum and cream of tartar until stiff peaks form. (A stand mixer does not give as good of a result—the crust becomes too dry for some reason.)

4. Gently fold the creamed cottage cheese into the beaten egg whites with a spatula. Don't stir like mad and deflate the egg whites. Now sprinkle on the dry mix in stages, folding it in gently.

5. Spread this mixture about ⅓ inch thick onto the prepared baking sheets or stone using a moistened spatula. Bake for 40 minutes. Remove from the oven, let cool a little, then top with your favorites. Return to the oven, place directly on an upper rack, and broil until the cheese is melty.

OPTION B

2. Place the dry mix and wet mix ingredients in a blender and blend.

3. Spread the mixture on the baking sheets and bake as directed in Option A.

NOTE: We think pizza should be a Drive-Thru-Sue, no-fuss experience, something that you go for when you don't want a lot of crazy cooking steps at dinnertime. So make a quadruple batch of the dry mix and divide it into 4 bags so you can easily whip one out, massage the lumps away, and avoid a step.

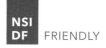
salad bar night

S OR **E** (OR CROSSOVER FOR THE KIDS)

FAMILY SERVE—FEEDS 6 TO 8 WITH INTENDED LEFTOVERS (HALVE IF YOUR FAMILY IS SMALLER)

SERENE CHATS: *Colorful and fresh with plenty of filling options, Salad Bar Night at my home is always a hit! The older children love to help with all the veggie chopping as we joke around together in the kitchen, and the younger ones love to peel hard-boiled eggs or rip up leafy greens. This all comes together quickly when everyone works together, and the enjoyment of dinner has already begun before we take our first bites. We lay all the options on the table, then everyone who is old enough grabs what they want for their own bowls. Our family likes to prep a huge bunch of salad bar items so that we are set with quick lunch or snack options for the next day or two. The blessings of Salad Bar Night are the leftovers that make your family eat more fresh veggies during the week.*

Come on, let's build a Trim Healthy Salad Bar in a few easy steps:

STEP 1: **GET YOUR GREENS ON**

1. Fill a super-large bowl with plenty of ripped or sliced greens and other fresh veggies that don't get soggy after a couple days in the fridge.

   OPTIONS: loads of romaine; a few good handfuls of spinach or kale; a generous smattering of mixed baby greens; ½ head cabbage, finely sliced; a bag of baby sweet peppers, sliced into colorful rings; a few large carrots, diced; a bunch of fresh cilantro or parsley. Do you love jicama? Okay, throw it in there. Snow peas or sugar snap peas, anyone? Sure.

STEP 2: **MAKE ROOM FOR MOIST VEGGIES**

1. Fill a few smaller bowls with moister veggie treasures.

   OPTIONS: sliced tomatoes, sliced cucumber, avocado slices, sliced mushrooms, or sliced red onion. Anything else you can think of? The idea is to keep them separate from the drier veggies for leftover meals.

STEP 3: **PREPARE YOUR PROTEIN**

1. Feature 1 or more protein options to anchor your meal.

   OPTIONS: a pulled rotisserie chicken or 2; diced cooked chicken (see page 45 for cooking methods); or a couple dozen hard-boiled eggs are easy. Are you a tuna-loving house? Go for it! Or maybe more of a steak strip family? Pre-packaged, cooked steak strips are easy. Another quick option is to cut up some smoked sausage and quickly brown it in a skillet.

STEP 4: **FIX THE FIXIN'S**

1. Tasty toppings are what this is all about—put them in bowls or on platters.

   S OPTIONS: feta cheese; grated cheddar; Parmesan cheese or 100% Parmesan crisps; goat cheese; toasted walnuts (toss with a teensy bit of soy sauce, a dash of cayenne, and broil for a few mins on a baking sheet); sliced almonds; toasted or raw pumpkin or sunflower seeds; toasted sesame seeds; hemp seeds; sliced olives (green, black, stuffed, or gourmet); flax seeds freshly ground in a coffee grinder; tahini to drizzle; or jarred labneh balls in olive oil (a Middle Eastern treat my family loves).

   E OPTIONS: brown rice; quinoa; black beans; chickpeas; baked sweet potato slices; toasted sprouted-grain bread croutons; baked corn chips (or the organic regular kind for Crossover children); apple or pear slices coated with lemon juice; mandarin orange segments, a little unsweetened dried fruit for children; or crumbled Wasa crackers.

   FP OPTIONS: fresh or thawed berries (my family loves thawed raspberries for their tart pop; fresh cranberries in season; artichoke hearts; steamed peas; crumbled Savory Sesame Crackers (page 504); or homemade or store-bought ferments or pickles.

STEP 5: **DRESS THE SALAD**

1. Celebrate the night with at least a couple yummy options.

   OPTIONS: Try one of the Trimmy Dressings (pages 527 to 533) or any store-bought on-plan family favorite. Or set out bottles of olive oil and balsamic vinegar for a simple vinaigrette. Also, set out final sprinkle touches: a salt shaker, a bottle of Bragg liquid aminos, a black pepper grinder, dried parsley flakes, Italian seasoning, red pepper flakes, and Tajín Clásico (lime and chili pepper seasoning). And if you are like me, you also have Middle Eastern za'atar and sumac, for sprinkling.

STEP 6: **DIG IN!**

1. Everyone grabs big sundae-size bowls and digs in to build their own creative flair salad.

STEP 7: **PACK UP INTO ZIPPIES**

1. Hopefully you'll have a bunch of leftovers for a couple quick and easy meals for the next day or two.

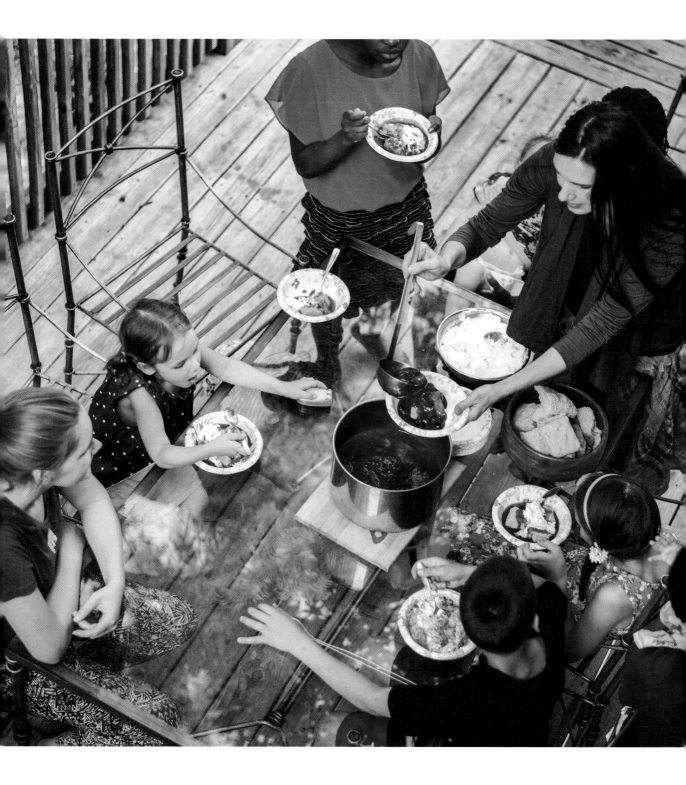

scones, jam, and cream night

FAMILY SERVE–FEEDS 6 TO 8 (HALVE IF YOUR FAMILY IS SMALLER)

SERENE CHATS: *There is one food tradition in my home that trumps all others . . . Scones, Jam, and Cream Night. It is what my children plead me to make on their birthdays or any special celebration. In fact, I am sworn by a pinkie promise to have Scones, Jam, and Cream Night for them when Pearl and I finish with this crazy, ginormous book. You see, it is more than a recipe. It is an event . . . a special night of decadent, sweet comfort.*

I can't claim to be the instigator of this special tradition. I am just one sibling among others who carry on the baton from our mum, and she carried it on from her mother before that. When I think of my nana, her famous scones appear in my mind. She always had a batch steaming fresh from the oven when guests would visit.

I have to admit, though, that the scone recipe that we share here is not our historic family tradition. Scones are usually blood-sugar igniters that pile on the fat since they contain lots of starch and lots of butter. We put our thinking caps on and came up with this delicious scone that rocks and rolls with the jam and cream all the while Trimming you a pretty waist.

Down Under, where we come from, scones are more like biscuits. But we don't call them biscuits because biscuits are our cookies . . . get it? Also don't expect to put a firm little plop of jam on your scone like you may have seen in a British movie. The jam that we are talking about for this celebration night is more like jam soup. Don't say "Blech!" or "Yuk!" or "I'll just skip that part and put on a dab of 'all-fruit' or sumpin." No no no! If you do this night you have to do it RIGHT! The jam is literally the best part. It is tart, sweet, and simmering hot and you ladle it generously over your scones like a berry gravy so it becomes the scone swimming pool, then top off your gorgeous bowl with cold whipped clouds of fresh cream. Oh, the joy! And you fill up much better this way.

Many hands make light the work, and when you have a crowd to feed you usually have a crowd to help. I usually get nagged at by quite a few of my children about who gets to whip the cream. They all want that job as the one who whips gets the whipper doodads to lick afterward. Making the jam is super simple and is easily taught and farmed out to a willing helper.

STEP 1: **MAKE YOUR SCONES**

Bake up a batch or two of Plain Flower Scones (page 249). These scones are crispy on the outside and soft and steaming in the center. One batch makes 16 scones (see Note, page 288). Nobody is allowed to go away from Scones, Jam, and Cream Night hungry and any very hungry person will want 3 or 4 scones (we're talking dinner portions here), so if your family is large, you'll need 2 batches. I always make a double batch. If your oven won't do two at a time, put 1 baking sheet in the fridge to keep firm while you wait for the other to bake.

STEP 2: **MAKE THE JAM GRAVY**

1 (12-ounce) bag frozen raspberries
1 (12-ounce) bag frozen blueberries
1 (16-ounce) bag frozen
   strawberries (or use 3 [12-ounce]
   bags mixed berries)
4 cups just off the boil water
2 teaspoons Gluccie
2 tablespoons Baobab Boost
   Powder (optional)
Juice of 3 large lemons, or ¾ cup
   bottled lemon juice
4 teaspoons Super Sweet Blend, or
   4 tablespoons Gentle Sweet

While the scones are baking, make your Jam Gravy. You want everything ready to go once the scones are done. You can bake the scones earlier in the day if you want, but be sure to do a quick 5- to 10-minute reheat in a 350°F oven so they are crisp with steaming centers.

1. Place the frozen berries in a soup pot and add 2 cups of the boiled water. Cover and bring to a boil. Uncover and simmer, stirring from time to time. After a few minutes, when the berries are melting, reduce the heat to medium-low.

2. Put the remaining 2 cups boiled water in a blender with the Gluccie and blend until smooth. Add this to the berries and stir the pot well. If using baobab powder, stir it into the lemon juice and stir out all the lumps. Add the lemon juice (with or without baobab) and the sweetener to the jam. As soon as the jam is lovely and hot and all the berries are heated through, it is ready to serve.

STEP 3: **WHIP THE CREAM**

1 quart heavy cream
2 to 3 teaspoons Super Sweet
   Blend, 3 tablespoons Gentle
   Sweet, or 4 doonks Pure Stevia
   Extract Powder, or to taste
1 to 2 teaspoons pure vanilla extract

Get the cream whipped before the scones come out of the oven.

1. Put the cream, sweetener, and vanilla in a large bowl and beat with an electric mixer until fluffy.

STEP 4: **FILL YOUR BOWL**

Not a plate! A plate won't do at all! There is a traditional order to how we assemble this meal. Place a couple hot-from-the-oven scones in the bottom of your bowl. (Some like to rip them up into chunks and others keep them whole.) Ladle a generous serving of jam over your scones so they start swimming in it, then top the center of your bowl with cream.

NOTE: If you have an army-size family (like I do) and have lots of growing children without weight issues, you may want to make just 1 batch of Plain Flower Scones for family members on the Trimming side of the plan along with a much bigger batch of regular scones using sprouted-wheat flour for growing, hungry tummies (look up a recipe online).

tootsie bell night
(hilltop famous burritos)

E (XO FOR GROWING CHILDREN)

FAMILY SERVE—FEEDS 6 TO 8 (HALVE IF YOUR FAMILY IS SMALLER)

SERENE CHATS: *Tootsie (my husband's mom) lives on the hilltop with us. The "hilltop" is the name we all gave to the hundreds of acres our family (and some extended family) have made homesteads on. Don't worry, we are not a freak-out commune of weirdos. I mean we all have our own land and our own husbands (ha ha) and our own personal mailboxes, but a whole bunch of us live on the top of these woodsy hills as close-knit neighbors. Pearl's tribe as well as our sister Vange and her fam live right next to Tootsie. They love her almost as much as my own children do.*

In case you were wondering about the name Tootsie, it isn't actually her name. It was the name she got saddled with when her first grandchild, Arden (my oldest son), was born and it has stuck ever since. She just didn't suit Granny or Gran as she is an artist who carries a trendy, modern kinda vibe, so Tootsie it was and Tootsie it is.

There are dozens of children (all cousins) who run the wilds of this "hilltop," including our cousin Melissa's huge family who are building a living earth home out here. Strangely, while these children have homes with fridges that are laden with food and mothers who are there to prepare it, many times they seem suspiciously full when they return home from gallivanting the land. Too full for dinner . . . Hmmm! We put two and two together and realized they all stop over at Tootsie's, who makes the meanest burritos in the world. I have taken a stroll past her front porch on occasion and have seen an actual line of cousins waiting for their Mexican fix.

The word around CNN (what we call Cousin News Network) is that her burritos taste better than Taco Bell, which is really saying something for our children. Cousins will do any kind of yard work or earth moving project for Tootsie and ask to get paid in Tootsie Bell Burritos instead of cash. So the name Tootsie Bell was born and it is how the children refer to her house and the burritos that come out of it. Our sister Vange's children even asked if they could have Tootsie Bell for Christmas Eve, which is their most special night of the year.

Tootsie raised her family on a sagebrush-covered mesa in New Mexico just a mile or so from the majestic cavernous Rio Grand Gorge Bridge. Her food carries the New Mexican flair of celebrating jalapeños. She does beans better than anyone I know and they were a staple of her children's diet. To this day my husband Sam's favorite comfort food is a bowl of his mom's beans. These burritos are all about the beans, so that's why they are a hearty E for our weight-loss crowd and a Crossover for everyone else.

We wanted to share this Tootsie Bell experience beyond the "hilltop." So here you have it!

STEP 1: MAKE THE BEANS (THE STAR OF THE SHOW)

Tootsie's secret is to cook them long and slow in a crockpot so they become super soft. She keeps flavorings simple with just one special touch of pickled jalapeño juice and that simple addition rocks the bean house!

TOOTSIE'S MEAN BEANS Ⓔ

1 pound dried pinto beans (soaked overnight with a generous amount of water so all are still submerged in the morning)

Enough water for cooking to perfectly cover the beans

1 rounded teaspoon Mineral Salt

½ cup pickled jalapeño juice (from a jar or can, simply drain out the juice and leave the pickles to use as toppings)

1. Place the soaked beans in a crockpot with enough water to just cover them (no beans poking out saying peekaboo, but the water should not sit way above the beans). Do not add the salt or pickled jalapeño juice until the end.

2. Cover and cook on low for 8 hours while you get to forget about dinner and leave the kitchen for the day. (Alternatively, you could soak the beans all day instead of overnight and stick them in the crockpot overnight on low, then have the meal ready for a Sunday brunch or any-day family lunch.)

3. Once the beans are soft, use a potato masher to smash them into mush with their liquid. Now add the salt and pickled jalapeño juice and stir well.

STEP 2: ANCHOR WITH PROTEIN (CHOOSE AND PREPARE YOUR PROTEIN)

Since this is primarily an E meal with a few Crossover sides for children, you want only ultra-lean protein choices: shredded or diced cooked chicken breast; or minimum 96% lean browned ground turkey, venison, or grass-fed beef (see Note). Flavor your protein choice with Mineral Salt and pepper and optional cumin to taste.

NOTE: If your ground meat is not that lean, brown it up, then rinse it extremely well in a colander under very hot (best boiling) water to get the extra fat out. That will make it E-friendly.

STEP 3: ASSEMBLE BURRITO FIXIN'S

The following are Tootsie's suggestions:

• Place diced pickled jalapeños in a "Mexican-y" looking bowl (or an ugly paper plate, we aren't checking).

• Fill a bowl with a generous amount of grated sharp white or Mexican cheese for Crossover family members.

The following are our suggestions:

• Put out a bowl of plain 0% Greek yogurt for "on-plan E peeps" and sour cream for "Crossies."

• Get your favorite homemade or store-bought hot sauces out of the fridge.

- Put out bowls (or paper plates . . . who cares) of sliced avocado or guacamole dip for Crossover family members.

- Include a small bowl of diced cilantro.

- Pearl says you can use a Laughing Cow Light cheese wedge or two smeared on your burrito to stay on plan and not feel like you are missing out on cheese. She has her hand clamped down on my purist lips so I can't respond.

STEP 4: GRAB YOUR TORTILLAS

- Ezekiel sprouted-grain wraps

- Wonder Wraps 2 (page 251)

- Pearl wants me to suggest low-carb tortillas for a Drive-Thru fix (I wash my hands of this)

- Good ol' whole-grain wraps for growing Crossover children (as they're cheaper)

STEP 5: CHOOSE SIDES AND DIG IN

- Baked organic blue corn chips with your favorite salsa (if you can't find the blue kind, regular baked corn chips are still on-plan and children can sometimes eat the regular kind)

- A large quick throw-together family salad with crunchy romaine, succulent tomatoes, crisp sweet peppers, and a light massage of MCT oil, a pinch or 2 of Mineral Salt and black pepper, and a splash of lime juice or apple cider vinegar

Now fill, fold, roll, and chomp on your burritos. Smile, talk, and laugh and make memories.

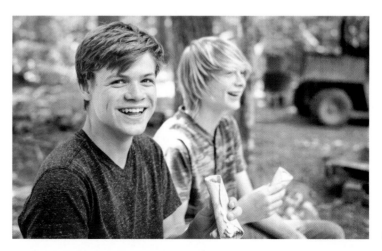

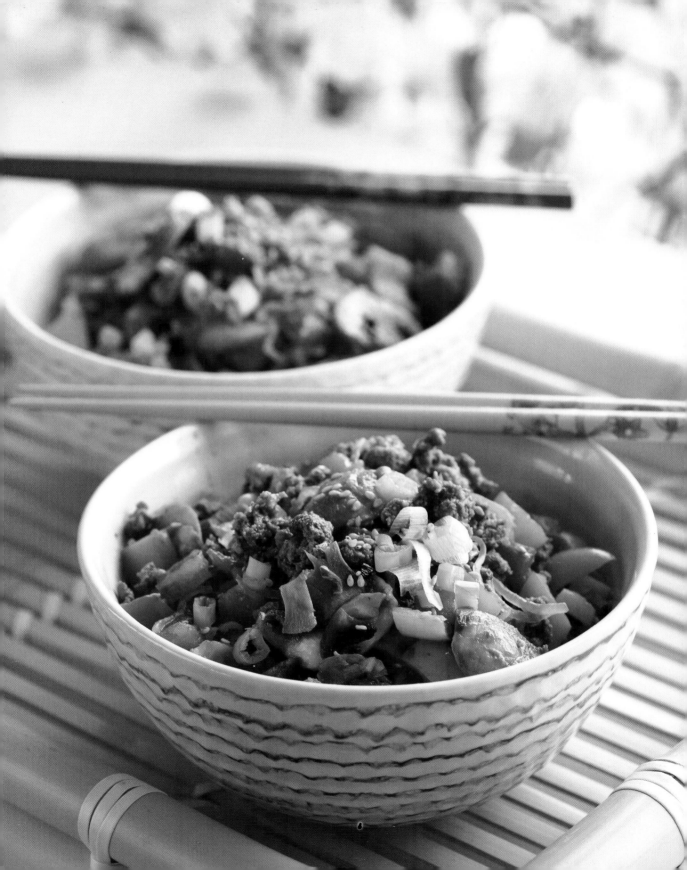

Hangry
Meals
for One

This chapter is chock-full of 5- to 10-minute single-serve meals that don't use any special ingredients (or if they do, we list easy subs). These meals will save you from a state of hangriness . . . you know, that dreadful hungry/angry state. When you have the "hangries" you are more likely to cave in to unhealthy choices because you can barely think straight and you sure don't have the time or the temper for a bunch of kitchen prep. The only recipe here that requires longer than 10 minutes before you can eat is Hangry Pockets (page 320), but all you have to do there is shove something that is already premade in your oven for about 15 minutes . . . couldn't be easier.

All the meals in this chapter make quick single-serve lunches or dinners that kick hangriness to the curb in record speed! Driving thru to grab a waist-exploding burger and fries will take you longer than whipping one of these up. For lots more Hangry Meals, check out our member site where we make them on video for you and visually show you just how easy they are.

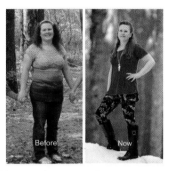

One of the top resolutions every year is to lose weight and be healthy! I made that resolution four years ago when I started Trim Healthy Mama and am happy to say that I don't have to keep making that same resolution every year now, as I'm still going strong! This is not a diet to me, it is a lifestyle. It is a way of eating where I do not feel deprived, can feed my whole family this way, can go to a restaurant and have plenty to choose from, can eat some "unhealthy" foods here and there but not get completely derailed! This really is food freedom to me! So, if you have this resolution this year, I would highly recommend this way of eating. I will never turn back. —CELINA S.

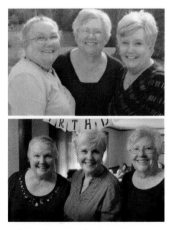

THM sisters over sixty! I have lost sixty pounds, one sister lost thirty and reduced her blood sugar to normal (unable to regulate diabetes prior to THM), and one sister lost twenty. We love to eat together and live this lifestyle! I started THM three years ago, weighing over two hundred pounds and turning sixty. My family has a history of heart disease and high blood pressure, and I knew I needed to make changes. After praying for God's help, I noticed a dear friend was shrinking before my eyes and kept posting decadent desserts on Facebook . . . how cruel! She introduced me to Trim Healthy Mama, and loving my sisters so much, I introduced them. We now have family dinners with THM-ified dishes, seasoned veggies, and a healthy sprinkling of my favorite sugar-free desserts. Just about anything we love, we find a way to make it healthy. Diabetes, heart disease, and hypertension no longer rule in this THM group of sisters!!! Thank you, God, and thank you to our other sisters, Pearl and Serene! —THERESA G.

blt wraps

S OR FP

4 slices turkey or other bacon (for S), or 2 slices turkey bacon (for FP)

4 large lettuce leaves, for wrapping (romaine works well)

Mayonnaise, for smearing (for S), or 1 wedge Laughing Cow Light cheese (for FP)

Small tomato, chopped

Black or cayenne pepper

½ avocado, sliced (optional; for S)

4 slices lean all-natural turkey deli meat (optional; for either version)

This is too easy! You gotta try.

1. Cook the bacon in a skillet until browned. Set aside.

2. Smear each lettuce leaf with some mayo (for S) or divide the Laughing Cow cheese among the 4 lettuce leaves (for FP).

3. **TO ASSEMBLE AN S WRAP:** Layer the chopped tomato on the lettuce, sprinkle with pepper, add 1 slice bacon for each wrap followed by avocado (if using) and deli meat (if using).

   TO ASSEMBLE AN FP WRAP: Layer the chopped tomato on the lettuce, sprinkle with pepper, and add ½ slice crumbled bacon to each wrap followed by deli meat (if using).

NOTE: Fill up further and get more protein with Speedy Chocolate Milk (page 457) or a baby-size S- or FP-friendly shake from the Shakes and Smoothies chapter (page 468).

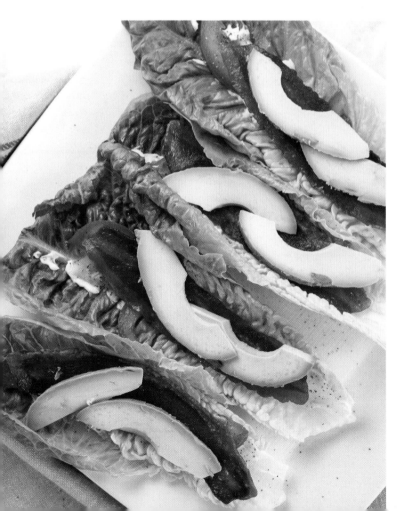

open-face tuna pizzazz

Ⓔ

2 slices sprouted-grain or true whole-grain sourdough bread

1 teaspoon tahini (sesame paste) or almond butter

2 to 3 tablespoons salsa

Pinch each of Mineral Salt and black pepper

Generous ¼ teaspoon chipotle powder (optional, for heat lovers)

¼ teaspoon mesquite liquid smoke

1 (5-ounce) can water-packed tuna, drained

½ lemon

Simple, super quick, and full of flavor PIZZAZZ! Tuna gets a flavor punch and you get to enjoy it on toast! When you are in a hurry and in need of E 'nergy, count the time it takes to toast your bread, then smear on this protein-rich deliciousness. We predict you'll be eating this meal within 5 minutes, and that's important when you are hangry! Have some celery or cucumber on the side or enjoy leftover Freshy Bowl (page 265) or throw together a quick side salad . . . your meal is ready.

1. Toast the bread and lay both pieces open on a plate.

2. Mix together the tahini, salsa, salt, pepper, chipotle powder, and liquid smoke in a bowl. Add the tuna and mix well. If you would like this mixture to be a little moister, add another tablespoon of salsa.

3. Spread half the mixture on 1 piece of toast, then do the same to the other. Squeeze a generous drizzle of lemon juice onto each piece.

NOTĖ: Fill up further with a cup of crisp, fresh cherries or Speedy Chocolate or Strawberry Milk (page 457) or a baby-size, E-friendly shake from the Shakes and Smoothies chapter (page 468). If gluten-free, use WWBB (page 242). Your meal will be an FP, or add a side of fruit to make it an E.

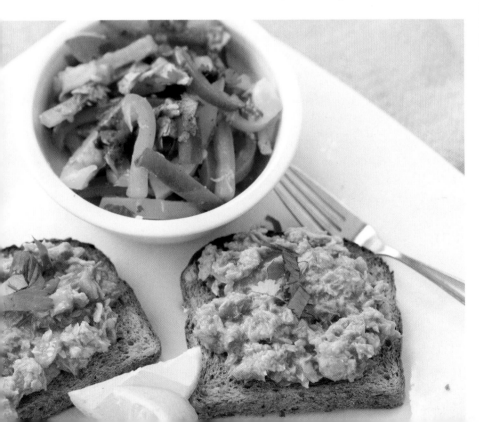

pizza grilled cheese

E OR S

2 slices sprouted-grain bread for E, or WWBB (page 242) or Nuke Queen's Awesome Bread (page 245) for S

2 wedges Laughing Cow Light cheese for E; or several thin slices of your favorite cheese for S

2 tablespoons sugar-free pizza sauce (we use Walmart Great Value brand) or Perfect Pizza Sauce (page 516)

3 slices turkey pepperoni, diced (you can use pork pepperoni for the S version but we use turkey for both)

1 to 2 teaspoons diced onion (optional)

Red pepper flakes or a sprinkle of cayenne pepper for a boost

Coconut oil cooking spray

½ teaspoon butter (for E), or 2 to 3 teaspoons butter (for S)

This sandwich merges grilled cheese with pizza . . . the perfect, quick, craving-soothing lunch. We're putting the E option here first for three reasons: 1. E meals work great for daytime meals like lunches (they can be wonderful dinner meals, too, but we have most of our E meals during the daylight hours). 2. Too many Mamas don't eat enough E meals, and this is a quick yummy way to eat one. 3. The E option requires no special ingredients so that's a no-brainer. Having said all that, the S option for this grilled cheese is equally Ah-mazing . . . so go ahead and enjoy that sometimes, too.

1. Make a sandwich with the bread and all the fillings and seasoning. Spray a skillet with coconut oil, set it over medium heat, and add the butter to melt. Place a sandwich in the skillet and brown on both sides, until the cheese is melty.

NOTE: Fill up further with either Speedy Chocolate Milk (page 457) or a baby-size shake from the Shakes and Smoothies chapter (page 468). If having your grilled cheese E style, enjoy with a side of fruit (like cherries). We love a cup of cherries on the side of any E sandwich . . . gives a nice crunchy satisfaction. For S, enjoy a side of berries or sliced cucumbers.

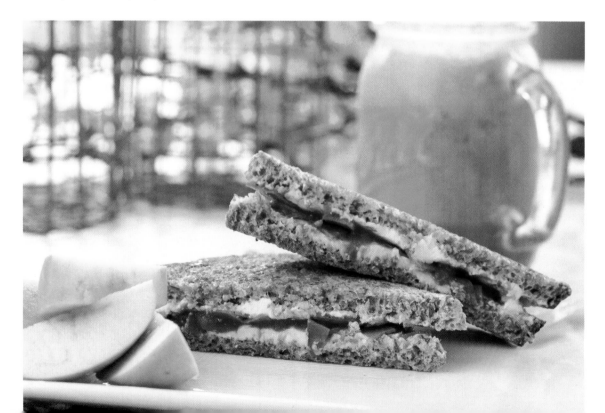

open-face turkey crunch lunch

E OR **S**

3 to 4 Wasa light rye or Ryvita crackers or 3 brown or wild rice cakes for E; 3 to 4 large-size Savory Sesame Crackers (page 504) for S

1 to 2 wedges Laughing Cow Light cheese for E; mayo for S

4 to 6 slices lean all-natural turkey deli meat

Dill pickles

Thin slices cheese (optional; for S)

Cayenne pepper, for sprinkling (optional)

You get a big savory crunch fix with this quick lunch.

FOR E STYLE: Smear crackers or rice cakes with the cheese wedges, then layer on the turkey, pickles, and cayenne (if using).

FOR S STYLE: Spread the crackers with mayo, then layer on the turkey, pickles, cheese (if using), and cayenne (if using).

NOTE: Fill up further with either Speedy Chocolate Milk (page 457) or a baby-size shake from the Shakes and Smoothies chapter (page 468). Have some sliced cucumber or carrot sticks on the side if desired.

* FOR DF: USE HELLO CHEESE RECIPE (FOUND FREE ON OUR WEBSITE) OR ANOTHER DAIRY-FREE, SPREADABLE CHEESE IN PLACE OF LAUGHING COW WEDGES.

NSI

chicken salad delight

E

⅓ cup plain 0% Greek yogurt

1 wedge Laughing Cow Light cheese

⅛ teaspoon garlic and/or onion powder

Black pepper and Mineral Salt

Red pepper flakes

1 (5-ounce) can chicken breast or similar amount diced cooked chicken breast (see page 45 for cooking methods)

1 to 2 tablespoons diced red or yellow onion

½ cup grapes, halved, or ½ apple, chopped

1 teaspoon very finely chopped walnuts (or any nuts)

1 to 2 slices sprouted-grain bread or lettuce leaves

PEARL CHATS: Now you can enjoy chicken salad the slimming way. This is deliciously creamy with sweet pops of grape or apple and a just right crunch of nuts. Enjoy open-face piled on sprouted-grain bread or wrapped in lettuce leaves. While Serene doesn't use Laughing Cow Light cheese, I sure love it. Blended with the Greek yogurt, it makes this dressing creamier and cuts down the tartness of the yogurt, but you can leave it out if it doesn't fit your purist approach to THM.

1. Put the yogurt and cheese wedge in a small bowl along with garlic and/or onion powder, and black pepper and salt to taste. Blend with a stick blender until smooth (or whisk really well with a hand whisk).

2. Add pepper flakes to taste, the chicken, onion, grapes (or apple), and nuts and stir well. Serve open-face on the bread or wrap in lettuce.

NOTE: Add some cut veggies like red bell pepper or cucumber to the side of your plate. Feel free to fill up further with Speedy Chocolate Milk (page 457) or an E-friendly baby-size shake from the Shakes and Smoothies chapter (page 468).

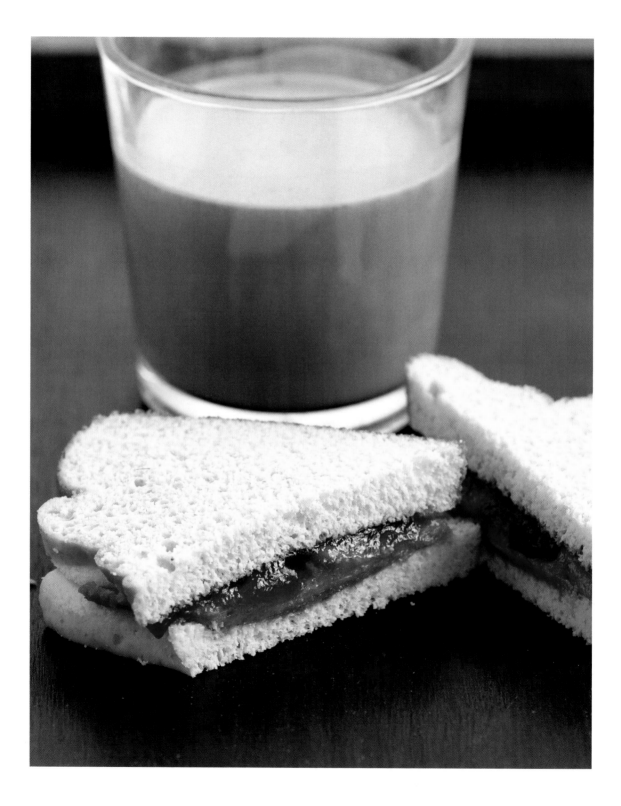

good ol' pb&j

E, **FP**, OR **S**

2 slices bread: sprouted-grain bread for E; store-bought Joseph's pita, WWBB (page 242; used in photo), or Nuke Queen's Awesome Bread (page 245) for FP or S

1 to 1½ tablespoons quick peanut spread (see Note) for E and FP; or sugar-free natural-style peanut butter for S

2 to 3 teaspoons all-fruit jelly for E; 1 to 2 teaspoons for FP; 1 teaspoon for S

½ banana, sliced (optional; for E)

Life is not life without the comfort of a peanut butter and jelly sandwich. You can make it three different ways . . . either E, FP, or S. No missing out! If you have *Trim Healthy Mama Cookbook* and keep Peanut Junkie Butter around, you can use that for the peanut spread on the E and FP versions. If not, we have a quick peanutty spread here for you that is E and FP friendly and takes only a minute to whip together. We love the option of including half a sliced banana for the E version, but that is up to you.

FOR AN E SANDWICH: Use sprouted-grain bread and spread it with quick peanut spread, 2 to 3 teaspoons jelly, and banana slices (if using).

FOR AN FP SANDWICH: Use one of the FP-friendly breads listed and spread with the quick peanut spread and 1 to 2 teaspoons jelly.

FOR AN S SANDWICH: Use one of the S-friendly breads listed and spread with the peanut butter and just 1 teaspoon jelly (or use more stevia-sweetened jelly—you can find some online) or the Slim Belly Jelly from our previous books.

NOTE: To make a quick peanut spread, mix together 2 tablespoons Pressed Peanut Flour*, ½ teaspoon sugar-free natural-style peanut butter, 3 to 4 small pinches Mineral Salt, and 1½ tablespoons water (or enough to form a nut butter consistency).

LAST NOTE: To fill up further, have Speedy Chocolate Milk with your meal (page 457) or a baby-size shake from the Shakes and Smoothies chapter (page 468).

* FOR NSI: USE GROCERY STORE SUGAR-FREE DEFATTED PEANUT FLOUR.

zingy zangy tuna salad

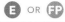 **E** OR **FP**

1 (5-ounce) can water-packed tuna, drained

1 apple, diced, for E; or ¼ green apple (see Note), finely diced, for FP

1 celery stalk, diced

¼ cup diced red bell pepper

¼ cup diced carrot

About 1 tablespoon diced sweet onion

Handful of finely diced fresh parsley (preferred), or 1 teaspoon dried parsley flakes

⅛ teaspoon red pepper flakes

Juice of 1 lemon

2 teaspoons apple cider vinegar

2 teaspoons hot sauce (less if you don't like heat)

2 teaspoons soy sauce, a squirt of Bragg liquid aminos or coconut aminos, or ¼ teaspoon Mineral Salt

2 doonks garlic powder

SERENE CHATS: *I love this mouthful-of-flavor fireworks salad, as it is so versatile and budget friendly. The apple brings that perfect burst of sweetness! This is a nice bowl of goodness on its own if you use the full apple. You'll be perfectly full pairing it with a baby-size shake or Speedy Chocolate Milk (page 457). Or use less apple for the FP version and slap it into Wonder Wraps 2 (page 251) or lettuce wraps or sprouted-grain bread for an awesome tuna sandwich. It also easily becomes the perfect side to a baked or boiled and smashed sweet potato. Make this in a jiffy for your hangry meal, or double or even quadruple the recipe so you have several quick lunch or dinner options for your week.*

1. Stir all the ingredients together well to combine the flavors. Taste and adjust to "own it." Eat the E version with the full apple in a bowl or slap the FP version in casings of your choice, such as sprouted-grain bread, lettuce, or other on-plan wraps.

NOTE: Use a little of the lemon juice for the leftover apple and store it in a baggie in the fridge for later use. Apple pieces make a great snack with the quick peanut spread described on page 301.

LAST NOTE: If you desire more filling power, pair with Speedy Chocolate Milk (page 457) or a baby-size E- or FP-shake or smoothie from the Shakes and Smoothies chapter (page 468).

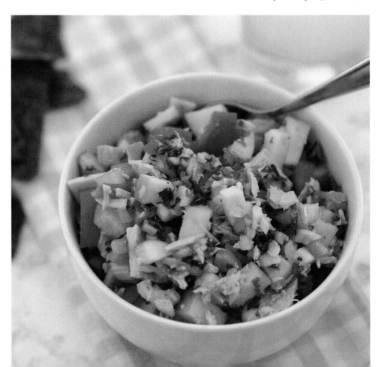

fast nachos or tostadas

E OR S

Tostadas: 2 to 3 Mission brand baked tostadas for E; 3 to 4 Savory Sesame Crackers (page 504) in larger shapes for E or S

Nachos: Baked corn chips for E; Savory Sesame Crackers (page 504), broken into chip-size pieces, for E or S

Greek yogurt for E or S, or sour cream for S

Salsa

Finely shredded lettuce

3 to 6 ounces diced or shredded cooked chicken breast (or canned chicken breast), seasoned with Mineral Salt, black pepper, and cumin for E or S; 3 to 6 ounces well-seasoned cooked beef for S

Fat-free refried beans

OPTIONAL TOPPINGS

Chopped tomato

Diced pickled jalapeños

Grated cheese or diced avocado for S

Nothing like the crunch of nachos or tostadas with the zesty flavors of Mexican goodies piled on top. There is no reason why you can't enjoy all of that on THM. While corn is not a big part of the plan (as it can be a spiker for your blood sugar and is used to fatten animals up), baked products made with corn traditionally soaked in lime can be used occasionally for E as this soaking process helps lower the glycemic index of the corn. While we prefer baked blue corn products, since they are not GMO, they are not always available. If you are not too concerned about GMO, here in the US, Mission brand has recently released baked tostadas that can be used on plan for E. If you can't find those, you can use baked corn chips for E nachos. Another (even healthier) option that works fabulously for both E and S versions of nachos or tostadas is to use the Savory Sesame Crackers (page 504). You get to eat one-sixth of that recipe as an FP, which is a nice amount; but if you include more than that, make sure your nachos are an S.

FOR E TOSTADAS: Smear the tostadas with a generous layer of refried beans, followed by yogurt. Top with salsa, shredded lettuce, and chicken. If desired, top with diced tomatoes and jalapeños.

FOR S TOSTADAS: Spread cracker shapes with a very thin layer of refried beans (see Note), followed by sour cream or Greek yogurt. Top with salsa, shredded lettuce, and chicken or beef. If desired, top with diced tomatoes, jalapeños, and grated cheese or avocado.

FOR E NACHOS: Put a pile of chips on a plate and pile on all the ingredients listed above for E tostadas.

FOR S NACHOS: Put a pile of broken crackers on a broiler-proof plate and cover with grated cheese. Broil for a couple minutes to melt the cheese, then pile on all the other S toppings.

NOTE: While beans are an E fuel, you can use a thin smear of refried beans if making the S-style tostadas, as up to ¼ cup beans can be used in S meals sometimes. Just don't pile the beans on for S.

LAST NOTE: Feel free to fill up further and get a little more protein with either Speedy Chocolate Milk (page 457) or a baby-size shake from the Shakes and Smoothies chapter (page 468).

* FOR NSI: USE E VERSION WITH STORE-BOUGHT BAKED CHIPS OR TOSTADAS.

turkey tacos

S OR FP

Coconut oil cooking spray

5 to 6 slices lean all-natural turkey deli meat (or other deli meat such as chicken)

Handful of fresh spinach, chopped

½ tomato or 1 small Roma tomato, chopped and drained of excess liquid

Handful of grated cheese of choice for S; or 2 wedges Laughing Cow Light cheese (divided among the tacos) for FP

Sliced onion (optional)

Favorite herbs and seasonings (optional)

The cutest, quickest tacos! Grab some all-natural deli turkey and you'll have lunch or a quick dinner within minutes. Tia is a Trim Healthy Mama who shared this idea on our Beginners' Facebook group. She had just started the plan and was in full-blown sugar detox! This recipe was so quick and tasty it saved her from going off plan.

1. Spray a large skillet with coconut oil and set over medium-high heat.

2. Put the deli meat slices into the pan without folding (if you can't fit 6, start with just 4). Top each "taco" with the fillings and allow the bottom side of the meat to brown for a couple minutes. Fold half of each taco over and let cook for a couple minutes, until the cheese is melty.

NOTE: If you'd rather use pico de gallo and cilantro in place of spinach and tomatoes, feel free. If desired, add Speedy Chocolate Milk (page 457) or a baby-size shake from the Shakes and Smoothies chapter (page 468) to fill up further and for more protein.

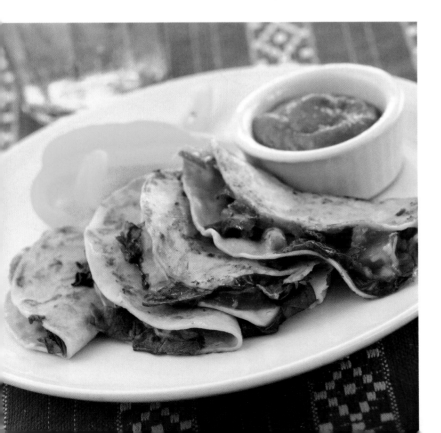

cherries on top chicken salad

(E)

FOR THE CHERRY DRESSING

¼ cup frozen or fresh pitted cherries

1 tablespoon water

2 teaspoons balsamic vinegar

½ teaspoon MCT oil or extra-virgin olive oil

½ to ¾ teaspoon Super Sweet Blend*

2 pinches Mineral Salt

Dash of black pepper and cayenne pepper

2 teaspoons Baobab Boost Powder (optional; for an added vitamin C and extra anti-inflammatory boost)

FOR THE SALAD

1 small heart romaine lettuce, chopped

1 (5-ounce) can chicken breast, drained, or 5 to 6 ounces diced cooked chicken breast (see page 45 for cooking methods)

¾ cup frozen or fresh pitted cherries, halved (we use frozen because they are already pitted, just take them out ahead of time to thaw . . . or you can pit your own fresh cherries)

¼ to ⅓ cup cooked rice or quinoa

1 heaping teaspoon slivered almonds

Eat this salad not just for its scrumptious taste but because it will help the inflammation in your body go down! Cherries are one of the most potent inflammation fighters on God's green earth and we can thank our caring heavenly father for also making them delicious! The little bit of rice or quinoa in this salad is the perfect addition as it helps sop up all the delicious cherry-flavored dressing. Please make this salad before we arrive on your doorstep to make it for you!

1. Make the dressing. Put all the ingredients in a bowl and use a stick blender to mix well. (Or you can just mix with a fork, mashing the cherries as best you can; it doesn't matter if the dressing stays a little chunky.)

2. Assemble the salad. Put the chopped lettuce on a large dinner plate and top with the chicken, cherries, and rice or quinoa. Pour the dressing over the salad and top with the almonds.

NOTE: Fill up further with Speedy Chocolate Milk (page 457) or an E-friendly baby-size shake from the Shakes and Smoothies chapter (page 468).

* FOR NSI: USE A GROCERY STORE ON-PLAN SWEETENER.

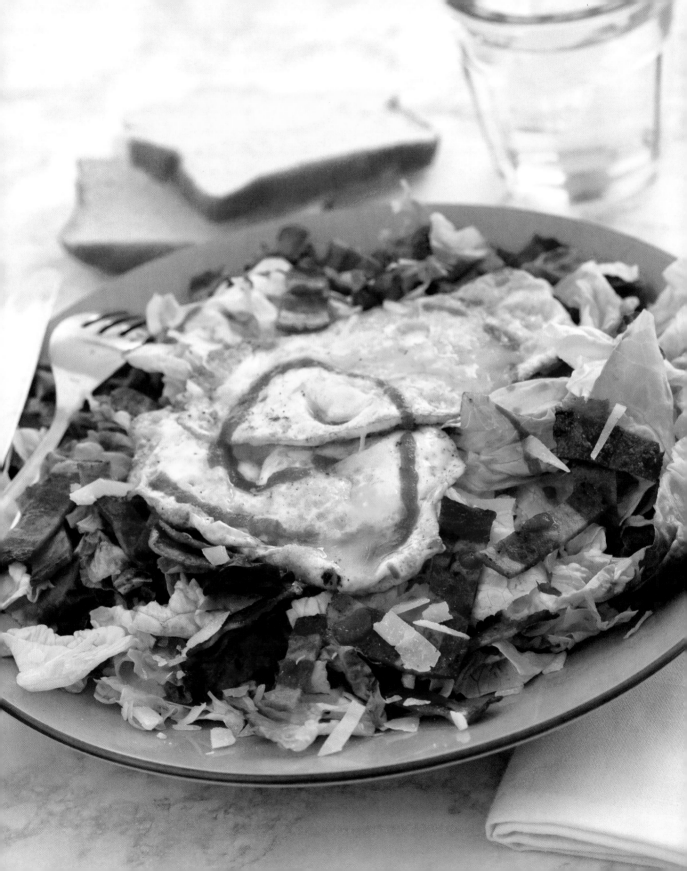

hot bacon and egg salad ⓢ

3 slices bacon, diced (I use turkey bacon, but you can use any kind; optional)

1 or 2 teaspoons butter* (optional; only needed for turkey bacon)

A dinner plate FULL of leafy greens (really pile them on as they'll wilt)

2 to 3 large eggs (use only 2 if including bacon)

Mineral Salt and black pepper

Nutritional Yeast

2 teaspoons MCT oil or extra-virgin olive oil (optional)

Sprinkle of grated Parmesan cheese* (the green can kind is fine)

Couple small dashes hot sauce (optional)

PEARL CHATS: This salad has saved me lots of times. You might think of bacon and eggs as breakfast foods, but this is my go-to lunch when I need something quick, filling, and tasty. In fact, as I write this, I am finishing up this very meal and thinking how yummy it was and how blessed I am to eat it! I think many people shy away from salad because they think "cold food" when it comes to salads. Their body craves warm and hearty to feel satisfied. My body cries out for warm food all the time, too; there are many days when I can't bear the thought of cold food. I find this helps me eat more salads as it doesn't make me say "Brrrrr." The bacon part here is really optional. I include it only as a now and then because I don't always have it and it takes a couple extra minutes that I sometimes don't have. So more often I just do 2 or 3 fried eggs and am just as happy.

1. If using turkey bacon, melt the butter in a large skillet over medium-high heat. Otherwise, just put the bacon in the pan. Toss the bacon around to brown, then remove it to the plate of greens.

2. Crack the eggs into the skillet (adding more butter only if needed). Season the eggs with salt, pepper, and nutritional yeast. Let the eggs crisp on the bottom, then flip them over. Keep cooking for a few minutes if you want hard eggs but I love them softer.

3. Transfer the eggs to the salad plate. If your eggs have soft yolks, prick them with a fork to let the yolks become part of the dressing for the greens. Stir the yolks into the greens just a little. Now drizzle any hot leftover grease from the pan over the top of the salad greens to help them wilt a little. If there is not enough grease left over, add the optional MCT oil or olive oil, followed by the Parmesan, a sprinkle of nutritional yeast, and a very small dash or two of hot sauce (if using). Toss a little, then enjoy.

NOTE: Fill up further with Speedy Chocolate Milk (page 457) or an S-friendly add-on shake from the Shakes and Smoothies chapter (page 468).

* FOR DF: LEAVE OUT THE PARMESAN CHEESE AND BUTTER.

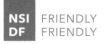
quick rip hearty kale salad

E WITH **FP** AND **S** OPTIONS

FOR THE QUICKER THAN QUICK DRESSING

2 teaspoons balsamic vinegar

2 teaspoons soy sauce

2 tablespoons water

1 teaspoon MCT oil or extra-virgin olive oil (or toasted sesame oil for Asian flair)

1 teaspoon Integral Collagen* (optional)

2 doonks Gluccie*

¼ teaspoon Super Sweet Blend*

FOR THE SALAD

2 to 3 large handfuls kale leaves, ripped into bite-size pieces

½ large green apple, diced

1 slice sprouted-grain or sourdough bread, toasted and ripped into crunchy chunks (if you are out of apples, use 2 pieces toast instead of 1)

½ to 1 cup low-fat cottage cheese* (Nancy's 1% is my favorite for this salad)

SERENE CHATS: *I know most of us hangry folk don't think "salad" when we are famished and ready to eat the car we are driving home in. Salad sounds lacy and light and plainly put, "NOT RIGHT FOR THE HANGRY TIMES IN LIFE." But you see, we hangry peeps need salad. I agree we don't need a dieter's insipid salad. We need one hearty enough to stick to our ribs.*

This salad is big and beautiful and has the hearty thing down like a boss. It has a good crunch and chew factor and a bunch of protein to tame the wild, hangry food thoughts scurrying through your brain like mad geese. There are no light leaves in this here hangry salad. I use curly kale, which carries more boldness for your poor hangry mouth. My favorite part is how the scrumptious dressing gets trapped in the little pockets of crumply toast texture and bursts in your mouth with each chomp.

1. Make the dressing. Shake all the ingredients super well in a small jar with a lid . . . do the rumba with it, or whisk in a bowl.

2. Assemble the salad. Put the kale in a large single-serve salad bowl . . . no teensy dainty bowl, K? Toss in the apple and toast chunks. Pour the dressing over. Now dollop your cottage cheese in a beautiful mound in the center.

3. The next pointer is super important, so listen up . . . don't mixy mixy the cottage cheese into your other treasures in your bowl. Just fork it into your salad bites from time to time as your whim and heart lead. Some bites may choose to go cottage cheese-less and others may get a good 'n' hearty dunk in the yummy stuff.

NOTE: For FP, leave off the toast and add broken-up Savory Sesame Crackers (page 504). Reduce the apple to ¼. Add diced fresh tomatoes and cucumber. For S, leave off the apple but include the tomatoes and cucumber. Throw in a handful of walnuts (you could even toss 'em quickly in a small amount of tamari and cayenne pepper and put under the broiler for a bit to toast them while you are ripping your kale). Up the oil amount to 1 to 2 tablespoons.

* FOR NSI: OMIT THE COLLAGEN, USE A GROCERY STORE ON-PLAN SWEETENER, AND SUB XANTHAN GUM FOR THE GLUCCIE.

* FOR DF: LEAVE OFF THE COTTAGE CHEESE AND GET YOUR PROTEIN INSTEAD THROUGH ADDED COOKED CHICKEN BREAST OR OTHER LEAN MEAT.

stupid simple zucchini alfredo FP

Coconut oil cooking spray

1 medium to larger zucchini, spiralized into Troodles (you want enough to give you a big plateful)

Mineral Salt and black pepper

2 wedges Laughing Cow Light cheese

3 to 4 tablespoons unsweetened almond or cashew milk

Garlic powder

1 teaspoon turkey bacon bits (optional)

3 to 4 ounces diced cooked or canned chicken breast (optional)

PEARL CHATS: So ridiculously easy and quick, but so so good! Zucchini noodles (or what we call Troodles . . . standing for Trim Noodles) get coated with an instant creamy Alfredo sauce. You'll smack your lips, never believing this is an FP meal . . . but oh indeedy it is!

1. Set a large skillet over medium-high heat and spray it with coconut oil. Put the zucchini noodles in the hot pan, sprinkle lightly with salt and pepper, and toss for a couple/few minutes, or until they are almost tender.

2. Reduce the heat to medium-low, move the noodles to the far side of the pan, and put the cheese wedges in the pan. Mash them with a fork until close to smooth. Add 1 tablespoon of the nut milk and mash and stir until a sauce starts to develop. Add the remaining 2 to 3 tablespoons milk, a sprinkle of garlic powder, and a little more salt and pepper. Stir the sauce well, then toss the noodles in the sauce. If desired, add the bacon and/or chicken, then taste and adjust for flavors until you love!

NOTE: If desired, enjoy with Speedy Chocolate Milk (page 457) or with a baby-size shake from the Shakes and Smoothies chapter (page 468) or with WWBB Garlic Bread (page 245), which would make your meal an S.

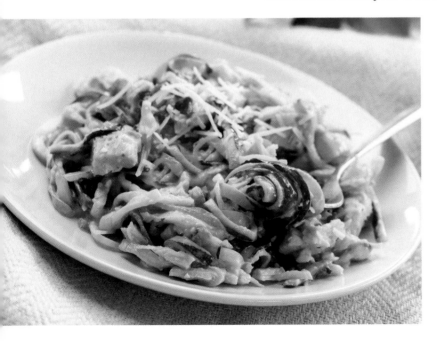

personal pan pizza

S

Batter from WWBB for One
(page 244)
¼ teaspoon Italian seasoning
¼ teaspoon garlic powder
1 tablespoon butter or coconut oil
Sugar-free pizza sauce, either
store-bought or Perfect Pizza
Sauce (page 516)
Grated part-skim mozzarella cheese
and your favorite S-friendly pizza
toppings

What happens if your family orders in pizza with that white crust stuff that you know will send your blood sugar through the roof and explode your waistline? Don't cave! Bless yourself with your very own pan of pizza for any quicky lunch or dinner. You can whip this up in about 10 minutes in a skillet. It is phenomenally good; you'll fill up and you won't feel a bit deprived. (You need a skillet that can go in the oven for this one.)

1. Preheat the oven to high broil.
2. Make the WWBB batter according to directions, but add the Italian seasoning and garlic powder.
3. Heat the butter in a skillet over medium-high heat. Place the pizza batter in the hot fat and spread out (using the back of a spoon) into the size you want your personal pizza to be (about 6 inches across). Let it get golden brown on the bottom, then flip and cook the other side for another minute or so.
4. Remove the skillet from the heat (but keep the crust in the skillet) and top with pizza sauce, cheese, and toppings of your choice. Put under the broiler until the cheese is melty and the toppings are crisping.
5. Transfer to a large dinner plate, cut into pieces, and let them sit for about a minute to firm up. After a minute or so, your pieces won't be bendy at all and will hold up to picking up with your hands.

NOTE: Fill up further with Speedy Chocolate Milk (page 457) or a baby-size S-friendly shake from the Shakes and Smoothies chapter (page 468).

* FOR NSI: USE THE FRUGAL FLOUR OPTION (SEE PAGE 40) IN THE WWBB BATTER.

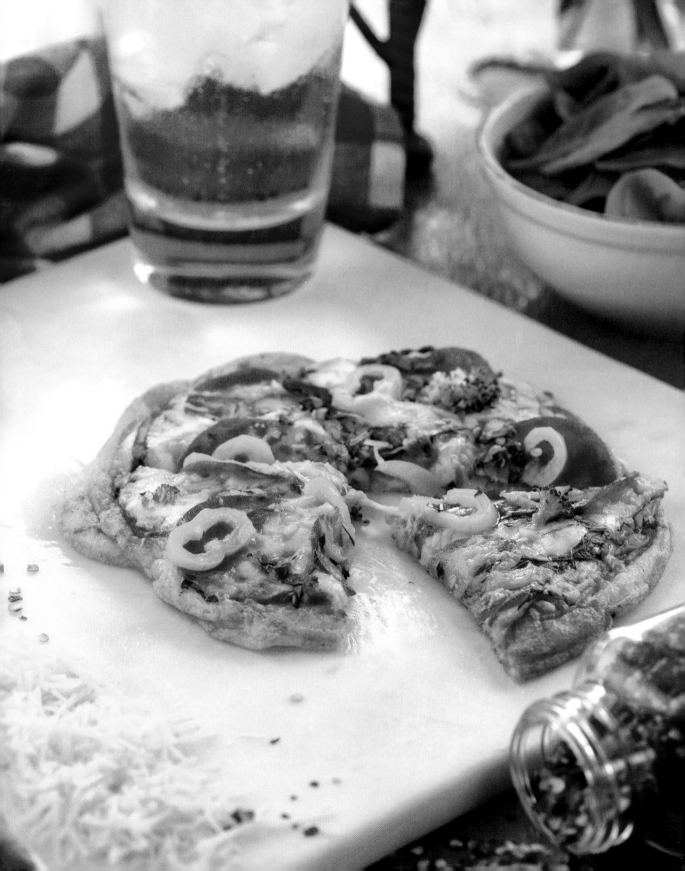

smoked sausage noodle stir-fry

S

2 teaspoons butter

¼ onion, coarsely chopped

2½ to 3 ounces smoked sausage, diced

1 small to medium zucchini, diced (½ green bell pepper, diced, if using Troodles; see below)

1 single-serve bag Trim Healthy Noodles or Not Naughty Noodles,* drained, rinsed well, and cut smaller (or 1 medium to large zucchini, spiralized into Troodles)

Creole seasoning (we use MSG-free Tony Chachere's)

Red pepper flakes (optional)

2 tablespoons heavy cream

1 tablespoon grated Parmesan cheese (the green can kind is fine)

Takes you all of 6 to 8 minutes and is slap your . . . no . . . don't slap your Mama . . . good!

1. Melt 1 teaspoon of the butter in a large skillet over medium-high heat. Add the onion, sausage, and diced zucchini (or bell pepper) and brown for 2 to 3 minutes.

2. Move the veggies and sausage to the very edge of the pan. Add the remaining 1 teaspoon butter to the skillet, followed by the noodles or Troodles. Allow the noodles to brown over high heat, tossing them for a couple minutes. Now toss all the ingredients in the pan together for another minute or so over high heat. Sprinkle with Creole seasoning and pepper flakes (if using) to taste. Add the cream and Parmesan, reduce the heat to medium, and toss for 1 more minute. Taste to "own it."

* FOR NSI: USE GROCERY STORE KONJAC NOODLES (SEE PAGE 43) (OR GO FOR THE TROODLE OPTION).

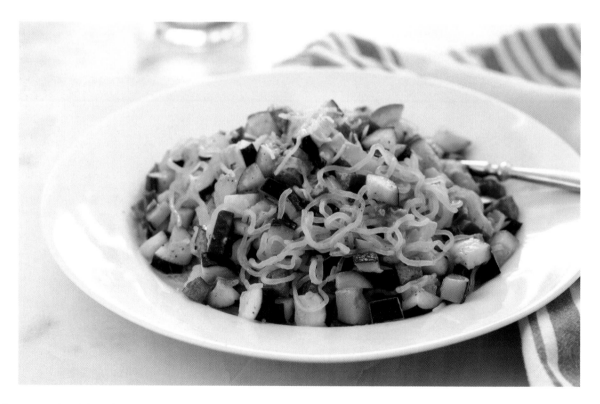

melty tuna pepper poppers Ⓢ

Coconut oil cooking spray

5 to 6 colorful mini peppers, or 1 large red or orange bell pepper

1 (5-ounce) can water-packed tuna, drained

2½ tablespoons mayonnaise (or 1 tablespoon mayo plus 1 heaping tablespoon ⅓ less fat cream cheese or plain 0% Greek yogurt)

Optional add-ins: 1 or 2 tablespoons chopped celery, finely diced white or green onion, finely diced dill pickle, 1 to 2 garlic cloves (minced), red pepper flakes

Grated part-skim mozzarella cheese, for topping

1. Preheat the oven to 425°F. Spray a baking sheet with coconut oil.

2. Cut the peppers into canoe shapes: If using mini peppers, just halve them, but you'll get several canoes from the large pepper.

3. Mix together the tuna, mayo (or mayo mixture), and any optional add-ins in a bowl. Stuff the mixture into the pepper canoes, top with mozzarella, and place on the baking sheet. Bake for 10 to 12 minutes.

NOTE: Enjoy with a baby-size shake from the Shakes and Smoothies chapter (page 468) or a piece of on-plan bread such as Wonderful White Blender Bread (page 242) and butter and a side salad.

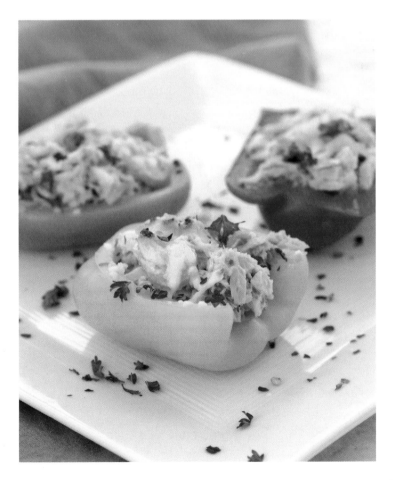

cream and crunch apple tuna salad Ⓔ

1 generous cup shredded cabbage, angel hair coleslaw, or coleslaw mix

1 apple, diced

⅓ cup plain 0% Greek yogurt

¾ teaspoon mayonnaise

1 teaspoon apple cider vinegar

½ teaspoon Super Sweet Blend, or 1 teaspoon Gentle Sweet*

1 (5-ounce) can tuna (or canned chicken if you don't like fish)

Seasonings: Mineral Salt, black pepper, and red pepper flakes

This makes for a quick, filling lunch that comes together in less than 5 minutes. The cabbage gives it a crunch while the sweet creamy yogurt dressing creams it up perfectly.

1. Put the cabbage and apple in a ceramic cereal bowl.

2. In another small bowl, put the yogurt and mayo, then add the vinegar to the side of the bowl. Put the sweetener into the vinegar to dissolve, then mix all together.

3. Add the dressing to the cabbage and apple. Stir together, then add the tuna and seasonings to taste.

NOTE: Fill up further with Speedy Chocolate Milk (page 457) or Speedy Strawberry Milk (page 457) or a baby-size shake or smoothie from the Shakes and Smoothies chapter (page 468).

* FOR NSI: USE A GROCERY STORE ON-PLAN SWEETENER.

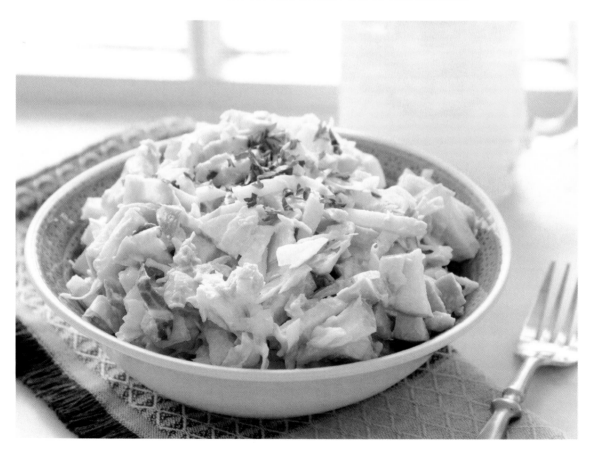

zucchini pizza bites S

Coconut oil cooking spray

1 medium to large zucchini, cut crosswise into ¼-inch-thick rounds

Mineral Salt and black pepper

1 to 2 tablespoons sugar-free pizza sauce, store-bought or Perfect Pizza Sauce (page 516)

Grated part-skim mozzarella cheese

Diced pepperoni (we use turkey, but you can use any kind)

Diced onion and other fixin's of your choice, such as diced olives (optional)

Italian seasoning

You got 5 minutes? You got pizza . . . along with a nice amount of slimming veggies! Trim down while you enjoy every bite.

1. Preheat the oven to high broil.

2. Spray a large skillet with coconut oil and heat over medium-high heat. Add the zucchini rounds and sprinkle lightly with salt and pepper. Lightly brown each side for just a minute or so, then transfer to a baking sheet.

3. Smear each zucchini round with pizza sauce, followed by mozzarella, pepperoni (and any other topping options), and a sprinkle of Italian seasoning. Broil for a couple minutes, or until the cheese is bubbling. (Watch that they don't burn as this happens very quickly.)

NOTE: Fill up further with Speedy Chocolate Milk (page 457) or a baby-size S-friendly shake from the Shakes and Smoothies chapter (page 468) or WWBB Garlic Bread (page 245).

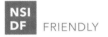

chimichanga come to mama S

2 Wonder Wraps 2 (page 251), or 1 medium (or 2 small) store-bought low-carb wraps

3 to 6 ounces precooked ground meat or shredded cooked chicken (seasoned with Mineral Salt, pepper, garlic, cumin, and paprika)

2 tablespoons canned Ro-tel-style diced tomatoes and green chilies (mild or medium)

Grated cheddar or mozzarella cheese*

1 to 2 tablespoons coconut oil or butter*

Sour cream,* for topping

Sorry if you are a guy reading this and thinking, Hey, I'd like to eat that. You can call it Chimichanga Come to Papa.

1. Stuff the wraps with the meat, tomatoes, and cheese. Fold or roll. Heat the oil in a skillet over medium-high heat, add the chimichangas, and brown. Top with sour cream and get it in your mouth! Enjoy with a side salad.

VARIATION

PIZZA POCKETS: Make pizza pockets using this idea. Put pepperoni, spinach, and cheese into the wraps and sauté in the same manner. Perfect for dipping into sugar-free pizza sauce.

* FOR DF: LEAVE OUT THE CHEESE, BUTTER, AND SOUR CREAM.

succulent fish and veggies

FP WITH S AND E OPTIONS

Coconut oil cooking spray

1 small or ½ very large zucchini, grated

1 medium tomato, diced

2 teaspoons apple cider vinegar

4 pinches Mineral Salt (more if needed after final tasting)

⅛ teaspoon black pepper

1 doonk cayenne pepper, or ¼ teaspoon chipotle powder (optional, for heat lovers)

1 tablespoon Nutritional Yeast

1 large or 2 smaller tilapia or other thin whitefish fillets

Seasonings: dried parsley flakes, Mineral Salt, and black pepper

Lemon wedge (optional)

SERENE CHATS: *This super-quick single-serve recipe is not only delicious, but wields super slimming powers. You would never believe the luscious mouthfeel of this dish belongs to a meal that falls safely within the FP boundaries. This is one of my favorite quick lunches or (if doubled) an easy healthy dinner for hubby and me when the kids are having a movie night and eating popcorn.*

I want you to enjoy this meal as a true FP sometimes, because we all need a lighter FP meal now and then, but feel free to also try it as an S by using butter or coconut oil to cook the fish. Or for a delightful E, toss in some cooked brown rice with the veggies.

1. Heat a small skillet over medium-high heat and spray with coconut oil. Add the zucchini and tomato. Add the vinegar, salt, black pepper, and cayenne (if using) and sauté for 2 to 3 minutes, until the veggies start to become soft and delicate. Reduce the heat to low and allow the veggies to simmer for another minute or 2. Add the nutritional yeast, stir well, then taste and adjust the flavors to "own it!" Plate the veggies and cover them to keep warm while you cook the fish.

2. Spray the skillet with coconut oil once again and increase the heat to medium-high. Sprinkle the fish with the seasonings to taste and place it sprinkled side down in the hot pan. Lightly sprinkle the top side of the fish with seasonings and cook about 2 minutes, or until the bottom side is nicely crisped. Flip the fillet over and cook until opaque, another 1 to 3 minutes (depending on the thickness of the fish). Lay the fish on top of your plated veggies. Squeeze on lemon juice (if desired).

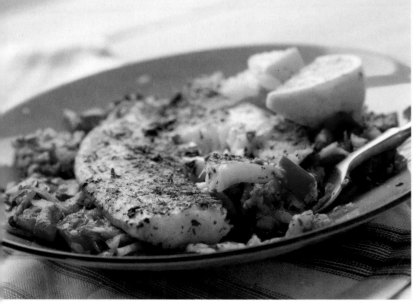

ramen bowl

S WITH FP OPTION

1 teaspoon coconut oil

2 teaspoons toasted sesame oil

1 garlic clove, minced

1 thumbnail-size piece of fresh ginger, minced, or ¼ teaspoon ground ginger

1 single-serve bag Trim Healthy Noodles or Not Naughty Noodles,* well rinsed and drained

2 teaspoons Nutritional Yeast

4 to 5 pinches Mineral Salt

Sprinkle of red pepper flakes

Sprinkle of cayenne pepper (optional)

½ teaspoon dried parsley flakes

1 doonk Pure Stevia Extract Powder, 1 teaspoon Gentle Sweet, or ½ teaspoon Super Sweet Blend*

Squirt or two of Bragg liquid aminos or soy sauce

1½ to 2 cups chicken broth

2 to 3 ounces cooked diced chicken breast or canned or pouch-packed salmon

Takes all of 5 minutes to make this amazing, Asian-inspired fat-blitzing soup.

1. Heat the coconut oil and 1 teaspoon of the sesame oil in a small saucepan over medium-high heat. Add the garlic and ginger and toss in the oil for a minute or so. Add the noodles, increase the heat to high, and add the nutritional yeast, salt, pepper flakes, cayenne (if using), parsley flakes, stevia powder, and liquid aminos and cook for 2 to 3 minutes.

2. Add the broth and chicken or salmon. Bring it to a boil, then simmer for another minute or so. Stir in the remaining 1 teaspoon sesame oil, then taste test to adjust the flavors to "own it."

NOTE: For an FP meal, omit the coconut oil and use only 1 teaspoon sesame oil.

* FOR NSI: USE GROCERY STORE KONJAC NOODLES (SEE PAGE 43) AND A GROCERY STORE ON-PLAN SWEETENER.

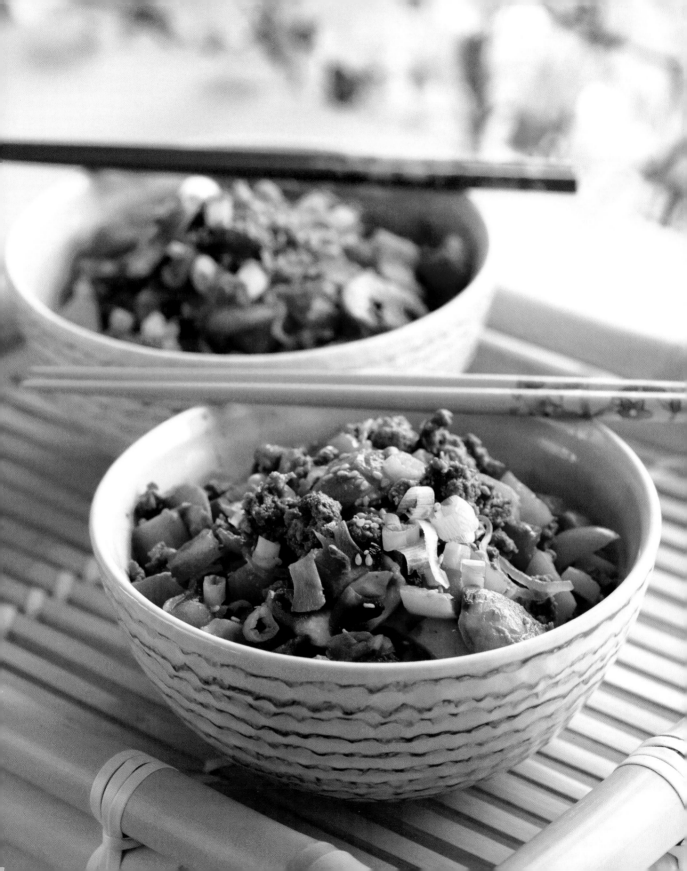

big 'n' beefy noodle bowl

MAKES 2 SUPER-LARGE HANGRY SERVINGS

FOR THE QUICK SAUTÉ

½ pound ground beef (I use grass-fed, but you can use whatever)

2 single-serve bags Trim Healthy Noodles or Not Naughty Noodles,* well rinsed and drained

2 bell peppers, diced (whatever color you want to splash on your dish)

2 tomatoes, diced

Couple green onions, finely diced

2 to 4 garlic cloves, minced

2 cups sliced mushrooms

½ teaspoon Mineral Salt

FOR THE QUICK SAUCE

1 tablespoon tomato paste

2 teaspoons yellow miso

2 teaspoons Nutritional Yeast

2 teaspoons Integral Collagen*

⅛ teaspoon Sunflower Lecithin (optional)

1 tablespoon soy sauce

2 teaspoons MCT oil (or toasted sesame oil for a more Asian flair)

1 tablespoon rice vinegar, or ½ tablespoon apple cider vinegar

1 teaspoon liquid smoke (optional)

Chunk of fresh chili pepper (I use ½ habanero with seeds for a real heat kick, but you may only want half a jalapeño without seeds if you don't like a lot of spice)

¾ cup boiling water

Toasted sesame seeds, for garnish (optional)

SERENE CHATS: *Have you been rushing about today and now you are beyond the normal parameters of hungry? Are you ready to eat the head off of the person next to you, not necessarily because they'd be tasty but because your blood sugar has taken a dive and you're now Mrs. Hangry Pants (or Mr. if you're a guy)? Stop a second and let's plan this wisely. Don't grab the Doritos or a whole box of Cheez-Its and chow down with reckless abandon. I've got something for you . . . it's big, it's beefy, and it is beautifully kind to your waistline.*

You might think this "puristy" recipe looks a little too detailed to belong in the Hangry chapter, but it is just a few steps and it makes two servings for the time it takes to make one. That's right, if you don't have another hangry human wanting to gobble up the extra portion, all the better; put it in the fridge for a "heat-up quickie" meal tomorrow. So I'm watching you . . . don't you turn up your nose at the ingredient list thinking it looks long and involved because it really is not.

1. Make the quick sauté. Brown the beef in a skillet over medium-high heat. Drain the excess fat from the browned beef and put the beef in a bowl. Throw the drained noodles into the skillet and fry them over high heat for a minute or two to soak up some of the beef flavor. Push them to one side of the pan.

2. Reduce the heat to medium-high. Add the bell peppers, tomatoes, green onions, garlic, mushrooms, and salt and start sautéing again. (If you used very lean grass-fed beef, you might need a little spritz of coconut oil or some butter to moisten the pan.)

3. Make the quick sauce. Blend all the ingredients using a stick blender (or a blender).

4. Return the browned beef to the skillet, pour on the sauce, and cook for just 2 to 4 minutes, until the veggies are cooked. Stir, taste, and adjust the flavors to "own it" (you may need more salt).

5. Divide between 2 bowls, toss on your sesame seeds (if using), give one bowl to someone else or put it in the fridge for tomorrow. Shove your fork in your bowl and chow down.

* FOR NSI: THE COLLAGEN SEEMS TO MAKE THE SAUCE A LITTLE CREAMIER, BUT YOU CAN SUB IT OUT WITH A GROCERY STORE PLAIN GELATIN. FIND KONJAC NOODLES AT YOUR GROCERY STORE (SEE PAGE 43).

hangry pockets

S, **E**, OR **FP**

Think of Hangry Pockets as your THM frozen dinners. Extreme hangry moments are not the time to be fixin' and fiddling with food prep. Sumpin's gonna blow if you have to prepare a "start from scratchy" meal. Now thanks to Hangry Pockets, it won't be your temper or waistline blowing up, only these delicious pockets as they steam in the oven. They literally blow up with steam and lock in all the goodness of your food while quickly cooking a moist and succulent gourmetfest of flavors in a pouch.

It is a great idea to take a Saturday once a month and fill some large gallon zippies with these pouches to put in your freezer. Just throw a couple pockets in the fridge to thaw the night before and you will have a hangry meal or two ready to go the next day. All Hangry Pockets are a one-dish meal with protein, lots of veggies, and include a grain or sweet potato for E versions. Try our example recipes, but then branch out into your own "besties." Thin fish fillets work the fastest and are soooo scrumptious. We think even people that turn up their noses at fish will be astounded at the yum factor. Chicken tenderloins and even ground meat work fab, too, so the sky is the limit with these Hangry Packets of flavor-bomb goodness.

In France they call this method of cooking *en papillote,* which actually means "in a butterfly." Isn't that fitting for a THM meal? The parchment pocket is cut in the shape of a butterfly (or a heart) so the modern meaning of *en papillote* means "baked in parchment." While baking with aluminum foil seems to be all the rage these days, we try to avoid heating food with foil due to the health hazards of metal toxicity. Parchment paper does not pose the same potential health issues and this pocket idea allows for beautiful, moist, flavorful oven-steamed meals.

Below is our tutorial for how to make these pockets in four easy steps, followed by our example Hangry Pocket recipes. If you are more of a visual person, please see our video on how to make Hangry Pockets free on our website or also on our member site.

STEP 1: CHOOSE YOUR PROTEIN

OPTIONS: frozen or fresh white fish or salmon; frozen or fresh chicken tenderloins; frozen or fresh ground beef for S or at minimum 96% ground lean turkey; venison or grass-fed beef for E or FP; frozen or fresh diced stew meat for S

STEP 2: CHOOSE YOUR VEGGIES
AND OPTIONAL GRAIN OR SWEET POTATO

NOTE: Choose quick-cooking veggies. If you'd like to include some veggies that are a bit tougher, you can do a quick steam to get a head start.

VEGGIE OPTIONS: thinly sliced or diced zucchini or summer squash; handfuls of fresh or frozen spinach, kale, or other

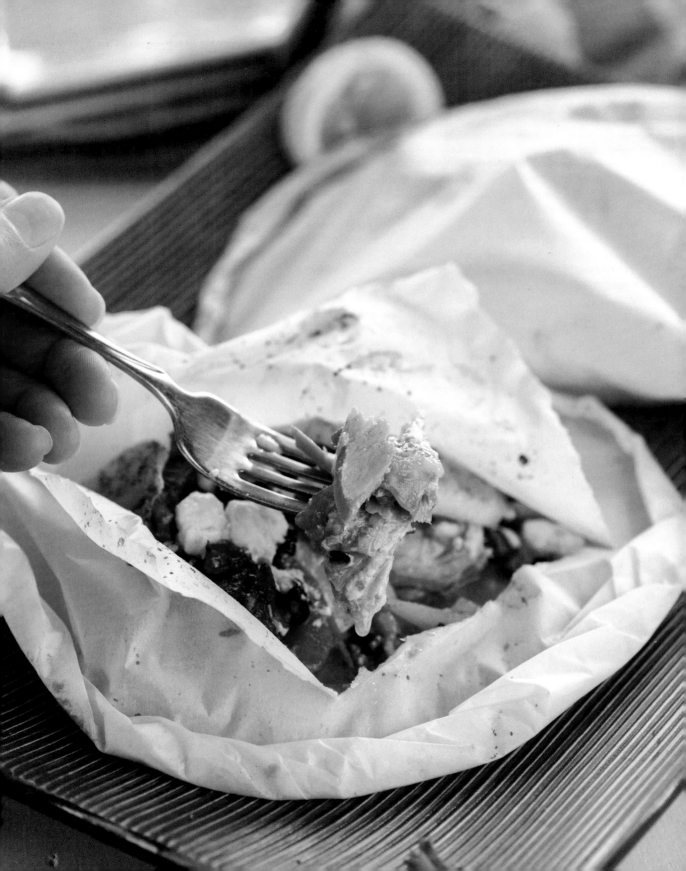

dark leafy greens; julienned bell peppers; sliced tomatoes or cherry tomatoes; diced green onions; thinly sliced cabbage (or bagged shredded cabbage or coleslaw); sliced mushrooms; sliced onion; green beans; or cauli rice (or broccoli or cauli florets cut into much smaller pieces)

GRAIN/SWEET POTATO OPTIONS (FOR E): ½ to ¾ cup cooked brown rice, wild rice, or quinoa; or a small to medium sweet potato, thinly sliced or diced

STEP 3: CHOOSE YOUR FLAVORINGS AND HEALTHY FATS

FAT OPTIONS: 1 tablespoon butter or coconut oil or MCT oil for S (use only 1 teaspoon for FP and E)

FLAVORING OPTIONS: ¼ teaspoon Mineral Salt (go down from here if using other salty spices); soy sauce, tamari, Bragg liquid aminos or coconut aminos; dried parsley flakes or minced fresh parsley; minced fresh cilantro; minced garlic or a sprinkling of dried garlic; feta or other favorite cheeses for S (you can use a sprinkling of Parmesan for FP and E); diced chili peppers, cayenne pepper, or red pepper flakes; hot sauce; chipotle powder; Cajun seasoning; Nutritional Yeast; liquid smoke; cumin; lemon slices; apple cider vinegar; mustard; Italian seasoning or oregano

STEP 4: **FOLD AND BAKE**

Coconut oil cooking spray

HANGRY POCKET S EXAMPLE

1 salmon fillet or 2 to 3 chicken
   tenderloins

4 slices tomato

2 garlic cloves, minced

2 to 3 tablespoons feta cheese

5 Kalamata or black olives, diced

1 tablespoon butter or coconut oil

Small sprinkling sun-dried tomatoes
   (optional)

2 lemon rounds

¼ teaspoon Mineral Salt

Handful of sliced bell peppers and/
   or 2 extra-large handfuls of
   spinach (frozen or fresh)

HANGRY POCKET E EXAMPLE

1 large or 2 small tilapia or
   other white fish fillets, or
   2 to 3 chicken tenderloins

3 tablespoons favorite salsa

2 tablespoons diced green onions

1 teaspoon butter or coconut oil

4 slices tomato

¼ teaspoon Mineral Salt

1 to 2 garlic cloves, minced

1 teaspoon diced chili peppers
   (optional, for hotties)

2 lemon rounds

1 or 2 very large handfuls of fresh
   spinach or kale (optional)

½ to ¾ cup cooked rice or quinoa

1. Fold a 15-inch square of parchment paper in half and place it in front of you like a book, spine side facing left. Using scissors, cut a half heart shape around the open right side (like the wing of a butterfly), rounding the corner at the top and cutting down to a point to the spine at the bottom of your book shape. Open up your heart (or butterfly wings) and lightly coat it with coconut oil cooking spray.

2. Place the fish or meat protein choice at the right side of the crease in the middle. Now add all the other ingredients into one huddle on the right side of the crease. Fold the left parchment page over the right, then working from the top open end, begin tightly folding the edges of the paper. Continue folding the edge, working downward to form a seal until you get to the bottom point, which you will tuck underneath the pouch. This is super quick and easy; just make sure it is tight so no air can escape. Use the examples to make a whole bunch of pouches and then put them in the freezer for future use, keeping a few in the refrigerator that you'll want to use during the next few days.

3. Bake the pocket in a preheated 400°F oven for 15 minutes for thin fish fillets or 20 minutes for thicker salmon fillets, chicken tenderloins, or ground or stew meats. (You can bake from frozen, but give it 40 to 45 minutes.) Remove from the oven, place the pouch on a dinner plate, and let it steam for another 5 minutes in the pocket before opening.

HANGRY POCKET FP EXAMPLE: Easy, just build your E pocket but leave out the carb option.

NOTE: To fill up further, add a side salad or Speedy Chocolate Milk (page 457) or a baby-size shake or smoothie from the Shakes and Smoothies chapter (page 468).

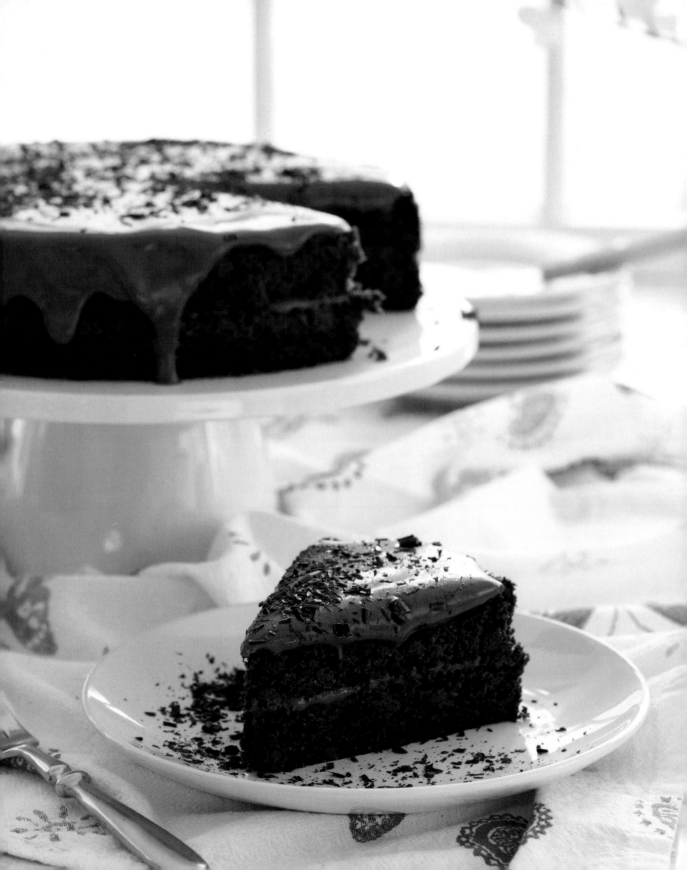

Breakfasts & Baked Goods

Blood Sugar–Balancing Breakfasts

Here's how you set the tone for the success of your day. . . . In fact, the success of your entire Trim Healthy journey depends on your breakfasts! Grab you one of these quick protein-centered morning meals and it will balance your blood sugar and cause your body to release a hormone called glucagon. Glucagon releases fat from your cells and helps control glucose levels in your bloodstream. If you don't have a protein-centered breakfast, that is not going to happen. You'll store fat and have blood sugar highs and lows for the rest of your day. Why do that to yourself? No more! It is a cinch to make a few of the recipes in this chapter and keep them in rotation. Watch yourself change! Watch your fat melt!

(Go to our Trim Healthy Podcast page or find it at our website and listen to podcast number 12 called "The Importance of Breakfast" for more encouragement, tips, and information on protein-centered breakfasts.)

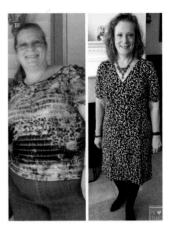

So did you hear the scream about 9:00 Central time today? That was me when my doctor told me I AM OFF ALL MEDS . . . including diabetic meds!!! No more cholesterol, blood pressure, diabetic, or rheumatoid arthritis meds! I have lost 108 pounds, gone from a size 26 to a size 10, can run distances I could not even walk before, and I feel FABULOUS. On January 3, 2015, the day I started Trim Healthy Mama, my fasting sugar level was 435, A1C was 8.9, cholesterol was 225, and BP was moderately high and climbing. My C Reactive Protein (a cardiac/inflammatory marker) was 18 to 22. 1 is normal, 3 is "not IF you will have a heart attack, but WHEN will you have one"! Now, my cholesterol and blood pressure are normal, my A1C is 5.9, and my CRP is now 1.3!!!!! The weight loss is great, but I would take reclaimed health over that ANY day!!! This Drive-Thru Sue has a message for you: THM works! You just have to believe you can do it. Yes, it involves work, change, planning, and learning to like new things and learning many new things, but it is so worth the effort!! I have said this before, but THANK YOU, PEARL AND SERENE!! THM ROCKS!! #108lbsandcounting #thmforlife #nomoremedsforme. –KIM M.

easiest breakfast casserole

S

LARGE FAMILY SERVE OR MULTIPLE SINGLE SERVES

Coconut oil cooking spray

4 to 6 ounces fresh spinach

1 pound breakfast sausage meat (we use turkey, but you can use any kind), thawed if frozen

1 (10-ounce) bag frozen small-cut seasoning blend (see page 35)

8 ounces mushrooms, sliced

6 large eggs

1½ cups egg whites (carton or fresh)

2 cups (8 ounces) grated cheese

½ teaspoon Mineral Salt

⅛ teaspoon black pepper

Find yourself on the run in the morning and need some grab-and-go options? Make this simple casserole, portion it out, and you'll have plenty of breakfasts for the week. It freezes well, too. Or let your whole family at it for a lovely weekend S breakfast.

1. Preheat the oven to 365°F. Spray a 9 × 13-inch baking dish with coconut oil.

2. Place the spinach in the baking dish.

3. Brown the sausage in a large skillet over high heat. Once browned, add the seasoning blend and mushrooms and cook the veggies with the sausage until tender. Some liquid may develop, but keep cooking on high, tossing the ingredients until it evaporates.

4. While the veggies are cooking with the sausage, whisk together the whole eggs, egg whites, 1 cup of the cheese, the salt, and pepper in a bowl.

5. Pour the sausage and veggies over the spinach in the baking dish. Add the egg mixture, then sprinkle on the rest of the cheese. Bake for 30 minutes.

eggalicious muffin cups

S

MAKES AS MANY AS YOU WANT

Coconut oil cooking spray
2 slices lean all-natural natural
    turkey deli meat or ham
2 large eggs
Seasonings: Mineral Salt, black
    pepper, Nutritional Yeast, and
    Parmesan cheese

PEARL CHATS: My twelve-year-old daughter, Autumn, makes these for the whole family about once a week and we all love them . . . so cute and tasty! Two or three of these warm from the oven with a handful of berries on the side makes a beautiful breakfast. (Although my teenage sons eat three or four at a time and a bunch of sprouted-grain toast for a Crossover, so if you have a big eating husband, two might not be enough.) Or you can keep these refrigerated and either reheat or eat cold on your way out the door. You can choose how many you want to make. Autumn makes lots at a time to feed our big eating family, but if you only want to make a couple or a few, that is just as easy. The ingredients are for making just two.

1. Preheat the oven to 350°F. Spray 2 cups of a muffin tin with coconut oil.

2. Place a slice of deli meat in each cup and push them in. The meat will be the base and sides of your "muffin." Crack an egg into each cup and sprinkle with the seasonings. Bake for 18 to 20 minutes if you want the eggs to be slightly soft and delicious on top (our favorite way) or bake for 20 to 25 minutes if you want firm eggs.

* FOR DF: LEAVE OFF THE PARMESAN CHEESE.

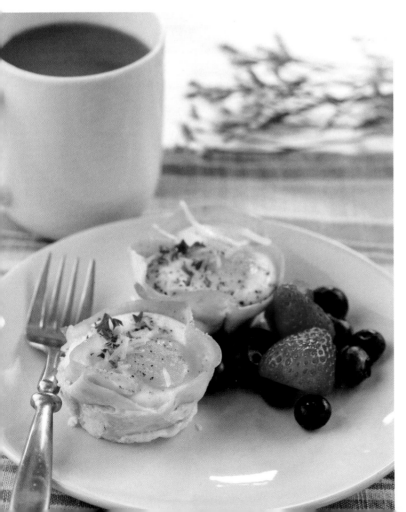

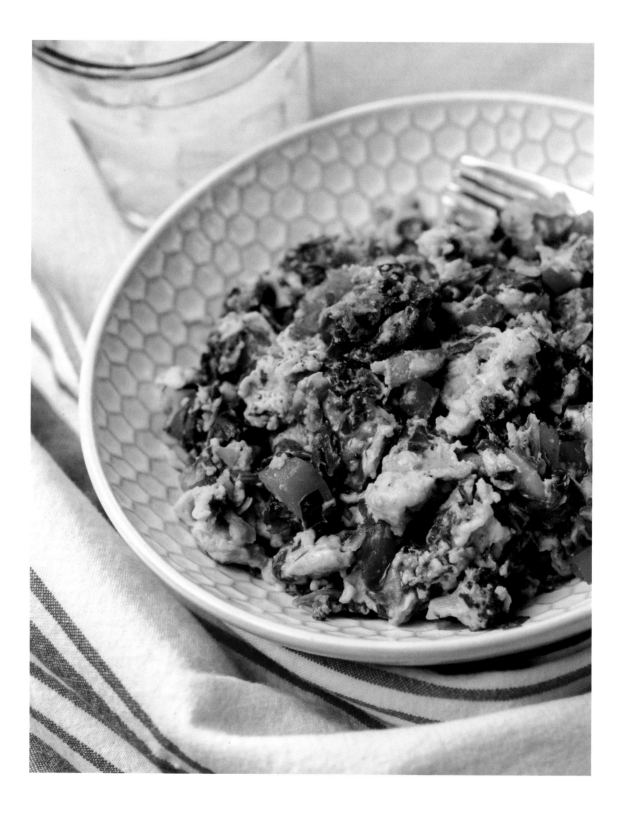

big bowl egg scram

S

SINGLE SERVE

Coconut oil cooking spray

Veggie options (2 to 3 cups): use
1 to 3 choices or combinations of
greens like kale or spinach, very
finely chopped onion, very finely
chopped rainbow bell peppers,
sliced mushrooms, very finely
diced zucchini, very finely diced
tomatoes, very thinly sliced
cabbage

4 pinches Mineral Salt

2 large eggs (or 1 egg and ½ cup
whites for an even lighter version)

½ teaspoon miso (optional, but
ultra-yummy; add Mineral Salt to
taste if not using)

1 teaspoon Nutritional Yeast

1 to 2 teaspoons apple cider
vinegar (basically a small drizzle)

A little squirt of mesquite liquid
smoke (optional)

Sprinkle of onion and garlic
powders (optional)

1 tablespoon water

1 rounded teaspoon extra-virgin
coconut oil

Chipotle powder (optional)

Small amount grated Pecorino
Romano or Parmesan cheese
(optional; this is a light S
breakfast, so don't go piling on
heaps of cheddar cheese, turning
this into heavy S)

Sesame seeds (optional)

SERENE CHATS: *As soon as I open my eyes in the morning, I turn into a Starvin' Marvin . . . or perhaps that's for a guy . . . okay, I am a Starved Marve! As a nursing Mama whose baby drinks all night on tap, once the sun rises I am beelinin' it to the kitchen. A couple of fried eggs look so measly on my eagerly awaiting large and lonely breakfast plate, so I created this egg breakfast for big eating! My Big Bowl Egg Scram was born to fill me up without filling me out. This recipe is incredibly Trimming. It helps me get back to my prebaby body very quickly after pregnancies, so I sometimes make a Crossover out of it by adding a piece of fruit or slice or two of bread so I don't go underweight.*

This is loaded with nonstarchy veggies. You really need to eat more of those in the morning, and here's a scrumptious way to do it. I love the way I feel so super satisfied without the heavy Jabba the Hutt feeling I get when I don't balance my meals with some nonstarchies. Always remember that Trim Healthy Mama works best to whittle pounds away when nonstarchy veggies stay in the limelight. Don't scrimp on your veggies in this breakfast. They cook down, so you'll want to start with a cutting board full of them and, although not mandatory, try to include kale, which is a leafy green low in oxalates. It is important to chop any veggies other than spinach or kale very fine, as they cook much more quickly that way and add more moist succulence. Let the big bowl begin.

1. Spray a large skillet with coconut oil and set it over medium-high heat. Add the veggies, sprinkle with the salt, and stir. Once they start to sizzle, reduce the heat to low and cover while you prepare the eggs. (Just stir now and then to check that your nonstarchies are not sticking.)

2. Blend the eggs, miso (if using), nutritional yeast, vinegar, liquid smoke (if using), onion and garlic powders (if using), and water in a small bowl or jar using a stick blender (or whisk very well).

3. Uncover the skillet, pour the eggs over the veggies, and increase the heat to medium. Stir well while the egg coats and cooks among the soft and caramelized veggies.

4. Place your scram in a bowl and drizzle your rounded tea-spoon of coconut oil on top and sprinkle the top with the (optional but absolutely AMAZING and highly recom-mended) chipotle powder. For the final topping, sprinkle with the cheese and sesame seeds (if using).

quick-fix egg white muffins

FP WITH **E** AND **S** OPTIONS

MAKES AS MANY AS YOU WANT

Coconut oil cooking spray
Fresh spinach, coarsely chopped
Baby tomatoes, halved or quartered
Turkey bacon bits (optional)
Egg whites (carton or fresh)
Seasonings: Mineral Salt, black
  pepper, and a light sprinkling of
  grated Parmesan cheese

These muffins are level 1 easy and make a fantastic E protein-centered breakfast paired with a piece of fruit such as an orange, sliced peach, or a large handful of cherries. Or just stick to an FP breakfast and eat a couple alone or pair with a baby-size FP, E, or S shake or smoothie. As with the Eggalicious Muffin Cups (page 329), you can choose how many you want to make. A few or a lot . . . it's up to you, but we think the best idea is to make up a bunch for your week so you can just grab from the fridge when needed (or freeze some for quick reheating). A couple of these muffins also make a quick lunch paired with a very large salad.

1. Preheat the oven to 350°F. Spray the cups of a muffin tin with coconut oil or use cupcake liners (the parchment kind work best).

2. Put some spinach and tomatoes and bacon bits (if using) in the muffin cups. Pour in the egg whites and sprinkle on the seasonings. Bake for 15 to 20 minutes.

* FOR DF: LEAVE OFF THE PARMESAN CHEESE.

pepper hole eggs

S

SINGLE SERVE

1 tablespoon butter or coconut oil
2 to 3 red or green bell pepper
  rings, ⅓ to ½ inch thick
2 to 3 large eggs
Seasonings: Mineral Salt, black
  pepper, Nutritional Yeast,
  Parmesan cheese (optional), and
  cayenne pepper

Peppers are bursting with vitamin C and disease-fighting flavonoids and antioxidants. They are a perfect partner for protein-rich eggs. As written, this is a single-serve breakfast for yourself, but you might be inspired to make more as this is a fun way to serve up fried eggs to your children!

1. Melt the butter in a skillet over medium heat. Add the pepper rings to the pan and cook for about 1 minute to start softening.

2. Add an egg to each "pepper hole." Season well and cook for a couple minutes, then flip the eggs (or cover the pan and steam them, no need to flip). Cook until the eggs are the desired consistency, either still yolky or hard.

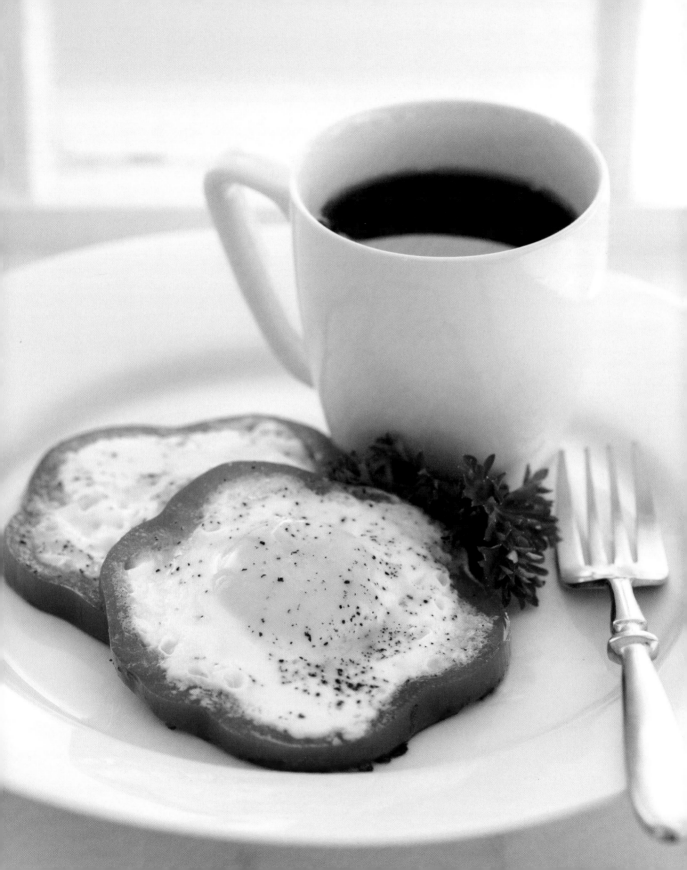

no-bake breakfast cheesecakes (S)

MAKES 12 MINI CHEESECAKES (RECIPE CAN BE HALVED)

1½ tablespoons Just Gelatin*

¼ cup cool water

¼ cup just off the boil water

1½ (8-ounce) packages ⅓ less fat cream cheese

1½ cups plain 0% Greek yogurt

Juice of ½ to 1 lemon (depending on your lemony preference)

2½ to 3 tablespoons Super Sweet Blend, or about ⅓ cup Gentle Sweet, or several doonks Pure Stevia Extract Powder*

1 to 2 scoops (¼ to ½ cup) unflavored (or perhaps strawberry) Pristine Whey Protein Powder (optional; if using strawberry whey, reduce sweetener by half)

1 to 2 handfuls of blueberries or diced strawberries (optional)

These are a lovely, cheesecakey way to start your day. Enjoy a couple for breakfast with coffee . . . mmm, perfection! The whey protein is completely optional since you already have a nice amount of protein in your Greek yogurt and gelatin, but it adds a nice little extra. Feel free to use the option of strawberry whey protein for a berry twist in your cheesecake breakfast.

1. Put the gelatin in a mug, pour the cool water over, and stir until dissolved. Add the boiled water and stir. Pour this into a blender.

2. Add the cream cheese, yogurt, lemon juice, and sweetener. Blend well. Finally, if using the whey protein, add it and blend for just 10 more seconds. Stir in the berries (if using).

3. Line 12 cups of a muffin tin with cupcake liners (parchment kind work best). Fill the cups with the cheesecake mixture. Place in the fridge and let set for 3 to 4 hours. Or put into 4-ounce mini jars if you want a grab-and-go option.

* FOR NSI: USE A GROCERY STORE ON-PLAN SWEETENER AND GROCERY UNFLAVORED PLAIN GELATIN.

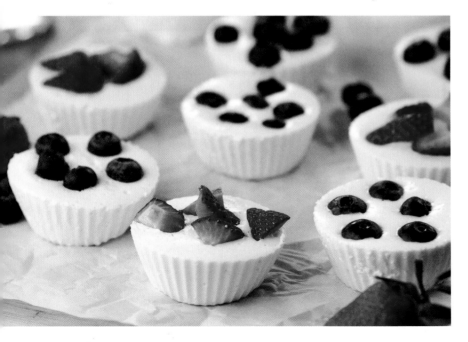

hash 'n' eggs

S

SINGLE SERVE

3 teaspoons butter or coconut oil

1 medium to large summer squash
  or zucchini, finely diced

Seasonings: Mineral Salt, black
  pepper, and Nutritional Yeast

2 large eggs (use 3 if you are super
  hungry or if you are a guy)

Hot sauce (optional)

PEARL CHATS: When I am on vacation, my favorite Crossover breakfast to order at a restaurant is fried eggs over skillet potatoes (hash browns). I just love the taste and textures and how the soft eggs mingle messily with the potatoes. But that is for sure not a weight-loss meal due to the starchy potatoes mixing with the fat from the whole eggs. I found I can get the same satisfaction making this an S-style meal using a yellow squash or a zucchini as the hash. This way is so good and so slimming!

1. Heat 2 teaspoons of the butter in a large skillet over medium-high heat. Add the squash, sprinkle with the seasonings, cover, and cook. Cover the pan for a minute or 2 to get the squash cooked more quickly.

2. Uncover, push the squash to one side of the pan, and add the remaining 1 teaspoon butter. Crack the eggs into the melted butter, season them, and fry according to how you like them. Once the squash is tender, put it on a large dinner plate and top with the eggs, then drizzle on hot sauce if desired.

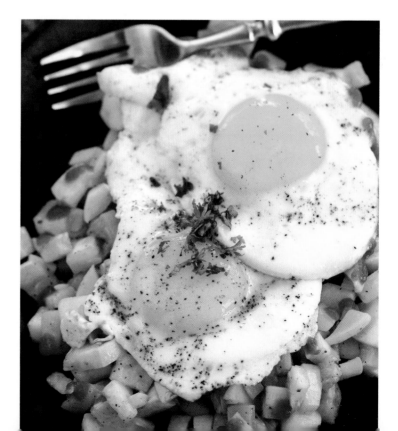

blender freezer waffles

(S)

MAKES 13 TO 16 WAFFLES

Coconut oil cooking spray

1½ (8-ounce) packages ⅓ less fat cream cheese

3 large eggs

¾ cup egg whites (carton or fresh)

1 tablespoon aluminum-free baking powder

3 generous tablespoons coconut oil (use the flavorless kind if you don't want a coconut flavor, but I love using extra-virgin coconut oil in these)

¼ cup plus 2 tablespoons unflavored Pristine Whey Protein Powder*

¼ cup plus 2 tablespoons THM Baking Blend*

1½ tablespoons Super Sweet Blend, or ¼ cup Gentle Sweet* (or more if you like sweeter waffles)

2 teaspoons pure vanilla extract

⅔ cup unsweetened cashew or almond milk or water

1½ teaspoons Gluccie*

PEARL CHATS: Just like the white toaster waffle kind . . . turn your family on to these waffles and you won't turn back. Kids and grown-ups alike love them. I have Serene's children coming to my house to ask me for these . . . (she better start making them!). Make up a batch, store in the freezer, then all you have to do is pop them in the toaster and smear with butter or peanut butter and syrup. Yum! We have included the easy recipe for Basic Pancake Syrup (page 516) from *Trim Healthy Mama Cookbook* in case you don't have that, but some of us Drive-Thru Sue's sometimes use a sugar-free grocery store syrup and hope Serene is not watching.

1. Turn on your waffle iron and spray it well with coconut oil cooking spray.

2. While the iron is heating, put all the ingredients in a blender and blend for about 30 seconds. Let the mixture rest for 10 seconds, then blend again for another minute. Leave the batter to rest for about 10 minutes to thicken up.

3. Put a generous ¼ cup batter in each waffle square and cook according to your waffle iron's instructions. You should get between 13 and 16 waffles, depending on the size of your iron. Freeze the waffles, 2 to 3 in each baggie, and toast to heat. Serve with Basic Pancake Syrup (page 516) if desired.

* FOR NSI: USE A GROCERY STORE ON-PLAN SWEETENER AND WHEY PROTEIN (SEE PAGE 43). USE THE FRUGAL FLOUR OPTION (SEE PAGE 40) AND SUB XANTHAN GUM FOR THE GLUCCIE.

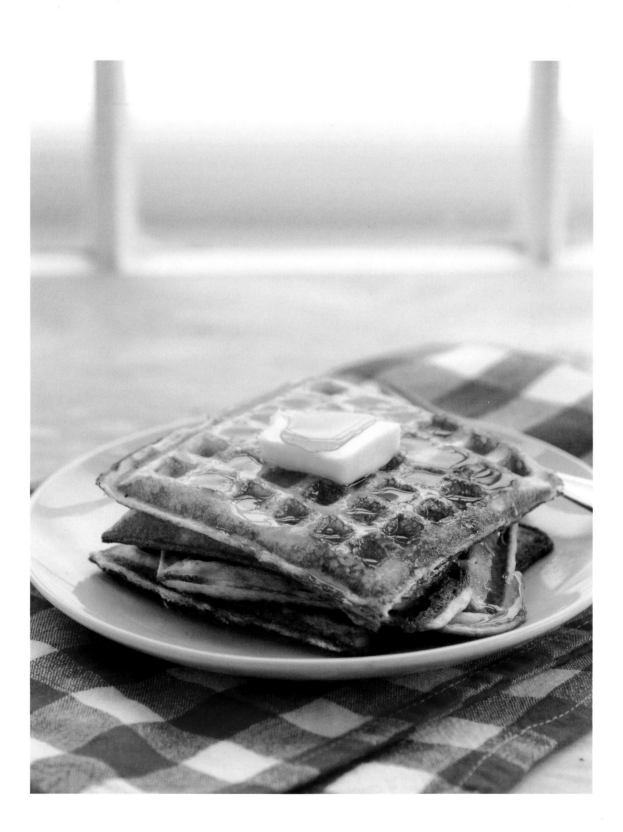

cinnamon pecan baked pancake

(S)

LARGE FAMILY SERVE OR MULTIPLE SINGLE SERVES

Coconut oil cooking spray

6 large eggs

2 cups THM Baking Blend*

1½ cups unsweetened cashew or almond milk

2½ to 3 tablespoons Super Sweet Blend, or ⅓ cup Gentle Sweet*

1½ to 2 teaspoons ground cinnamon, plus more for sprinkling

4 teaspoons aluminum-free baking powder

¼ teaspoon Mineral Salt

2 to 3 teaspoons pure vanilla extract or other extract of choice (Natural Burst caramel or butter extract is amazing)

½ cup chopped pecans

Smear on the butter and pour on the syrup . . . breakfast just got easy and amazing. Now you can bake only once and have breakfasts for days! Or the whole family can enjoy this together and scarf it all down.

1. Preheat the oven to 350°F. Spray a 9 × 13-inch baking dish with coconut oil.

2. Whisk the eggs well in a large bowl, then add all the other ingredients. Pour into the baking dish, sprinkle the top with a little cinnamon, and bake for 30 minutes. Cut into 6 servings.

* FOR NSI: USE THE FRUGAL FLOUR OPTION (SEE PAGE 40) AND A GROCERY STORE ON-PLAN SWEETENER.

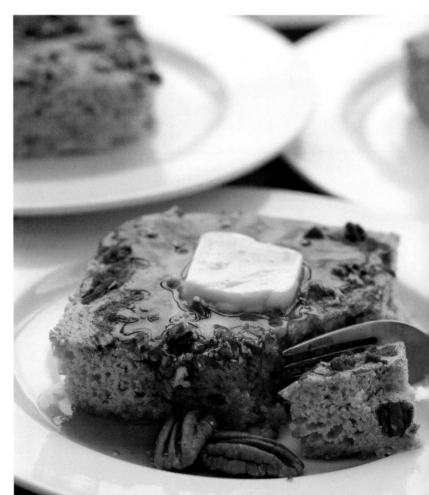

fluffy white banana pancakes   Ⓔ

MAKES 12 PANCAKES (4 SERVINGS OF 3 PANCAKES EACH)

⅔ cup old-fashioned rolled oats

⅔ cup THM Baking Blend*

1 banana

¾ cup 1% cottage cheese

½ cup plain 0% Greek yogurt (optional, but if you leave out, increase the cottage cheese by ½ cup)

1¼ cups egg whites (carton or fresh)

2½ to 3 teaspoons Super Sweet Blend*

1 teaspoon pure vanilla extract

1 teaspoon Natural Burst banana extract*

2½ teaspoons aluminum-free baking powder

Coconut oil cooking spray

These are a new twist on our original Trim Healthy Pancakes. The banana and the addition of Baking Blend brings them to a whole new sweet and fluffy level. But don't worry if you don't have THM Baking Blend, there are a couple of no worries, no special ingredients options (see "For NSI," below). Top with berries, Basic Pancake Syrup (page 516), or a close to plan-approved store-bought syrup, and an optional dollop of Greek yogurt. Make up a batch of these, eat three for your meal, and then refrigerate leftovers between paper towels for the rest of your week (or freeze leftovers in baggies).

1. Put the rolled oats in a blender and blend until they become a powder. Add all the other ingredients (except the cooking spray) and blend well. Allow the batter to set up for 5 minutes.

2. Turn an electric griddle to medium heat. Once hot, spray the griddle with coconut oil. Spoon the batter onto the griddle to make 3 pancakes. Cook on one side for about 3 minutes, then flip to cook on the second side for a couple of minutes.

* FOR NSI: REPLACE THE BAKING BLEND WITH EITHER ANOTHER ⅔ CUP GROUND ROLLED OATS (GROUND INTO A POWDER) OR A MIXTURE OF HALF COCONUT FLOUR AND HALF OAT FIBER. USE A GROCERY STORE ON-PLAN SWEETENER AND BANANA EXTRACT.

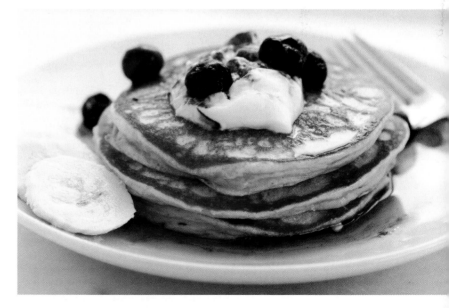

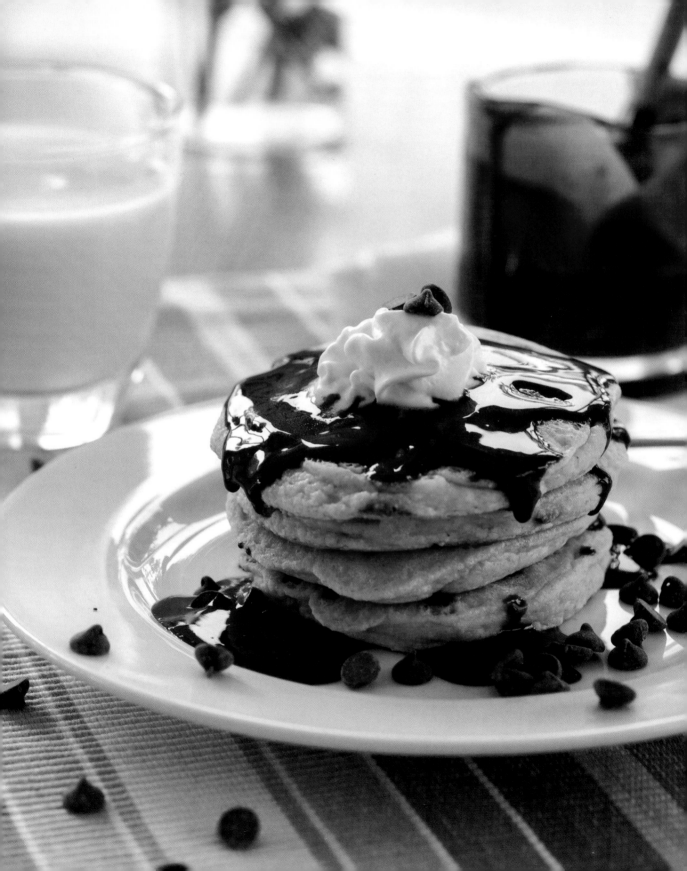

chocolate chip pancakes

S

SINGLE SERVE (3 TO 4 PANCAKES)

1 large egg

⅓ cup THM Baking Blend*

1 teaspoon Super Sweet Blend*

⅓ cup unsweetened almond or cashew milk, plus more as needed

½ teaspoon aluminum-free baking powder

Dash of pure vanilla extract (optional)

2 teaspoons melted coconut oil or butter (optional, but delightful)

2 tablespoons Trim Healthy Chocolate Chips*

Coconut oil cooking spray or butter, for cooking

Coconut oil or butter, for serving

Basic Pancake Syrup (page 516) or Handy Chocolate Syrup (page 371), for serving (see Note)

PEARL CHATS: My daughter Meadow created these. Chocolate chip pancakes were her very favorite special breakfast as a child, but once she became an adult she realized they were very hard on her waistline. She has been happily eating these pancakes ever since, staying slender while doing so.

1. Mix together the egg, Baking Blend, sweetener, nut milk, baking powder, vanilla (if using), and coconut oil (if using) in a small bowl, stirring with a whisk or fork. Add a couple more tablespoons nut milk if needed to get the perfect batter consistency. Add the chocolate chips and stir again. Let sit for a few minutes while you heat the griddle.

2. Turn an electric griddle to medium heat. Once hot, coat with coconut oil cooking spray or a smear of butter. Ladle on the pancake batter to make 3 or 4 pancakes. Cook on one side for about 3 minutes, then flip to brown the other side for a couple minutes.

3. Top with a dollop of extra butter (or coconut oil if dairy-free) and pancake syrup or chocolate syrup.

NOTE: If you are a Drive-Thru Sue, find a store-bought sugar-free syrup as close to plan as possible. An erythritol/stevia-sweetened syrup would be optimum but harder to find in stores (until we release our own brand . . . hopefully soon!), but you can get away with some sorbitol-sweetened syrup here and there. Avoid maltitol if you can.

* FOR NSI: USE THE FRUGAL FLOUR OPTION (SEE PAGE 40) AND A GROCERY STORE ON-PLAN SWEETENER. SUB ANOTHER STEVIA-SWEETENED CHOCOLATE CHIP, OR USE CHOPPED 85% CHOCOLATE.

bam waffles

E

MAKES 8 WAFFLES (ENJOY 2 WAFFLES FOR A SERVING, PERHAPS 3 IF YOU ARE SUPER HUNGRY)

Coconut oil cooking spray
1¼ cups old-fashioned rolled oats
1 large banana
⅛ teaspoon Mineral Salt
1 teaspoon aluminum-free baking
   powder
½ teaspoon baking soda
¼ cup Gentle Sweet, or
   1½ tablespoons Super Sweet
   Blend*
½ cup plain 0% Greek yogurt
½ cup egg whites (carton or fresh)
½ teaspoon pure vanilla extract
½ teaspoon Natural Burst banana
   extract*

Delicious banana cake–style waffles for your energizing break-fast! We discovered the popular Bust-a-Myth Banana Cake from *Trim Healthy Mama Cookbook* makes amazing waffles. Top with syrup and berries . . . oh my!

1. Preheat a waffle iron and spray it with coconut oil.
2. Measure out ¼ cup of the oats and set aside. Grind the remaining 1 cup oats to a flour in a blender. Mash the banana in a bowl, then add the ground oats, whole oats, and remaining waffle ingredients and stir together.
3. Scoop the batter into each waffle square and cook according to the manufacturer's instructions.

* FOR NSI: USE A GROCERY STORE ON-PLAN SWEETENER AND BANANA EXTRACT.

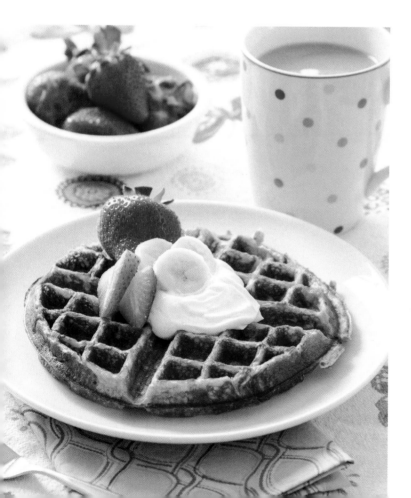

pint jar oats

E

MAKES 3 PINT JARS

1½ cups unsweetened cashew or almond milk

4½ tablespoons unflavored Pristine Whey Protein Powder*

1 cup unsweetened applesauce

¾ cup plain 0% Greek yogurt

1½ teaspoons apple pie spice

2¼ to 3 teaspoons Super Sweet Blend*

1½ cups old-fashioned rolled oats

Making up these jars ahead of time can save your sanity on busy mornings. Just 5 to 10 minutes of prep in the evening will give you three E breakfasts for your week, all ready to go. That leaves four other days where you can juggle up between S or FP breakfasts so your body doesn't adapt to the same thing all the time or you can use these as a nice E afternoon snack. This idea is similar to Sweet Dreams Oatmeal from *Trim Healthy Mama Cookbook*, but with Pint Jar Oats you don't have to cook anything, just pull your jar out of the fridge and eat! (You can warm them if you prefer though.) Enjoy with a Healing Trimmy (page 463) or Lazy Collagen Coffee (page 466) or some scrambled, seasoned egg whites if you feel like you need more food.

1. In each pint jar put ½ cup cashew milk and 1½ tablespoons whey protein. Stir.

2. Now to each jar add ⅓ cup applesauce, ¼ cup Greek yogurt, ½ teaspoon apple pie spice, ¾ to 1 teaspoon sweetener, and ½ cup oats. Stir. Screw on the lids and refrigerate until breakfast time. If you don't like ice-cold oatmeal, pull the jar out as soon as you wake up so it gets to room temperature by the time you are ready to eat.

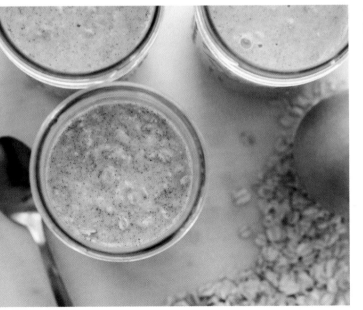

VARIATIONS

PUMPKIN PINT JAR OATS: Replace the applesauce with canned pure pumpkin puree and sub pumpkin pie spice for the apple pie spice.

BERRY PINT JAR OATS: Replace the applesauce with ⅓ cup berries and replace the apple pie spice with ½ teaspoon pure vanilla extract.

* FOR NSI: LEAVE OUT THE WHEY PROTEIN, BUT ADD ANOTHER ¼ CUP GREEK YOGURT; OR LOOK FOR A GROCERY STORE MINIMALLY PROCESSED SUGAR-FREE WHEY PROTEIN ISOLATE. USE A GROCERY STORE ON-PLAN SWEETENER.

wake up trim down banana bars

E

MAKES 5 BREAKFASTS

Coconut oil cooking spray

2 cups egg whites (carton or fresh)

1 banana

1 cup old-fashioned rolled oats

5 oolong tea bags (opened and finely ground in a coffee grinder)

6 tablespoons (4 scoops) Integral Collagen

3 tablespoons THM Baking Blend

2 tablespoons Whole Husk Psyllium powder

½ cup Gentle Sweet plus 2 doonks Pure Stevia Extract Powder (or use Serene's original measly ¼ cup Gentle Sweet if you're strange like her –Pearl)

2 teaspoons pure vanilla extract

1 teaspoon Natural Burst banana extract

1 teaspoon Natural Burst butter extract

1 heaping tablespoon ground cinnamon

1 tablespoon aluminum-free baking powder

1 teaspoon Sunflower Lecithin (optional, but makes them all the more amazing)

1 to 2 teaspoons ghee (clarified butter), extra-virgin coconut oil, or butter

½ teaspoon Mineral Salt

SERENE CHATS: *Good morning, Mama (or perhaps you're a Papa). I am gonna burn the fat off you for breakfast! Wake up the waist-whittling way and grab yourself a generous square of energizing awesomeness. The gentle but steady flow of caffeine from oolong tea leaves contained in these bars will not only put a spring in your step but also ignite a fire under your metabolism. Oolong tea is a powerful fat burner. These ancient tea leaves of the Orient brew inside the moist mixture while it steams in the oven, infusing every morsel of these bars with fat-melting power.*

The balanced amino acid profile of this breakfast pairs perfectly with the gentle carbohydrates and provides an adrenal-nurturing, body-repairing, and anti-aging breakfast. These squares are moist and almost springy in texture and proudly flaunt their banana flavor mixed with the earthiness of the tea leaves.

Since they are so easy to bake ahead for grab 'n' go, they work perfectly for in-the-car "rush hour" breakfasts as well as afternoon pick-me-up snacks for out of the house afternoons. They also freeze well, which makes this Trimming breakfast easy peasy perfect. (Oh BTW, Pearl and I had a big FIGHT about how sweet these should be . . . I only use ¼ cup Gentle Sweet and that is it. I hate breakfast bars that are too sweet, but Pearl, the bossy big sister, said she much prefers them sweeter . . . she does the final editing of our books, so her version is the one written in . . . boo to her!)

1. Preheat the oven to 350°F. Lightly spray 3 standard loaf pans or one 9 × 13-inch baking dish with coconut oil. (They cook faster in the loaf pans and I prefer the texture this way.)

2. Place the egg whites and banana in a food processor and process well. Add all the other ingredients and process just to the point where most of the oats are in smaller pieces but not processed to smithereens! Scrape this mixture into the prepared pans or baking dish. Bake until the top is just done, 40 minutes for the larger pan, or 25 to 30 minutes for the smaller loaf pans. For the bars made in the loaf pans, remove from pans and cut each one in half, then cut one of the halves into 5 pieces (that way you have 1 large piece and a mini piece for your breakfast). For the large pan version, simply cut into 5 squares or bars inside the pan, and then remove.

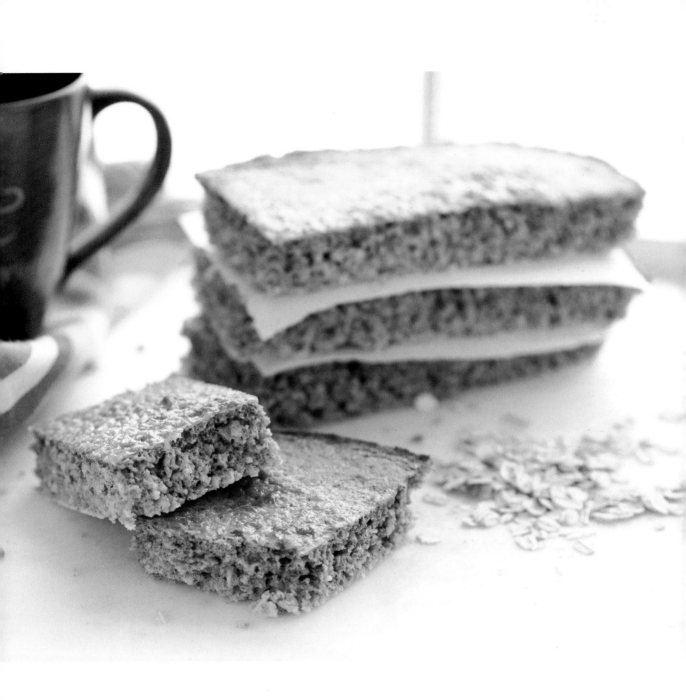

NOTE: These are delicious as is or top them with creamed 1% cottage cheese (blended quickly with a stick blender) or 0% plain Greek yogurt. Add a doonk of stevia or a squirt of vanilla extract and/or a squeeze of lemon.

wake up trim down carrot cake bars

E

MAKES 5 BREAKFASTS

2 cups egg whites (carton or fresh)

1½ packed cups grated carrot

1 cup old-fashioned rolled oats

5 oolong tea bags (opened and ground finely in a coffee grinder)

6 tablespoons (4 scoops) Integral Collagen

1 tablespoon ground cinnamon

½ teaspoon grated nutmeg (optional)

½ teaspoon Mineral Salt

2½ tablespoons Whole Husk Psyllium Flakes

1 teaspoon Sunflower Lecithin

7 tablespoons THM Baking Blend

1 teaspoon Natural Burst butter extract

3 doonks Pure Stevia Extract Powder

¾ cup Gentle Sweet

4 teaspoons aluminum-free baking powder

Another yummy variation on the Wake Up Trim Down bars.

1. Process and bake in the same manner as for Wake Up Trim Down Banana Bars (page 344). Top if desired with a similar topping.

can-do cereal

MAKES MULTIPLE SINGLE SERVE MEALS

OPTION A:
Coconut oil cooking spray

FOR THE SPONGE
2⅔ cups egg whites (carton or fresh but easier with carton)
1¼ teaspoons xanthan gum
1¼ teaspoons cream of tartar
2 cups THM Baking Blend
6 to 8 pinches Mineral Salt
1½ tablespoons Super Sweet Blend
1 tablespoon plus 1 teaspoon aluminum-free baking powder
6 tablespoons (4 scoops) Integral Collagen
1 tablespoon ground cinnamon
5 teaspoons Whole Husk Psyllium Flakes

FOR THE SLURRY
1 tablespoon MCT oil
⅛ teaspoon Sunflower Lecithin
4 tablespoons Gentle Sweet
2 teaspoons Super Sweet Blend
2 teaspoons ground cinnamon
2 tablespoons Integral Collagen
Scant ¼ teaspoon Mineral Salt
1¼ cups water
6 tablespoons chia seeds

OPTIONAL INGREDIENTS (FOR S)
1 cup walnuts, chopped
1 to 2 cups unsweetened shredded coconut
½ cup your favorite seeds (or a mix of hemp, sunflower, and pumpkin seeds)

SERENE CHATS: *We say "don't" to most store-bought cereal because it can pretty much be summed up as fat in a box. Yes, even if it is the pretend whole-grain type. The problem is not just the added sugar, fructose, and corn syrup, but the highly processed and refined flours pushed through extrusion machines into all kinds of crazy shapes. Processed flour like this ignites your blood sugar like dried kindling in a fire. Don't get down in the dumps though. We're giving you a can-do cereal. It is beautifully balanced in protein, rich in fiber, and is even a Fuel Pull to top off its saintliness.*

Don't be put off by the longish directions. This really is a simple process and only needs to be made in bulk once a month. You make the sponge, then make the slurry, then bake. Growing children who do not have weight problems can have homemade granola made with honey. Keep this cereal for those in the family who need slimming. This way it lasts longer and serves its purpose of slimming down the folks who need it.

There are two versions of this cereal below. Option A has an extra puffing step, but those that love it think it is worth it. Option B is quicker but denser. If you are missing cereal like crazy, try both and see which becomes your fave.

1. Position a rack at the bottom of the oven and preheat to 350°F. Spray 2 regular-size rimmed baking sheets or 1 ultra-large baking sheet with coconut oil.

2. Make the sponge. Put the egg whites, xanthan, and cream of tartar into a glass bowl and beat with an electric mixer until stiff peaks form.

3. Place the Baking Blend, salt, sweetener, baking powder, collagen, cinnamon, and psyllium flakes in another bowl and whisk. Gently fold the dry mixture into the stiff egg whites in several additions, stirring gently with a spatula until all the dry ingredients are stirred in.

4. Spread the mixture onto the baking sheets. Moisten a spatula with water (and keep moistening when necessary) and use the flat top to spread the mixture across the pan. Bake for 40 minutes. Take the baking sheets out to cool slightly and reduce the oven temperature to 170°F.

5. Meanwhile, make the slurry. Add everything (except the chia seeds) to a large jar. Blend until smooth with a stick

(continues)

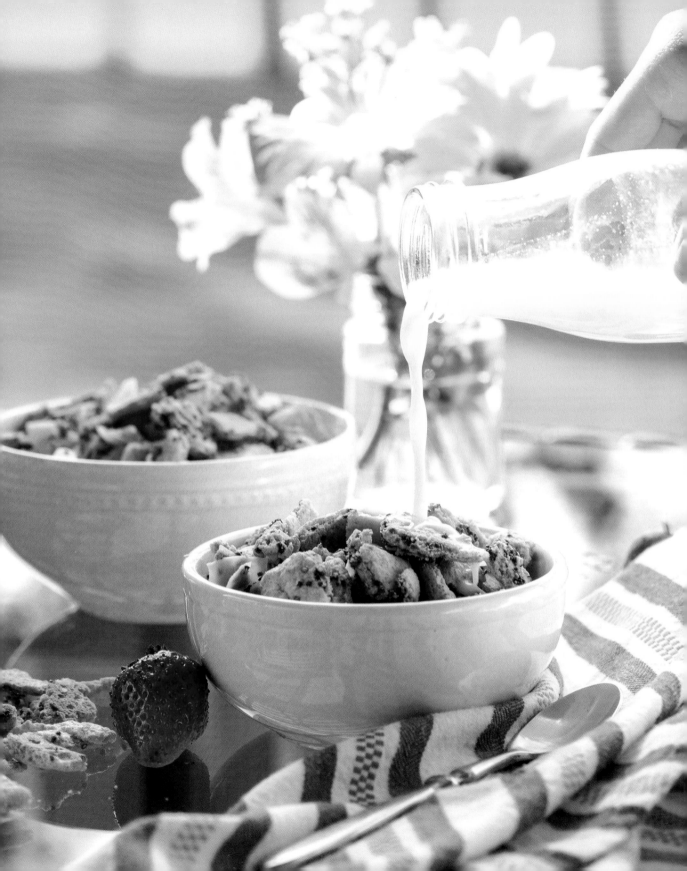

blender (or do this in a blender). Once smooth, add the chia seeds and stir well. Set aside to thicken while your sponge is cooling.

6. Crumble the cooled sponge in your hands in the baking sheets. Don't crumble to the size of rice. Shoot for a variation of crouton-ish and maybe a few smaller-size crumbles. If making this S style, add your optional S ingredients to the crumbles. Pour the slurry over the top and gently combine everything well. Don't massage it into mush, just combine until it forms a clustery-like mix over your baking sheet.

7. Bake in the low oven all night (or 7 to 8 hours) and continue until crisp (works best in an oven that has a convection setting). Once cooled, store in zippy bags in the freezer to preserve the best crunch. To eat, pour a generous amount into a bowl, top with unsweetened cashew or almond milk, and add a teaspoon or so Gentle Sweet to the milk for more of a pop of sweetness.

OPTION B:

FOR THE SPONGE

2⅔ cups egg whites (carton or fresh but carton is easier)

½ cup water

2 cups THM Baking Blend

6 tablespoons (4 scoops) Integral Collagen

1 tablespoon plus 1 teaspoon aluminum-free baking powder

1 tablespoon ground cinnamon

6 to 8 pinches Mineral Salt

1½ teaspoons Super Sweet Blend

FOR THE SLURRY

Same as Option A, but sub flax seeds for chia seeds and reduce the water to ½ cup plus 2 tablespoons

OPTIONAL INGREDIENTS (FOR S)

Same as Option A

1. Make the sponge. Whisk the egg whites and water in a large bowl. Then stir in all the dry ingredients. Bake and cool as in Option A.

2. Make the slurry as for Option A.

3. Crumble the sponge, add the optional S ingredients, combine with the slurry, and slow-bake as in Option A.

oatmeal on the go cups

E

Coconut oil cooking spray

2½ cups old-fashioned rolled oats

½ cup Gentle Sweet* (plus 2 doonks of Pure Stevia Extract Powder for a sweeter tooth)

2 bananas

1 generous cup frozen or fresh blueberries

¾ cup egg whites (carton or fresh)

½ cup unsweetened almond or cashew milk (or water)

1½ teaspoons aluminum-free baking powder

2 pinches Mineral Salt

1 teaspoon Natural Burst banana extract*

1 teaspoon pure vanilla extract

¼ cup Integral Collagen (optional, for added protein)

Perfect for busy mornings. Grab and go! Enjoy 2 or even 3 for your E breakfast.

1. Preheat the oven to 425°F. Line 12 cups of a muffin tin with cupcake or muffin liners and coat with coconut oil cooking spray.

2. Combine all the ingredients in a large bowl, then divide among the 12 muffin cups and bake for 17 to 18 minutes.

* FOR NSI: USE A GROCERY STORE ON-PLAN SWEETENER AND EXTRACT AND LEAVE OUT THE COLLAGEN.

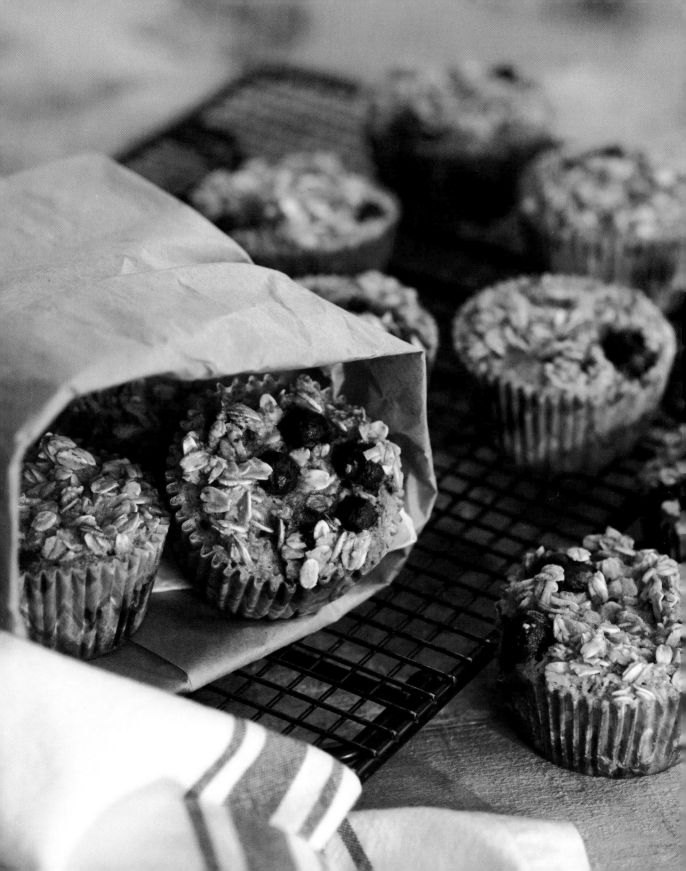

pint jar chia

S

MAKES 3 PINT JARS

3¾ cups unsweetened cashew or
  almond milk

1 tablespoon heavy cream or
  MCT oil

Generous ¾ teaspoon Gluccie

6 to 9 doonks (about scant
  ¼ teaspoon) Pure Stevia Extract
  Powder*

1½ teaspoons pure vanilla extract

¾ teaspoon ground cinnamon

4½ tablespoons chia seeds

3 tablespoons old-fashioned rolled
  oats (see Note)

¾ cup frozen or fresh raspberries or
  blueberries

A nice change-up to oatmeal in the morning is chia! This incredible superfood hydrates your cells and offers sustained energy and powerful nutrients. Take one of these jars out of the fridge in the morning to sit on the counter, then go take your shower and get ready. Once you're back it won't be as ice-cold to eat . . . unless you love an icy cold breakfast. This also makes a great afternoon snack or enjoy half a serving for a dessert.

1. Put the nut milk, cream, Gluccie, sweetener, vanilla, and cinnamon in a blender and blend well for about a minute. Divide this mixture among 3 pint jars. Add 1½ tablespoons chia seeds, 1 tablespoon oats, and ¼ cup berries to each jar. Stir well. Screw the lids on the jars and put them in the refrigerator overnight or for several hours.

NOTE: While oats are an E food, the very small amount of 1 tablespoon per jar won't be enough to cause a significant fuel collision.

* FOR NSI: USE A GROCERY STORE ON-PLAN SWEETENER.

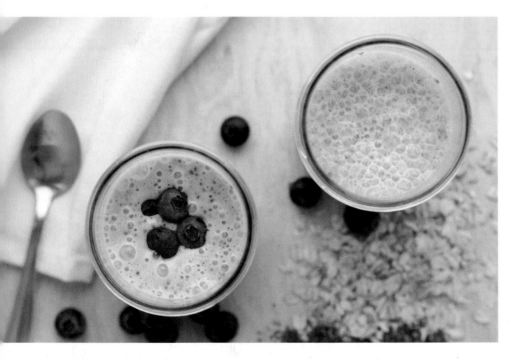

cream of treat hot porridge

FP WITH S AND E OPTIONS

SINGLE SERVE

½ cup unsweetened almond milk

½ cup plus 2 tablespoons water

⅓ cup THM Baking Blend*

2 teaspoons Gentle Sweet (or on-plan sweetener to taste)

¼ teaspoon pure vanilla or maple extract

2 to 3 generous pinches Mineral Salt

Sprinkle of ground cinnamon (optional)

1 to 2 tablespoons unflavored Pristine Whey Protein Powder or Integral Collagen (optional, to increase protein)

OPTIONAL TOPPINGS

Generous pat of coconut oil or butter, or a good splash of heavy cream, for S; handful of berries or cut fruit such as apple for FP or E

PEARL CHATS: I actually do love Serene's cream of wheat knock-off (page 357). You should go make it as it really doesn't take long to whip up. But here is a super-quick, 2-minute version of cream of wheat that our photographer Rohnda passed along to me, and I adore it because of its ease.

1. Put the almond milk, water, Baking Blend, sweetener, vanilla, salt, cinnamon (if using), and whey protein (if using) into a saucepan and mix well. Heat to a gentle boil until the porridge thickens, 1 to 2 minutes. (Or heat in a microwave-safe bowl for 1 minute, if you are the hardcore Drive-Thru Sue type.)

NOTE: For FP, omit the oil, butter, or cream but include the berries. For S, include the oil, butter, or cream and berries. For E, omit the added fat and add diced apples and cinnamon.

* FOR NSI: USE THE FRUGAL FLOUR OPTION (SEE PAGE 40), BUT NOTE THAT WILL CHANGE THE PORRIDGE TO A LIGHT S.

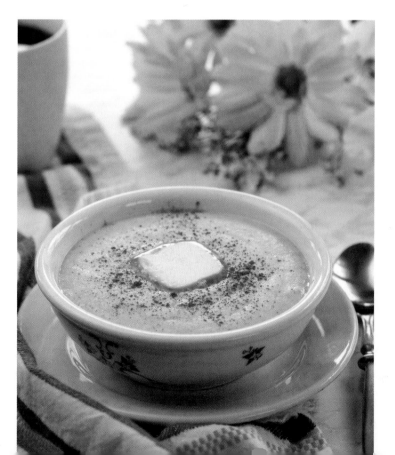

big bowl cinnamon oatmeal

(E)

SINGLE SERVE

½ cup old-fashioned rolled oats

¾ cup unsweetened cashew or
   almond milk

1 cup water

½ teaspoon ground cinnamon

4 teaspoons Gentle Sweet, or
   1½ teaspoons Super Sweet Blend*

1 or 2 pinches Mineral Salt

Dash pure vanilla extract (optional)

2 teaspoons Baobab Boost Powder
   (optional)

Cinnamon sugar (optional; from
   Cinnamon Sugar Toast, page 358),
   for serving

PEARL CHATS: If Serene can have her Big Bowl Egg Scram (page 331), I can have a big bowl oatmeal version. I love oatmeal, but most of the time I feel I don't get enough to eat when I have it. With this recipe, just 10 minutes and ½ cup oats cooks up into big eats! The trick here is to use a lot of liquid. If you give oats enough time, they magically swell and soak up the liquid. You don't have to stand over the stove for 10 minutes, just cover the pot, go brush your teeth or make your bed or scurry around finishing getting ready for your day. When you come back you'll have a HUGE steaming bowlful.

Did you know oats are one of the rare grains that contain a nice amount of protein? The 5 grams per ½ cup is part of the reason they are a slow-burning grain and perfect for the Trim Healthy Plan. You can up the protein two ways: either mix ½ scoop whey protein with 2 tablespoons unsweetened nut milk and add after cooking, or stir in a scoop of collagen before cooking your oats. Or you can always put collagen into your coffee instead. If you don't have collagen or whey protein, having some Greek yogurt with your oatmeal is another great way to get more protein in.

1. Put all the ingredients (except the cinnamon sugar) into a small saucepan and bring to a quick boil. Reduce the heat to low, remove from the heat for about 30 seconds while it cools down, then return to low heat, cover the pot, and allow to steam for 10 minutes. Come back to the pot, remove from the heat, stir, and allow to cool and thicken even more for about a minute. If desired, top with cinnamon sugar (page 358).

VARIATIONS

CHOCOLATE BIGGIE OATMEAL: Omit the cinnamon and pull back the Gentle Sweet to 1 to 2 teaspoons. Add 1 teaspoon unsweetened cocoa powder before cooking. Once cooked, mix 2 tablespoons chocolate Pristine Whey Protein Powder with 2 tablespoons almond milk and stir in. Sprinkle the top of the oatmeal with extra Gentle Sweet if you have a sweet tooth.

STRAWBERRY BIGGIE OATMEAL: Omit the cinnamon and stir in a handful of chopped frozen strawberries before cooking. Once cooked, mix 2 tablespoons strawberry Pristine Whey Protein Powder with 2 tablespoons almond milk and stir in.

* FOR NSI: USE A GROCERY STORE ON-PLAN SWEETENER.

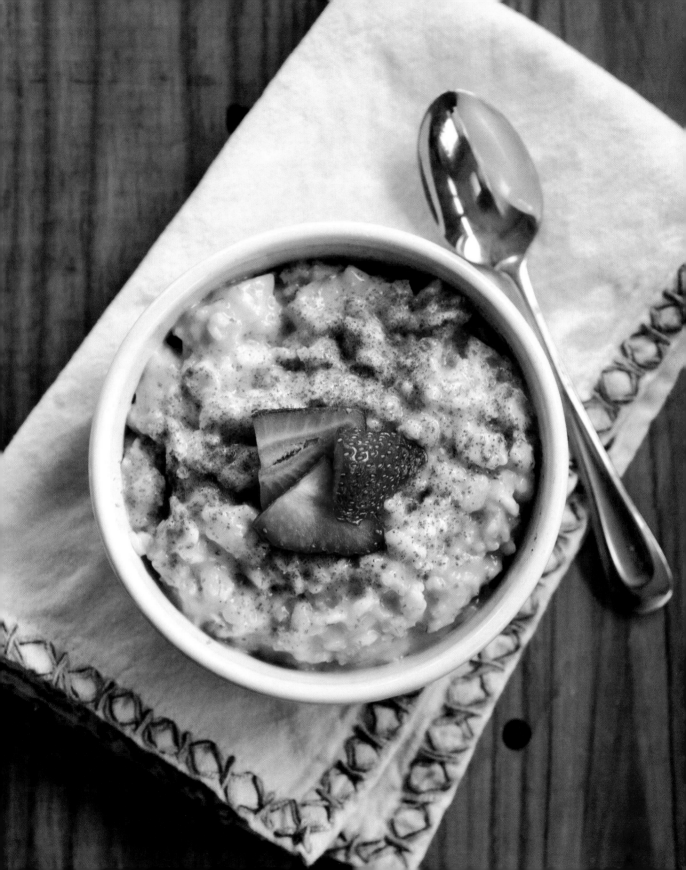

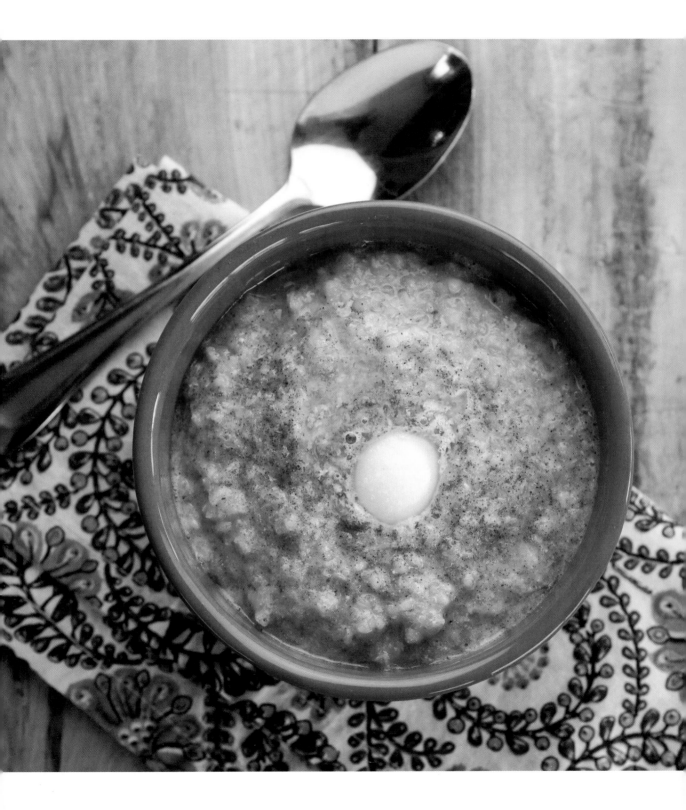

cream of buckwheat

E

SINGLE SERVE

½ cup buckwheat groats

¾ to 1 cup just off the boil water for blending

1 teaspoon extra-virgin coconut oil or butter

1 teaspoon Just Gelatin

1½ tablespoons (1 scoop) Integral Collagen

1 doonk Sunflower Lecithin (optional)

1½ teaspoons Super Sweet Blend

¾ teaspoon ground cinnamon

4 pinches Mineral Salt

2 tablespoons (½ scoop) unflavored Pristine Whey Protein Powder

SERENE CHATS: *I love cream of wheat. I don't eat it as it is starchy, refined, and hybridized wheat stuff, but I think of it fondly. So what's a cream of wheat lover like me to do? Wipe my eyes and curl that pout into a smile. This cream of wheat knockoff is not a close second, it is a total winner. Lately it has been my husband's favorite breakfast, too. So we sit and eat Cream of Buckwheat in the morning and stare into each other's eyes in peaceful bliss. Ha ha . . . actually the house is blowing up with the noise and clatter of boisterous children frying up eggs, breaking dishes, and running through our little cream of wheat world, making it all the more wonderful.*

Buckwheat is not a variety of wheat at all. It cannot even be classified as a grain. It is a seed of a fruit related to sorrel. It is loaded with a rich supply of flavonoids, which protect us against the onslaught of disease and are most famous for their antioxidant and anti-inflammatory powers. Buckwheat helps lower glucose levels, insulin responses, and bad cholesterol.

1. Soak the buckwheat groats overnight in a bowl with enough water to cover generously. In the morning, drain in a fine-mesh sieve and rinse well. Put the soaked buckwheat in a small saucepan with just enough water to be even with the groats (not over the groats–equal is key). Bring to a boil, then simmer over low heat for just a few minutes, until the water is mostly absorbed and the buckwheat becomes gelatinous. Remove the saucepan from the heat.

2. Now make a Trimmy to cream up your buckwheat. Put the boiled water and all the Trimmy ingredients–coconut oil, gelatin, collagen, and lecithin (if using)–in a blender with the sweetener, cinnamon, and salt and blend until creamy. Dump in the whey protein and blend for only 3 seconds more (you don't want to make a lot of froth).

3. Pour this over your buckwheat inside the saucepan and blend with a stick blender until the texture is a bit smooth but still a little textured and grainy. (Note: If this is not thick enough for you and you used a full cup of boiled water in your Trimmy, use just ¾ cup next time.)

4. If desired, you can top with thawed berries, Gentle Sweet, and a little unsweetened almond milk, or leave out the coconut oil from the Trimmy blend and instead top your bowl with a teaspoon of butter, shaking more cinnamon and sweetener over top.

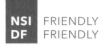
cinnamon sugar toast

S WITH E AND FP OPTIONS

MAKES ANY AMOUNT OF TOAST FOR YOU AND YOUR FAMILY

FOR THE CINNAMON SUGAR
1 cup Gentle Sweet*
3 tablespoons ground cinnamon

FOR THE TOAST
Slices of sprouted-grain or artisan sourdough bread (for E)
Laughing Cow Light cheese or coconut oil spray (for E or FP)
Slices of Wonderful White Blender Bread (page 242) or Nuke Queen's Awesome Bread (page 245), for S or FP
Butter or coconut oil (for S)

You can always make Cinnamon Swirl WWBB (page 256), but if you don't want to do that, here's a superquick way to get your cinnamon fix in the morning. Kids love this, too! Keep some of this cinnamon sugar in a shaker jar and you can use it not only for toast but also to top waffles, pancakes, and whatever else you love cinnamon on.

1. Make the cinnamon sugar. Mix together the Gentle Sweet and cinnamon and put in a sprinkle jar.

   FOR E-STYLE TOAST: Smear sprouted-grain or sourdough toast with Laughing Cow Light cheese or spray with coconut oil, then sprinkle on the cinnamon sugar.

   FOR FP TOAST: Use WWBB or Nuke Queen's Awesome Bread and use Laughing Cow Light cheese or coconut oil spray before sprinkling with cinnamon sugar.

   FOR DELICIOUS S-STYLE TOAST: Slather on plenty of butter or coconut oil, then sprinkle on your cinnamon sugar.

NOTE: If using WWBB bread, you don't have to worry too much about getting extra protein in, as that bread is protein rich so you can enjoy it alone as a simple breakfast. However, you can always add a Lazy Collagen Coffee (page 466) or a Trimmy (page 463) or a baby-size shake or smoothie from the Shakes and Smoothies chapter (page 468), or have a small side of eggs or egg whites for a little more protein.

* FOR NSI: USE A GROCERY STORE ON-PLAN SWEETENER.

* FOR DF: USE COCONUT OIL IN PLACE OF BUTTER.

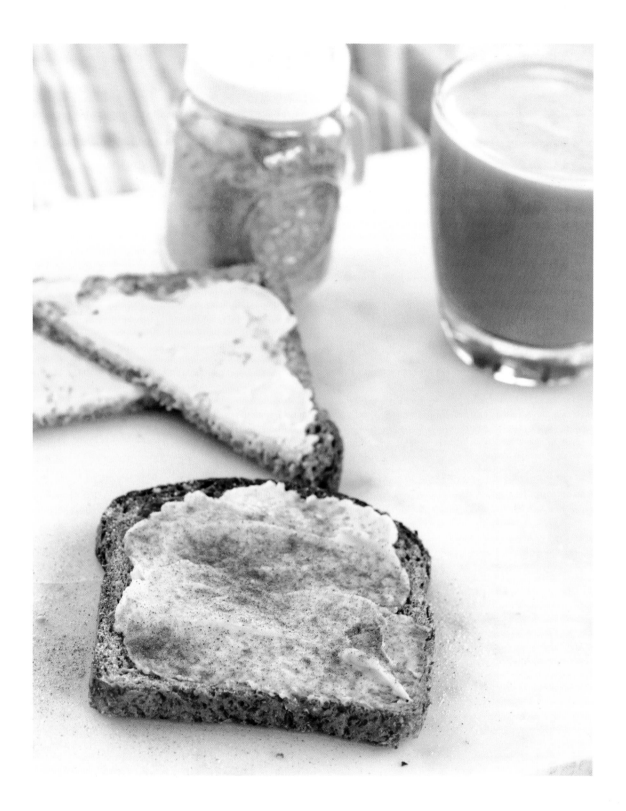

wwbb french toast S

SINGLE SERVE

1 large egg
⅛ to ¼ teaspoon ground cinnamon
⅛ teaspoon grated nutmeg
1 to 2 teaspoons butter or
  coconut oil
2 to 3 slices Wonderful White
  Blender Bread (page 242)
Gentle Sweet and/or Basic Pancake
  Syrup (page 516) or plan-
  approved syrup

1. Whisk the egg, cinnamon, and nutmeg in a small bowl. Melt the butter in a skillet over medium heat. Dip the bread in the egg mixture so it coats both sides well, then brown in the hot skillet on both sides. Top with a generous sprinkle of sweetener and pancake syrup.

* FOR NSI: USE A GROCERY STORE ON-PLAN SWEETENER.

sausage and cheese breakfast biscuits S

MAKES 16 BISCUITS

4 to 6 ounces sausage meat
  (mild, medium, or hot), thawed
  if frozen
¾ cup frozen small-cut seasoning
  blend (optional; see page 35)
Batter from Cheesy Flower Biscuits
  (page 248)

Here is another great grab-and-go breakfast for ya! Have two or three even. If you're still hungry, add on an S-friendly baby-size shake from the Shakes and Smoothies chapter (page 468), but you might not need that as these stick to your ribs. Kids love them, too, but if your kids are picky about onions, just leave out the seasoning blend and use only the sausage as they are just as good without the onions and peppers. Keep these biscuits in a large baggie in the fridge. Warm up in a hot oven for a few minutes or slice in half and toast to warm and crisp, then pat on some butter and you have brekky! Another delish way to enjoy these biscuits is to break one into pieces and put in the pan as you fry two eggs and some added egg whites if you are very hungry. No need for a breakfast meat that way.

1. Brown the sausage and seasoning blend (if using) in a skillet over medium-high heat. Keep cooking until all the liquid from the seasoning blend has evaporated.
2. Make the batter for the biscuits and add the cooked sausage and seasoning blend. Bake as directed in the biscuit recipe.

crunchy granola

MAKES 8 SERVINGS (¾ CUP EACH)

Coconut oil cooking spray

6 cups old-fashioned rolled oats

¾ cup THM Baking Blend*

¾ cup unflavored Pristine Whey Protein Powder*

1 teaspoon Mineral Salt

1½ to 2 tablespoons ground cinnamon

¾ cup Gentle Sweet plus rounded ¼ teaspoon Pure Stevia Extract Powder*

¾ cup egg whites (carton or fresh)

1½ tablespoons pure vanilla extract (or 2 teaspoons vanilla plus 2 teaspoons Natural Burst maple extract)

2 tablespoons MCT oil or coconut oil

Freeze-dried berries (optional)

Keeping on-plan granola in your cupboard (or freezer) will make quick breakfasts or snacks an absolute breeze! It's kid friendly, too! This granola contains a nice amount of protein, but you can always feel free to add on Lazy Collagen Coffee (page 466) or a Healing Trimmy (page 463) for a little more. Totally hits the spot! To serve, just measure out ¾ cup granola into a bowl and top with chilled unsweetened nut milk. If it is not quite sweet enough for you, simply put ½ to 1 teaspoon Gentle Sweet in the bowl with your milk and stir. For a snack, make a parfait and top Greek yogurt with a generous handful of granola and some berries.

1. Preheat the oven to 300°F. Spray a large rimmed baking sheet with coconut oil.

2. Combine the dry ingredients in a large bowl. Add the egg whites, vanilla, and MCT oil and stir well so all the oats get fully dampened. Stir in the freeze-dried berries (if using).

3. Spread the granola out on the baking sheet and bake for 45 to 50 minutes, tossing every 15 minutes.

* FOR NSI: USE A FRUGAL FLOUR OPTION OF HALF COCONUT FLOUR, HALF OAT FIBER TO STAY E FRIENDLY. USE A GROCERY STORE ON-PLAN WHEY PROTEIN (SEE PAGE 43) AND AN ON-PLAN SWEETENER.

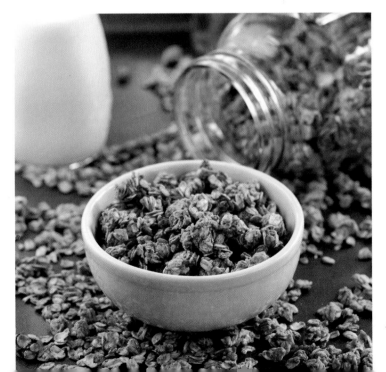

Muffins

Muffins make great breakfasts and snacks, or perhaps a dessert now and then. But there is one muffin in this chapter that can be your go-to dessert anytime, the Incredible Peanut Butter Cookie Muffins (page 371). They are Fuel Pull–decadent in taste but light in fuel, so they make for a wise dessert muffin, especially for the evening when it doesn't make sense to be snacking on heavy foods. Freeze some and pull one out to thaw when the sweet tooth comes a knocking.

Twenty-two months ago, I started on Trim Healthy Mama. I downloaded the Kindle version and jumped in headfirst. To say this has been life changing is an understatement. I'm five pounds away from what I weighed 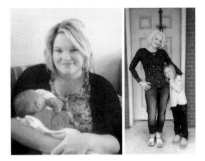 my senior year in high school, and I'm forty-four years old and I've birthed eight babies. It's not like I had a measly twenty pounds to lose. I didn't just look a little bloated. No, I was technically morbidly obese. Not just obese . . . morbidly so.

I've lost more than 105 pounds, which is awesome. More importantly, though, I've regained my health! I'm not too tired to shop anymore (poor hubby)!! I have energy to keep up with my kids, and I am just all-around much happier. I enjoy exercising and look forward to dancing at the gym whenever I can.

I can't say enough great things about Trim Healthy Mama. I don't work for them, so I have nothing to gain by singing their praises. I just want to encourage people who might feel like losing weight is hopeless: It's not!!! It's definitely doable and sustainable. **–LEA T.**

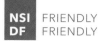
blueberry muffins with lemon glosting ⓢ

MAKES 12 MUFFINS

Coconut oil cooking spray

3 large eggs

½ cup egg whites (carton or fresh)

¾ cup unsweetened almond or
  cashew milk

3 tablespoons coconut oil or butter,
  melted

1 teaspoon pure vanilla extract

1½ cups THM Baking Blend*

½ cup Gentle Sweet, or
  3 tablespoons Super Sweet Blend*

⅛ teaspoon Pure Stevia Extract
  Powder*

1½ teaspoons aluminum-free
  baking powder

½ teaspoon baking soda

1 generous cup frozen blueberries

FOR THE GLOSTING*

2 tablespoons butter

2 tablespoons cream cheese
  (⅓ less fat works well)

2 tablespoons lemon juice

⅛ teaspoon lemon extract

2 to 2½ tablespoons Gentle Sweet*

A "glosting" is a delicious, drippy cross between a glaze and a frosting. Perfect over these muffins, or you can try the dairy-free Lemon Boost Glosting (page 368).

1. Preheat the oven to 375°F. Spray 12 cups of a muffin tin with coconut oil.

2. Whisk together the whole eggs, egg whites, nut milk, coconut oil, and vanilla in a large bowl. Incorporate the Baking Blend, sweeteners, baking powder, and baking soda. Whisk until you have a smooth batter. Allow the batter to sit and thicken a little, 2 to 3 minutes, then fold in the blueberries and combine gently.

3. Fill the muffin cups with batter and bake for 20 to 25 minutes, until the tops are just firm.

4. Remove the muffins from the tin and while they are cooling, make the glosting. Combine the butter and cream cheese in a small bowl. Whisk until smooth, then add 1 tablespoon of the lemon juice and the lemon extract. Whisk until completely smooth, then add the remaining 1 tablespoon lemon juice, followed by the sweetener. Keep whisking until combined properly.

5. Drizzle the glosting all over the tops of the muffins . . . it should be messy and drippy and not perfect at all.

* FOR NSI: USE THE FRUGAL FLOUR OPTION (SEE PAGE 40) AND A GROCERY STORE ON-PLAN SWEETENER.

* FOR DF: USE LEMON BOOST GLOSTING (PAGE 368).

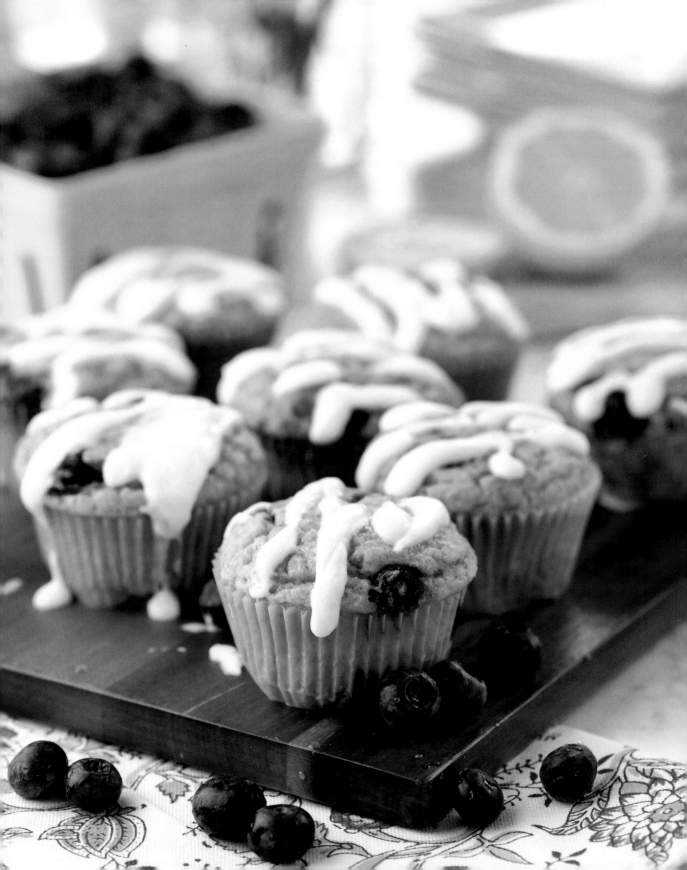

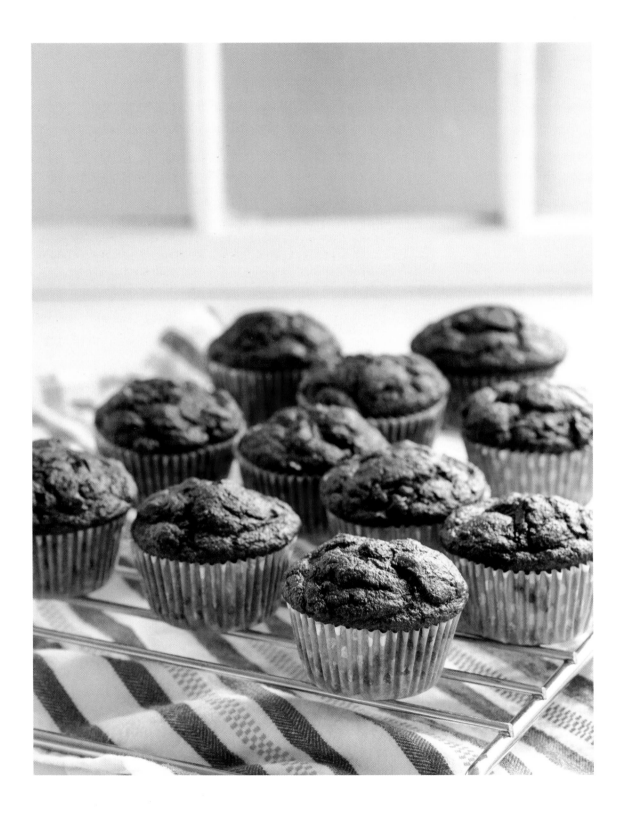

chocolate-covered cherry muffins

E

MAKES 12 MUFFINS

Coconut oil cooking spray

1½ cups frozen pitted cherries

2 cups plus 3 tablespoons old-fashioned rolled oats

3 large egg whites (carton or fresh)

⅓ cup unsweetened cocoa powder (equal mix of extra-dark and regular is awesome)

¾ cup Gentle Sweet*

Generous ¼ teaspoon Mineral Salt

1½ teaspoons aluminum-free baking powder

½ teaspoon baking soda

1 cup plain 0% Greek yogurt

½ cup water or unsweetened almond or cashew milk

1 teaspoon Natural Burst cherry extract*

1 teaspoon pure vanilla extract

Moist and chocolaty, these muffins bring you all the delicious taste and health benefits of cherries. Did you know that cherries are one of the most anti-inflammatory foods on this planet? They can help with conditions like arthritis and gout. They are also high in beta-carotene, containing 19 times more than even blueberries or strawberries. They protect your heart, help fight cancer, and enable a good night's sleep. Round of applause for cherries! Get some more in your E meals!

We like to split each muffin and top with just a smear of butter or coconut oil to stay in E mode, or if you are not a purist, squirt on a little fat-free Reddi-wip. You could also top with some Handy Chocolate Syrup (page 371).

1. Preheat the oven to 350°F. Line 12 cups of a muffin tin with parchment cupcake liners or lightly coat the muffin cups with coconut oil spray.

2. Put the frozen cherries in a food processor and process until they are broken down into smaller pieces but not all the way to mush. Measure out 3 tablespoons oats and set aside. Grind the remaining 2 cups oats to a flour in a blender.

3. Lightly beat the egg whites with a hand whisk in a large bowl. Add the ground oats, whole oats, cocoa powder, sweetener, salt, baking powder, baking soda, yogurt, water, and extracts. Stir in the cherries.

4. Spoon the batter into the muffin cups and bake for 20 minutes. Best eaten once fully cooled.

* FOR NSI: USE A GROCERY STORE ON-PLAN SWEETENER AND CHERRY EXTRACT. OR OMIT THE CHERRY EXTRACT AND INCREASE THE VANILLA TO 1½ TEASPOONS TOTAL.

* FOR DF: OMIT THE YOGURT AND USE UNSWEETENED APPLESAUCE.

lemon poppy boost muffins

S

MAKES 12 MUFFINS

Coconut oil cooking spray
¾ cup THM Baking Blend*
¼ cup Baobab Boost Powder*
5 tablespoons Gentle Sweet*
4 teaspoons Super Sweet* (if you don't have this, use more Gentle Sweet or a couple/few doonks Pure Stevia Extract Powder)
2 teaspoons aluminum-free baking powder
4 pinches Mineral Salt
1½ to 2 tablespoons poppy seeds
2 large eggs
⅓ cup plus 3 tablespoons egg whites (carton or fresh)
2 tablespoons extra-virgin coconut oil
3 tablespoons plus 2 teaspoons hot water
3 tablespoons lemon juice
1 tablespoon pure vanilla extract
Lemon Boost Glosting (optional; recipe follows)

These muffins are a lovely light S with a moist crumb structure and a citrus burst to tickle the tongue. They feature the super-food baobab, which boosts them with vitamin C, antioxidants, and satiating fiber. So delicious sliced and slathered with butter or glosted with the dairy-free Lemon Boost Glosting below. Each scrumptious bite drenches your body with health.

1. Preheat the oven to 350°F. Spray 12 cups of a muffin tin with coconut oil.

2. Combine all the dry ingredients in a large bowl. In a smaller bowl, whisk the whole eggs with the egg whites. Put the coconut oil into a mug, pour the hot water over it, and stir so it melts. Let it cool a little, then stir into the egg mixture. Add the lemon juice and vanilla.

3. Combine the wet and dry mixes and pour the batter into the muffin cups. Bake for 25 minutes. Remove from the tin and then enjoy a muffin or two with a pat of butter, or spread some of the dairy-free glosting over each muffin.

* FOR NSI: FIND BAOBAB POWDER LOCALLY. USE THE FRUGAL FLOUR OPTION (SEE PAGE 40) AND A GROCERY STORE ON-PLAN SWEETENER. OMIT THE GLOSTING.

LEMON BOOST GLOSTING

MAKES ENOUGH FOR 1 BATCH MUFFINS OR 1 CAKE

5 teaspoons cold water
2 teaspoons lemon juice
¼ teaspoon Just Gelatin
⅓ cup just off the boil water
1 tablespoon flavorless coconut oil
⅛ teaspoon Sunflower Lecithin
1½ tablespoons (1 scoop) Integral Collagen
1 tablespoon Baobab Boost Powder
1 teaspoon pure vanilla extract
1 tablespoon Gentle Sweet
Pinch of Mineral Salt

1. Put the cold water, lemon juice, and gelatin in a small bowl and stir until dissolved. Add the boiled water and coconut oil and let the oil melt. Add the lecithin, collagen, baobab powder, vanilla, sweetener, and salt. Blend with a stick blender or whisk super well.

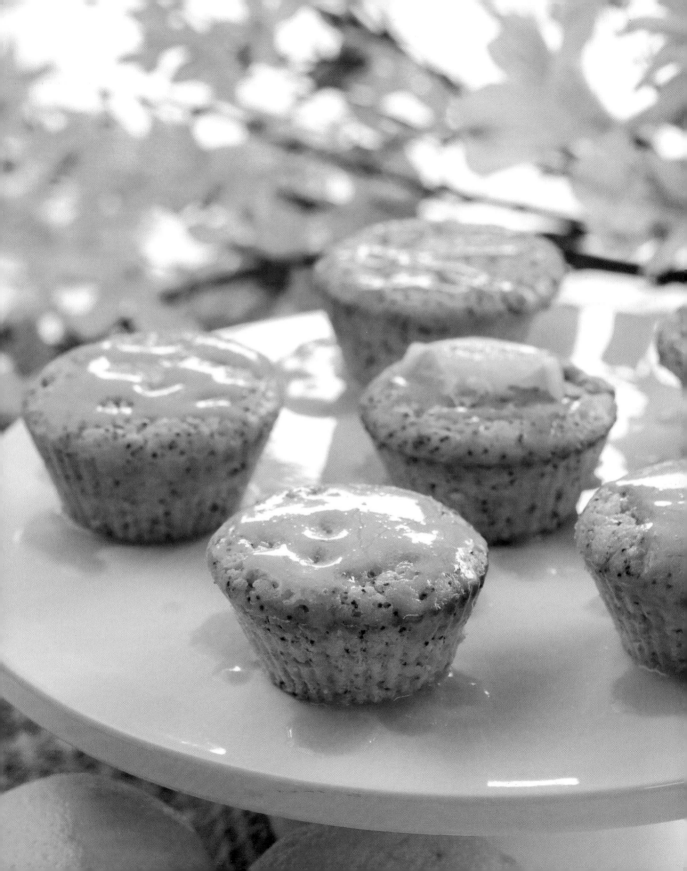

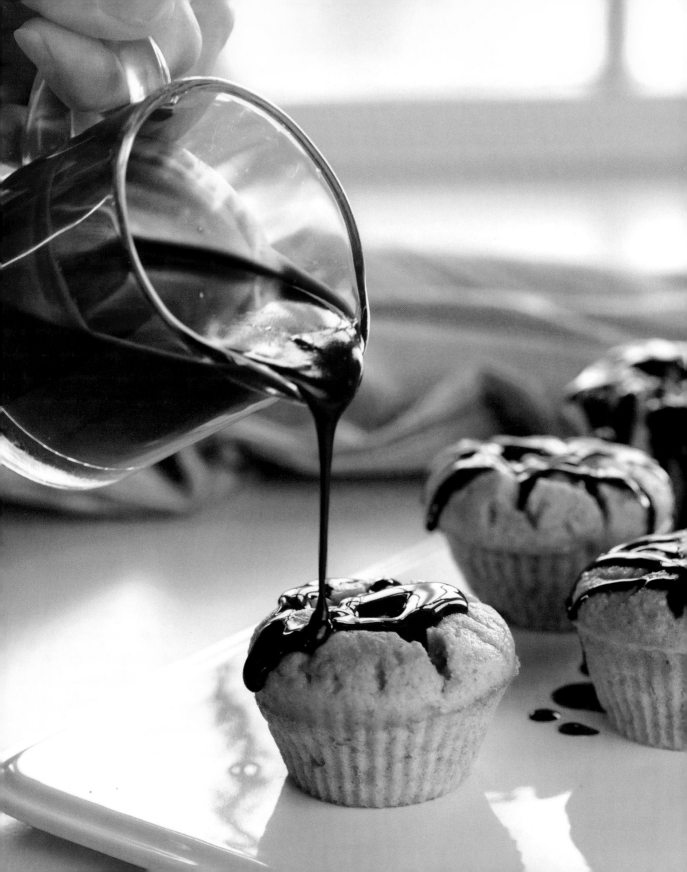

incredible peanut butter cookie muffins

FP

MAKES 12 LARGE MUFFINS

Coconut oil cooking spray
1⅓ cups THM Baking Blend*
¾ cup Pressed Peanut Flour*
½ cup Gentle Sweet* (plus optional 2 doonks Pure Stevia Extract Powder)
1 tablespoon aluminum-free baking powder
½ teaspoon Mineral Salt
1½ cups egg whites (carton or fresh)
1½ cups water
1½ teaspoons pure vanilla extract
Handy Chocolate Syrup (recipe follows)

You need a sweet Fuel Pull treat for those times when you know you've already had a big meal but you're still craving that moist, sweet baked good afterward. These hit the spot and they're incredible because it is hard to believe they are FP. Freeze them in baggies and pull out to heat or thaw for breakfast, a snack, or dessert.

We adapted this recipe from a single-serve muffin that one of our creative admins, Raye Pankratz, put in our membership site recipe database. She paired the muffin with the chocolate syrup from *Trim Healthy Mama Cookbook* (which we've included below) for an over-the-top chocolate/peanut butter kick. Raye also has a helpful blog with lots of other THM recipes. You can find it at rayesplace.blogspot.com.

1. Preheat the oven to 400°F. Line 12 cups of a muffin tin with cupcake liners (parchment liners work best) and spray the liners with coconut oil.

2. Put all the dry ingredients in a large bowl and whisk together. Add the wet ingredients and stir well. Allow the mixture to set up for 10 minutes (as it will be very wet at first).

3. Ladle the batter to the top of the muffin cups and bake for 22 minutes. (While the muffins are baking, make the chocolate syrup; see below.)

4. Remove the muffins from the pan, let them cool enough to remove the liners, then place on a tray. Drizzle the muffins with chocolate syrup (if you have leftover sauce, put it in a small jar with a lid and store in the fridge for other purposes, such as topping pancakes or waffles).

* FOR NSI: USE THE FRUGAL FLOUR OPTION (SEE PAGE 40), BUT NOTE THIS WILL CHANGE THE MUFFINS TO A LIGHT S. OR YOU CAN MAKE AN FP-FRIENDLY FRUGAL OPTION OF HALF COCONUT FLOUR, HALF OAT FIBER. USE GROCERY STORE SUGAR-FREE DEFATTED PEANUT FLOUR AND AN ON-PLAN SWEETENER.

HANDY CHOCOLATE SYRUP

MAKES ABOUT ¾ CUP

½ cup water
¼ cup unsweetened cocoa powder
5 tablespoons Gentle Sweet
3 generous pinches Mineral Salt
½ teaspoon pure vanilla extract

1. Put all the syrup ingredients in a small saucepan and bring to a boil over medium-high heat, whisking often. Reduce the heat to low and whisk while the mixture simmers gently for a couple more minutes. Remove from the heat.

Cakes

Below are a few tips on how to have the most success with your THM cakes:

Enjoy cake for breakfast! This is our mantra and we're not kidding about this. These cakes are all protein rich (if using our THM Baking Blend) and they help you get a balanced blood sugar start to your day. There is not one unhealthy ingredient in them! And honestly, what could be more undiet-y than cake and coffee for breakfast . . . we're living here! Of course, you won't want cake for brekkie every morning, but feel free to do it a couple mornings a week.

Sweeten up right! Gentle Sweet is the listed ingredient for all these cakes since it tastes closest to sugar and is the best option for your taste buds if you are new to a sugar-free lifestyle. (If you are concerned about your dog snatching a bite of cake, we also have a xylitol-free version of Gentle Sweet.) For budgeting Mamas and for those whose tastes have already adjusted to stevia—feel free to use Super Sweet blend, but be sure to use only one-third as much as what is called for with Gentle Sweet. Super Sweet is by far a more cost-effective option, but if used in too high amounts it can taste bitter. Or, if you have your own favorite on-plan sweetener, check the sweetener conversion chart on our website at www.trimhealthymama.com.

Don't sweat the Baking Blend! Check out Magic Salted Caramel Cupcakes (page 379) and the BAM Cakes, which don't use Baking Blend, but please read page 39 on why we list it in our other cakes. If you can't afford our blend, use the frugal flour option on page 40. Copycat versions of our Baking Blend can also give you a reasonable result (although some copycat versions are drier, we hear). Please don't use all almond flour in our cakes—that stuff is simply ground up nuts, and while nuts are wonderful on-plan foods, you can get into calorie abuse when using straight almond flour all the time. It's like pouring hundreds of nuts down your throat!

Lighten up! Some people can eat our cakes as written for dessert after a big meal every single night and still Trim down just fine. For others (our turtle Mamas), doing that too often will be too much fuel tacked onto the end of a meal and may stall weight loss. If that's true in your case, it may be wiser for you to eat cake as dessert less often and more often for an afternoon snack or breakfast, as we described earlier. Your body can process the fuel better that way. Having said that, there is a way to make frequent cake for actual dessert more doable. All of our Trimtastic cakes can be lightened up in these ways:

• Replace the eggs with egg whites. If a cake calls for 4 eggs, you would use 1 cup whites.

• Cut the butter or oil amounts in half. The zucchini in these Trimtastic cakes keeps the batter so moist, the extra fat is not really missed.

• Replace heavy cream icings with any glaze option listed or our Handy Chocolate Syrup (page 371).

And don't forget the baby-size shakes and smoothies (page 469 to page 494) as a smart, sweet treat option for you as an everyday dessert, not to mention the Peanut Butter Cookie Muffins (page 371), which are a Fuel Pull.

Serving sizes. These are all family-size cakes. Sorry, we are not going to tell you exactly how big of a piece you can eat or whether you can eat one or two pieces. As you mature in this lifestyle you will begin to tune in to your own body. Your serving size may vary depending on how hungry you are or whether you are enjoying it as a mini meal or as a dessert. For common sense's sake, don't go crazy and eat three giant pieces, but do enjoy a nice piece or two.

frappuccino cake

(S)

MULTIPLE SERVE

Coconut oil cooking spray

1½ cups THM Baking Blend*

½ cup Gentle Sweet*

¼ teaspoon Mineral Salt

2 teaspoons aluminum-free baking powder

3 large eggs

½ cup egg whites (carton or fresh)

4 tablespoons (½ stick) butter or coconut oil, melted

1 cup of your favorite strong brewed coffee, cooled

FOR THE FROSTING

3 tablespoons ⅓ less fat cream cheese

½ cup heavy cream

¾ teaspoon pure vanilla extract

¼ teaspoon coffee extract

¼ cup Gentle Sweet*

2 pinches Mineral Salt

Ground espresso beans, for sprinkling

Take this to any function, be it a baby shower, wedding shower, or potluck, and see how many requests you get for the recipe. It is super easy to make, tastes like the creamiest coffee creation ever, and is always a winner!

1. Preheat the oven to 350°F. Thoroughly spray an 8-inch square cake pan with coconut oil.

2. Whisk together the Baking Blend, sweetener, salt, and baking powder in a large bowl. In another bowl, mix the whole eggs, egg whites, melted butter, and coffee well. Add the wet ingredients to the dry and whisk all together well. (Or put all the ingredients in a food processor and process well, which in our minds is just easier.)

3. Pour the batter into the cake dish and bake for 30 minutes.

4. Meanwhile, make the frosting. Put all the ingredients (except the ground espresso) in a blender and blend until thickened. Place the frosting in the fridge.

5. Cool the cake in the pan, then frost inside the pan. Sprinkle ground espresso beans over the top.

* FOR NSI: USE THE FRUGAL FLOUR OPTION (SEE PAGE 40) AND A GROCERY STORE ON-PLAN SWEETENER.

* FOR DF: USE COCONUT OIL IN THE CAKE BATTER. OMIT THE FROSTING AND MAKE A DF RUNNY GLAZE BY HEATING TOGETHER 4 TABLESPOONS COCONUT OIL, 3 TABLESPOONS GENTLE SWEET, 2 TABLESPOONS NUT MILK, ¼ TEASPOON COFFEE EXTRACT, AND A COUPLE PINCHES OF SALT IN A SAUCEPAN.

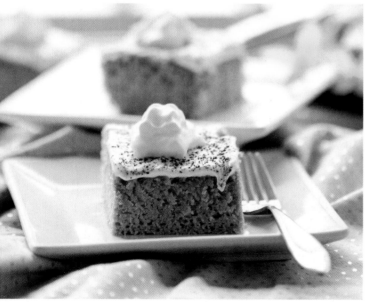

carrot cake deluxe

MULTIPLE SERVE

Coconut oil cooking spray
1½ cups THM Baking Blend*
¼ cup unflavored Pristine Whey
  Protein Powder*
⅓ cup unsweetened shredded
  coconut
⅓ cup walnuts, chopped
¾ cup Gentle Sweet*
2 teaspoons ground cinnamon
1 teaspoon grated nutmeg
½ to ¾ teaspoon ground allspice
¼ teaspoon ground cloves
  (optional)
¼ teaspoon Mineral Salt
2 teaspoons aluminum-free baking
  powder
3 large eggs, lightly beaten
½ cup egg whites (carton or fresh)
⅓ cup coconut oil
¾ cup unsweetened almond milk
1½ cups grated carrots, grated on
  the finest grating option (2 small
  to medium carrots)

FOR THE DELUXE FROSTING
4 ounces ⅓ less fat cream cheese
4 tablespoons (½ stick) softened
  butter
⅓ cup Gentle Sweet*
½ teaspoon pure vanilla extract
  (optional)

1. Preheat the oven to 350°F. Spray an 8-inch square cake pan with coconut oil.

2. Whisk together the Baking Blend, whey protein, coconut, walnuts, sweetener, spices, salt, and baking powder. Add the beaten eggs, egg whites, coconut oil, almond milk, and carrots and stir well.

3. Pour the batter into the prepared pan and bake for 40 to 45 minutes, until the top of the cake is no longer soggy. Let cool.

4. Make the frosting. Beat or whisk the ingredients together. Frost the cake once cooled.

* FOR NSI: USE THE FRUGAL FLOUR OPTION (SEE PAGE 40) AND FIND A GENTLY PROCESSED GROCERY STORE WHEY PROTEIN ISOLATE WITH ONLY 1 GRAM CARB. USE A GROCERY STORE ON-PLAN SWEETENER.

* FOR DF: OMIT THE FROSTING AND MAKE A GLAZE BY WHISKING TOGETHER 2 TABLESPOONS NUT MILK, 1 TEASPOON LEMON JUICE, ¼ CUP GENTLE SWEET, AND ⅛ TEASPOON PURE LEMON EXTRACT (FOR AN ABSOLUTELY SMOOTH GLAZE, RUN THE GENTLE SWEET THROUGH A COFFEE GRINDER FIRST).

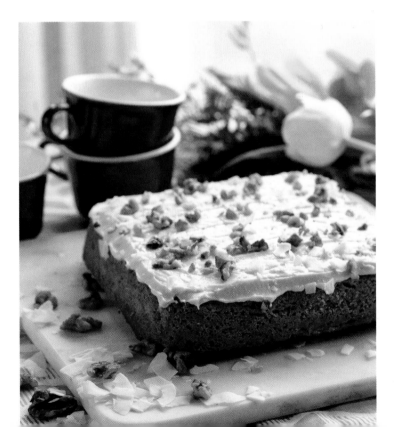

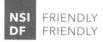
life by chocolate cake

S

MULTIPLE SERVE

Coconut oil cooking spray

1¾ cups THM Baking Blend*

½ cup unsweetened cocoa powder

1 cup Gentle Sweet*

⅛ to ¼ teaspoon Pure Stevia Extract Powder* (depending on your sweet tooth)

1 tablespoon aluminum-free baking powder

Rounded ¼ teaspoon Mineral Salt

4 large eggs

¾ cup egg whites (carton or fresh)

4 tablespoons (½ stick) butter or coconut oil, melted

1½ cups water

FOR THE GANACHE

2 ounces unsweetened baking chocolate

4 tablespoons coconut oil (use the flavorless kind if you don't want a coconut taste)

¼ cup heavy cream

½ cup unsweetened cashew or almond milk

¼ cup Gentle Sweet*

¼ teaspoon Pure Stevia Extract Powder*

4 pinches Mineral Salt

½ teaspoon Natural Burst chocolate extract, pure vanilla extract, or any kind of extract you love (optional)

You've heard of Death by Chocolate Cake. We're about to turn that all upside down and back to front. You *can* gain life and health by eating chocolate cake! This cake is sweet and rich and tastes like the bad-for-you stuff, but it is oh so good for you. Enjoy for life!

1. Preheat the oven to 350°F. Line the bottoms of two 9-inch springform pans with rounds of parchment paper. Spray the pans with coconut oil.

2. Mix together the Baking Blend, cocoa powder, sweeteners, baking powder, and salt in one bowl. In a second bowl, mix the whole eggs, egg whites, butter, and water. Combine the wet and dry ingredients and whisk well.

3. Pour the batter into the 2 prepared pans and bake for 25 to 30 minutes, until the tops of the cakes are done. Allow the cakes to cool on your counter.

4. Meanwhile, make the ganache. Put the baking chocolate and coconut oil in a small heatproof bowl and set over a small saucepan of simmering water (making sure the water doesn't touch the bowl). Allow to melt completely, then reduce the heat under the saucepan to low. Whisk in the heavy cream, then the nut milk. Keep whisking as you add the sweeteners, salt, and extract of choice (if using).

5. Place the bowl of ganache in the freezer. Check it every 10 minutes and give it a whisk as it thickens. It should be ganache consistency after about 30 minutes.

6. Remove the cakes from the pans and place one layer on a cake plate. Ice the top of the layer with some of the ganache, then place the other layer on top. Frost the top, then put a thin smear of the ganache around the sides of the whole cake. Keep refrigerated until ready to eat. Store leftovers in the fridge.

* FOR NSI: USE THE FRUGAL FLOUR OPTION (SEE PAGE 40) AND A GROCERY STORE ON-PLAN SWEETENER.

* FOR DF: OMIT THE HEAVY CREAM FROM THE GANACHE AND REPLACE WITH ¼ CUP MORE NUT MILK.

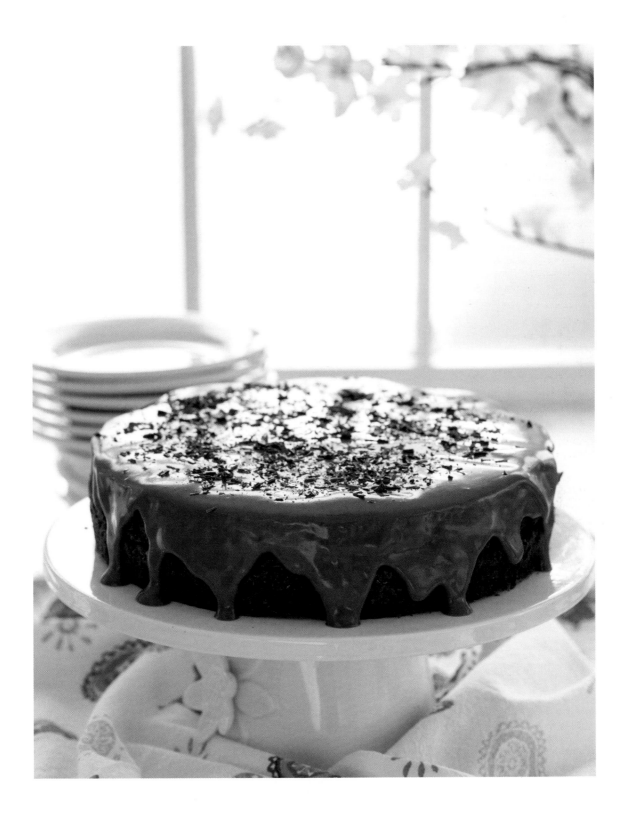

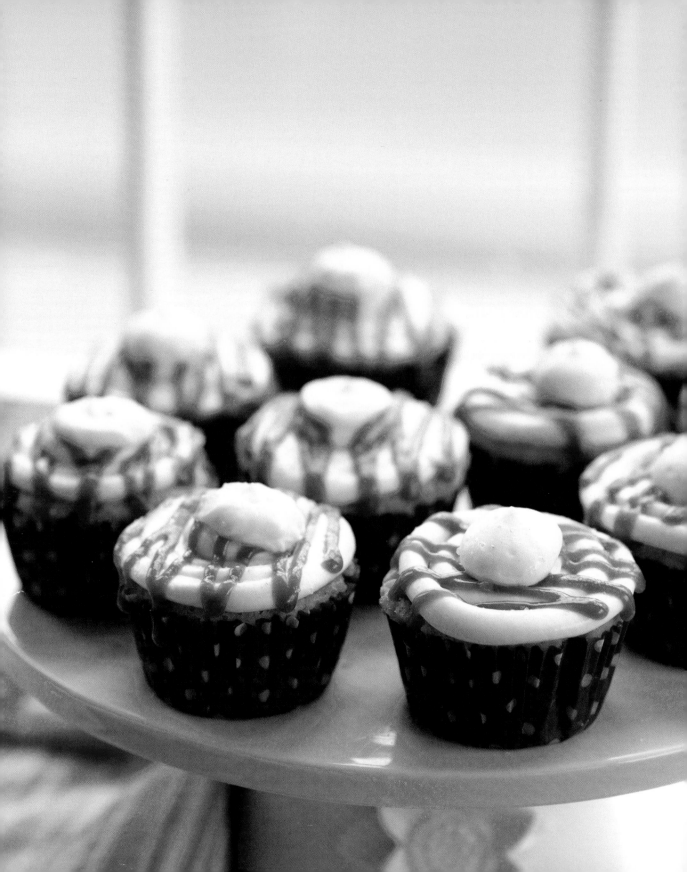

magic salted caramel cupcakes

S

MAKES 16 CUPCAKES

Coconut oil cooking spray

FOR THE CUPCAKES

2 (15-ounce) cans white beans, rinsed and drained, or 3 cups home-cooked white beans

3 large eggs

¾ cup egg whites (carton or fresh)

¾ cup Gentle Sweet*

2 teaspoons aluminum-free baking powder

1 teaspoon baking soda

1 teaspoon pure vanilla extract

¾ to 1 teaspoon Natural Burst caramel extract*

¼ teaspoon Mineral Salt

2 tablespoons coconut oil

FOR THE FROSTING

3 ounces ⅓ less fat cream cheese

½ cup heavy cream

¼ cup Gentle Sweet*

½ teaspoon pure vanilla extract

¼ teaspoon Natural Burst caramel extract*

5 pinches Mineral Salt

FOR THE OPTIONAL CARAMEL SAUCE TOPPING

2 tablespoons butter

2 tablespoons Gentle Sweet*

½ teaspoon blackstrap molasses (optional, for a brown sugar effect)

⅛ teaspoon Mineral Salt

2 tablespoons heavy cream

⅛ teaspoon xanthan gum or Gluccie*

The magic lies in the fact that no flour is needed for these babies. Don't tell any picky family members, but white beans create the moist and lovely texture! The key is to refrigerate the cupcakes for at least 4 to 6 hours before eating to get rid of any beany taste (even better overnight).

1. Preheat the oven to 350°F. Line 16 cups of muffin tins with cake liners (the parchment kind work best). Lightly spray the insides with coconut oil.

2. Put all the cupcake ingredients in a food processor and process well. Using a spoon, drop the batter into the muffin cups and bake for 25 minutes. Remove the cupcakes from the pans and allow the muffins to cool on the counter for a little while, then refrigerate until ready to frost.

3. Make the frosting. Put all the frosting ingredients in a blender and blend until thickened. If choosing to make the caramel sauce, put butter, sweetener, and molasses in a small saucepan. Heat until bubbly over medium-high heat and allow to bubble for about 2 minutes, whisking constantly. Remove from the heat and add the salt and cream while whisking. Gently sprinkle in xanthan or Gluccie while continuing to stir. Allow the sauce to cool and thicken. Frost the cupcakes, drizzle the sauce over the top, then refrigerate for several hours (or overnight) before eating.

NOTE: You'll notice these are an S recipe, yet we use beans here. You can get by with having about ¼ cup beans in some of your S meals. Each of these cupcakes has well less than ¼ cup beans, so you're fine. Also, beans are full of resistant starch, so they are one very gentle E fuel that is not as clashy when mixed with S foods. If having as a dessert after an S meal, best to stick to 1 cupcake, otherwise you'll be piling on too many carbs. We much prefer to enjoy them for breakfast or an afternoon snack so we can squeeze 2 in.

* FOR NSI: USE A GROCERY STORE ON-PLAN SWEETENER AND CARAMEL EXTRACT.

* FOR DF: OMIT THE FROSTING AND MAKE A DF RUNNY GLAZE BY HEATING TOGETHER 4 TABLESPOONS COCONUT OIL, 3 TABLESPOONS GENTLE SWEET, 2 TABLESPOONS NUT MILK, AND ¼ TEASPOON CARAMEL EXTRACT IN A SAUCEPAN.

cinnamon butter bundt cake Ⓢ

MULTIPLE SERVE

Coconut oil cooking spray and
  ground cinnamon for the pan
8 tablespoons (1 stick) softened
  butter
1 cup Gentle Sweet*
3 large eggs
½ cup egg whites (carton or fresh)
2 cups THM Baking Blend*
1 tablespoon aluminum-free baking
  powder
1½ teaspoons ground cinnamon
½ teaspoon Mineral Salt
1 cup unsweetened cashew or
  almond milk
¼ cup heavy cream or half-and-half
1 teaspoon pure vanilla extract
1 teaspoon Natural Burst butter
  extract

FOR THE CINNAMON BUTTER GLAZE
4 tablespoons (½ stick) butter
3 tablespoons Gentle Sweet*
1 teaspoon ground cinnamon
¼ to ½ teaspoon Natural Burst
  butter extract
2 tablespoons unsweetened cashew
  or almond milk

PEARL CHATS: Take one bite of this succulent cake and you'd swear it contains 2 cups of butter, it is so buttery and moist. Nope, just a sensible ½ cup butter in the batter, the pure butter extract helps do the trick without abuse of calories. I think this might be my favorite cake from this book. It's hard to pick favorites but I'm eating this right now and I can't stop saying "Mmmm."

1. Preheat the oven to 350°F. Spray a 10-inch Bundt pan thoroughly with coconut oil or grease it very well with butter. Sprinkle cinnamon liberally all over the pan so it sticks to the oil or butter.

2. With an electric mixer, cream together the butter and sweetener in a large bowl. Beat in the whole eggs until smooth, then beat in the egg whites. Keep beating for another 30 seconds. Add the Baking Blend, baking powder, cinnamon, and salt and beat again until the mixture is well combined. Add the nut milk, heavy cream, and extracts, and beat for another half minute or so.

3. Scrape the batter into the prepared pan, smooth the top with a spatula, and bake for 40 minutes. Once the cake is close to cool, use a knife to pull the edges away from the sides of the pan and invert it onto a cake plate (if only half comes out at once, it is not the end of the world . . . just loosen the other half out and sort it back together on the plate—you'll be poking holes in it, anyway).

4. Meanwhile, make the glaze. Melt the ingredients together in a small saucepan (it will look runny and swirly, not smooth, that's fine).

5. Poke lots of holes all over the cake with a chopstick or other utensil, then spoon the glaze all over the cake, allowing it to drizzle into the holes and smear around the edges of the cake. The cake is lovely eaten still slightly warm, but once it's refrigerated, the glaze sets and is amazingly yummy.

NOTE: If you don't have a Bundt pan, you can make these into 12 to 16 cupcakes. Bake them for 20 minutes at 350°F.

* FOR NSI: USE A GROCERY STORE ON-PLAN SWEETENER, THE FRUGAL FLOUR OPTION (SEE PAGE 40), AND GROCERY STORE EXTRACTS.

* FOR DF: REPLACE THE BUTTER WITH COCONUT OIL AND THE HEAVY CREAM WITH UNSWEETENED NUT MILK.

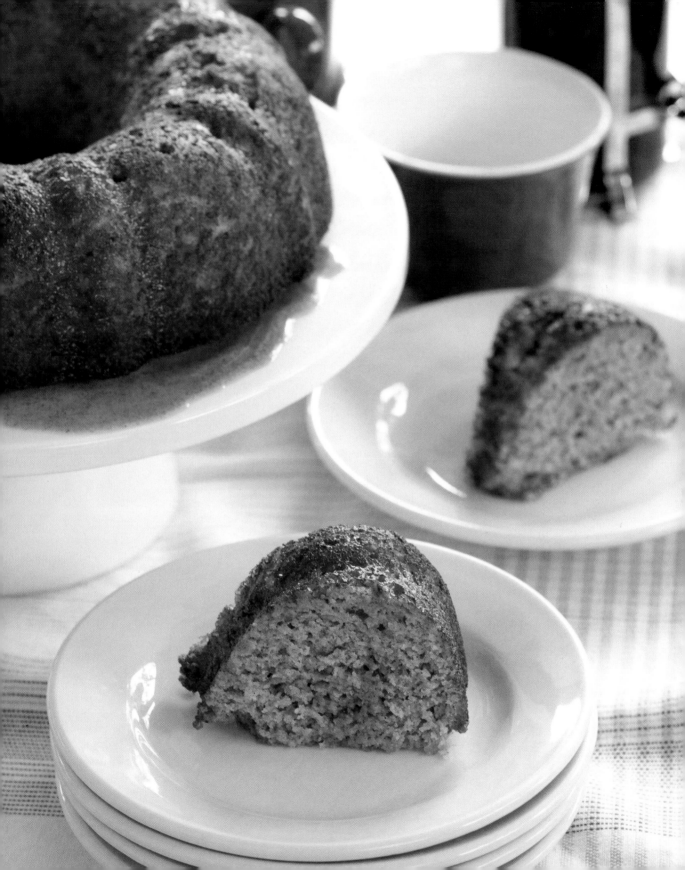

chocolate treeces poke cake

S

MULTIPLE SERVE

Coconut oil cooking spray

FOR THE CAKE

1 cup THM Baking Blend*
½ cup unsweetened cocoa powder
¾ cup Gentle Sweet*
⅛ teaspoon Pure Stevia Extract Powder*
3 large eggs
½ cup egg whites (carton or fresh)
4 tablespoons coconut oil or butter
1 cup water
¼ teaspoon Mineral Salt
1 teaspoon pure vanilla extract
2 teaspoons aluminum-free baking powder

FOR THE FROSTING

½ cup coconut oil
¼ cup Pressed Peanut Flour*
¼ cup sugar-free natural-style peanut butter (we love chunky for this)
4 to 5 pinches Mineral Salt
1 tablespoon Super Sweet Blend (ground in a coffee grinder), or 3 tablespoons Gentle Sweet*

Moist and chocolaty . . . topped with gooey peanutty goodness . . . come to Mama! Instead of sugar-laden, waist-exploding Reese's, do it the Trimming Healthy way and you have . . . Treeces! This Treecified frosting drips down into the cake and makes you sigh with pleasure. All this goodness and the cake is completely dairy-free! You're welcome, dairy-free Mamas.

1. Preheat the oven to 350°F. Generously spray an 8-inch square cake pan with coconut oil.

2. Make the cake. Place all the ingredients in a food processor and process well for about 30 seconds. Pour the batter into the cake pan and bake for 35 minutes, or until the top of the cake is just done but not too firm. While the cake is cooling inside the pan on the counter, use a knife or chopstick to poke holes all over the top of the cake.

3. Make the frosting. Place all the ingredients in a food processor and process (or stir all the ingredients together in a bowl, making sure your coconut oil is liquid before doing so). Pour the frosting all over the cake, then refrigerate the cake until you want to eat it.

NOTE: If you have an allergy to peanuts, the frosting can be made with almonds. You would use ⅓ cup almond butter to replace the peanut flour and peanut butter.

* FOR NSI: USE THE FRUGAL FLOUR OPTION (SEE PAGE 40), A GROCERY STORE ON-PLAN SWEETENER, AND SUGAR-FREE DEFATTED PEANUT FLOUR.

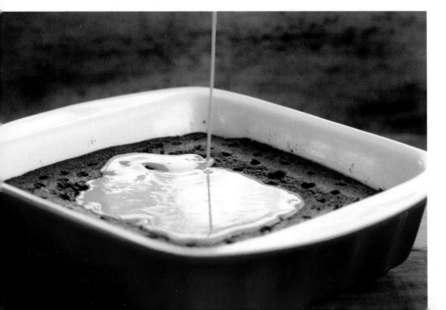

peanut butter banana bam cake

E

MULTIPLE SERVE

Coconut oil cooking spray

2 cups old-fashioned rolled oats

1 cup egg whites (carton or fresh)

¾ teaspoon cream of tartar, or
   ½ teaspoon xanthan gum
   (optional; see Note)

2 large bananas

½ cup Pressed Peanut Flour*

½ teaspoon Mineral Salt

2 teaspoons aluminum-free baking
   powder

1 teaspoon baking soda

½ cup Gentle Sweet plus 2 to
   4 doonks Pure Stevia Extract
   Powder*

1 cup plain 0% Greek yogurt

1 teaspoon Natural Burst banana
   extract

1 teaspoon pure vanilla extract

One of the popular cakes from *Trim Healthy Mama Cookbook* was Bust-a-Myth Banana Cake, which got shortened to BAM Cake by everyone. A couple of very smart ladies had the brilliant idea to beat the eggs whites first, which took the cake to a whole new world of fluffier texture! This recipe and the following two are awesome new versions of BAM cake. Enjoy BAM for an energizing breakfast or for a snack.

1. Preheat the oven to 350°F. Lightly coat an 8-inch square baking pan or a 9 × 13-inch baking dish with coconut oil spray.

2. Measure out ½ cup oats and set aside. Grind the remaining 1½ cups oats to a flour in a blender.

3. In a bowl, beat the egg whites and cream of tartar (if using; or xanthan gum) until soft peaks form.

4. Mash the bananas in another bowl, then add the ground oats, whole oats, peanut flour, salt, baking powder, baking soda, sweetener, yogurt, and extracts and mix well. Finally, fold in the egg whites.

5. Pour the batter into the prepared pan and bake until golden brown on top, 40 minutes in the smaller pan, or 30 minutes in the baking dish.

NOTE: You can also prepare this the original way and not bother to beat the egg whites. Simply mash the bananas and add all the other ingredients—still great.

* FOR NSI: USE A GROCERY STORE SUGAR-FREE DEFATTED PEANUT FLOUR, EXTRACTS, AND AN ON-PLAN SWEETENER.

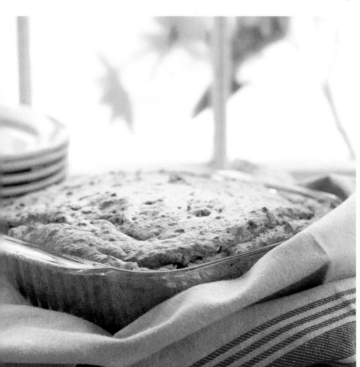

FRIENDLY

caramel apple bam cake
with optional caramel glosting

Ⓔ

MULTIPLE SERVE

Coconut oil cooking spray

1 cup egg whites (carton or fresh)

¾ teaspoon cream of tartar, or
  ½ teaspoon xanthan gum
  (optional; see Note)

2½ cups old-fashioned rolled oats

1 small apple, diced

1 cup unsweetened applesauce
  (if you don't have applesauce,
  increase the diced apples to 2)

2 teaspoons ground cinnamon or
  apple pie spice

1 teaspoon Natural Burst caramel
  extract*

Scant ¼ teaspoon Mineral Salt

2 teaspoons aluminum-free baking
  powder

1 teaspoon baking soda

½ cup Gentle Sweet plus 2 to
  4 doonks Pure Stevia Extract
  Powder*

1 cup plain 0% Greek yogurt

1 to 2 teaspoons pure vanilla extract

**FOR THE OPTIONAL CARAMEL
GLOSTING**

2 tablespoons ⅓ less fat cream
  cheese

2 heaping tablespoons plain
  0% Greek yogurt

¼ teaspoon Natural Burst caramel
  extract*

2 to 3 tablespoons Gentle Sweet*

2 teaspoons unsweetened cashew
  or almond milk

1. Preheat the oven to 350°F. Lightly spray an 8-inch square baking pan or a 9 × 13-inch baking dish with coconut oil.

2. In a bowl, beat the egg whites and cream of tartar (if using; or xanthan gum) until soft peaks form.

3. Measure out ½ cup of the oats and set aside. Grind the remaining 2 cups oats to a flour in a blender. In another bowl, add the whole oats, ground oats, diced apple, applesauce, cinnamon, caramel extract, salt, baking powder, baking soda, sweetener, yogurt, and vanilla and mix well. Finally, fold in the egg whites.

4. Pour the batter into the prepared pan and bake until golden brown on top, 40 to 45 minutes in the smaller pan, or 30 to 35 minutes in the larger pan. Let the cake cool.

5. Make the glosting. Whisk the ingredients together. Frost the cooled cake.

NOTE: You can also prepare this the original BAM way and not bother to beat the egg whites. Simply mix all the ingredients together in a bowl.

* FOR NSI: USE A GROCERY STORE ON-PLAN SWEETENER AND EXTRACTS.

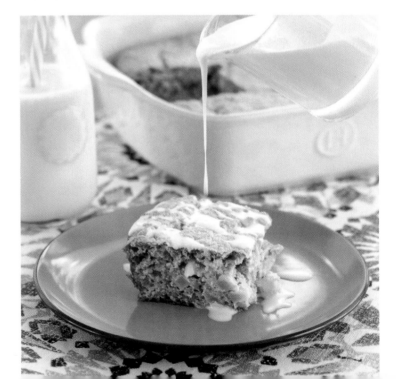

pumpkin bam cake

MULTIPLE SERVE

Coconut oil cooking spray

1 cup egg whites (carton or fresh)

¾ teaspoon cream of tartar, or
½ teaspoon xanthan gum
(optional; see Note)

2½ cups old-fashioned rolled oats

1 (15-ounce) can pure pumpkin
puree

2 teaspoons pumpkin pie spice

1 teaspoon pure vanilla extract

Scant ¼ teaspoon Mineral Salt

2 teaspoons aluminum-free baking
powder

1 teaspoon baking soda

½ cup Gentle Sweet plus 2 to
4 doonks Pure Stevia Extra
Powder*

1 cup plain 0% Greek yogurt

FOR THE GLOSTING

2 tablespoons ⅓ less fat cream
cheese

2 heaping tablespoons plain
0% Greek yogurt

½ teaspoon pure vanilla extract

2 to 3 tablespoons Gentle Sweet*

2 teaspoons unsweetened cashew
or almond milk

1. Preheat the oven to 350°F. Lightly coat an 8-inch square baking pan or a 9 × 13- inch baking dish with coconut oil.

2. In a bowl, beat the egg whites and cream of tartar (if using; or xanthan gum) until soft peaks form.

3. Measure out ½ cup of the oats and set aside. Grind the remaining 2 cups oats to a flour in a blender. In another bowl, add the whole oats, ground oats, pumpkin, pumpkin pie spice, vanilla, salt, baking powder, baking soda, sweetener, and yogurt and mix well. Finally, fold in the egg whites.

4. Pour the batter into the prepared pan and bake until golden brown on top, 40 to 45 minutes in the smaller pan, or 30 to 35 minutes in the larger pan. Let cool.

5. Make the glosting. Whisk the ingredients together. Frost the cooled cake.

NOTE: You can also prepare this the original BAM way and not bother to beat the egg whites. Simply mix all the ingredients together in a bowl.

* FOR NSI: USE A GROCERY STORE ON-PLAN SWEETENER.

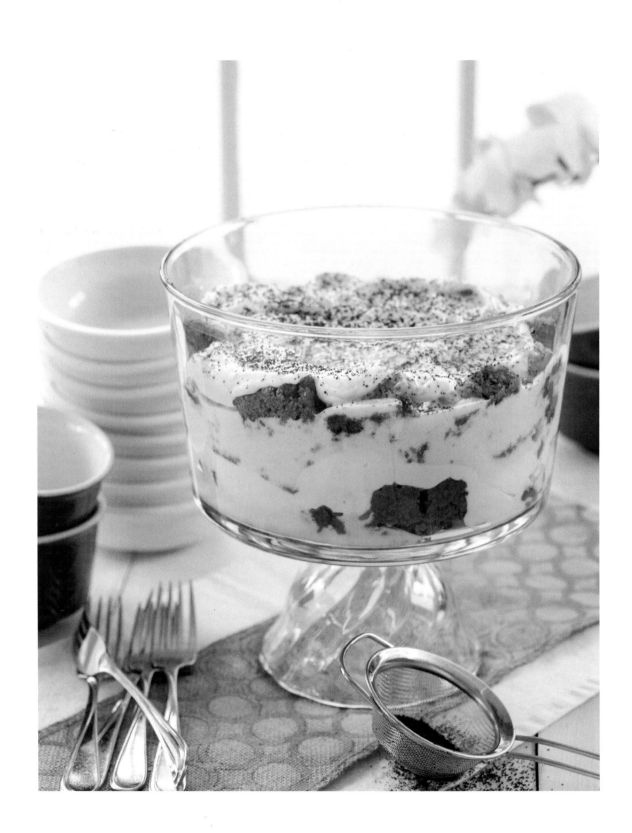

tiramisu trifle cake

MULTIPLE SERVE

S

Frappuccino Cake (page 374)
¾ cup strong brewed coffee

FOR THE PUDDING LAYER
1 teaspoon Just Gelatin*
¼ cup water
1 teaspoon coconut oil
1½ cups unsweetened cashew or almond milk
2 pinches Mineral Salt
1½ teaspoons unsweetened cocoa powder
1½ teaspoons Super Sweet Blend, or 2 tablespoons Gentle Sweet*

FOR THE CREAM LAYER
1 (8-ounce) package ⅓ less fat cream cheese
1½ cups heavy cream
⅛ teaspoon rum extract (or you can use a couple splashes of the real thing!)
¼ teaspoon coffee extract
⅓ cup Gentle Sweet*

Unsweetened cocoa powder, for sprinkling

Oh, how we love thee, tiramisu. . . . Come and layer yourself into our lives! Although this has layers, it is not horribly time consuming. Take it to parties or any sort of get-together.

1. Make the Frappuccino Cake (page 374) and brew your favorite coffee.

2. While the cake is baking, make the pudding layer. Put the gelatin and water in a very small saucepan and whisk until there are no lumps. Heat the mixture over medium-high heat until hot. Add the coconut oil and allow it to melt. Put this mixture into your blender. Add the nut milk, salt, cocoa powder, and sweetener and blend well. Pour into an 8-inch square dish and place in the freezer to chill for 10 minutes, then transfer to the refrigerator.

3. Dice the cake up into small pieces while it is still inside the cake pan. Pour the coffee all over it and set aside.

4. Make the cream layer. Put all the ingredients into the blender and blend until thickened.

5. To assemble the trifle: Put half the cubed cake into the bottom of a medium glass bowl. Cover with about one-third of the cream layer, followed by half of the pudding. Make a layer of the remaining cake pieces, add another third of the cream, then top with the remaining pudding. Top with a final cream layer. Sprinkle a little cocoa powder on top.

NOTE: If you have made Trimmy Choco Pudding (page 439), you can use a generous serving of that for the pudding layer here.

* FOR NSI: USE A GROCERY STORE ON-PLAN SWEETENER, GROCERY STORE EXTRACTS, AND THE FRUGAL FLOUR OPTION (SEE PAGE 40) FOR THE CAKE AND CREAM LAYERS. USE GROCERY STORE UNFLAVORED GELATIN FOR THE PUDDING.

peanut lovers trimtastic cake

S

MULTIPLE SERVE

(CHECK OUT PAGE 373 FOR WAYS TO MAKE THIS A LIGHTER S CAKE)

Coconut oil cooking spray

2 very small or 1 medium yellow squash (to yield 1½ cups processed)

4 large eggs

4 tablespoons (½ stick) butter

½ cup THM Baking Blend*

½ cup Pressed Peanut Flour*

¾ cup Gentle Sweet*

⅛ teaspoon Pure Stevia Extract Powder*

1½ teaspoons Natural Burst butter extract or pure vanilla extract

4 to 5 generous pinches Mineral Salt

FOR THE FROSTING

¾ cup heavy cream

3 tablespoons Pressed Peanut Flour*

1 tablespoon sugar-free natural-style peanut butter

2 to 3 pinches Mineral Salt

¼ cup Gentle Sweet*

Handful of chopped peanuts, for sprinkling (optional)

This cake is incredibly peanutty with a moist crumb, but the frosting . . . oh boy! It is the stuff dreams are made of. This is the first of six Trimtastic cakes here. Our original Chocolate Zucchini Trimtastic cake was one of the most made recipes in the *Trim Healthy Mama Cookbook*. We couldn't help coming up with more.

1. Preheat the oven to 350°F. Lightly spray an 8-inch square baking pan with coconut oil.

2. Trim the squash on both ends, chop into a few pieces, and process in a food processor until broken down into very tiny pieces. Add the eggs, butter, Baking Blend, pressed peanut flour, sweeteners, butter extract, and salt and process until well combined.

3. Pour the batter into the prepared pan and bake for 35 to 40 minutes. Let the cake cool.

4. Meanwhile, make the frosting. Place all the ingredients in a blender and blend on high until thickened. Place in the refrigerator while the cake cools.

5. Frost the cooled cake and sprinkle with the peanuts (if using).

* FOR NSI: USE THE FRUGAL FLOUR OPTION (SEE PAGE 40), GROCERY STORE SUGAR-FREE DEFATTED PEANUT FLOUR, AND AN ON-PLAN SWEETENER.

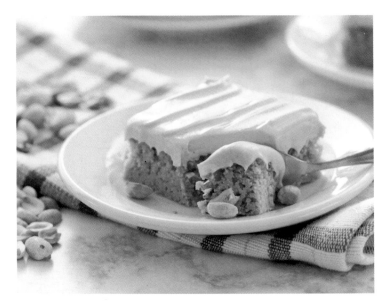

strawberry trimtastic cake

S

MULTIPLE SERVE

(CHECK OUT PAGE 373 FOR WAYS TO MAKE THIS A LIGHTER S CAKE)

Coconut oil cooking spray

1 small yellow squash (to yield ¾ to 1 cup processed)

1 cup frozen or fresh sliced strawberries

4 large eggs

4 tablespoons (½ stick) butter or coconut oil

1¼ cups THM Baking Blend*

¾ cup Gentle Sweet*

¼ teaspoon Pure Stevia Extract Powder,* or to taste

1 teaspoon aluminum-free baking powder

1 teaspoon baking soda

2 teaspoons pure strawberry extract

FOR THE FROSTING

4 ounces heavy cream

4 ounces ⅓ less fat cream cheese

¼ cup Gentle Sweet plus 2 to 3 doonks Pure Stevia Extract Powder*

½ teaspoon pure strawberry extract

½ cup frozen or fresh sliced strawberries

Sliced fresh strawberries, for decoration (optional)

If you are a strawberry cake lover . . . you're welcome!

1. Preheat the oven to 350°F. Lightly spray an 8-inch square baking pan or 8- or 9-inch round cake pan with coconut oil.

2. Trim the yellow squash on the ends (no need to peel), then cut into a couple of chunks and throw into a food processor and process to the size of rice. Add the strawberries, eggs, butter, Baking Blend, sweeteners, baking powder, baking soda, and strawberry extract and process until well combined.

3. Pour the batter into the prepared pan and bake for 35 to 40 minutes. Let the cake cool in the pan or remove to a wire rack.

4. Meanwhile, make the frosting. Blend all the ingredients in a blender on high until thickened. Place the frosting in the fridge until the cake is cool.

5. Frost the cooled cake, just on top if still in the pan, or on the top and sides if unmolded.

* FOR NSI: USE THE FRUGAL FLOUR OPTION (SEE PAGE 40) AND A GROCERY STORE ON-PLAN SWEETENER.

* FOR DF: USE THE GLAZE FROM SUPER MOIST TRIMTASTIC LEMON CAKE (PAGE 392) FOR A STRAWBERRY LEMON CAKE.

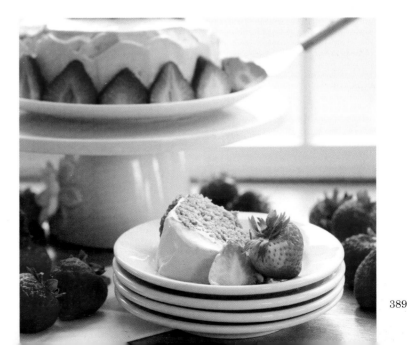

peppermint cream chocolate trimtastic cake   Ⓢ

MULTIPLE SERVE

(CHECK OUT PAGE 373 FOR WAYS TO
MAKE THIS A LIGHTER S CAKE)

Coconut oil cooking spray

1 large or 2 small zucchini or yellow
squash (to yield 2 cups processed),
or 1 (15-ounce) can pure pumpkin
puree

3 large eggs

½ cup egg whites (carton or fresh)

1 cup THM Baking Blend*

½ cup unsweetened cocoa powder

4 tablespoons (½ stick) butter

1 cup Gentle Sweet*

⅛ teaspoon Pure Stevia Extract
Powder*

2 teaspoons pure vanilla extract

2 teaspoons aluminum-free baking
powder

1 teaspoon baking soda

¼ teaspoon Mineral Salt

**FOR THE PEPPERMINT CREAM
FROSTING**

⅔ cup heavy cream

6 ounces ⅓ less fat cream cheese

¼ cup Gentle Sweet*

1 teaspoon pure peppermint extract
plus an optional drop or 2 of
peppermint essential oil

**OPTIONAL CHOCOLATE-PEPPERMINT
TOPPING**

¼ cup melted coconut oil (use
flavorless kind if desired)

2 tablespoons unsweetened cocoa
powder

1¼ teaspoons Super Sweet Blend*
(ground in a coffee grinder)

¼ teaspoon pure peppermint
extract

This is a large, gorgeous layer cake that is perfect for holiday parties. Or don't even wait for a party . . . just make it if you are a peppermint freak.

1. Preheat the oven to 350°F. Line the bottoms of two 9-inch springform pans with rounds of parchment paper. Spray the pans sides and parchment with coconut oil.

2. **IF USING ZUCCHINI OR SQUASH:** Don't bother peeling, cut into a couple of chunks, and process in a food processor until broken down into rice-size pieces. Add the whole eggs, egg whites, Baking Blend, cocoa powder, butter, sweeteners, vanilla, baking powder, baking soda, and salt and process until well combined.

   IF USING PUMPKIN: Just process everything together.

3. Divide the batter between the 2 pans and bake for 25 minutes (if using pumpkin, be sure it is done as the baking time may be a tad longer). Let the cakes cool.

4. Meanwhile, make the frosting. Blend all the frosting ingredients together until thickened, then place the frosting in the fridge.

5. Once the cakes have cooled, remove 1 of the cakes from the pan. Place the layer on a cake plate. Spread with a thin layer of frosting, top with the second layer, and frost the top and all the sides. Place the cake in the fridge to chill.

6. If desired, while the cake is chilling, make the optional chocolate-peppermint topping. Stir the ingredients together well in a small bowl.

7. Drizzle the chocolate topping all over the cake, allowing some to drip down the sides, then return the cake to the refrigerator until the topping hardens. Store any leftover cake in the refrigerator.

NOTE: In any of the chocolate Trimtastic Cakes you have the option of using zucchini or canned pumpkin. Zucchini is our preferred choice since it is the lower-carb option, but pumpkin is quicker and some people prefer it, so change it up if you like.

* FOR NSI: USE THE FRUGAL FLOUR OPTION (SEE PAGE 40) AND A GROCERY
STORE ON-PLAN SWEETENER.

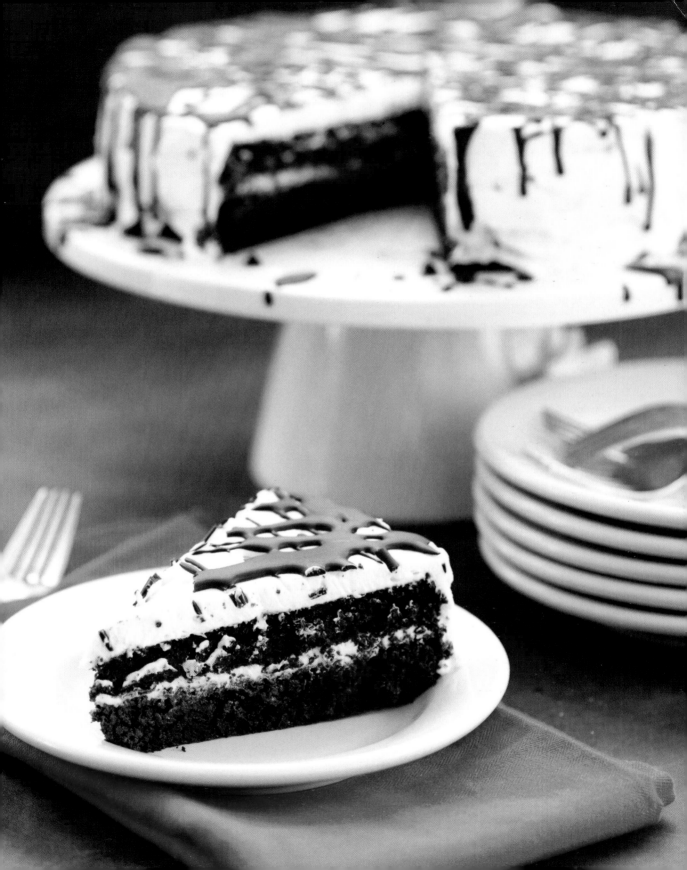

super moist trimtastic lemon cake **S**

MULTIPLE SERVE

(CHECK OUT PAGE 373 FOR WAYS TO MAKE THIS A LIGHTER S CAKE)

Coconut oil cooking spray

1 small yellow squash (to yield 1 cup processed)

4 large eggs

4 tablespoons (½ stick) butter or coconut oil

Juice of 2 lemons (about ¼ cup)

1 cup THM Baking Blend*

¾ cup Gentle Sweet, or ¼ cup Super Sweet Blend*

2 pinches Mineral Salt

2½ teaspoons aluminum-free baking powder

1 teaspoon pure lemon extract

1 teaspoon pure vanilla extract

2 teaspoons grated lemon zest (optional)

OPTIONAL CREAMY FROSTING

⅓ cup heavy cream

3 ounces ⅓ less fat cream cheese

¼ cup Gentle Sweet*

Juice of 1 lemon

OPTIONAL DAIRY-FREE LEMON GLAZE

1 tablespoon unsweetened cashew or almond milk

Juice of ½ lemon

¼ cup Gentle Sweet*

⅛ teaspoon pure lemon extract

Get your lemon fix with this lovely moist cake. The texture and taste will take you back to the days of refrigerator jello poke cakes . . . mmmm! Take your pick with the frostings—we couldn't leave our dairy-free peeps out! Even if you are not dairy-free, the glaze is awesome!

1. Preheat the oven to 350°F. Lightly coat an 8-inch square glass baking dish or 9-inch round cake or pie plate with coconut oil spray.

2. Trim the squash, chop into a few pieces, and process well in a food processor so it is not mush but broken down into tiny pieces. Add the eggs, butter, lemon juice, Baking Blend, sweetener, salt, baking powder, extracts, and lemon zest (if using) and process well.

3. Pour the batter into the prepared pan and bake for 30 to 35 minutes. Let the cake cool in the pan. While the cake is cooling, make either the frosting or the dairy-free glaze.

4. **FOR THE CREAMY FROSTING:** Blend all the ingredients in a blender until thickened. Frost the cake in the pan or invert the cake onto a plate and frost it.

   FOR THE DAIRY-FREE GLAZE: Whisk the glaze ingredients together (if you want an absolutely smooth glaze, run the Gentle Sweet through your coffee grinder first). Spread the glaze over the cake.

5. Keep the cake refrigerated until ready to eat.

* FOR NSI: USE THE FRUGAL FLOUR OPTION (SEE PAGE 40) AND A GROCERY STORE ON-PLAN SWEETENER.

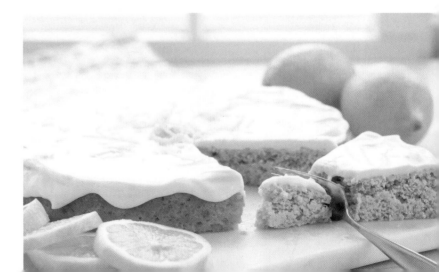

holiday pumpkin trimtastic roll

S

MULTIPLE SERVE

Gentle Sweet,* for sprinkling

½ medium or 1 very small zucchini (to yield ½ to ¾ cup processed)

¾ cup canned pure pumpkin puree

4 large eggs

4 tablespoons (½ stick) butter

¾ to 1 cup THM Baking Blend*

¾ cup Gentle Sweet*

⅛ teaspoon Pure Stevia Extract Powder,* or to taste

1½ teaspoons pure vanilla extract

1 teaspoon aluminum-free baking powder

1 teaspoon baking soda

2 pinches Mineral Salt

1 tablespoon pumpkin pie spice

¾ cup walnuts or pecans, chopped (optional)

FOR THE CREAM CHEESE FILLING

1 (8-ounce) package ⅓ less fat cream cheese

4 tablespoons (½ stick) softened butter

3 to 4 tablespoons Gentle Sweet,* to taste

1 teaspoon pure vanilla extract

1. Preheat the oven to 350°F. Line a 15 x 10-inch jelly-roll pan with parchment paper. Sprinkle a clean thin tea towel (or thin dish towel) with Gentle Sweet and set aside for rolling the cake.

2. Trim the zucchini and chop into a few chunks. Pulse in a food processor so it is not mush, but broken down well into very tiny pieces. Add the pumpkin, eggs, butter, Baking Blend, sweeteners, vanilla, baking powder, baking soda, salt, and pumpkin pie spice and process until well combined.

3. Spread the batter evenly onto the prepared jelly-roll pan. If opting to use the nuts, sprinkle over the batter. Bake for 15 to 20 minutes, until the top of the cake springs back when touched. (Dark-colored pans tend to cook faster.)

4. Immediately turn the cake onto the prepared towel. Carefully peel off the parchment paper. Roll the cake and towel together, starting at a narrow end. Allow to cool completely on a wire rack. (You'll want to allow the cake to cool completely as to avoid cracking later while filling.)

5. While the cake is cooling, make the filling. Beat together the cream cheese, butter, Gentle Sweet, and vanilla until smooth. Set aside.

6. Carefully unroll the completely cooled cake and spread the cream cheese mixture over the cake. Reroll the cake. Wrap in plastic wrap and then in foil. Best if placed in the freezer.

7. Remove from the freezer a couple hours before serving. Cut the roll into slices.

* FOR NSI: USE THE FRUGAL FLOUR OPTION (SEE PAGE 40) AND A GROCERY STORE ON-PLAN SWEETENER.

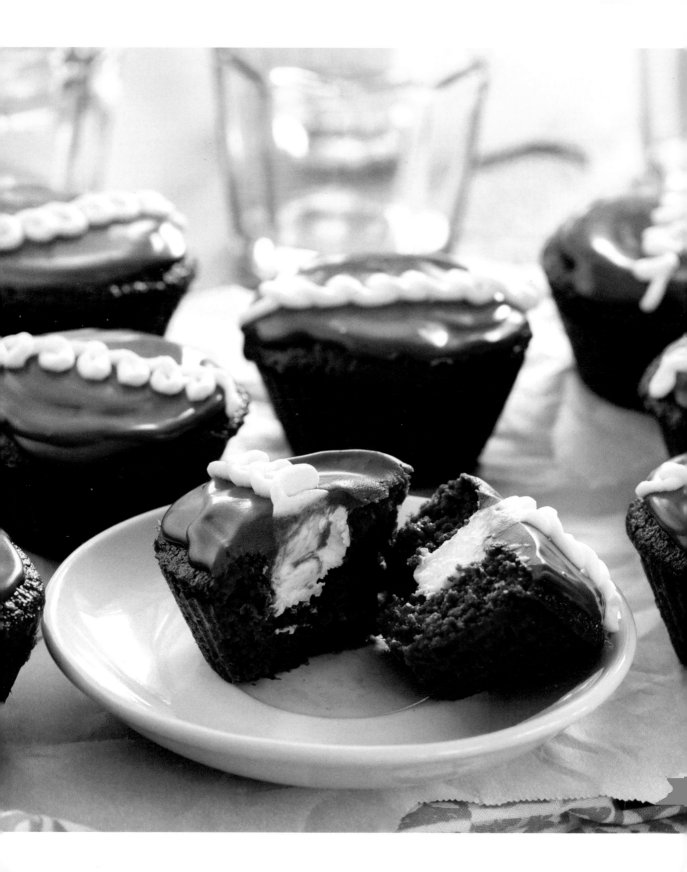

trimtastic mostess cupcakes (S)

MAKES 12 CUPCAKES

(CHECK OUT PAGE 373 FOR WAYS TO MAKE THIS A LIGHTER S CAKE)

Coconut oil cooking spray

1 medium zucchini (to yield 1½ cups processed), or 1 cup canned pure pumpkin puree

4 large eggs

¼ cup (½ stick) butter

¾ cup THM Baking Blend*

¾ cup Gentle Sweet*

⅛ teaspoon Pure Stevia Extract Powder*

1 teaspoon baking soda

1 teaspoon aluminum-free baking powder

2 pinches Mineral Salt

¼ cup unsweetened cocoa powder

FOR THE WHIPPED CREAM FILLING

1¼ teaspoons Just Gelatin*

1 tablespoon cool water plus 2 tablespoons just off the boil water

¾ cup cold heavy cream

1 tablespoon Gentle Sweet*

FOR THE GANACHE TOPPING

¼ cup Trim Healthy Chocolate Chips*

½ cup heavy cream

2 pinches Mineral Salt

You'll be the Hostess with the Mostess when you take these to any event or serve them up to your family.

1. Preheat the oven to 350°F. Line 12 cups of a muffin tin with cupcake liners and spray them with coconut oil. Put a glass bowl and the metal beaters of an electric mixer in your freezer to chill.

2. IF USING ZUCCHINI: Cut it into chunks and process it in a food processor until rice-size. Add the eggs, butter, Baking Blend, sweeteners, baking soda, baking powder, salt, and cocoa powder and process until well combined.

   IF USING PUMPKIN: Just process everything together.

3. Scoop the batter into the muffin cups and bake for 15 to 20 minutes (a few minutes longer if using pumpkin). Remove the cupcakes from the tin and let them cool.

4. Meanwhile, make the whipped cream filling. Put the gelatin in a little cup, cover with the cool water, stir to dissolve, then add the boiled water. Transfer to the fridge so it can cool down. Put the cream and sweetener in the chilled bowl and whip until gentle peaks form. Once the gelatin mix has cooled to room temperature, pour it into the whipped cream while beating. Continue beating until stiff peaks form.

5. Make the ganache. Melt the chocolate chips in a small heatproof bowl set over a saucepan of simmering water. Once melted, slowly whisk in the heavy cream and salt until smooth. Remove from the heat.

6. Once the cupcakes have cooled, use an apple corer and push it down into the middle of each cupcake. Use a knife to take this cylindrical piece of cake out (save the pieces in a baggie and freeze for when you want a quick trifle). Fill the hole with the whipped cream mixture up to the top, then ice over with the ganache. You can decorate the top of the cupcakes with leftover whipped cream by putting some in a zippy baggie, cutting the corner, and squirting it on.

NOTE: In any of the chocolate Trimtastic Cakes you can use either zucchini (lower-carb) or canned pumpkin.

* FOR NSI: USE THE FRUGAL FLOUR OPTION (SEE PAGE 40), A GROCERY STORE ON-PLAN SWEETENER AND UNFLAVORED GELATIN, AND SUB ANOTHER STEVIA-SWEETENED CHOCOLATE CHIP OR CHOPPED 85% CHOCOLATE.

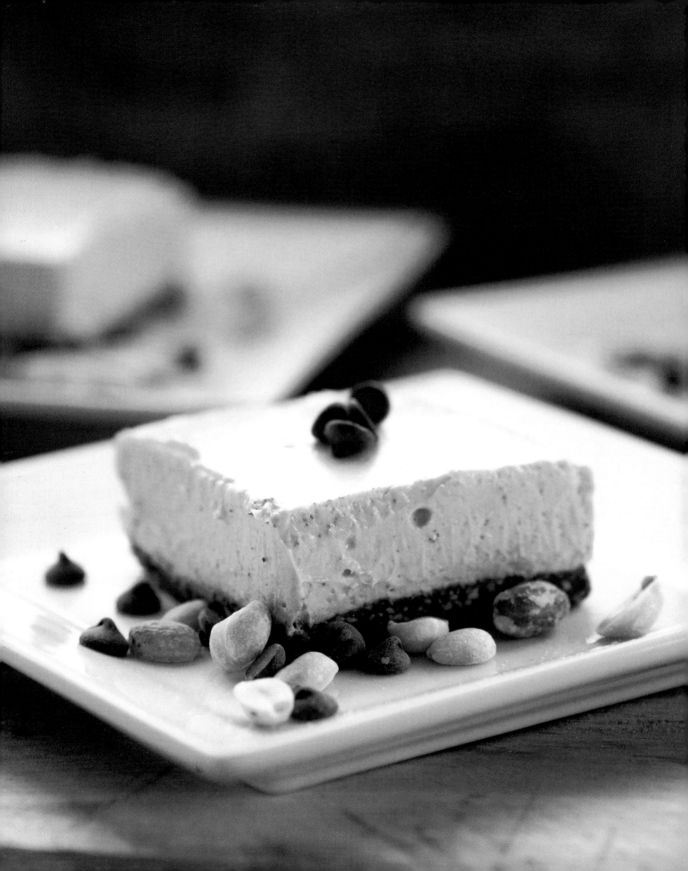

Delicious Desserts & Treats

Cookies,
Brownies
&
Pies

Enjoy all the recipes in this chapter, but don't miss out on all the Beauty Blend recipes, too (starting on page 502). In that chapter you will find more cookies, along with graham crackers and blondies.

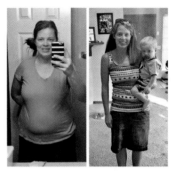

I just can't thank Pearl and Serene enough for this wonderful plan! Today, seven months and three days after I started Trim Healthy Mama, I have reached my goal weight.

I've had people ask if I'm smaller now than at my wedding five years ago. Nope, actually 20 pounds heavier, but I'm healthy! I started at 187.5 pounds. This morning the scale said 139.8 pounds. My goal was 140. Went from a size large/X-large to a medium shirt. Size 14 pants to size 6 and 8.

I have two kids, ages 3½ and 17 months. I need to be healthy for myself, my husband, and them. I want to encourage you all to keep going. Don't let excuses deter you from starting. I have two kids, I teach second grade, and my husband sometimes works twenty-four-hour shifts and is in school. Everyone is busy. Make time for yourself and your health!

–KERRI V.

soft double chocolate chip cookies

(S)

MAKES 30 TO 32 COOKIES

Coconut oil cooking spray

8 tablespoons (1 stick) butter

1 cup Gentle Sweet*

1 teaspoon blackstrap molasses
(optional, for a brown sugar effect)

1 large egg

1 teaspoon pure vanilla extract

¾ cup THM Baking Blend*

⅓ cup unsweetened cocoa powder

½ teaspoon baking soda

¼ teaspoon Mineral Salt

¾ cup Trim Healthy Chocolate
Chips*

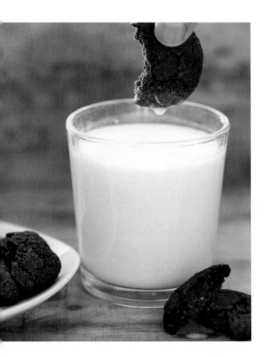

We got a message from K.B., a Trim Healthy Mama who loves taking "regular, bad for your bod" treats and modifying them into healthy ones. She encouraged us to put these cookies in this cookbook, saying, "My kids scarfed them down faster than I could blink!" We tried them on our own children and the same thing happened . . . these are keepers. They are oh-so-perfect with a glass of chilled unsweetened cashew milk, even better when that milk has a teaspoon of heavy cream added to it for extra indulgence.

1. Preheat the oven to 350°F. Line 2 large baking sheets with parchment paper and spray with coconut oil.

2. With an electric mixer (handheld or stand), cream the butter, sweetener, and molasses (if using) together for about 2 minutes. Add the egg and vanilla and continue mixing until combined, about another 30 seconds. Turn off the mixer and scrape down the sides of the bowl. Using a fork or spoon, stir in the Baking Blend, cocoa, baking soda, and salt until incorporated. Stir the chocolate chips into the dough.

3. Form the dough into scant 1-tablespoon balls and place them 2 inches apart on the baking sheets. Press them down to flatten just a little.

4. Bake the cookies for 11 minutes, or until the tops are just set. Remove from the oven. They will fall apart at first, so let them cool on the baking sheets.

VARIATION

CHEWY PEANUT BUTTER COOKIES: Sub in Pressed Peanut Flour (or other sugar-free defatted peanut flour) for the cocoa and add 2 tablespoons sugar-free natural-style peanut butter to the dough.

* FOR NSI: USE A GROCERY STORE ON-PLAN SWEETENER, THE FRUGAL FLOUR
  OPTION (SEE PAGE 40), AND ANOTHER STEVIA-SWEETENED CHOCOLATE CHIP
  OR CHOPPED 85% CHOCOLATE.

pay off day brownies

MULTIPLE SERVE

Coconut oil cooking spray

2 ounces unsweetened baking chocolate

6 tablespoons (¾ stick) softened butter

2 large eggs

½ cup plus 2 tablespoons Gentle Sweet*

½ cup THM Baking Blend*

¾ teaspoon pure vanilla extract

Generous ¼ teaspoon Mineral Salt

¼ cup plus 1 tablespoon water

½ teaspoon baking soda

FOR THE PRALINE TOPPING

¼ cup Gentle Sweet*

2 doonks Pure Stevia Extract Powder* (optional, only if you like things sweeter)

2 tablespoons butter

2 tablespoons heavy cream

2 to 3 pinches Mineral Salt

⅛ teaspoon Natural Burst caramel extract*

¾ cup chopped nuts of any kind

Pay Off Day Candies are one of the most popular sweets from our *Trim Healthy Mama Cookbook.* Now they are paired off with a brownie and the marriage is wonderful.

1. Preheat the oven to 350°F. Spray an 8-inch square baking dish with coconut oil.

2. Melt the chocolate chips in a small glass or ceramic bowl set over a saucepan of simmering water (the bowl shouldn't touch the water). Pour the melted chocolate into a large bowl and beat with the butter until creamed. Add the remaining ingredients and beat until smooth.

3. Pour the batter into the prepared pan and bake for 15 to 20 minutes, until just cooked on top. Let cool.

4. Meanwhile, make the praline topping. Combine the sweeteners and butter in a saucepan and melt over medium-high heat. Add the cream, salt, and caramel extract and let come to a boil. Reduce the heat to medium-low and cook for about 4 minutes, stirring frequently. Remove from the heat and pour over the brownies. Evenly spread out the topping, then refrigerate the brownies.

* FOR NSI: USE A GROCERY STORE ON-PLAN SWEETENER, THE FRUGAL FLOUR OPTION (SEE PAGE 40), AND GROCERY STORE PURE CARAMEL EXTRACT.

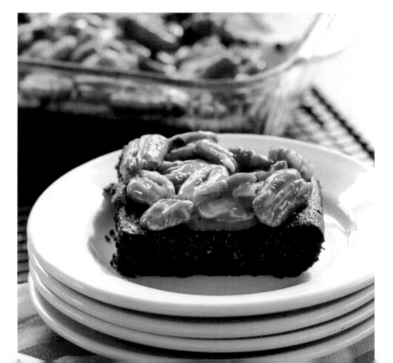

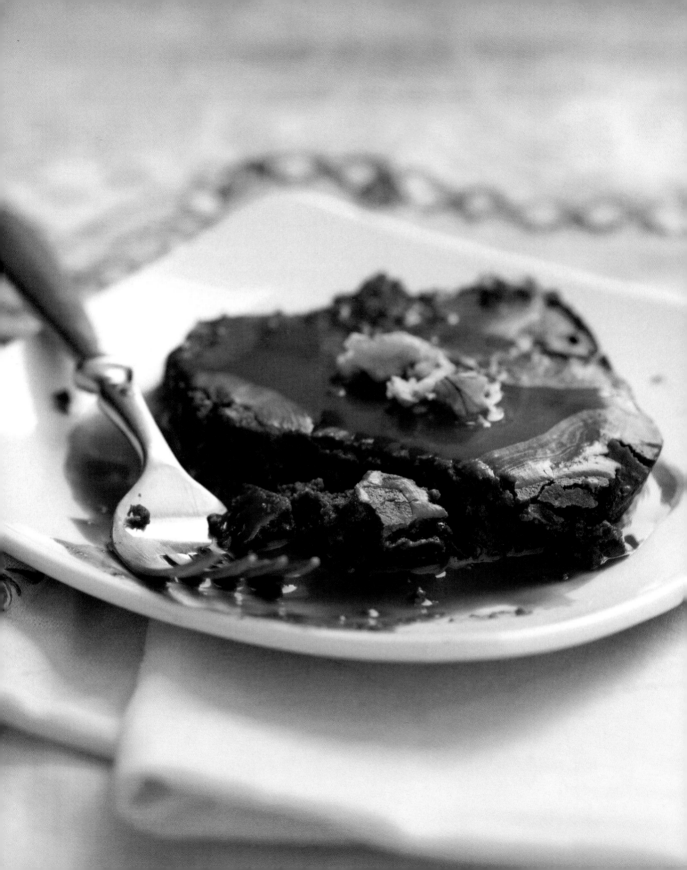

transformer fudge brownies

S

MULTIPLE SERVE

Coconut oil cooking spray

8 tablespoons (1 stick) butter

2 ounces unsweetened baking chocolate

¾ cup Gentle Sweet*

2 large eggs

½ teaspoon Natural Burst chocolate extract* (optional)

⅛ to ¼ teaspoon Natural Burst caramel extract*

¼ teaspoon Mineral Salt

¼ cup THM Baking Blend*

⅓ cup finely chopped walnuts (optional)

FOR THE CHOCOLATE CARAMEL TOPPING

1 ounce unsweetened baking chocolate

2 tablespoons coconut oil (use the flavorless kind if you don't want a coconut taste)

2 tablespoons heavy cream

¼ cup unsweetened cashew or almond milk

2 pinches Mineral Salt

2 tablespoons Gentle Sweet*

2 to 3 doonks Pure Stevia Extract Powder* (optional, for added sweetness)

⅛ to ¼ teaspoon Natural Burst caramel extract*

A lot of chocolate with a little caramel makes for happiness in a pan! The delishimo topping for this brownie is adapted from the ganache that goes with Life by Chocolate Cake (page 376), but with a hint of caramel. Hot from the pan, the topping oozes all over the brownies and they are a thing of yumminess.... Once you refrigerate them, they transform, thicken up to get all fudgy, and become a totally different treat. So two ways to enjoy these brownies. Pick your joy!

1. Preheat the oven to 350°F. Spray an 8-inch square baking dish with coconut oil.

2. Melt the butter and chocolate in a saucepan over medium heat. Remove from the heat, add the sweetener, and beat all together with an electric mixer. Beat in the eggs one at a time. Add the chocolate extract (if using), caramel extract, salt, and Baking Blend and beat until smooth. Stir in the nuts (if using).

3. Scrape the batter into the pan and bake for 35 minutes.

4. Meanwhile, make the topping. Melt the chocolate and coconut oil in a small heatproof bowl set over a saucepan of simmering water (the bowl shouldn't touch the water). Reduce the heat under the pan to low. Add the heavy cream and whisk well, then whisk in the almond milk. Keep whisking as you add the salt, sweeteners, and caramel extract. Remove from the heat and set aside.

5. When the brownies are done, pour the liquid ganache over the brownies and spread out messily. The ganache will stay rather runny while the brownies are hot . . . but it will thicken more as the brownies cool and even more once refrigerated. Enjoy both ways!

* FOR NSI: USE A GROCERY STORE ON-PLAN SWEETENER AND EXTRACTS. USE THE FRUGAL FLOUR OPTION (SEE PAGE 40).

brownie fudge

MULTIPLE SERVE

S

4 ounces unsweetened baking chocolate

8 tablespoons (1 stick) butter

2 large eggs

1 cup water

½ cup canned pure pumpkin puree

½ cup THM Baking Blend or coconut flour

¾ cup Gentle Sweet*

2 to 3 doonks Pure Stevia Extract Powder* (optional, if you have a sweeter tooth)

Rounded ¼ teaspoon Mineral Salt

½ teaspoon baking soda

We didn't know whether to call this Fudge Brownies or Brownie Fudge and whether to put it in the candy section or the brownie section. What a dilemma! Either way, this is a delicious, rich, chocolaty treat. Don't you dare eat it right out of the oven though! It is not to be eaten warm—it has to set into fudgy form in the refrigerator for several hours, or best overnight.

1. Preheat the oven to 350°F. Lightly coat an 8-inch square or 7 x 9-inch baking pan with coconut oil spray.

2. Put the chocolate in a small ceramic bowl and set it above a saucepan of simmering water to melt.

3. In a food processor, put the butter, eggs, water, pumpkin puree, Baking Blend, Gentle Sweet, stevia powder (if using), salt, and baking soda, then add the melted chocolate. Process well. Pour the batter into the baking pan and bake for 35 minutes. Let the brownies cool, then place in the refrigerator for several hours to form into a fudge.

* FOR NSI: USE THE FRUGAL FLOUR OPTION (SEE PAGE 40) OR PLAIN COCONUT FLOUR AND A GROCERY STORE ON-PLAN SWEETENER.

* FOR DF: USE COCONUT OIL IN PLACE OF THE BUTTER.

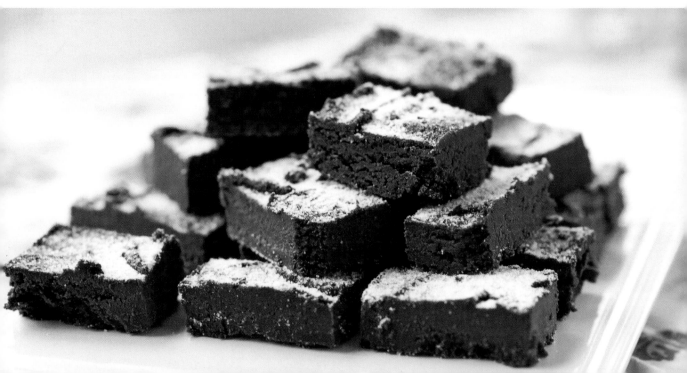

brownie batter in a mug

S

SINGLE SERVE

1 tablespoon coconut oil

3 tablespoons unsweetened vanilla almond milk

½ teaspoon pure vanilla extract

1 to 1½ tablespoons unsweetened cocoa powder (use the smaller amount if you don't want it to be as intense)

1 rounded tablespoon Gentle Sweet*

2½ tablespoons THM Baking Blend*

¼ teaspoon aluminum-free baking powder

2 pinches Mineral Salt

1 to 2 tablespoons Trim Healthy Chocolate Chips (optional)

PEARL CHATS: This quick, ooey gooey brownie for one is too good not to share. Jennifer Mason is a THM vet, who has been doing the plan successfully for years now and has a helpful blog to encourage others on their Trim Healthy Journeys: www.workingathomeschool.com. She came up with this quick-as-a-flash (and egg-free) brownie recipe, and it is going to save many a Drive-Thru Sue's day! To our purists . . . we have plenty of awesome from-scratch baked goods for you, but we gotta give our struggling Drive-Thru Sue's what they need sometimes, too, and sometimes that means using a microwave!

1. Melt the coconut oil in a microwave-safe mug. Stir the almond milk and vanilla into the melted coconut oil.

2. Mix the dry ingredients well in a small bowl. Add the dry ingredients to the wet ingredients in the mug and mix thoroughly. Stir in the chocolate chips (if using).

3. Microwave for 35 to 45 seconds. It should puff up a bit, but still look a bit undercooked. It may take your microwave a tad longer, but don't go more than 1 minute. You are shooting for molten-lava-cake-type texture in the middle.

* FOR NSI: USE A GROCERY STORE ON-PLAN SWEETENER AND THE FRUGAL FLOUR OPTION (SEE PAGE 40).

no-bake peanut butter cheesecake
with chocolate crust

S

MULTIPLE SERVE

FOR THE NO-BAKE CHOCOLATE CRUST (MAKES ENOUGH FOR A 9-INCH ROUND OR 8-INCH SQUARE PAN)

1 cup peanuts

¼ cup unsweetened cocoa powder

2 pinches Mineral Salt

½ teaspoon Super Sweet, or
   2 tablespoons Gentle Sweet*

4 tablespoons (½ stick) butter, melted

FOR THE FILLING

1 cup unsweetened cashew or almond milk

2½ teaspoons Just Gelatin*

2 (8-ounce) packages ⅓ less fat cream cheese

½ cup sugar-free natural-style peanut butter

¼ cup Pressed Peanut Flour*

¼ teaspoon Mineral Salt

¾ cup Gentle Sweet*

¼ teaspoon Pure Stevia Extract Powder*

Chocolate and cheesecake together . . . calls for a happy dance! Make the crust first, and then add the filling and refrigerate—simple but oh so succulent.

1. Make the crust. Put the peanuts, cocoa powder, salt, and sweetener into a food processor. Pulse until well combined and the nuts are finely chopped but not like flour. Pour the mixture into the bottom of a 9-inch round or an 8-inch square baking dish. Pour the melted butter into the mixture. Mix well, then flatten the mixture out so it covers the entire bottom of the dish. Refrigerate the crust.

2. Make the filling. Put the nut milk in a small saucepan and sprinkle on the gelatin. Set aside for a couple minutes so the gelatin can dissolve.

3. Put the cream cheese, peanut butter, peanut flour, salt, and sweeteners in the food processor and process well until smooth. Heat the gelatin/milk mixture over medium heat until it comes to a simmer, then immediately take it off the heat and pour into the processor. Process well for a minute or so.

4. Scrape the filling onto the crust and refrigerate again for a couple of hours until set.

* FOR NSI: USE GROCERY STORE ON-PLAN SWEETENER, SUGAR-FREE DEFATTED PEANUT FLOUR, AND UNFLAVORED GELATIN.

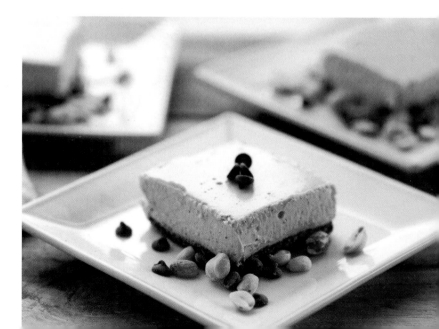

no moo cheesecake

S

Beauty Blend Base Pie Crust
(page 508) or Traditional Pie
Crust (page 408), or any other
on-plan crust

6 oolong tea bags

1¾ cups just off the boil water

1 tablespoon plus ¼ teaspon plus
⅛ teaspoon Just Gelatin (I'm not
crazy, had to be precise here)

½ cup extra-virgin coconut oil

1½ tablespoons (1 scoop) Integral
Collagen

2 doonks Sunflower Lecithin

3 tablespoons Gentle Sweet

1 tablespoon Super Sweet Blend
(if you don't have Super Sweet,
double the Gentle Sweet)

6 tablespoons Baobab Boost
Powder

10 pinches Mineral Salt

1½ teaspoons pure vanilla extract

1 scoop unflavored Pristine Whey
Protein Powder

Juice of 1 lemon

½ teaspoon Natural Burst butter
extract

⅛ to ¼ teaspoon pure lemon extract
(optional)

SERENE CHATS: *Adapted from our No Moo Cream Cheese Bites (page 440), this full-size cheesecake will please those who can't say "moo" and even those who "doo"! Dairy-free Mamas . . . time to celebrate big time! You have cheesecake again! But even if you are someone who can indulge in desserts made from real cream cheese, it is good to take a break from the pasteurized heavy-cal stuff in exchange for a dessert plate of superfoodiness sometimes. Foods like real cream cheese are on plan, of course, but overdoing them can sometimes cause weight-loss stalls. I promise nobody ain't gonna miss nothin' in this indulgent treat—sorry to my mother for my lack of grammar, but I'm excited!*

This cheesecake is easy no-bake style and is brewed with fat-blasting, anti-aging, and beautifying oolong tea. It also contains a nice dose of Baobab Boost powder to infuse your body with vitamin C so you can lose weight more easily. So cut a giant slice and savor each mouthful while you revitalize and revolutionize inside and out. Now let's play Eye Spy. If you've been making my Trimmy Bisques and Trimmy Dressings, can you find the basic Trimmy ingredients here? Trimmies are at the heart of many of our dairy-free Trimmifying recipes. In case you can't, I put them in color.

1. Line a standard (9-inch) pie pan with one of the pie crusts.
2. Place the tea bags in the boiled water and let brew for 5 minutes in an insulated coffee cup so it will stay hot (or cover a regular mug with a saucer).
3. Measure out 1½ cups plus 2 tablespoons of the tea and put in a blender. Add the **gelatin** and blend for a few seconds. Turn off the blender, add the **coconut oil,** and blend for a few seconds so it all melts nicely. Add the **collagen, lecithin,** sweeteners, baobab powder, salt, vanilla, whey protein, lemon juice, butter extract, and lemon extract (if using) to the blender and blend well on high.
4. Pour the mixture into the pie crust. Place in the refrigerator until "sliceably" set, which takes 3 to 4 hours.

NOTE: If you eat this after a few hours, it will be perfect, but if you wait a day or eat as leftovers, it will set up harder than you may want. Still yummy, but more jello-ish. To remedy this, just use ½ teaspoon less of the gelatin.

LAST NOTE: For a pumpkin version, add ½ cup of canned pure pumpkin puree and ½ teaspoon grated nutmeg (use the full amount of gelatin).

lemon cream pie

S

MULTPLE SERVE

FOR THE TRADITIONAL PIE CRUST

1 cup THM Baking Blend*

5 tablespoons cold butter

2 teaspoons Super Sweet Blend*

2 large egg yolks

1 tablespoon cold water

FOR THE FILLING

1 tablespoon Just Gelatin*

¼ cup cold water

1 cup 1% cottage cheese

1 (8-ounce) package ⅓ less fat cream cheese

5 tablespoons plus 5 teaspoons Gentle Sweet*

⅓ cup lemon juice

¼ cup hot water

⅔ cup heavy cream

SERENE CHATS: *Here's an amazing dessert from my daughter-in-law Esther Allison. We call her the hilltop dessert wizard. If there is a family function, you can bet Esther brings this and it is devoured in a few seconds flat! You'll make the crust first and you can use the traditional pie crust listed here or instead the Light 'n' Luscious No-Bake Crust (page 412) or the lighter Beauty Blend Base Pie Crust (page 508).*

1. Preheat the oven to 350°F.

2. Make the pie crust. Put the Baking Blend, butter, and sweetener in a food processor and process until a coarse meal forms. Add the egg yolks and pulse to mix. Add the cold water and pulse again.

3. Roll out the dough between 2 pieces of parchment paper and invert into a standard (9-inch) pie plate by slowly peeling off the bottom paper. Or simply press the dough into the bottom and up the sides of the pan.

4. Bake for 10 to 15 minutes, until just slightly toasted. Let cool before filling.

5. Make the filling. Put the gelatin into a small bowl and add the cold water. Let sit. While it sits, put the cottage cheese, cream cheese, 5 tablespoons of the sweetener, and the lemon juice in a blender and blend well. Put the hot water into the bowl of gelatin and mix with a spoon. Put it into the blender and blend until dissolved. Pour the mixture from the blender into the cooled pie crust and refrigerate for 2 hours or until set.

6. With an electric mixer, beat the heavy cream and the remaining 5 teaspoons Gentle Sweet until soft peaks form. Spread on top of the pie and store in the refrigerator.

* FOR NSI: USE THE FRUGAL FLOUR OPTION (SEE PAGE 40), AND A GROCERY STORE ON-PLAN SWEETENER FOR THE CRUST, AND UNFLAVORED GELATIN AND A GROCERY STORE ON-PLAN SWEETENER FOR THE FILLING.

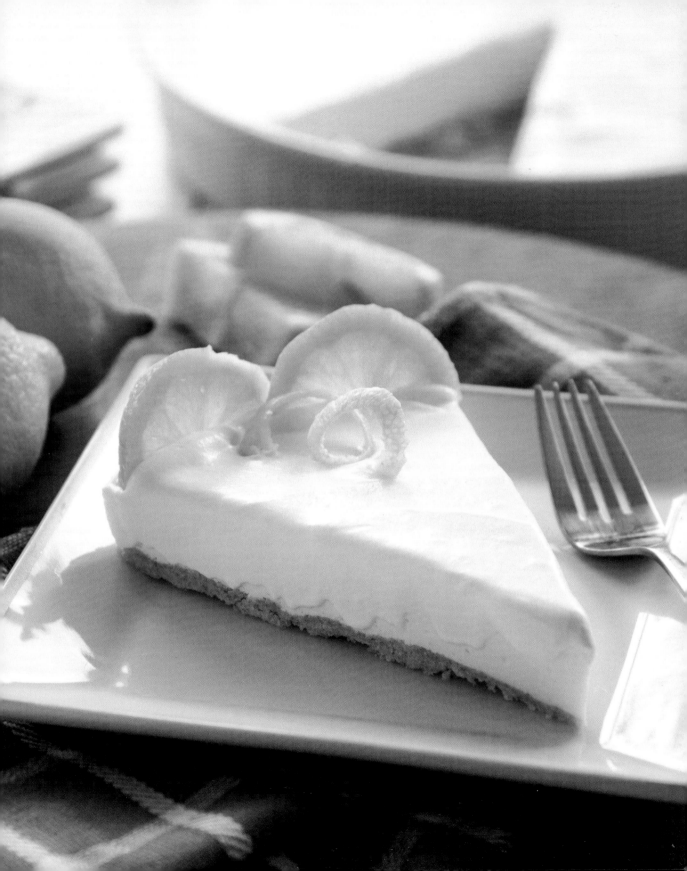

pumpkin custard silk squares or pie

(S)

FOR THE CRUST

¾ cup almond flour (see Note)

½ cup unsweetened shredded coconut

½ cup THM Baking Blend

½ teaspoon coconut oil

2 pinches Mineral Salt

1 teaspoon Super Sweet, or 1 tablespoon Gentle Sweet

⅛ teaspoon pure almond extract

¼ cup water

¾ teaspoon aluminum-free baking powder (optional, if baking the crust)

FOR THE FILLING

1½ tablespoons Just Gelatin

2 tablespoons cool water plus 2 tablespoons just off the boil water

¾ teaspoon Gluccie

⅓ cup Gentle Sweet (plus a doonk or 2 of Pure Stevia Extract Powder and/or more Gentle Sweet if you like things sweeter)

2 rounded teaspoons (½ scoop) Integral Collagen (optional)

2 tablespoons (½ scoop) unflavored Pristine Whey Protein Powder

¼ teaspoon grated nutmeg

½ teaspoon ground ginger

1 teaspoon ground cinnamon

6 pinches Mineral Salt

1 teaspoon pure vanilla extract

1 tablespoon heavy cream (preferably raw if you are a purist)

1 tablespoon MCT oil

½ cup coconut oil

1 (15-ounce) can pure pumpkin puree

SERENE CHATS: *In Australia, where we spent part of our childhood, there was a delicious creamy treat called custard squares that you could buy from any local bakery. Here in the United States, custard is a little different. Here people think of it as a liquid filled with a lot of eggs but the custard squares Down Under are more like a creamy set pie filling . . . so so dreamy good!*

My version of these squares is holiday inspired. I make them for our big hilltop family get-togethers at Thanksgiving and Christmas, so I can happily stay on-plan, but my husband asks me to make them more often as he loves pumpkin treats any time. You have two versions here: As written it is a celebratory heavy S, which I indulge in on the holidays. When I make this year-round I use a version (Lightened-Up Pumpkin Custard Silk Squares, page 412) that lightens up both the crust and the filling. Still great, but more fuel-conscious. So if you are a pumpkin freak like me and want to make this frequently, lighten it up.

Oh by the way . . . you know by now I don't like things too sweet, right? Pearl doesn't find this quite sweet enough as written, so taste the batter and add more sweetener to your liking. Rohnda (our photographer) added double the Gentle Sweet and 2 teaspoons Super Sweet, along with the 2 doonks of Pure Stevia Extract. She said that was not too sweet for her, but that girl's sweet tooth is super strong!

1. If making a baked crust, preheat the oven to 350°F.

2. Make the crust. Process the almond flour, coconut, and Baking Blend in a food processor for a few minutes so they start releasing their oils. Add the coconut oil and process again for a minute or so. Add the salt, sweetener, almond extract, water, and baking powder (if using), and process one last time. Using water-dampened fingers, press the mixture into an 8-inch square glass baking dish (if making squares) or a regular pie plate (if making pie). Bake for 10 minutes, then allow to cool before using. (If not baking it, put in the fridge to firm up.)

3. Make the filling. Place the gelatin in the bottom of a 1-cup measuring cup. Add the cool water, stir well, then add the boiled water to melt it properly and stir again until dissolved. Add enough water to the cup to come to the 1-cup mark, then pour into a blender. Add the Gluccie and blend this mix for 30 seconds. Add the sweetener, collagen, whey protein, nutmeg, ginger, cinnamon, salt, vanilla, heavy cream, MCT oil, coconut oil, and pumpkin puree and blend until super silky and smooth.

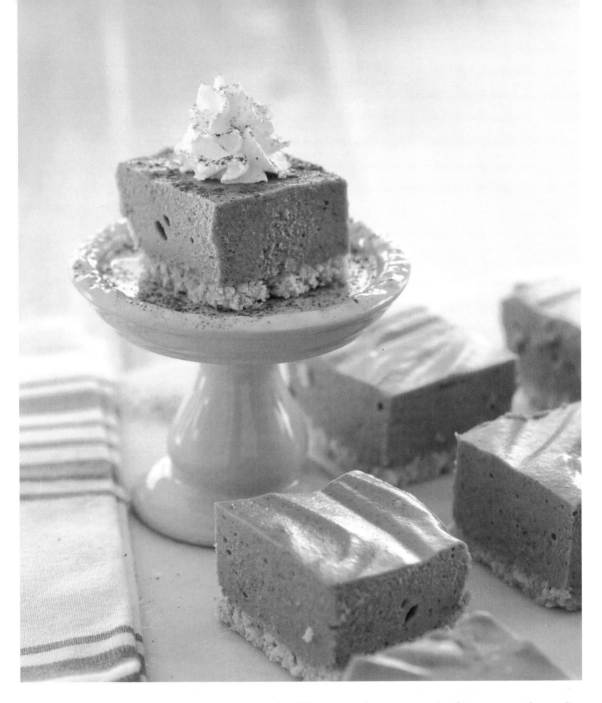

4. Pour the filling into the crust and refrigerate until set. Cut into squares or slices.

NOTE: For the crust, if you don't have almond flour, increase the shredded coconut to 1¼ cups and increase the coconut oil to ½ tablespoon. Omit the almond extract.

lightened-up pumpkin custard silk squares

(S)

MULTIPLE SERVE

(BUT MUCH LIGHTER S THAN ORIGINAL)

**FOR THE LIGHT 'N' LUSCIOUS
NO-BAKE CRUST**

½ cup unsweetened shredded
  coconut

½ cup almond flour

½ cup THM Baking Blend

½ teaspoon extra-virgin coconut oil

¼ cup unflavored Pristine Whey
  Protein Powder

2 pinches Mineral Salt

½ teaspoon Super Sweet Blend

¼ cup water

⅛ teaspoon pure almond extract

FOR THE FILLING

2½ tablespoons Just Gelatin

2 tablespoons cool water plus
  2 tablespoons just off the boil
  water

¼ cup plus 2 teaspoons Gentle
  Sweet (you will probably need
  more if you have a sweet tooth,
  so throw in a couple doonks
  stevia, too)

¼ teaspoon Gluccie

¼ teaspoon Sunflower Lecithin

2 rounded teaspoons (½ scoop)
  Integral Collagen

2 tablespoons (½ scoop) unflavored
  Pristine Whey Protein Powder

¼ teaspoon plus 2 doonks grated
  nutmeg

½ teaspoon plus ⅛ teaspoon
  ground ginger

1¼ teaspoons ground cinnamon

6 pinches Mineral Salt

1½ teaspoons pure vanilla extract

¼ cup extra-virgin coconut oil

1 (15-ounce) can pure pumpkin
  puree

1 more cup water

1. Make the crust. Process the coconut, almond flour, and Baking Blend in a food processor for a couple minutes so they start releasing their own oils. Add the coconut oil and process again for a minute or so. Add the whey protein, salt, sweetener, water, and almond extract, and process one last time. Press with water-dampened fingers into an 8-inch glass baking dish or a regular pie plate. Refrigerate. You are done with the crust!

2. Make the filling. Place the gelatin in the bottom of a 1-cup measuring cup. Add the cool water, stir well, then add the boiled water to melt it properly and stir again until dissolved. Add enough water to the cup to come up to ⅔ cup, then pour into a blender. Continue to make in the exact same way as for Pumpkin Custard Silk Squares or Pie (page 410) by blending all the other ingredients, but be sure to add the extra cup of water to the filling.

strawberries and cream pie

MULTIPLE SERVE

Ⓢ

1 premade pie crust,* such as Traditional Pie Crust (page 408), Light 'n' Luscious No-Bake Crust (page 412), Beauty Blend Base Pie Crust (page 508), or No-Bake Chocolate Crust (page 406)

¼ cup water

1 tablespoon plus 1 teaspoon Just Gelatin*

2 cups frozen sliced strawberries

½ cup unsweetened cashew or almond milk

½ cup heavy cream

½ cup Gentle Sweet* (plus 2 doonks Pure Stevia Extract Powder if you are more of a sweet lover)

1 teaspoon pure strawberry or vanilla extract

This is like level 1 easy! Go make it!

1. Make whatever crust you are using, letting it cool if it's a baked crust.
2. Put the water in a small saucepan. Sprinkle the gelatin over it and allow to sit for a few minutes while the gelatin dissolves.
3. Place the strawberries, nut milk, heavy cream, and sweetener in a food processor and process well until smooth.
4. Turn the heat under the gelatin to medium-high and bring to a simmer, stirring to dissolve. Pour the mixture into the food processor along with the extract and process well for another minute or 2. Pour the pie filling into the crust, quickly spreading it with a spatula, then refrigerate for an hour or 2 before eating.

* FOR NSI: USE THE NO-BAKE CHOCOLATE CRUST (PAGE 406) USING ALMONDS INSTEAD OF PEANUTS, AND USE A GROCERY STORE ON-PLAN SWEETENER AND UNFLAVORED GELATIN.

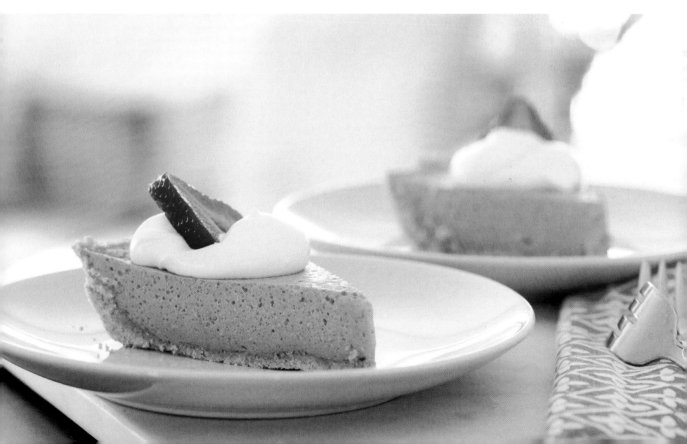

french silk pie

S

MULTIPLE SERVE

Beauty Blend Base Pie Crust*
(page 508), baked and cooled
as directed

3 ounces unsweetened baking
chocolate

⅔ to ¾ cup Gentle Sweet* (¾ cup is
a tad too sweet for me but may be
just right for people like our
photographer, Rohnda . . . chuckle)

8 tablespoons (1 stick) softened
butter

¼ cup plus ⅔ cup heavy cream

1½ teaspoons pure vanilla extract

3 pinches Mineral Salt

¾ cup egg whites (from a carton)

Flaked stevia-sweetened or shaved
85% chocolate, for decoration
(optional)

PEARL CHATS: French Silk Pie has always been a favorite of mine, but I had never made it because I was sure it would be too involved and time consuming, but I was wrong. If a lazy cook like me can make this rich chocolate dessert, so can you. Wow your family with it or take it to a gathering! You can even eat it for breakfast if you're feeling inclined. Traditionally, French Silk Pie uses raw eggs, but since many people are concerned about getting sick from eating raw eggs I used carton egg whites and it worked beautifully. The whites also bring a wiser fuel balance since this is very fat heavy. For this same reason, it is best that you use the lighter Beauty Blend Base Pie Crust (page 508) for this unless you are determined to use a no special ingredient version, then you can use the No-Bake Chocolate Crust (page 406). We're not afraid of fat or calories, but keep in mind that it is best not to abuse them either!

1. Press the pie dough into a 9-inch pie plate and bake and cool as directed.

2. Melt the chocolate in a glass or ceramic bowl set over a saucepan of simmering water (the bowl shouldn't touch the water). Once just melted, stir, take the bowl off the heat, and set the chocolate aside to cool to room temperature.

3. Meanwhile, put the Gentle Sweet in a blender and blend until it becomes an even finer powder. Leave about 1 tablespoon of the Gentle Sweet in the blender and pour the rest into a large bowl. Add the butter and, with an electric mixer, cream the Gentle Sweet and butter for about 2 minutes.

4. Once the melted chocolate is close to room temperature (you don't want it to melt the butter), add it to the bowl along with the ¼ cup heavy cream and beat for another 2 to 3 minutes. Beat in the vanilla and salt. Beat in the egg whites ¼ cup at a time, beating well, about a minute or 2, after each addition. Then beat the mixture for at least another couple minutes, or until the mixture is nicely thickened.

5. Pour the ⅔ cup heavy cream into the blender (with the reserved Gentle Sweet) and blend until thickened.

6. Scrape the chocolate mixture into the baked pie crust, top with the whipped cream and optional chocolate flakes, and chill in the refrigerator for at least a couple hours.

* FOR NSI: USE THE NO-BAKE CHOCOLATE CRUST (PAGE 406) USING ALMONDS INSTEAD OF PEANUTS, AND USE A GROCERY STORE ON-PLAN SWEETENER.

Candies
&
Bars

Truffles, gummies, and bites of sweet goodness are all coming
your way! And we couldn't leave out bars that you can throw
into your purse to stay THM strong when you're out and about.

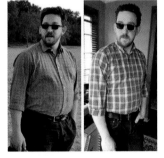

We're a Trim Healthy Couple who have removed 145 pounds between us! THM was an answer to a prayer for help. When we began the plan, we took baby steps and gave up the four "whites" (white flour, white rice, white potatoes, and sugar). I tried at least one new recipe a week. I also made sure we were getting at least five E meals in every week. One thing that I've found most helpful is to read the Plan book more than once. I read it completely through the first time, just like it says to do, then I read it a second time and highlighted parts that I figured I would be referring back to often. I have since reread the book two to three more times. I am going through the book study with a group of ladies from my church, so I needed to read it again so I would be able to answer their questions. After getting rid of 105 pounds, I have been at a standstill for a few weeks. I'm not worried. I have learned to be patient on this plan. The numbers aren't moving, but my clothes are looser. **—LINDA R.**

When my wife and I started THM, I have to admit that I was pretty non-committal. My willingness to stay on-plan extended as far as it took to help her stay on-plan and no further. But even with that little effort, I started to lose weight. Once I saw that it was really working for both of us, I got a lot more gung-ho. Now, I'm down forty-three pounds, I feel great, and I'm seeing muscle definition that I haven't seen since college and fitting into clothes from high school. I still joke about the name, but now it's always a lead-in to telling people that they need to give Trim Healthy Mama a try. **—DAVE J.**

singing canary truffles

S

MULTIPLE SERVE

1¼ teaspoons Just Gelatin*

1 tablespoon cool water

⅓ cup plus 1 tablespoon just off the boil water

½ cup plus 2 tablespoons extra-virgin coconut oil

2 doonks Sunflower Lecithin (optional)

½ teaspoon pure vanilla extract

4 tablespoons Baobab Boost Powder*

2 teaspoons ground turmeric

2 pinches Mineral Salt

Juice of 1 lemon

1 to 2 tablespoons Gentle Sweet (use 2 if you have a sweet tooth), or 1½ to 2 teaspoons Super Sweet Blend*

We introduced you to the Singing Canary sipper in *Trim Healthy Mama Cookbook*. That golden drink helps worn-out, adrenal-fatigued Mamas by supporting thyroid and adrenals and boosting the immune system. But what if you don't feel like chuggin' liquid? Get all the goodness of the Singing Canary in a decadent and creamy truffle. Now with baobab powder added, they have even more natural vitamin C healing power. Let these tart and zingy golden morsels of sunny scrumptiousness delight your taste buds and support your adrenal interplay. Be sure to keep them around as decadent defenders during cold and flu season.

1. Put the gelatin and cool water in a mug and stir to dissolve. Add the boiled water and stir again. Place this mixture in a blender and blend for just a few seconds. Let it sit for a little bit until warm but not "ouch!" hot (you are going to add virgin coconut oil and don't want to kill the medicinal effects). Add the coconut oil and all the other ingredients and blend until creamy.

2. Pour into ice cube trays or pretty molds and freeze. Once frozen, pop them out of the molds and store in the fridge in zippies and do not eat them till they completely thaw and become that perfect smooth truffle texture. Half-frozen truffles are not ready yet!

* FOR NSI: USE A GROCERY STORE UNFLAVORED GELATIN AND AN ON-PLAN SWEETENER. YOU CAN FIND BAOBAB POWDER AT GROCERY STORES, TOO, SOMETIMES.

singing canary gummies

MULTIPLE SERVE

Juice of 3 large lemons (if you can't handle too strong a lemon flavor, use 2 lemons and add 2 tablespoons water to the blend)

½ to 1 tablespoon Gentle Sweet (use the full tablespoon for a sweeter tooth)

1 teaspoon Super Sweet Blend (see Note)

½ teaspoon pure vanilla extract

2 pinches Mineral Salt

½ teaspoon ground turmeric (you may have to work up to this amount; start with less if you are not used to it)

1 teaspoon MCT oil (turmeric needs a little fat to be absorbed properly)

2 doonks Sunflower Lecithin

2 rounded teaspoons (½ scoop) Integral Collagen

1 teaspoon Baobab Boost Powder

2½ tablespoons Just Gelatin

Why not gummies, too? There are so many ways to enjoy the medicinal goodness of the Singing Canary. Check out Singing Canary Pops (page 446) and Singing Canary Sherbet (page 446), too.

1. Place everything (except the gelatin) in a blender and blend on low until smooth. (If your blender is huge and won't turn, use a stick blender.) With the blender on low, slowly stir in the gelatin and blend for around 10 seconds.

2. Place the blended gummy mix in a small saucepan and bring it to "just hot" to your finger over medium-low heat while stirring constantly. Pour this lovely warm golden goo into gummy molds or shallowly fill ice cube trays and freeze for 10 minutes. Place in the refrigerator if they are not firm after the freezer time. Once firm, pop them out and store in zippies in the fridge.

NOTE: If you don't have Super Sweet Blend, just use double amounts of Gentle Sweet and taste the mixture to see if you need more.

good girl moonshine gummies

(FP)

MULTIPLE SERVE

½ cup cold water

2½ tablespoons Just Gelatin* (use 2½ teaspoons for soft gummies)

½ cup just off the boil water

1 teaspoon Super Sweet Blend*

½ to 1 tablespoon Gentle Sweet* (use the full tablespoon for a sweeter tooth)

1 tablespoon Baobab Boost Powder*

¼ to ½ teaspoon ground ginger (depending on your love of the moonshine bite)

4 teaspoons apple cider vinegar

We couldn't leave your other favorite All Day Sipper out of the gummy fun. Pop them for health, for fun, and for taste!

1. Place the cold water and gelatin in a big mug and stir to dissolve, then pour in the boiled water and stir again. Add the sweeteners, baobab powder, and ground ginger and blend until smooth with a stick blender (or use a stand mixer).

2. Once the gelatin mix is no longer superhot (too high a heat will kill the live enzymes in the vinegar), blend in the vinegar, then pour the mixture into cute molds or shallowly into ice cube trays and freeze for 10 minutes. Take out and keep in the fridge until they are firm enough to pop out of the molds and store in zippies in the fridge, if they last that long.

* FOR NSI: USE A GROCERY STORE UNFLAVORED GELATIN AND AN ON-PLAN SWEETENER. SOME GROCERY STORES ALSO HAVE BAOBAB POWDER.

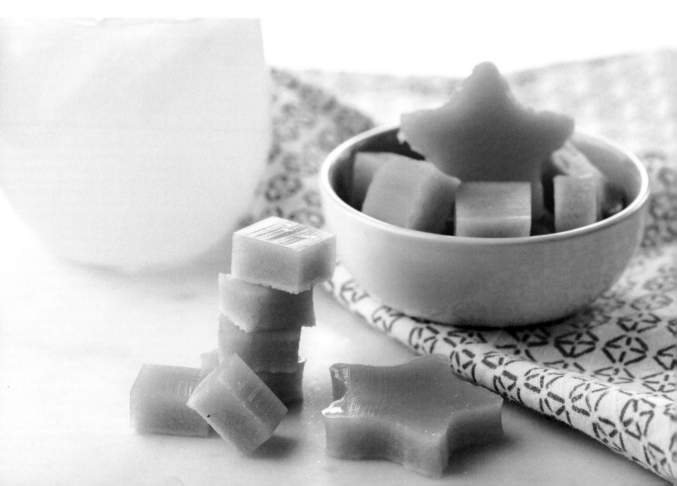

shrinker gummies

MULTIPLE SERVE

2½ tablespoons Just Gelatin

½ cup cool water

1 oolong tea bag

½ cup plus 2 tablespoons just off
  the boil water

1 doonk cayenne pepper

¼ teaspoon ground cinnamon

2 teaspoons pure vanilla extract

1 teaspoon Super Sweet Blend

1 tablespoon Gentle Sweet

2 rounded teaspoons (½ scoop)
  Integral Collagen

1 teaspoon MCT oil

2 doonks Sunflower Lecithin

2 pinches Mineral Salt

These gummies pack a punch of powerful sweet chai flavor but that's not all these little babies do. Anything with oolong tea is a metabolic-boosting, fat-stripping missile. These candies mean fat-shrinking bidness!

1. Dissolve the gelatin in the cool water in a mug. Brew the oolong tea in the boiled water in an insulated coffee mug to keep the heat in (or use a regular mug and cover it) for 3 to 5 minutes. Once brewed, squeeze out the medicinal dregs of oolong and discard your tea bag. Pour the tea into the mug of dissolved gelatin and stir well.

2. Place this gelatin tea mixture into a blender along with the rest of the ingredients and blend until smooth (or for ease use a stick blender). Pour into molds or pour shallowly into ice cube trays and freeze for 10 minutes. Transfer to the fridge until they are firm enough to pop out of the molds and store in zippies in the fridge.

two-minute truffles

S

SINGLE SERVE

2 tablespoons Pressed Peanut Flour*

½ tablespoon unsweetened cocoa powder

½ tablespoon Gentle Sweet*

1 tablespoon coconut oil

1 teaspoon water

Pinch of Mineral Salt

Dash of pure vanilla extract (optional)

½ tablespoon Trim Healthy Chocolate Chips (optional)

More Gentle Sweet, for rolling (optional)

Got a chocolate craving that must be fulfilled? These truffles will be the quick fix! Sarah Montana is the one to thank for this recipe creation. She shares THM-inspired recipe creations on her blog www.mymontanakitchen.com. We love these truffles so much we asked Sarah if we could share them with all of you.

1. Place all the ingredients in a bowl and stir to mix.
2. Shape into small balls and roll in a little more Gentle Sweet or just eat with a spoon (tastes like frosting)!

* FOR NSI: USE A GROCERY STORE SUGAR-FREE DEFATTED PEANUT FLOUR AND AN ON-PLAN SWEETENER.

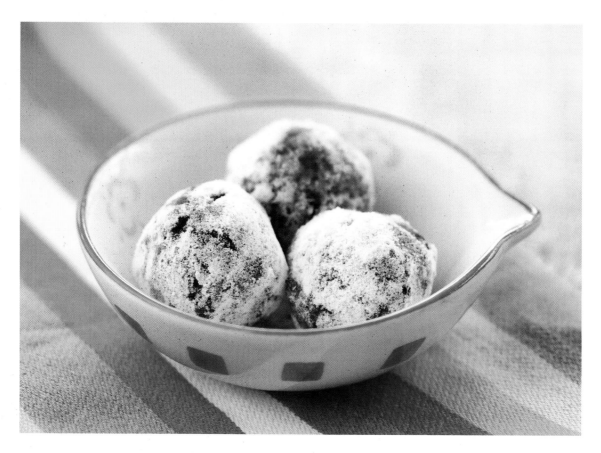

fudgaroons

(S)

MULTIPLE SERVE

5 tablespoons unsweetened cocoa
powder

1 (15-ounce) jar coconut cream
(such as MaraNatha or Let's Do . . .
Organic brand)

3 tablespoons extra-virgin
coconut oil

3 tablespoons Gentle Sweet plus
1 teaspoon Super Sweet Blend, or
2 doonks Pure Stevia Extract
Powder (or 5½ teaspoons Super
Sweet Blend and no stevia powder
if you don't have Gentle Sweet)*

1 to 2 teaspoons Natural Burst
chocolate extract (optional)

2 teaspoons pure vanilla extract

¼ teaspoon Mineral Salt

Fudgaroons are a delightful hybrid of rich fudge and maca-
roons. They are a decadent but waist-whittling melt-in-your-
mouth moment. They contain all the Trimming powers of the
MCT (middle chain triglycerides) found in coconut oil, but also
boast all the detoxifying and satiating fiber found in whole
coconut. Best of all they are so simple to make, with only a few
ingredients.

1. Place all the ingredients in a food processor (if the coconut butter is hard, break it up into smaller clumps with a
   fork or butter knife as you add it to your machine). Process
   until smooth, then place in a glass baking dish (or even better, use a plastic tray that can easily pop out your mixture
   when set).

2. Chill in the fridge until firm. Score into squares and eat a
   few pieces after letting it sit out for a few minutes to get a
   little softer. Store the remaining pieces in a zippy bag in the
   fridge.

* FOR NSI: USE A GROCERY STORE ON-PLAN SWEETENER.

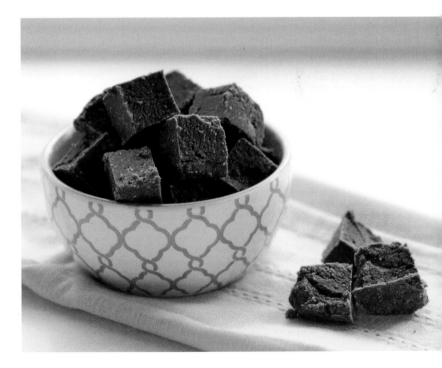

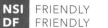
superfood mounds

MAKES ABOUT 3 DOZEN BITES

1 (15-ounce) can full-fat
coconut milk

1 tablespoon Just Gelatin*

¼ cup plus 3 tablespoons Gentle
Sweet* (or to taste)

½ teaspoon Mineral Salt

¼ cup Integral Collagen

1 tablespoon butter (optional)

1 teaspoon pure vanilla extract

⅛ teaspoon Natural Burst coconut
extract (optional)

⅛ teaspoon Natural Burst butter
extract (optional)

1 doonk Natural Burst maple extract
(optional)

3 cups unsweetened finely
shredded coconut

OPTIONAL CHOCOLATE TOPPING

Chocolate topping from Peppermint
Cream Chocolate Trimtastic Cake
(page 390), but omit the
peppermint extract (unless you
want chocolate peppermint
Mounds), or Trim Healthy
Chocolate Chips, melted

If you love Mounds candy bars, then you'll want to thank Ginger, one of the wonderful admins on our Trim Healthy Mama Facebook groups (and membership site chat group), who developed this recipe. She called in the help of many of her admin friends and they tweaked this superfood treat for weeks until they perfected the "Moundsiness." Ginger says: "The candy bar we all know relies on corn syrup (the first ingredient!) for its chewiness. Instead, this version owes its wonderful chewiness to health-promoting gelatin and collagen. Drizzling chocolate on top is very fast, or you can even skip the chocolate and just enjoy the coconut!"

1. Pour the coconut milk into a saucepan. Sprinkle the gelatin across the surface. Allow the gelatin to soften for several minutes before heating. Turn the heat to medium, then whisk in the sweetener, salt, collagen, and butter (if using). Simmer, whisking occasionally, for 15 minutes. Remove from the heat, then add the extracts and shredded coconut and stir.

2. Cover a baking sheet with wax paper or parchment paper. Form bites as desired (use a small cookie scoop or just roll the cooled mixture into balls with your hands). You could also use candy molds. Chill or freeze.

3. If desired, drizzle with melted chocolate, or dip in, or toss with. Put Mounds bites in baggies. Keep what you want for the week in the refrigerator and put the rest in the freezer.

* FOR NSI: USE A GROCERY STORE ON-PLAN SWEETENER, UNFLAVORED GELATIN, AND PURE EXTRACTS.

* FOR DF: LEAVE OUT THE BUTTER . . . PERFECTLY FINE WITHOUT IT.

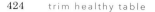

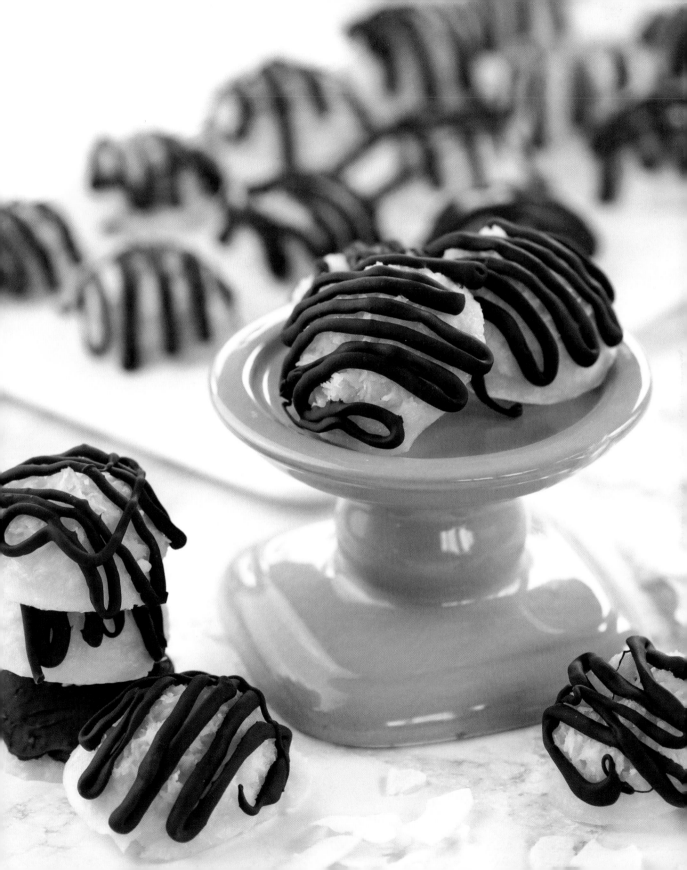

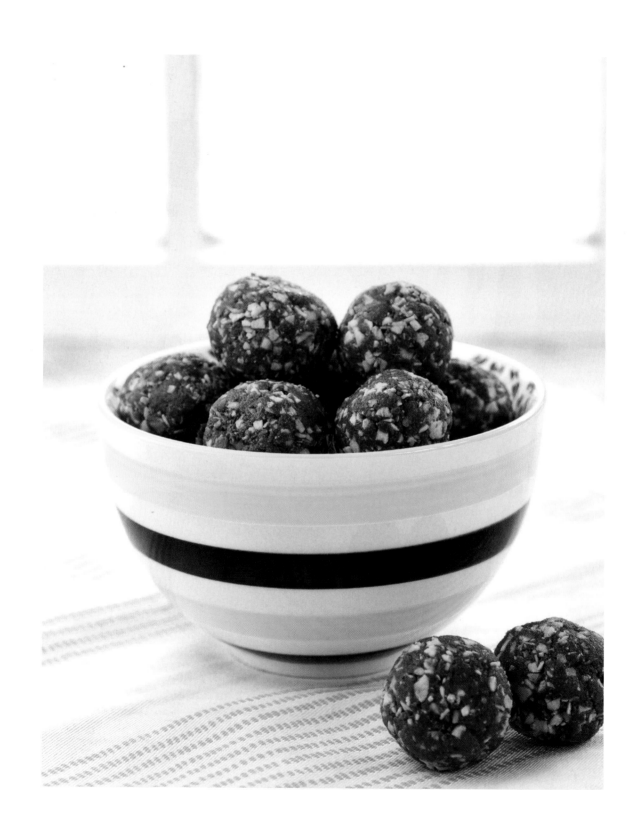

happy bites

MULTIPLE SERVE (MAKES LOTS OF BITES)

FOR TART STRAWBERRY BITES

¾ cup strawberry Pristine Whey Protein Powder

5 tablespoons Baobab Boost Powder

3 tablespoons (2 scoops) Integral Collagen

5 tablespoons fresh lemon juice

2 cups loosely packed coconut flakes (we use Great Value organic coconut flakes)

¼ teaspoon Mineral Salt

2 tablespoons Gentle Sweet

1 tablespoon extra-virgin coconut oil

FOR SALTED CHOCOLATE BITES

3 to 4 oolong tea bags (optional)

⅓ cup plus 2 tablespoons boiling water

¾ cup chocolate Pristine Whey Protein Powder

3 tablespoon (2 scoops) Integral Collagen

2 tablespoons unsweetened cocoa powder

3 tablespoons Baobab Boost Powder

2 cups loosely packed coconut flakes (we use Great Value organic coconut flakes)

⅛ teaspoon Mineral Salt

1 tablespoon Gentle Sweet

SERENE CHATS: *These bites are delicious morsels of metabolism-revving, thermogenic, fat-blasting, health-recharging, beautifying, flavor-drenching yumser stuff! Pop a Happy Bite in your mouth and you get a mouthful of bliss with the sensibleness of protein and superfoods. You have two choices here: a tart strawberry version and a salted chocolate version.*

Those who love their chocolate with a little salt will love these "edgy" treats. They go down smooth with the depth of oolong and cocoa but do a little baobab flavor cartwheel just for kicks and foodie funzies. The oolong tea adds to the thermogenic burn and takes regular chocolate to leaping newness, but you sure can leave it out and just use water . . . still great that way!

FOR TART STRAWBERRY BITES: Place all the ingredients in a food processor and process until they hold together when you press a little of the mixture firmly between your fingers. Transfer to a bowl, press together, then roll between your palms into snack-size balls. Refrigerate until all gobbled up.

FOR SALTED CHOCOLATE BITES: If using the oolong, brew the tea in a mug with the boiled water for 5 minutes. Squeeze the tea bags, place the mug of tea in the freezer to cool, then transfer to a food processor. If not using tea, place all the other ingredients in a food processor and process until the mixture holds together when you press a little of it firmly between your fingers. Transfer the mixture to a bowl, and press together, then roll between your palms into snack-size balls. Refrigerate.

VARIATION

HAPPY BARS: Instead of rolling the mixture into balls, divide it among 4 small zippy bags. Squeeze into a bar form and you have 4 bars that you'll keep in the refrigerator. Or just pull pieces off for bites.

instant cookie dough protein bar

FP (KINDA)

SINGLE SERVE

4 tablespoons (1 scoop) unflavored
Pristine Whey Protein Powder*

1 tablespoon Pressed Peanut Flour*

2 to 2½ teaspoons Gentle Sweet*

Dash Mineral Salt

1 teaspoon softened butter or
coconut oil

2 teaspoons water

1 teaspoon Trim Healthy Chocolate
Chips* or chopped nuts

This is the quickest protein bar you will ever make. It rushes to the rescue to curb cravings as the protein helps satiate out-of-control hunger. It makes for the perfect afternoon snack. Since it has a full serving of protein powder, we don't recommend eating this as a dessert if you already had sufficient protein in your meal, but you could eat half for dessert.

This just sorta squeaks into FP mode. If you do a rounded teaspoon of chocolate chips you may be heading into ultra-light S territory here. Nuts push it into S, but that is just fine, too.

1. Put the whey protein, peanut flour, sweetener, and salt in a bowl. Add the butter and smash with a fork to blend with the dry ingredients. Add the water 1 teaspoon at a time, mixing well with the fork. Add the chocolate chips or nuts, using your hands to press the mixture into a bar shape.

* FOR NSI: USE A GROCERY STORE ON-PLAN WHEY PROTEIN (SEE PAGE 43), SUGAR-FREE DEFATTED PEANUT FLOUR, AND AN ON-PLAN SWEETENER. USE CHOPPED 85% CHOCOLATE IN PLACE OF CHOCOLATE CHIPS.

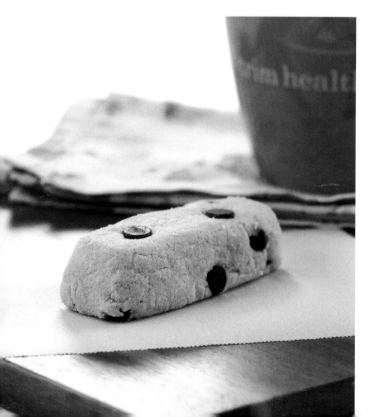

chocolate chip peanut butter cookie bars

(S)

MAKES 9 BARS

½ cup canned pure pumpkin puree

1 large egg

½ cup sugar-free natural-style peanut butter (or other nut butter)

½ cup plus 2 tablespoons THM Baking Blend

¼ cup Integral Collagen

¼ cup unflavored Pristine Whey Protein Powder

½ teaspoon Mineral Salt

¾ cup Gentle Sweet

2 to 3 doonks Pure Stevia Extract Powder (if you are a sweetie)

1 teaspoon pure vanilla extract

1 teaspoon baking soda

⅓ cup Trim Healthy Chocolate Chips, other stevia-sweetened chocolate chips, or chopped 85% chocolate

Look it's a cookie . . . no it's a bar . . . no it's a cookie! Whatever you call these, call them yummy!! They are a wonderful blood-sugar balancing afternoon pick-me-up, the perfect treat to toss in your bag in a zippy bag for a protein-based afternoon snack. Each bar gives you close to 10 grams of protein, which is a fine amount for a snack. If you're at home, have with a glass of chilled unsweetened almond milk, relax, and say "Ahhhh!" If you are not a big breakfast eater, they can work as a quick breakfast, too. Enjoy with a Healing Trimmy (page 463) or Lazy Collagen Coffee (page 466) for extra protein and you're set.

1. Preheat the oven to 350°F. Line a 17 x 11-inch baking sheet with parchment paper.

2. Stir together all the ingredients (except the chocolate chips) with a fork until well combined (or use a stand mixer). Stir in the chocolate chips.

3. Scrape the dough onto the parchment. The dough will be sticky, so use water-moistened fingers to spread it out into a skinny rectangle about 13 x 4 inches. Bake for 15 minutes.

4. Remove from the oven and score cross-wise into 9 bars. The bars will still be soft and will not appear fully cooked. This is fine. Leave them alone for 30 minutes while they set, then cut into bars. You can keep them out for several hours, but refrigerate after that in a zippy bag.

NOTE: If you have an allergy to peanuts, use almond or another nut butter and substitute equal parts collagen and whey for the peanut flour.

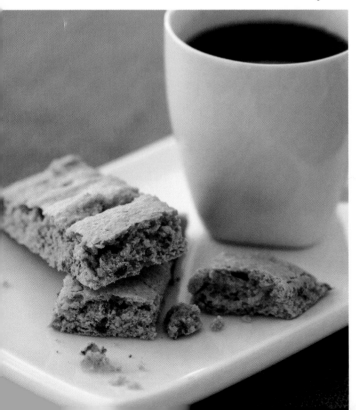

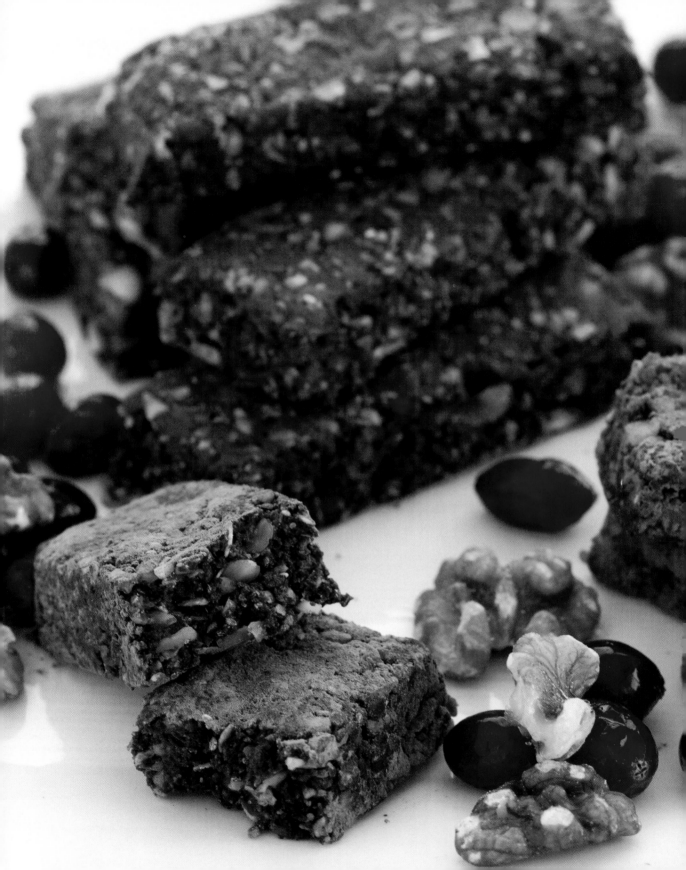

chocolate berry boost bars ⓢ

MAKES 14 BARS

1½ cups fresh cranberries (or frozen, thawed with juice drained)

½ cup unflavored Pristine Whey Protein Powder

¼ cup Integral Collagen

¼ cup Baobab Boost Powder

2 tablespoons flax seeds or chia seeds (not ground)

1 cup unsweetened shredded coconut

2 tablespoons extra-virgin coconut oil

½ cup raw or dry-roasted almonds

¼ to ⅓ cup Gentle Sweet, depending on your sweet tooth (our photographer and food tester, Rohnda, likes these with a full ¾ cup Gentle Sweet—shows how different we all are)

½ cup unsweetened cocoa powder

½ teaspoon Natural Burst apricot extract (this is awesome but you can use pure orange extract)

2 to 3 pinches Mineral Salt

½ cup raw walnuts, coarsely chopped

OPTIONAL DUSTING INGREDIENTS (GREAT WITHOUT, BUT ADDS A LITTLE SUMPIN')

½ tablespoon Gentle Sweet

½ tablespoon unsweetened cocoa powder

SERENE CHATS: *If you don't want to get addicted to these bars, then don't attempt to make them. Their tangy precious selves are soooooooo scrumptious they can get you into all sorts of good trouble. Trouble like eating a batch so quickly you have to make them again in a few days or making them as a gift for a friend and sneaking a few too many for yourself.*

Put them in zippies, toss one or two in your bag for the day, and you'll be able to stay on the THM wagon with yummy ease! Buy up a bunch of fresh cranberries in the fall and winter and keep them in your freezer all year long so you can always make this recipe.

1. Place the cranberries in a food processor and process until finely textured. (During the processing you might need to stop your processor and break things apart with a fork and position some stuck parts back down toward the blades.) Add all the other ingredients (except the walnuts) and process for a while. Add the walnuts once the mixture is perfectly combined and forms into a thick ball of dough.

2. Use your hands and a table knife to shape the dough into a large flat square or rectangle on parchment paper or a silicone mat. Score into 14 bars. For the optional topping, mix the Gentle Sweet and cocoa powder on a flat plate and one at a time press the bars, front and back and on all sides, into the dust.

3. Store some in the refrigerator for near future use and others in the freezer for later use. You can transfer them to the refrigerator when you're ready to eat.

VARIATIONS

CHOCOLATE RASPBERRY BOOST BARS: When you cannot find cranberries in season or if you have run out of your frozen supply, you can use the same amount of frozen raspberries, thawed and drained.

COCONUT BERRY BOOST BARS: Omit the cocoa and add 2 tablespoons collagen, 2 tablespoons coconut flour, and 2 tablespoons whey protein. Dust with finely shredded coconut.

NOTE: To make the bars firmer and even easier to take in your purse, add ½ cup unflavored pea protein (I use Nutrasumma unflavored Fermented Pea Protein) and an additional 1 tablespoon coconut oil and 2 tablespoons Gentle Sweet.

ultimate e bars

8 oolong tea bags

½ cup just off the boil water

9 tablespoons (6 scoops) Integral Collagen

1½ cups (6 scoops) unflavored Pristine Whey Protein Powder

½ cup unsweetened cocoa powder

½ cup Baobab Boost Powder

½ cup Gentle Sweet

½ teaspoon Mineral Salt

2 teaspoons pure vanilla extract

½ teaspoon Natural Burst pecan extract (optional, or use another extract such as ¼ teaspoon almond)

2 tablespoons MCT oil

2 teaspoons raw honey (see Note)

2 tablespoons kombucha or kefir water (optional; see Last Note)

2 cups old-fashioned rolled oats

Pow Wow . . . these bars pack a powerful punch of filling concentrated energy! They have been formulated with your busy lifestyle in mind and carefully crafted for weight zapping while on the go. No more wondering what to eat when you're in a rush and out and about. No more energy slumps and sluggish mojo! Grab a bar from your purse while in afternoon rush hour traffic or even make a quick Ultimate E breakfast with one. They are perfect as a preworkout meal (or *Workin*, if you do our exercise DVDs) and are the ultimate fix for the person who has a hard time incorporating E meals.

These Ultimate E Bars will rev your metabolism, nourish tired adrenals, and strip fat. They will get to work burning calories through the proven "fat burn" of oolong tea, which also blocks fat-building enzymes. Oolong contains gentle amounts of caffeine that, combined with the catechins in this ancient tea, work together to keep a spring in your step, a perk in your posture, and a downward direction in your dress size (ahem . . . pant size if you are a dude). Along with the help of baobab powder, these bars will help lower too-high blood sugar and help keep wild cravings at bay. Slow-burning oats are thrown in the mix for easy-burn energy without any left over to store around your middle. A tad of MCT oil is used as immediately absorbed rocket fuel energy. Each of these perfectly balanced protein bars packs an awesome 22 grams of body-repairing protein.

Our favorite thing about them is that they take a long time to eat and are large and hefty. By the time you've chewed your way through one of these, your hand to mouth and teeth chomping desires have been well satisfied.

1. Brew 4 of the tea bags in a glass measuring cup with the boiled water for 5 to 10 minutes. After brewing, squeeze out the tea bags (and discard). If necessary, add enough water to the measuring cup to come up to ½ cup (some may have evaporated during brewing). Pour the tea into a food processor.

2. Open the remaining 4 tea bags and grind the tea leaves in a coffee grinder. Add to the processor. Then add the collagen, whey protein, cocoa powder, baobab powder, sweetener, salt, vanilla, pecan extract (if using), MCT oil, honey, and kombucha (if using) and process for a while until a nice gooey ball forms. Use patience, you may have to scrape

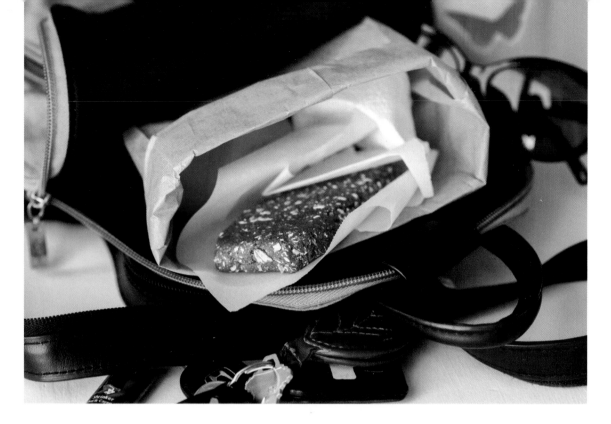

down the sides several times. Once the ball has formed, start adding the oats ½ cup at a time and process them to incorporate.

3. Once all the oats are added, process a bit more, then take the dough ball out and put it into a gallon zippy bag. Don't zip it up. Carefully massage the bar mixture inside the bag until it is nice and combined. While still in the bag, form a nice and even large log shape. Remove this log and place it on a cutting board and cut into 8 large Clif Bar–size bars. Put each one in a little zippy bag and refrigerate until needed.

NOTE: Raw honey is a superfood and welcome in small amounts, especially at goal weight. But honey can easily turn THM recipes from waist-whittling to waist-ruining when used without thought for its impact on blood sugar. For this reason, we do not normally add it to THM official recipes. However, we have carefully crafted this bar with the perfect amount of raw honey that will not sabotage your weight loss. It is used here primarily as a natural preservative so your bars last longer in your purse.

LAST NOTE: The kombucha or kefir water is optional, but it can also give more "purse life" to your bars so they have good bacteria to fight off any bad guy bacteria. It helps them last more than a day or two in your purse.

More Sweet Treats

We can't deprive you of cinnamon buns, creamy sweet puddings, whips, popsicles, sherbets, and Rice Krispies treats.

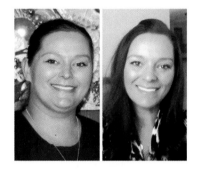

I have been overweight/ obese since I was around thirteen. Before I found THM, I was given one more chance from my doctor to do something or I would be put on high-cholesterol meds. A friend of mine let me know about a book she had ordered that looked like it would be a good option for me. I was reluctant, because I felt I couldn't grasp the S, E, and FP. Finally, I was added to the THM Facebook pages, and it was like a light came on. I loved seeing everyone's SV (scale victories) and NSV (nonscale victories). I wanted to be one of them someday. I decided to give it a try and the rest is history.

I truly believe God led me to this plan, because I had tried so many quick fixes and failed immediately. Not this time. I love what I eat and how I feel. My favorite on-plan foods are: Egg Roll in a Bowl, Ezekiel bread sandwiches with Light Laughing Cow cheese, veggies, and deli meat, Trimtastic cake with cream cheese icing, Creamy Chicken and wild rice soup, No-Bake Cookies, Pizza Casserole, fried cabbage and fried eggs for breakfast, instant pot oatmeal with fresh chopped apples, and many, many more!! –SARAH S.

cini-minis

S

MAKES 24 (YOU CAN HALVE RECIPE IF DESIRED)

FOR THE DOUGH

2 large eggs

⅔ cup egg whites (carton or fresh)

⅔ cup unsweetened almond milk

¼ cup Super Sweet Blend*

1½ cups THM Baking Blend*

2 teaspoons aluminum-free baking powder

½ teaspoon baking soda

FOR THE CINNAMON SWIRL

¼ cup Gentle Sweet*

2 tablespoons ground cinnamon

4 tablespoons (½ stick) butter

1 teaspoon blackstrap molasses (optional, for a brown sugar effect)

FOR THE FROSTING

4 tablespoons (½ stick) butter

6 tablespoons ⅓ less fat cream cheese

5 tablespoon Gentle Sweet*

1½ teaspoons pure vanilla extract

Sticky and sweet just like cinnamon buns should be. These are minis!

1. Preheat the oven to 375°F. Grease 24 cups of 2 standard muffin tins.

2. Make the dough. Mix together all the ingredients in a large bowl. Spread 1 tablespoon of dough into each of the 24 muffin cups.

3. Make the cinnamon swirl. Mix all the ingredients together. If it's too stiff, add just a teaspoon of hot water and stir so that it is thick, but can be scooped out with a measuring spoon. Drop ½ teaspoon of cinnamon swirl onto each muffin cup and give it a little swirl into the dough with a knife. Don't overmix it.

4. Bake for 10 minutes. Cool slightly on a wire rack.

5. Meanwhile, make the frosting. Mix together all the ingredients with a fork until there are no lumps.

6. Spread the frosting all over the warm cinnamon buns.

* FOR NSI: USE A GROCERY STORE ON-PLAN SWEETENER AND THE FRUGAL FLOUR OPTION (SEE PAGE 40).

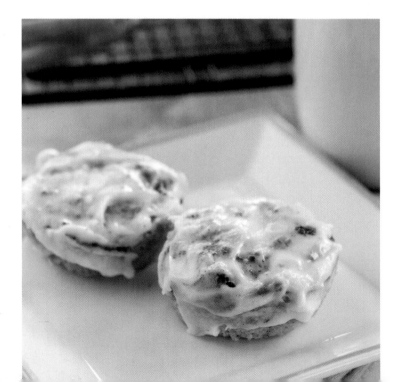

magic skinny chocolate nut clusters ⓢ

MULTIPLE SERVE

½ cup melted coconut oil (use the flavorless kind if you don't want a coconut flavor)

¼ cup unsweetened cocoa powder

4 to 6 teaspoons Gentle Sweet* (depending on your sweet tooth)

1 to 2 pinches Mineral Salt

½ teaspoon pure vanilla extract (optional)

1 cup frozen nuts of any kind

Watch the nuts magically turn into a chocolate-covered, to-die-for treat. Frozen nuts are the key to this super-speedy treat. They instantly set the Skinny Chocolate into a crunchy, nutty, chocolaty sensation. Nuts are a wonderful part of the THM plan—just be sure to treat them with the respect they deserve, because they are a heavy fuel. Enjoy this treat as a lovely afternoon snack with a cuppa coffee or tea (perhaps with some collagen added for protein), or have a few after dinner, but do remember to include some of the lighter treats in this section, too, for the perfect balance.

1. In a bowl, mix together the coconut oil, cocoa powder, sweetener, salt, and vanilla. Add the frozen nuts. Stir, then chill.

* FOR NSI: USE A GROCERY STORE ON-PLAN SWEETENER.

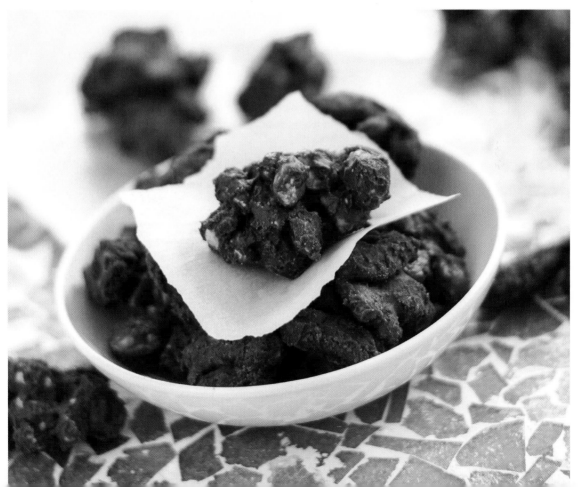

brown rice krispy treats

E

MULTIPLE SERVE

11 brown rice cakes, unsalted (we use Lundberg Family Farms brand)

2 tablespoons Just Gelatin*

1½ cups water

⅓ cup plus 3 tablespoons Gentle Sweet*

¼ teaspoon xanthan gum

1½ teaspoons pure vanilla extract

¼ teaspoon Mineral Salt

4 tablespoons (1 scoop) unflavored Pristine Whey Protein Powder

No need to rely on store-bought Rice Krispies Treats anymore with all of that sugar, corn syrup, margarine, and dextrose! Enjoy this Trim Healthy treat with all of the benefits of brown rice, gelatin, and whey protein! Throw them in your kids' lunch bags or take some along for a quick pick-me-up E snack for yourself!

1. Place the rice cakes in a gallon zippy bag. Seal the bag. Squeeze and crush the brown rice cakes until they turn into a nice-size crumble, about ¼- to ½-inch pieces.

2. Place the crumbled brown rice cakes into a 9 × 13-inch pan. Smooth them into the pan so they are distributed evenly.

3. Combine the gelatin with ½ cup of the water in a small bowl and stir. Allow to sit so the gelatin dissolves.

4. Place the remaining 1 cup water in a small saucepan over high heat and bring to a rapid boil.

5. In a large bowl, combine the sweetener, xanthan gum, vanilla, and salt. Add the softened gelatin, then slowly pour in the boiling water. Start beating on high speed with an electric hand mixer until the mixture gets thick and marshmallow-like. Be patient; it takes a while. After the first 5 minutes of beating, add the whey protein a little at a time, then beat for another 3 to 4 minutes.

6. Pour the marshmallow mixture on top of the crumbled brown rice cakes and use a small spatula to stir the mixture into the crumbles until all the pieces are covered. Smooth and pat the mixture down using your spatula and press firmly into the pan.

7. Refrigerate the pan for 4 hours. Cut into squares and serve. Store leftovers in a sealed container or baggie and keep in the refrigerator.

* FOR NSI: USE A GROCERY STORE ON-PLAN SWEETENER AND UNFLAVORED GELATIN.

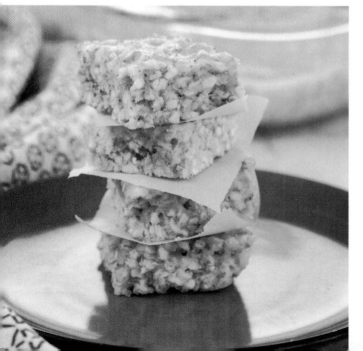

trimmy choco pudding

S

MAKES 2 SERVINGS

1 tablespoon extra-virgin coconut oil

½ cup hot (not boiling) water

1½ cups plus 2 tablespoons cold water

1 avocado

4 tablespoons unsweetened cocoa powder

3½ teaspoons Super Sweet Blend, or 3 tablespoons Gentle Sweet plus 1 to 2 doonks of Pure Stevia Extract Powder*

6 pinches Mineral Salt

2 teaspoons pure vanilla extract

½ teaspoon Natural Burst chocolate extract (optional)

⅛ teaspoon Sunflower Lecithin (optional)

1½ tablespoons (1 scoop) Integral Collagen (optional)

½ tablespoon Just Gelatin*

1 tablespoon just off the boil water

SERENE CHATS: *Dairy-free, super simple, and super-duper delicious. This makes two servings to keep on hand in the fridge when the snackies hit. Or take some to work with you, if you have access to a refrigerator, and enjoy for a delightful afternoon snack. You'll notice the Trimmy ingredients once again. I put them in color for you. They are what creams this pudding up so healthfully and perfectly so it is not jello-ish but smooth and creamy.*

1. Melt the coconut oil in the hot water and place it in a blender. Add the 1½ cups cold water, avocado, cocoa powder, sweetener, salt, vanilla, chocolate extract, lecithin (if using), and collagen (if using). Blend for about 30 seconds on high.

2. Add the gelatin to a mug with the 2 tablespoons cold water and stir, then add the boiled water and stir again. Turn the blender on low and add every drip of the gelatin mixture while the blender is whizzing. Place the lid back on and blend on high for 20 seconds.

3. Pour the mixture into 2 pint jars and refrigerate overnight. You need to wait the full night (or several hours) for the perfect setting. If it looks a little too set, just give it a good stir with your spoon and it will be thick, smooth, and creamy. This recipe is so simple and quick that you can keep making it in such a way that you have 1 batch setting while you are enjoying the other.

* FOR NSI: USE A GROCERY STORE ON-PLAN SWEETENER AND UNFLAVORED GELATIN.

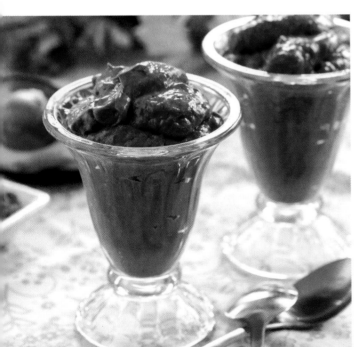

no moo cream cheese bites

S

MULTIPLE SERVE

4 oolong tea bags

1 cup just off the boil water

2¼ teaspoons Just Gelatin

1 cup extra-virgin coconut oil

⅛ teaspoon Sunflower Lecithin

1 teaspoon pure vanilla extract

4 pinches Mineral Salt

2 tablespoons Gentle Sweet

¾ teaspoon Super Sweet Blend
(or use another tablespoon
Gentle Sweet)

6 tablespoons Baobab Boost
Powder

SERENE CHATS: *Dairy-free but not yummy-free! These indulgent bites quench the mightiest sweet cravings while drenching your body with superfoods. Pour into pretty molds (or ice cube trays) and enjoy some for a snack or a couple for dessert. Or pour the mixture into a small plastic tub and use as you would any sweetened cream cheese. You can smear it on breads, muffins, Beauty Blend Graham Crackers (page 504) or onto pancakes, or just dip a spoon in and enjoy. If you want to go the extra mile, you can press one of our no-bake crust options into mini muffin tins, and then top with the cream cheese mix, making them the cutest cheesecake bites ever.*

For years I had tried to come up with a dairy-free or superfood-deep S alternative for pasteurized cream cheese. Pearl is fine using that stuff on her journey (you can see that from some of her recipes) and while I include it a time or two, it doesn't gel well in my crazy purist soul. I prefer my dairy raw and pastured on green grass. Even Pearl agrees with me that too much pasteurized dairy can cause weight stalls for some people. She's the first to tell people to scale back on pasteurized dairy a tad if they can't get the scale to move, so even if you are not dairy intolerant, shake things up and give these a try.

Most of my attempts at dairy-free cream cheese were total failure bombs that only the trash would swallow. Some were passable and others could only bring a halfhearted yippee. This recipe was a total accident. I was playing around with oolong tea recipes and fell upon this yummy stuff. I put my finger in the creamy mix, took a giant lick, and my feet sprang into a major dorky dance . . . this was No Moo Cream Cheese . . . at last! I poured it into some pretty flower molds and once set, I called Pearl over to taste. She declared them better than cheesecake itself!

1. Brew the oolong tea bags in the boiled water for 5 minutes in an insulated coffee mug to keep it nice and hot (or cover a mug with a saucer to help the tea stay hot). Squeeze and remove the tea bags, then pour the tea into a blender (adding a little more water to make the liquid come up to the 1-cup line on your blender, as the tea leaves absorb some of the water as they rehydrate).

2. Add the gelatin to the blender and blend for a few seconds. Add the coconut oil and blend for a few seconds again. Throw in the lecithin, vanilla, salt, sweeteners, and baobab powder and blend until smooth.

3. Pour into pretty molds or ice cube trays or any old kitchen plastic tub.

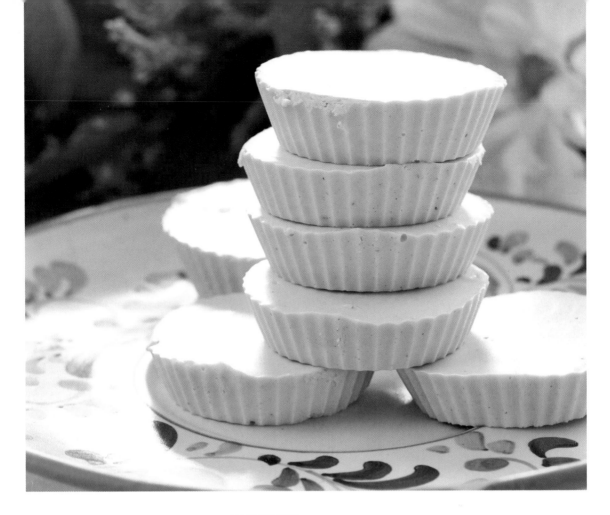

VARIATIONS

CRUSTED NO MOO BITES: For a no-bake version, make No-Bake Chocolate Crust (page 406) or Light 'n' Luscious No-Bake Crust (page 412). Press the dough into mini muffin tins, then top with a spoonful of the cream cheese mix. For a baked crust, make Beauty Blend Base Pie Crust (page 508) or Traditional Pie Crust (page 408). Press the dough into mini muffins tins and bake for a few minutes less than directed, then cool. Fill the cooled crusts with the cream cheese mix. Freeze until the bites can pop right out. Transfer the amount you will use for the week to the fridge and allow to thaw before eating for the perfect consistency. Freeze the rest in a zippy bag.

NO MOO CREAM CHEESE: If you would like to make an unsweetened version like regular Philly cream cheese, use only ½ teaspoon vanilla, up the salt by one more pinch, use only 2 teaspoons Gentle Sweet, and only 3 to 4 teaspoons baobab powder.

lemon lime burst whip (FP)

SINGLE SERVE

1 cup 1% cottage cheese
Juice of 1 lemon
Juice of 1 lime
3 doonks Pure Stevia Extract
    Powder*

The zingy flavors in this protein-packed snack (or even break-fast) wow your mouth! If you want some for dessert, just eat half and save half for later.

1. Put all the ingredients in a blender and blend well.

* FOR NSI: USE A GROCERY STORE ON-PLAN SWEETENER.

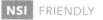 FRIENDLY

peanut chocolate whip (FP)

SINGLE SERVE

1 cup 1% cottage cheese
1 teaspoon MCT oil, butter, or heavy
    cream
2 level teaspoons unsweetened
    cocoa powder
2 rounded teaspoons Pressed
    Peanut Flour*
2 pinches Mineral Salt
2 tablespoons Gentle Sweet*

This is pure deliciousness in protein form. It's the perfect after-noon snack, or even breakfast, but if you'd rather eat it for a dessert, just eat half of it and save the rest for a smaller mid-morning snack tomorrow.

1. Put all ingredients in a small bowl and blend with a stick blender. (Or place all the ingredients in a mini food proces-sor or blender and process until smooth.)

* FOR NSI: USE A GROCERY STORE SUGAR-FREE DEFATTED PEANUT FLOUR AND AN ON-PLAN SWEETENER.

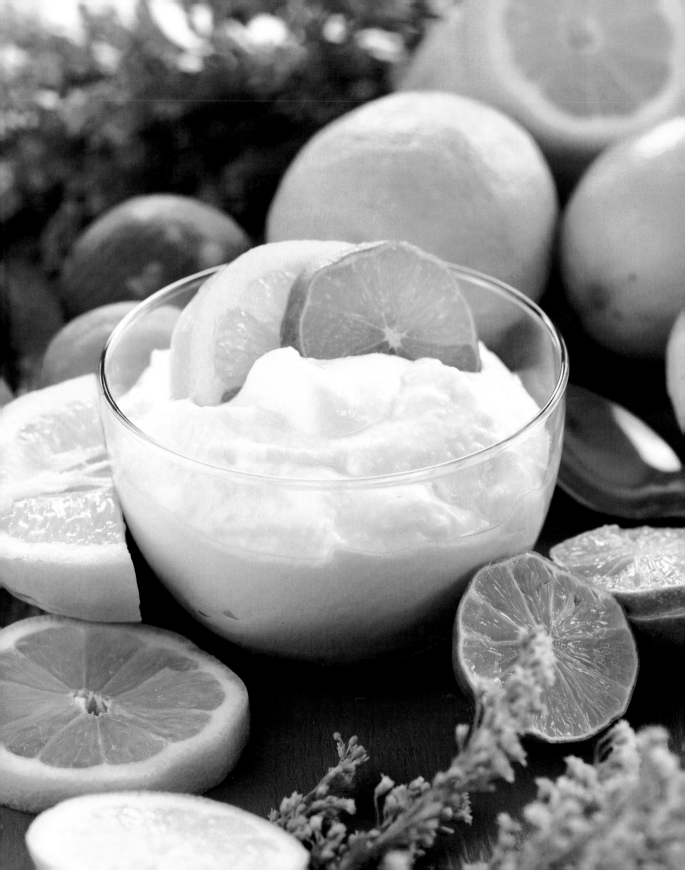

miracle mousse makeover

LARGE SINGLE SERVE

1 tablespoon Just Gelatin

¼ cup cool water

¼ cup just off the boil water

1 tablespoon extra-virgin coconut oil (1 teaspoon for FP)

½ teaspoon Sunflower Lecithin (optional)

2 rounded teaspoons (½ scoop) Integral Collagen

3 tablespoons unsweetened cocoa powder

1 teaspoon pure vanilla extract

1 tablespoon Super Sweet, or 3 tablespoons Gentle Sweet (plus an added doonk or 2 Pure Stevia Extract Powder if needed)

4 pinches Mineral Salt

2 tablespoons (½ scoop) unflavored Pristine Whey Protein Powder

2 cups ice cubes

Chocolate mousse just got a Trim Healthy makeover. This is a huge single serving of instant, magical, ultraslimming mousse that tastes similar to creamy chocolate ice cream. You can enjoy as a big snack or mini meal, but it is big enough that you might want to share with another family member or freeze leftovers as mousse pops since it will not hold its shape in the fridge. (Note the Trimmy ingredients in color again.)

1. Put the **gelatin** in a measuring cup, pour in the cool water, and stir, then add the boiled water and stir again. Put the hot gelatin mixture into a blender and add the **coconut oil, lecithin** (if using), **collagen,** cocoa powder, vanilla, sweetener, salt, and whey protein. Blend well.

2. Turn the blender to its lowest setting and dump in the ice while the blades are spinning. Let it crunch up a bit on low and then turn the blender up and keep whizzing until perfectly creamy. You might have to turn the blender off and push the mixture back into the blades once or twice with a spatula. Just make sure it is not crunchy with ice, but smoooooooth. Pour it into your bowl or parfait glass. At first it might be a tad runny, but it will set up before your eyes in the next 5 minutes or so.

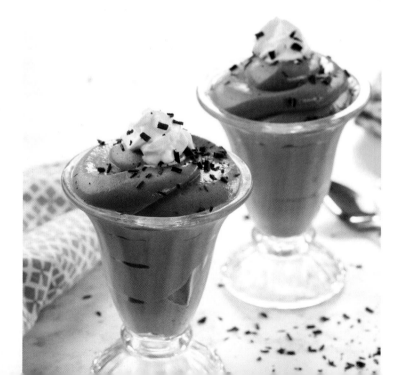

one-minute yogurt bowl

SINGLE SERVE

¾ cup plain 0% Greek yogurt

3½ tablespoons unsweetened cashew or almond milk

3 tablespoons strawberry or chocolate Pristine Whey Protein Powder

1 to 2 pinches Mineral Salt

OPTIONAL ADD-INS

Chopped berries (for FP)

Chopped fruit (for E)

Sprinkling of Crunchy Granola (page 361) or oats (for E)

2 teaspoons chopped nuts or chia seeds (for S)

2 teaspoons Trim Healthy Chocolate Chips (for S)

1 teaspoon heavy cream, for swirling in (for S, but can even fit into FP)

Stevia-sweetened Greek yogurt cups have turned up in grocery stores recently, which made a lot of Trim Healthy Mamas happy. But heads up . . . if you've been busy eating those and are now wondering why you feel bloated and gassy, sadly inulin is often used in the ingredients, and that can cause these symptoms for many of us. Also, they can get pricey. We prefer to make our own: It is less expensive and barely takes more time than taking the top off of a yogurt cup. Flavored whey protein makes slapping this creamy stuff together a speedy no-brainer. Chocolate is a hard-to-get-right flavor when paired with yogurt, so perhaps start with the strawberry version as that is the yummiest (we think). But our chocolate version beats the pants off store-bought versions. Enjoy for a snack or a breakfast (use a full cup of yogurt if having as a breakfast). You can enjoy as written as an FP or choose one or two of the add-ins for an optional E or S. The teaspoon of heavy cream swirled on top knocks this out of the park!

1. Whisk together the yogurt, nut milk, whey protein, and salt in a small bowl until smooth. Top with add-ins (if using).

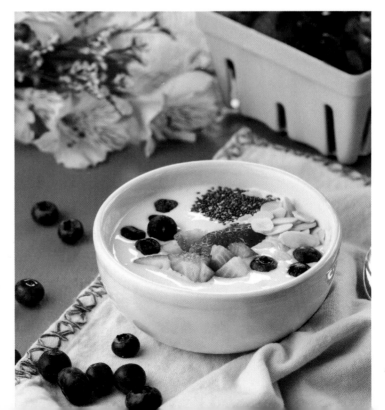

445

singing canary pops

MULTIPLE SERVE

2 teaspoons Just Gelatin

2 tablespoons cool water, for the gelatin

2 tablespoons just off the boil water, for the gelatin

2 cups plus 2 tablespoons water

Juice of 1 large lemon

½ teaspoon ground turmeric (you may need to work up to this amount; start with less)

1 teaspoon pure vanilla extract

2 teaspoons Super Sweet (or just slightly more to taste)

4 pinches Mineral Salt

1 tablespoon Baobab Boost Powder

1½ tablespoons (1 scoop) Integral Collagen

⅛ teaspoon Sunflower Lecithin

1 teaspoon MCT oil

1 to 2 tablespoons full-fat canned coconut milk or heavy cream (optional; for S)

4 tablespoons (1 scoop) unflavored Pristine Whey Protein Powder

Yet another refreshing way to enjoy the health benefits of the adrenal fatigue-fighting Singing Canary.

1. Put the gelatin in a mug, pour in the 2 tablespoons cool water, and stir to dissolve, then add the boiled water and stir again. Set aside.

2. In a blender, combine the 2 cups plus 2 tablespoons water, the lemon juice, turmeric, vanilla, sweetener, salt, baobab powder, collagen, lecithin, MCT oil, and coconut milk (if using) and whiz. Turn the blender to low and while it is whizzing, add the gelatin mixture. Blend for a few seconds, then add the whey protein and blend for about 10 more seconds. Pour into ice pop molds and freeze until solid.

VARIATION

SINGING CANARY SHERBET: To make a sherbet, pull the collagen back to 1 teaspoon and the whey protein to just 2 tablespoons. Follow the same directions, but pour into ice cube trays and freeze until solid. When ready to make your sherbet, process the cubes in a food processor until a yellow snow forms. For S, add 2 tablespoons full-fat coconut milk or cream; for FP, add unsweetened coconut, cashew, or almond milk. Process to sherbet consistency.

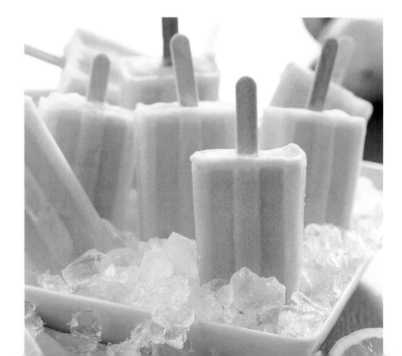

chocolate berry cream fluff

S

MULTIPLE SERVE

1½ to 2 cups heavy cream

1½ tablespoons Super Sweet Blend, or ¼ cup Gentle Sweet*

16 ounces fresh strawberries, sliced

1 cup fresh blueberries

1 cup fresh raspberries

¾ cup Trim Healthy Chocolate Chips*

Our sister Vange came up with this easy recipe. We stole it, of course. It is simply berries, chocolate chips, and whipped cream, but loved by everyone. Now one of us sisters never fails to bring this amazing dessert to our hilltop family gatherings. We ask each other, "Who's bringing the Fluff?" A family gathering without Fluff just won't do. Take this to any potluck or bridal or baby shower and watch it get gobbled up before your eyes. This makes a huge amount, so if you want to make it just for your family you should halve the ingredients.

1. Whip the cream with the sweetener until soft peaks form. Combine with the berries and chocolate chips. Chill until serving time.

* FOR NSI: USE A GROCERY STORE ON-PLAN SWEETENER AND CHOPPED 85% CHOCOLATE OR OTHER STEVIA-SWEETENED CHOCOLATE CHIPS.

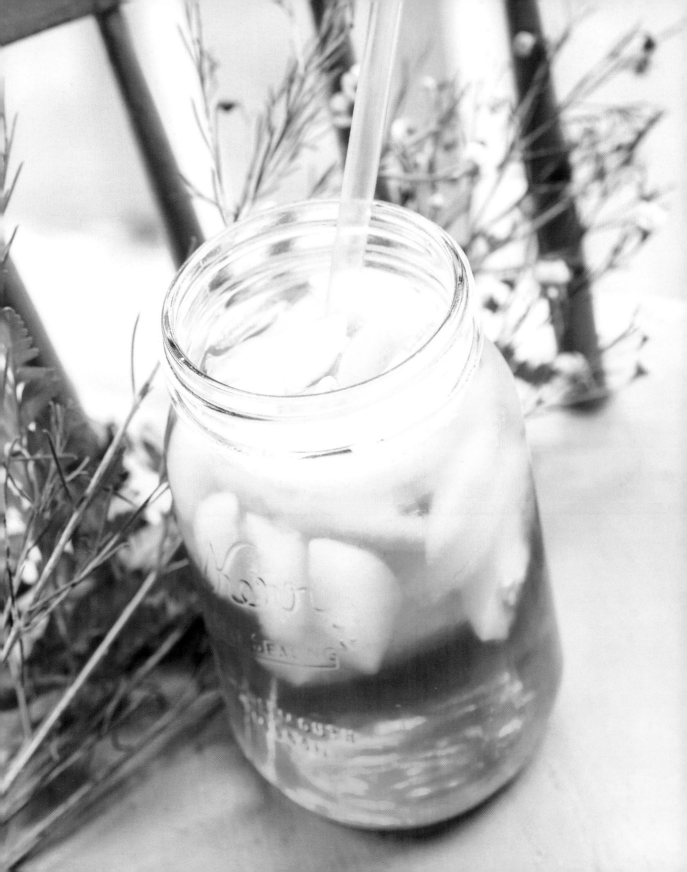

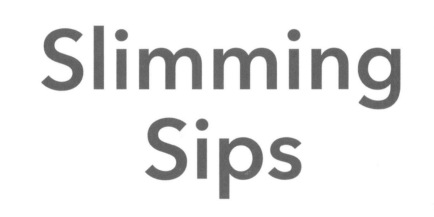

Slimming Sips

Drinks

Sip yourself trim! Quench your thirst and hydrate every cell with yummy goodness. Drink deep from the healing well. Bottoms up!

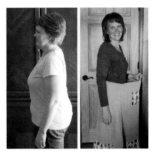

Two years ago I set a weight-loss goal. I did it because I had to, not because I really thought I would reach that number. I would have been tickled pink if I lost just half of that amount. After all, I had never succeeded in losing weight. Maybe a few pounds, but they always came roaring back with ten of their friends. But this time it was different. I had Trim Healthy Mama. No calorie counting, no exercising, no deprivation. Just a new way of eating and finding some healthy alternatives for the foods I craved.

I am not joking when I say THM gave me my life back. I've lost seventy pounds and I know they will never come back because I can eat this way for the rest of my life. I can't believe I'm here! When I started, I promised myself that I would reward myself with something big once I reached my goal. But now that I've gotten here, I realize the way I feel and the journey to get here is all the reward I could ever need or want. I feel so much better than I did two years ago. Good enough that I actually WANT to start exercising! Not earth-shattering, but true. So please, if you want to make changes, go for it! I have not exercised one bit, I am menopausal and hypothyroid, so I am serious when I say that if I can do it, anyone can! Even if it's slow, you will be better off than you are today. I'm so thankful for Trim Healthy Mama, and I smile for what tomorrow will bring. THANK YOU, Serene and Pearl. **–DONNA G.**

hello health sipper

MAKES 1 QUART FOR ALL-DAY SIPPING (CAN BE DOUBLED IF YOU ARE A 2-QUART-A-DAY TYPE)

Hello, energy. Hello, humming metabolism. Hello, glowing skin. Hello, strong bones. Hello, healthy hair. Hello, powerful immune function. Hello Health Sipper!

To our THM vets . . . time for a new sipper, don't you think? We gave you Good Girl Moonshine, The Shrinker, and the Singing Canary in *Trim Healthy Mama Cookbook*. Now welcome our new all-day sipper to the stage. It is good for your body to change up, so perhaps take a little break from the other sippers and let Hello Health boost your immune system and metabolism with its own unique powers. (To all our newbies, those drink recipes can be found for free on our website or in the cookbook—you don't have to drink them for plan success, but they help boost health and weight loss.)

Hello Health is a gorgeous, vibrant drink that is like sunshine and sherbet combined. It might remind you of tropical pineapples, with a hint of tart citrus. It has a creamy mouthfeel, yet you can sip your heart away on this FP delight all day long and not worry about excess calories, carbs, or fat. It satiates but masterfully helps to sculpt a Trim waist. Yippee!

The star of our new all-day sipper is a superfood powder made from the pulp of the baobab fruit (you can read more about it on page 42). When paired with its costar red capsicum, you have a vitamin C powerhouse drink to help slim you down! "What?" you say. Vitamin C helps weight loss? It is crucial for it actually. Baobab boasts one of the highest vitamin C contents of any food in the world. Red bell pepper, another costar in this drink, is also brimming with vitamin C, containing three times more than an orange!

Baobab fruit pulp slows the absorption of blood sugars dramatically. As you revel in the absolute yumminess of your Hello Health Sipper, the baobab powder will be going to work helping to keep your metabolic hormones and insulin levels in check. Baobab is loaded with pectin, which turns into a gel in your stomach and keeps you satiated longer, which in turn curbs the desire to overeat and snack like a crazy woman (or guy)! It reduces inflammation in the gut and helps friendly bacteria flourish to optimize digestion.

The weight-loss and blood-sugar benefits of this sipper are just the beginning. Even though it doesn't contain caffeine, over time Hello Health can work to improve your energy levels. Baobab has high iron content, in fact twice that of spinach. It supports hemoglobin production, which helps transport oxygen-rich blood throughout your body. That means energy . . . at last! Anemia is exhausting and can lead to adrenal fatigue. It afflicts loads of tired Mamas during childbearing years. Sipping on Hello Health will help restore lost iron stores and bring renewed vitality to your day. Red Bull and the like can go jump. Hello Health is true and lasting energy repair!

Since this sipper is caffeine free, it is great for evening hours, too. Often this time can be the most dangerous for mindless snacking, especially when we are sooo tired and just want to zone and eat for no good reason. Making Hello Health Sipper your "after dinner till bedtime" pacifier will help with the hand-to-mouth cravings.

We are addicts of this gorgeous drink and are sipping it as we write this to you. Join us and clink your jar to ours as we celebrate greater health and happiness! Cheers!

½ teaspoon Just Gelatin

1 tablespoon cool water, for the gelatin

1 tablespoon just off the boil water, for the gelatin

2 tablespoons Baobab Boost Powder

4 to 6 pinches Mineral Salt

½ to 1 teaspoon MCT oil

1 to 2 teaspoons Integral Collagen

⅛ teaspoon Sunflower Lecithin

2 to 3 doonks Pure Stevia Extract Powder

Juice of ½ lemon

2 red mini sweet peppers (or ¼ red bell pepper)

Chunk of a red jalapeño (optional, for us feisty tigers)

⅛ teaspoon Natural Burst apricot extract or pure orange extract (optional)

1. Place the gelatin in a 1-cup measuring cup. Add the cool water and stir until dissolved, then add the boiled water and stir. Fill the measuring cup with enough cool water to come to 1 cup and place in the blender. Now fill the measuring cup with 1 more cup cold water and add to the blender. Blend for a few seconds.

2. Add all the remaining ingredients and blend on high until all is creamy and the peppers are completely broken down. Pour this concentrate into a quart jar. Fill to the top with ice, add water only if needed to reach the top, and stir well. Taste and adjust the flavors to "own it" and sip your health into renewal.

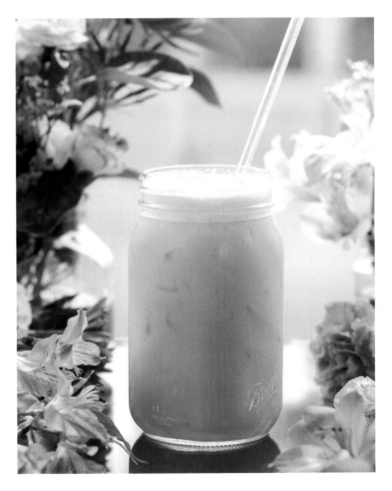

converted sailor toddy

MAKES 1 QUART FOR ALL-DAY SIPPING—IF YOU CAN HANDLE IT!

4-inch chunk fresh ginger (6 inches for absolute ginger psychos like Serene)

2 cups water, plus more if needed

Juice of 2 large lemons

2 to 3 doonks Pure Stevia Extract Powder

Ice, to top it off

SERENE CHATS: *Got a little scratchy throat? Maybe feeling a little under the weather? Or do you just want more pep in your step? Blast those gweebly germs and put a fire under your immune soldier troops. This ginger-flooded tonic is designed to make you holler like a sailor, hopefully a converted one. Four-letter words have been turned into a much nobler string of ten or more letters like BOOMDABBER BAFOODLEMUB!!! Of course, you might be more civilized in nature and restrain your whiskey-throated blast to a polite little "ahem" with a covered mouth. Either way we want this toddy to burn the nasties out of your system and build up your health so you can keep awhistlin' your favorite maritime tune. Don't get scared! This is fun pain. It really is an addictive, delicious swig of enjoyable intensity that can help decrease inflammation in your body. Get your toddy to fixin' what ails ya or just drink it cause it's good girl liquor and yew is a good girl!*

1. Coarsely chop the ginger and place it in a blender with the 2 cups water. Blend on low for 30 seconds to 1 minute. (Do not blend on too high a speed as the ginger fiber will become emulsified into the water.)

2. Strain the ginger juice through a fine-mesh sieve into a bowl and squeeze the ginger mash in your hands above the sieve to get every dreg of the medicinal juice. (If you don't want to use your hands, then just press the ginger with the back of a large spoon while it is in the sieve, but not too hard as you don't want to force any fiber through the mesh.) If this sounds complicated, it is not, it is simple and quick.

3. Now pour your ginger juice into a quart jar and add the lemon juice and stevia and stir. Add ice to the top of the jar and a little additional water if needed. Taste and adjust the flavors to "own it." It should grab your throat. Do you need more lemon? A touch more sweet? Get to feelin' better, Mama.

**Iced Vanilla
Fat-Burning Tea**
(page 456)

Speedy Chocolate Milk
(page 457)

Frozen Mocha
(page 458)

Converted Sailor Toddy
(opposite)

lemonade

FP

MAKES 1 QUART FOR ALL-DAY SIPPING (CAN BE DOUBLED)

Ice and water

Juice of 1 to 2 large lemons (depending on how lemony you like things), or 3 limes

2 to 3 doonks Pure Stevia Extract Powder

Don't overlook the simple power of a lemon. Your liver takes on a bigger job as you lose weight. It has to filter through all the toxins fat cells release as they are shed. Lemons stimulate your liver to work harder, so this can help your body break through weight-loss stalls a little sooner. Lemons also help dissolve uric acid and other poisons, and their sour flavor is an indication they are helping to regulate your blood sugar. Of course, lemonade is just yummy and you can sip on this all day.

1. Fill a quart jar with ice and water. Add the lemon juice and stevia. Stir, taste for sweetness, then sip the goodness!

NOTE: You can make a pink lemonade by replacing the water with Raspberry Zinger herbal tea.

iced vanilla fat-burning tea

FP

MAKES 1 QUART FOR ALL-DAY SIPPING (CAN BE DOUBLED)

2 oolong tea bags

½ cup just off the boil water

Ice and water

½ to 1 teaspoon pure vanilla extract

Pinch of Mineral Salt

2 to 3 doonks Pure Stevia Extract Powder (or to taste)

Try replacing your regular iced tea with this magical tea and see if stubborn weight doesn't start melting. Out of all teas on this planet, oolong has the most fat-burning power. Research shows that the polyphenols that are highest in oolong tea help activate thermogenesis, which increases fat oxidation in your body. Japanese scientists from the University of Tokushima found that oolong tea can double the amount of fat excreted by the body. They reported that 2 cups of oolong tea burned over 157% more fat than the same amount of green tea! Just 1 cup of this stuff can help burn off an extra 67 calories. Yeah!!

1. Steep the tea bags in the boiled water for about 5 minutes. Remove and discard the tea bags and put the tea into a quart jar. Fill with ice, then top off with water. Add the stevia, vanilla, and salt, then stir and taste for sweetness and your own preferred strength of vanilla.

NOTE: You can also drink this hot in winter months; simply omit the ice and use boiling water.

speedy chocolate milk FP

SINGLE SERVE

1 generous cup unsweetened cashew or almond milk

2 tablespoons (½ scoop) chocolate Pristine Whey Protein Powder (see Note)

A glass of this milk with a meal really helps give you extra filling mileage so you can more easily make it to that 3- to 4-hour mark before you eat again. But it does so in such a yummy way. Our children love this drink, and it is a great way to ensure they are getting plenty of protein.

1. Blend all the ingredients for a few seconds in a stand blender (or use a stick blender).

NOTE: If you don't have chocolate whey protein, no worries, you can use our original Slimming Chocolate Milk recipe to get a similar result. This is how we made the drink before we had chocolate-flavored whey: Blend together 1 cup unsweetened cashew or almond milk, 1 rounded teaspoon unsweetened cocoa powder, 1 rounded teaspoon Super Sweet, and 1 to 2 tablespoons unflavored Pristine Whey Protein Powder. If you have sufficient protein in your meal, you can leave off the whey . . . still tastes great.

* FOR NSI: USE VARIATION IN NOTE USING A GROCERY STORE ON-PLAN SWEETENER AND WHEY PROTEIN (SEE PAGE 43).

speedy strawberry milk FP

SINGLE SERVE

1 generous cup unsweetened cashew or almond milk

2 tablespoons (½ scoop) strawberry Pristine Whey Protein Powder

1 to 2 frozen strawberries (optional)

1. Blend all the ingredients in a stand blender (or use a stick blender).

frozen mocha

S

SINGLE SERVE

1 cup brewed coffee, cooled
1 generous cup ice (7 to 8 large cubes)
1 tablespoon heavy cream
2 to 4 tablespoons (½ to 1 scoop) chocolate Pristine Whey Protein Powder

This can be a full snack or very occasional full breakfast using the full scoop of protein powder. Stick to half a scoop if pairing it with a snack or meal that already contains protein. You may need to add a little on-plan sweetener at the end if half a scoop doesn't give enough sweetness for you.

1. Put the coffee, ice, and heavy cream in a blender and blend well until the ice is broken down. Add the whey and blend for another 10 to 20 seconds.

ruby sparkler

FP

SINGLE SERVE

½ cup ice
¼ cup Beautiful Beet Kvass (page 461)
½ cup sparkling water

1. Place the ice in a glass. Pour in the kvass, then top off with sparkling water.

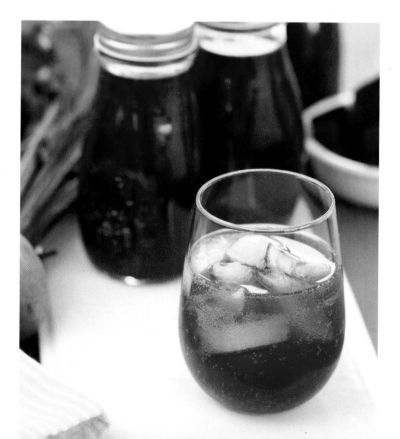

CULTURED DRINKS

NSI

shockingly simple milk kefir   FP OR S

MAKES CLOSE TO 1 QUART

1 (2-quart) canning jar

1 handful (¼ to ⅓ cup) kefir grains (get for free from a fermenting friend or online)

1 quart milk (whole milk for S, fat-free for FP)

1 (1-quart) jar with plastic lid

SERENE CHATS: *Kefir is a cultured (fermented) tangy, schweppy, and absolutely delicious milk drink. It is the perfect way to get the most nutrition from milk, but without the sugars, as the double fermentation eats them up. As you can tell from reading this book, Pearl and I have different approaches to Trim Healthy Mama even though our core beliefs are the same. While Pearl has never made kefir and probably never will, it is a huge part of my nutritional life. I live on the stuff in my Yuck Yum Bitty (page 497). We have milk goats and cows so I get to enjoy kefir made from raw milk, but you can definitely buy milk from the store. So join me in the art of kefir making if you like . . .*

1. In the 2-quart glass canning jar (with screw band), combine the kefir grains and milk. Put a coffee filter over the mouth of the jar and use the metal screw band to hold it in place. Let it ferment at room temperature for 24 hours. (If your home is super cold you might need to extend the first ferment for another 24 hours.) Uncover and stir well. Strain the kefir through a fine-mesh sieve into a bowl. Push the grains around the sieve with a big spoon to help the liquid go through while the grains stay in the sieve.

2. Pour your first-ferment kefir from the bowl into a clean quart jar, this time with a tight-fitting plastic lid, and put the strained kefir grains back in the original 2-quart jar (don't wash it). Let your kefir liquid ferment once more at room temperature for another 24 hours. Congrats! You have made a double-fermented kefir! (If you don't use it all up, then you can keep it fermenting for up to 3 days out of the refrigerator. Shake it occasionally to help it ferment evenly.)

3. Now let's go back in time a day to when you poured your first-ferment kefir liquid through the sieve and you put your kefir grains back in the jar. Fill the 2-quart jar with another fresh quart of milk and start the kefir process over again.

NOTE: Watch me make kefir in a free video on our website (and on our member site) if you are more of a visual person. We also have a video showing how to make the coconut kefir (page 460) on our member website starring our sister Vange.

vangibabe's coconut kefir

S

MAKES CLOSE TO 2 CUPS

1 (15-ounce) can full-fat (see Note) coconut milk (one with no weird preservatives)

1 (1-quart) canning jar

1 to 2 tablespoons milk kefir grains

1 (1-quart) jar with plastic lid

1. Place the coconut milk in a 1-quart glass canning jar (with a screw band) and stir to make it smooth and creamy. Add the kefir grains and stir well. Put a coffee filter over the mouth of the jar and use the metal screw band to hold it in place. Ferment at room temperature for 24 hours. (If your home is super cold, you might need to extend this first ferment for another 24 hours.) Uncover and stir well. Strain the kefir through a fine-mesh sieve, allowing the fermented elixir to pour into a bowl and the grains to stay in the sieve. Push the grains around the sieve with a big spoon to help out the process. Coconut kefir is thicker than milk, so massage the liquid through with a spoon.

2. Place the first ferment in another clean quart jar with a tight-fitting plastic lid and put the kefir grains back in the original 1-quart canning jar. Allow the kefir liquid in the new quart jar to ferment outside the refrigerator for another 24 hours. Congrats! You now have your zippy, zappy, tangy, wangy coconut kefir. Refrigerate after the second 24 hours.

3. Let's go back to when you put the kefir grains back into the original canning jar after the first ferment was poured out. Add another can of coconut milk to the grains and start the process over again. The kefir grains will be good for a few fermenting batches, but then you need to put them into a little dairy milk for a day to refresh them. Drain off the dairy milk and throw it away. This recharges your grains. Any dairy milk residue will be eaten up, so it usually doesn't pose allergen or sensitivity problems.

NOTE: Kefir grains prefer fatty coconut milk and do not perform as well with the watered-down versions.

beautiful beet kvass ⒻⓅ

MULTIPLE SERVE

3 to 4 medium beets, or 2 biggies
  (organic is best here)
1 tablespoon Mineral Salt
Purified water or natural spring or
  well water (not tap water)
Patience

SERENE CHATS: *No, it's not complicated. I see you, Drive-Thru Sue . . . turning your brain off and flippin' to the next page. Come back here! Have you ever cut a few veggies up for a salad? Not even a pretty salad, just a quick throw-together hodgepodge? Of course you have. Well, this is even simpler, with only one veggie to cut! If you have chopped a veggie before and have a jar in your cupboard, then you CAN make this revolutionary ruby red drink.*

This recipe is so simple but it comes with so much payback in health bucks. It is literally teeming with life and infuses your cells with vitality. Traditionally it is known as a blood and liver cleanser and rebuilder. Modern science is now revealing a substance known as betacyanin in beets that increases the oxygen levels of your blood dramatically. It balances the electrolytes in your body and floods it with vigor and mineral-rich hydration. When you ferment anything, the health benefits multiply, so this drink amps up the natural healing medicine in beets to intense levels.

1. Wash the dirt off the beets, but don't peel or scrub, as that will get rid of all the good bacteria that helps with proper fermentation. Cut them into 1- to 2-inch chunks.

2. Throw your beets in a 2-quart jar and plonk in the Mineral Salt (or split into two 1-quart jars if that is all you've got). Cover the beets with water until 1 inch from the top of the jar. Cover tightly with your jar lid and allow to ferment at room temperature for a full week. If your house is very cold, wrap it in a towel; it might still need a few more days. Very hot houses may have it ready in 2 days, or if you have fresh whey from homemade kefir or yogurt, you can add ½ cup of this to your jar. This will give you a shorter fermentation time of only 2 to 3 days as it inoculates the kvass with robust probiotic strains.

3. Once your kvass is a deep burgundy and has little effervescent bubbles rising from inside, then congrats . . . you are ready to move it to the refrigerator. Told you this was easy! You can begin to drink it at once, but leaving it for a week or so mellows the salty flavor and most people who make kvass say it gets more vibrantly wonderful if you let it sit a few weeks more in the back of your refrigerator.

4. You can choose to decant into smaller jars (such as cleaned out kombucha-size juice jars) as this will keep the efferves-

(continues)

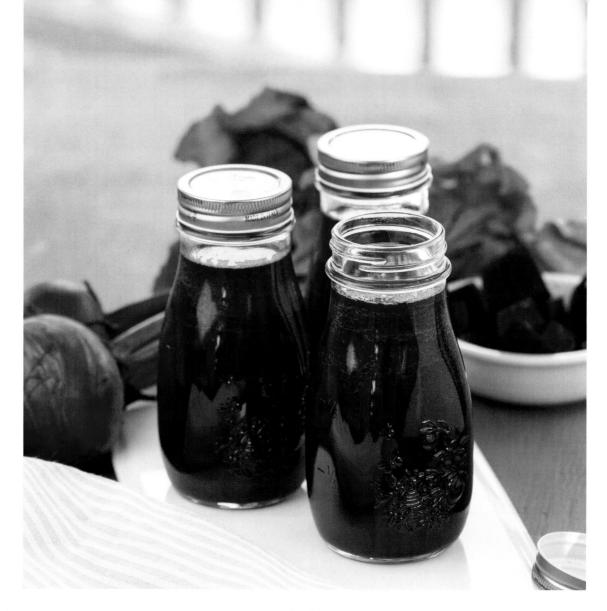

cent air building and make each sip more deliciously zingy and alive. When dividing into smaller jars, throw a few of the diced beet chunks into every jar. Keep the cut beets in your jar until the last drop is swigged. Then you will have lovely wild pickled beets to enjoy on salads.

NOTE: This is not an all-day sipper, but it has less natural sugar than kombucha, so you can drink a small glass with your meal—whether S, E, or FP—as it helps to aid digestion of any meal. Or drink some whenever you feel a need for intense refreshment. Use it to make a Ruby Sparkler (page 458) or Beet It Creamy Smoothie (page 493). You can also use it to replace the water content in your dressings or simply swig a shot like whiskey for a health pump.

HOT DRINKS

prep-ahead healing trimmy mix (FP) OR (S)

MAKES 30 TRIMMIES (1 FOR EACH DAY OF THE MONTH)

FOR THE MIX
¾ cup Integral Collagen

¾ cup unflavored Pristine Whey Protein Powder

3 tablespoons Sunflower Lecithin

1 teaspoon Pure Stevia Extract Powder (optional; see Note)

FOR THE TRIMMY
1½ cups freshly brewed coffee or any hot tea

1 teaspoon MCT oil, coconut oil, or butter for FP (use 2 to 3 teaspoons for S)

SERENE CHATS: *In* Trim Healthy Mama Cookbook *we showed you a healthy way to cream up your coffee or tea with the Healing Trimmy. That original hot Trimmy drink inspired my new line of Trimmy bisques (starting on page 162) and dressings (starting on page 527) since they use the same basic idea for creaminess in an ultrahealthy way. But back to coffee . . . sure you can use cream in your coffee on THM, but some of us can overdo the cream sometimes, ya know? Anyone's hand raised? And Trimmy ingredients allow you to have creamy coffee with an E or FP meal while at the same time going to work healing your gut and boosting your immune system. They are also more slimming than regular ol' cream in your coffee. Instead of having to make up a daily Trimmy, we now have a bulk mix version for you to keep on hand that will make your Trimmies much faster.*

1. Make the mix. Place the ingredients in a jar or container that has a lid. Shake or whisk to mix the ingredients. (Or put all the ingredients into your blender or food processor and swirl it for about 45 seconds to get a nice powdery mix.)

2. Make the Trimmy. Blend your hot coffee or tea with 2 rounded teaspoons of the mix and the oil or butter in a blender (holding the lid down tightly). Or use a stick blender.

NOTE: Leave out the stevia if you don't like sweetened coffee or tea. Using stevia in the mix gives a mildly sweet result, so if you prefer sweeter coffee or tea, add Gentle Sweet when making your Trimmy.

12 ounces freshly brewed coffee

1 tablespoon heavy cream

2 to 4 tablespoons (½ to 1 scoop) chocolate Pristine Whey Protein Powder

This might become your new favorite way to drink coffee . . . so frothy and creamy! You can use a full scoop of the chocolate whey if you want to have this for an occasional full breakfast (no other food required). Don't do that every day, of course, but it will be a protein-rich, on-the-go ultra-FP breakfast for occasional use. If eating other breakfast foods that contain protein with this drink, stick to the ½ scoop of whey and then you'll need to add a little more sweetener at the end, such as 2 to 3 teaspoons Gentle Sweet.

1. Blend all the ingredients in a blender for 10 seconds (holding the lid down tightly).

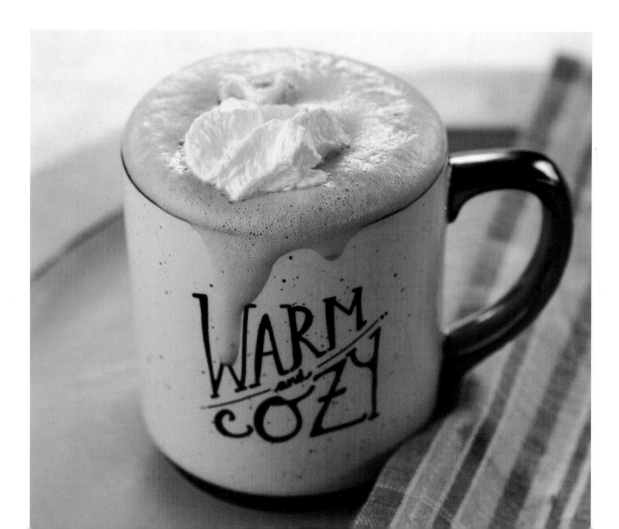

matcha spice trimmy

SINGLE SERVE

1½ cups just off the boil water
½ teaspoon matcha tea
¼ teaspoon ground turmeric
¼ teaspoon ground ginger
¼ teaspoon ground cinnamon
2 black peppercorns, or a dash of
   ground black pepper (optional)
2 pinches Mineral Salt
1 teaspoon Super Sweet Blend
1 teaspoon extra-virgin coconut oil
⅛ teaspoon Sunflower Lecithin
   (optional)
1 to 2 teaspoons Integral Collagen

And now for a new awesome Trimmy for you: This is a happy mug of latte-like, delicious, warming smoothness. Vivid green with matcha superfood goodness, this drink is brimming with antioxidants, including the powerful catechin EGCG, which is scientifically proven to target cancer cells. This Trimmy is medicine in a cup. It lights a bonfire under your metabolism, helps balance blood sugar, and burns calories for fun. Matcha can help a glum mood, calm a wound-up mind, and at the same time aid in concentration.

1. Blend everything up in a blender and you are done.

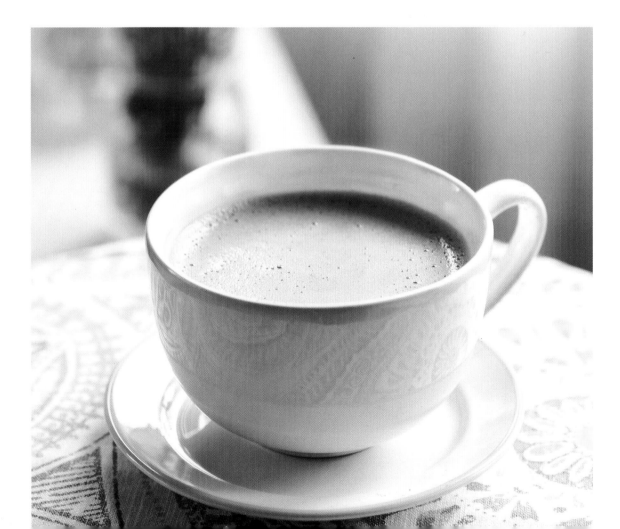

lazy collagen coffee

SINGLE SERVE

(FOR AN FP—STICK TO JUST
2 TABLESPOONS HALF-AND-HALF
OR LESS)

PEARL CHATS: I enjoy plenty of Trimmies, but sometimes I'm too lazy to even blend my coffee. Yep, I admit it, sometimes I just want good ol' cream in my coffee and don't want to worry about putting MCT oil or whey protein, or Sunflower Lecithin in the blender. So here's what I do on those mornings to still reap the benefits of collagen and to help balance the amino acid profile of my breakfast. This is my protein-rich, liver-cleansing, inflammation-fighting way to get collagen when I'm still half asleep and shudder at the thought of a loud blender.

1. Pour a little hot coffee into your mug.

2. Add 2 teaspoons (about ½ scoop) Integral Collagen and mix well with a fork.

3. Pour in the rest of your coffee, then add heavy cream or half-and-half.

4. Stir again. Now you have an awesome, protein-rich mug of coffee with no detectable collagen taste and no lumps—easy!

prep-ahead healing hot cocoa trimmy mix

MAKES 15 HOT COCOAS

FOR THE MIX

⅔ cup unsweetened cocoa powder

5 tablespoons Super Sweet Blend

4 teaspoons Sunflower Lecithin

¾ cup Integral Collagen

Generous ½ teaspoon Mineral Salt

5 tablespoons unflavored Pristine Whey Protein Powder (see Note)

FOR THE TRIMMY

1½ cups just off the boil water (or heated unsweetened cashew or almond milk)

1 teaspoon MCT oil, butter, or coconut oil for FP (use 2 to 3 teaspoons for S)

The perfect, healthy evening or anytime hot chocolate just got faster!

1. Make the mix. Place the ingredients in a jar or container that has a lid. Shake or whisk to mix the ingredients. (Or you can put all the ingredients into your blender or food processor and swirl it for about 45 seconds to get a nice powdery mix.)

2. Make a Trimmy. Blend the hot water or nut milk with 2 rounded teaspoons of the mix and the oil or butter in a blender (holding the lid down tightly). Or use a stick blender.

NOTE: You can use chocolate Pristine Whey Protein Powder in this mix but if you do, reduce the sweetener to 4 tablespoons and the cocoa powder to ⅓ cup.

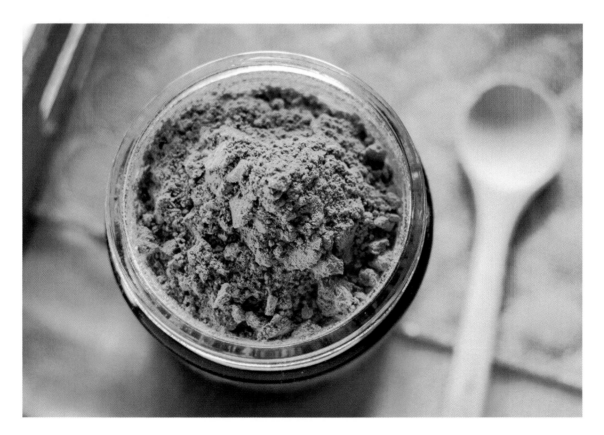

Shakes & Smoothies

Welcome to the chapter where you make best friends with large, creamy sweet drinks to bliss up your life! Our Biggie shakes and smoothies are massive. Most of them make close to 1 quart of good stuff that helps strip the weight off you! They can be a full meal, such as a lunch or a breakfast (although feel free to add more food if you are super hungry). Or they can be a filling afternoon snack. They are really too big to be dessert, but hey . . . now and then you may want a huge dessert to keep you satisfied on-plan, so you can break that rule occasionally.

The Baby shakes or smoothies are the perfect dessert size. They are that just right, sweet and creamy way to end your meal. Or if you just need a bit more filling power for any snack, feel free to add one on so you come away satisfied. They can stand alone as small snacks, too. Despite the name "baby," they are not tiny. A pint jar will be the perfect size of glass for you enjoy them in. (There are a couple snack-size-only smoothies at the end of the chapter. Those are too small for full meals.)

NOTE: You'll notice we use Super Sweet Blend as the chief sweetener in most of these recipes. We do this to help out your budget. Super Sweet is so much more economical than Gentle Sweet. It is easier to get a good sweet result using it in smoothies and shakes than in baking, when we have to rely more on Gentle Sweet. So having a bag of each makes your Gentle Sweet last much longer. If you want to use a grocery store on-plan sweetener, check the sweetener conversion chart on our website. If you don't want to order our whey protein, best to find one that is a cross-flow micro-filtered whey isolate. We don't use concentrates as they too easily oxidize. For those who cannot use whey protein, a similar creamy effect can be achieved combining collagen and egg white protein, or you can simply add more cottage cheese or Greek yogurt.

cinnamon bun shake

S

SINGLE SERVE

FOR THE BIGGIE SHAKE

1 cup unsweetened cashew or almond milk

½ cup 1% cottage cheese

2 tablespoons (½ scoop) unflavored Pristine Whey Protein Powder*

1 teaspoon ground cinnamon

½ teaspoon ground ginger

½ teaspoon pure vanilla extract

1 tablespoon Super Sweet Blend*

2 tablespoons ⅓ less fat cream cheese

¼ teaspoon Gluccie*

1½ to 2 cups ice

FOR THE BABY SHAKE

½ cup unsweetened almond milk

¼ cup 1% cottage cheese

1 tablespoon unflavored Pristine Whey Protein Powder*

½ teaspoon ground cinnamon

¼ teaspoon ground ginger

¼ teaspoon pure vanilla extract

1½ teaspoons Super Sweet Blend*

1 tablespoon ⅓ less fat cream cheese

⅛ teaspoon Gluccie*

¾ to 1 cup ice

PEARL CHATS: We're starting this shake and smoothie chapter off with our new personal favorite, okra-less shakes and smoothies, first mine then Serene's. Okrafied shakes come later in the chapter (read about them on page 478), but if you are new to this lifestyle, we didn't want to freak you out with okra shakes too soon. You can slowly ease your way into those. The only freaking out you will be doing when drinking this Cinnamon Bun Shake is from love and excitement. This is an ultracreamy shake that has all the flavor of a cinnamon bun with a little kick of ginger! Imagine waking up and enjoying this huge shake for breakfast or blessing yourself with a Biggie for an afternoon snack or a Baby for dessert. . . . You'll feel like you are on the un-diet!

1. Put all the ingredients in a blender and blend extremely well until smooth.

* FOR NSI: USE A GROCERY STORE ON-PLAN WHEY PROTEIN (SEE PAGE 43) AND SWEETENER. SUB XANTHAN GUM FOR THE GLUCCIE.

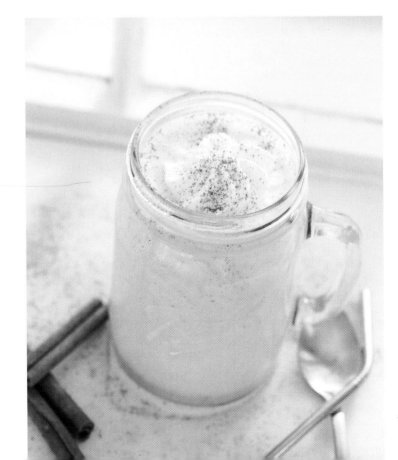

cheesecake shake down

SINGLE SERVE

FOR THE BIGGIE SHAKE

1 or 2 oolong tea bags

½ cup just off the boil water

1 teaspoon extra-virgin coconut oil

1 teaspoon Just Gelatin

1 to 2 tablespoons Baobab Boost Powder

⅛ teaspoon Sunflower Lecithin (optional, but preferred)

2 teaspoons Super Sweet Blend plus 2 tablespoons Gentle Sweet, or 3½ teaspoons Super Sweet

1 teaspoon pure vanilla extract

6 pinches Mineral Salt

1½ tablespoons (1 scoop) Integral Collagen

¼ to ½ teaspoon Natural Burst butter extract

Juice of 1 lemon (½ lemon if you prefer less tangy cheesecake)

⅛ teaspoon Gluccie

About 2 cups ice

2 tablespoons (½ scoop) unflavored Pristine Whey Protein Powder

FOR THE BABY SHAKE

1 oolong tea bag

¼ cup just off the boil water (plus more cold water)

½ teaspoon extra-virgin coconut oil

½ teaspoon Just Gelatin

1 tablespoon Baobab Boost Powder

1 doonk Sunflower Lecithin (optional, but preferred)

1 teaspoon Super Sweet Blend plus 1 tablespoon Gentle Sweet, or 2 teaspoons Super Sweet

½ teaspoon pure vanilla extract

3 pinches Mineral Salt

1 to 2 teaspoons Integral Collagen

About 1 cup ice

1 tablespoon unflavored Pristine Whey Protein Powder

SERENE CHATS: *Shake Down that scale while chuggin' a HA-UUUUGE shake that will remind you of cheesecake but contains no cream cheese. You're welcome, dairy-free Mamas! This shake does contain whey protein, but many (not all) dairy-free people can tolerate our Pristine Whey Protein isolate as it contains no lactose.*

Even if you can eat dairy with no issues, I want you to try this shake as it has fat-blitzing and blood sugar–controlling ingredients that shake up sluggish weight loss so you can shake down and celebrate success. Sure, enjoy Pearl's shakes that contain cream cheese, but don't stay in Pearl Land every day. Come over to Serene Land sometimes. Here I rarely use cream cheese, but visiting between us two sisters brings the best beautiful balance to your journey and ensures that you don't overdo certain foods. Oolong tea is one of the starring fat-blasting ingredients here. Just 1 cup of this tea helps your body burn off an extra 67 calories. I put 2 tea bags in this drink for double the slimming power! (If you are caffeine sensitive, feel free to go with just 1 tea bag.)

1. Place the tea bag(s) in a mug with the boiled water and brew for 5 minutes. Remove the tea bag(s) and squeeze to get all the goodness. Place the coconut oil in the warm tea to melt along with the gelatin and stir well. Place this mix in the blender and blend for a few seconds. Add cold water to reach the 1-cup line in the blender for a Biggie shake or the ½-cup line for a Baby shake.

2. Add all the other ingredients (except the ice and whey protein) and blend for another few seconds. Add the ice and blend again very well until all the ice is broken down. Add the whey and whip until a creamy Shake Down is born.

VARIATIONS

BERRY CHEESECAKE SHAKE DOWN: Add ½ cup favorite frozen berries.

PUMPKIN CHEESECAKE SHAKE DOWN: Add ½ cup canned pure pumpkin puree and ⅛ teaspoon pumpkin pie spice.

chocolate-covered cherry shake

E

SINGLE SERVE

FOR THE BIGGIE SHAKE

1 cup frozen pitted cherries

1½ to 2 tablespoons unsweetened cocoa powder

½ cup 1% cottage cheese

1 cup unsweetened cashew or almond milk

2 pinches Mineral Salt

1 tablespoon Super Sweet Blend*

¼ teaspoon Natural Burst cherry extract (optional)

1 teaspoon heavy cream (optional)

¼ to ½ teaspoon Gluccie*

Large handful of ice

2 tablespoons unflavored Pristine Whey Protein Powder* (see Note)

FOR THE BABY SHAKE

½ cup frozen pitted cherries

2 to 3 teaspoons unsweetened cocoa powder

¼ cup 1% cottage cheese

½ cup unsweetened cashew or almond milk

Pinch of Mineral Salt

1½ teaspoons Super Sweet Blend*

⅛ teaspoon Natural Burst cherry extract (optional)

½ teaspoon heavy cream (optional)

⅛ to ¼ teaspoon Gluccie*

Small handful of ice

1 tablespoon unflavored Pristine Whey Protein Powder* (see Note)

Cherries are a wonderful E fuel. They are packed with antioxidants, help with insomnia, fight inflammation, and powerfully wage war against belly fat. You can easily get them year-round in the frozen section of your grocery store.

1. Blend all the ingredients in a blender until completely smooth.

NOTE: You can use chocolate Pristine Whey Protein in this shake. If you do, pull back to 1 teaspoon sweetener and just 1 tablespoon unsweetened cocoa in the Biggie size, then taste at the end and adjust.

* FOR NSI: USE A GROCERY STORE ON-PLAN SWEETENER, SUB XANTHAN GUM FOR THE GLUCCIE, AND FIND AN ON-PLAN WHEY PROTEIN (SEE PAGE 43).

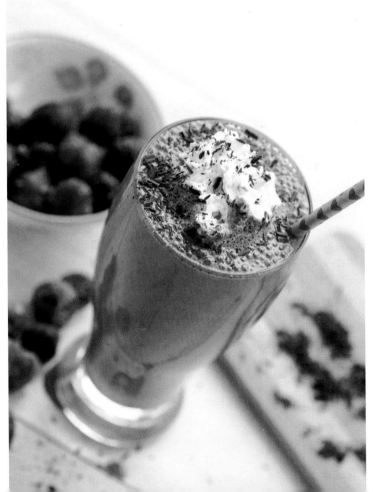

frisky

S OR E

SINGLE SERVE

FOR THE BIGGIE FRISKY

⅔ cup unsweetened cashew or
almond milk

2 tablespoons heavy cream,
or 1 heaping tablespoon peanut
butter (for S)

1 small or ½ large banana (for E)

2 generous tablespoons
unsweetened cocoa powder

4 pinches Mineral Salt

2½ teaspoons Super Sweet Blend
plus 2 to 3 teaspoons Gentle
Sweet* (this is the perfect combo
of sweeteners for people we've
tested these on, but you can try
your own sweetener combos)

½ teaspoon Gluccie*

½ teaspoon pure extract of choice

16 to 18 large ice cubes

4 tablespoons (1 scoop) unflavored
Pristine Whey Protein Powder*
(see Note)

FOR THE BABY FRISKY

⅓ cup unsweetened cashew or
almond milk

1 tablespoon heavy cream, or
½ tablespoon peanut butter (for S)

⅓ banana (for E)

1 tablespoon unsweetened cocoa
powder

2 pinches Mineral Salt

1¼ teaspoons Super Sweet Blend
plus 1 very rounded teaspoon
Gentle Sweet*

¼ teaspoon Gluccie*

¼ teaspoon pure extract of choice

8 to 10 large ice cubes

1 tablespoon unflavored Pristine
Whey Protein Powder* (see Note)

If you love a Wendy's Frosty, you are going to love this thick and creamy Frisky! As you shed the sugar bloat and gain energy, you may just start feeling a little more frisky in more ways than one! Oh yeah! We predict happy husbands galore! (If you want to read more on being a Foxy, Frisky Mama, go read chapter 34 in our original Trim Healthy Mama book. It just might change your life and marriage.)

It is best to use a powerful blender to get these smooth. Because friskies have less liquid, you really need to blend and blend, then blend some more until they are perfectly smooth and not icy. If you have to add another tablespoon or two of nut milk to help get it blended, you can do so. But don't give up . . . Friskies are worth it! They make a great ice cream replacement and the Baby size is a perfect dessert; or heck, indulge once in a while and even do the Biggie size for a huge dessert if that makes you happy. Feel free to add extracts to create awesome new flavors.

1. Put all the ingredients (except the ice and whey protein) in a blender and blend for 10 seconds. Add the ice and blend on high until completely smooth . . . no tiny bits of ice should be left, so keep on blending! Finally add the whey protein and blend for another 15 to 20 seconds.

NOTE: You can use chocolate Pristine Whey Protein in this shake. If you do, omit the sweetener and halve the cocoa amounts. Taste at the end to see if more sweetener is needed; it might be if you have a sweet tooth. Also feel free to add pressed peanut flour for a change-up.

* FOR NSI: USE A GROCERY STORE ON-PLAN SWEETENER AND WHEY PROTEIN (SEE PAGE 43) AND SUB XANTHAN GUM FOR THE GLUCCIE.

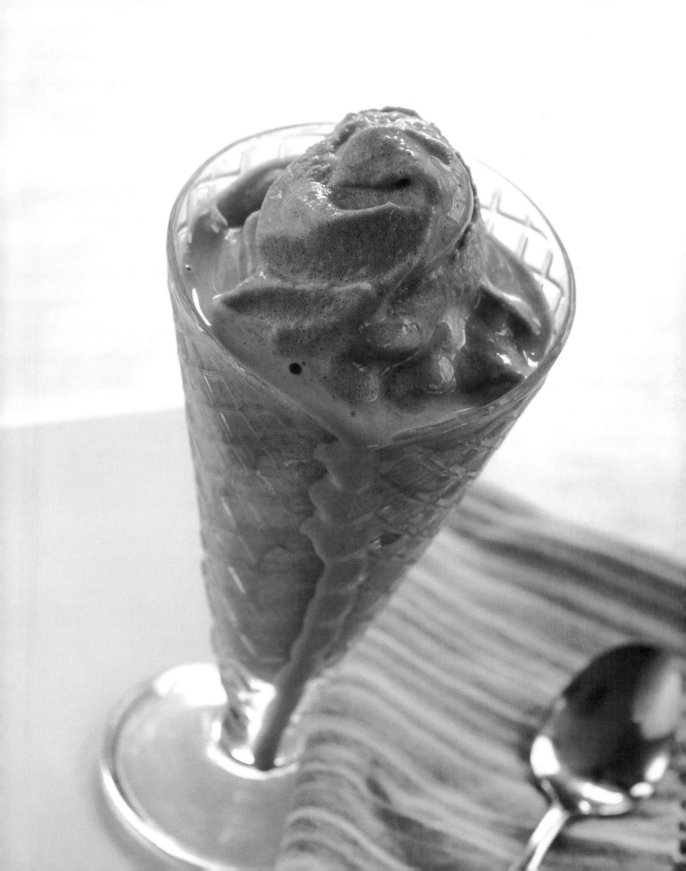

lemon-blueberry cheesecake shake

S

SINGLE SERVE

FOR THE BIGGIE SHAKE

⅓ cup frozen blueberries

½ cup 1% cottage cheese

½ cup unsweetened cashew or
  almond milk

⅓ cup water

Juice of 1 lemon (about
  2 tablespoons)

2 tablespoons (½ scoop) unflavored
  Pristine Whey Protein Powder*

1 tablespoon Super Sweet Blend*

1 very rounded tablespoon ⅓ less
  fat cream cheese

¼ to ½ teaspoon Gluccie*

1½ to 2 cups ice

FOR THE BABY SHAKE

2 heaping tablespoons frozen
  blueberries

¼ cup 1% cottage cheese

¼ cup unsweetened cashew or
  almond milk

2 to 3 tablespoons water

Juice of ½ lemon

1 tablespoon unflavored Pristine
  Whey Protein Powder*

1½ teaspoons Super Sweet Blend*

2 teaspoons ⅓ less fat cream
  cheese

⅛ to ¼ teaspoon Gluccie*

¾ to 1 cup ice

1. Place all the ingredients in a blender and blend until smooth.

* FOR NSI: USE GROCERY STORE ON-PLAN WHEY PROTEIN (SEE PAGE 43) AND
  SWEETENER. SUB XANTHAN GUM FOR THE GLUCCIE.

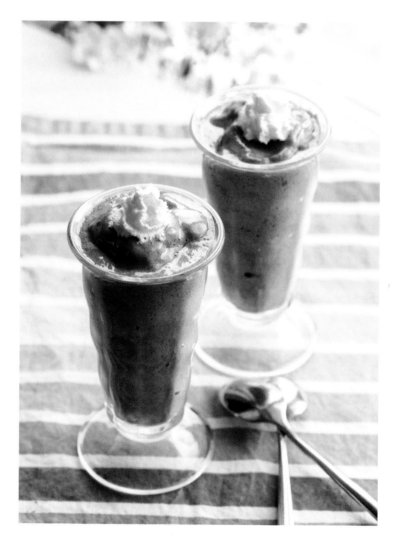

triple-berry power shake

S

SINGLE SERVE

FOR THE BIGGIE SHAKE

⅔ cup frozen berries (strawberries, raspberries, or mixed berries)

1 or 2 tablespoons frozen or fresh cranberries (optional)

⅓ cup 1% cottage cheese

3 tablespoons heavy cream

¼ to ½ teaspoon Gluccie*

1 cup unsweetened cashew or almond milk

2 to 3 tablespoons strawberry or unflavored Pristine Whey Protein Powder*

2 teaspoons Baobab Boost Powder (optional)

1 teaspoon Super Sweet Blend*

1½ to 2 cups ice

FOR THE BABY SHAKE

⅔ cup frozen berries (strawberries, raspberries, or mixed berries)

2 to 3 teaspoons frozen or fresh cranberries (optional)

3 tablespoons 1% cottage cheese

1½ tablespoons heavy cream

⅛ to ¼ teaspoon Gluccie*

½ cup unsweetened cashew or almond milk

1 to 2 tablespoons strawberry or unflavored Pristine Whey Protein Powder*

1 teaspoon Baobab Boost Powder (optional)

½ teaspoon Super Sweet Blend*

¾ to 1 cup ice

This is a lovely creamy shake that uses frozen berries, our strawberry whey protein powder (if you have it), and optional cranberries along with Baobab Boost Powder (read about that on page 42) for a triple-berry, powerful vitamin C hit. If you don't have strawberry whey protein or baobab powder, no worries, just use regular whey protein and leave out the baobab, and it will still be a really yummy berry shake. Just be sure to double the sweetener amounts.

1. Place all the ingredients in a blender and blend until smooth.

* FOR NSI: USE A GROCERY STORE ON-PLAN WHEY PROTEIN (SEE PAGE 43) AND SWEETENER, AND SUB XANTHAN GUM FOR THE GLUCCIE.

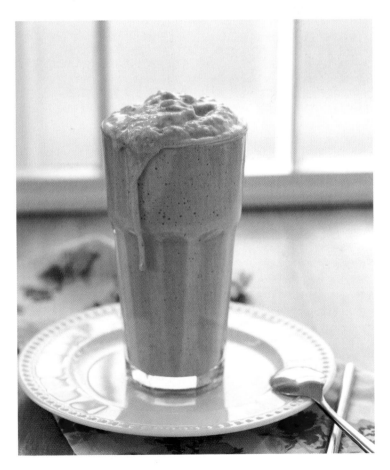

chai chaga smoothie

SINGLE SERVE

FOR THE BIGGIE SMOOTHIE

1 cup cold water or unsweetened nut milk

½ teaspoon chaga extract (I use VitaJing Herbs brand)

½ teaspoon pure vanilla extract

2 teaspoons Super Sweet Blend

4 pinches Mineral Salt

¼ teaspoon ground cinnamon

3 black peppercorns, or a small sprinkle ground black pepper (optional)

1½ tablespoons (1 scoop) Integral Collagen

⅛ teaspoon Sunflower Lecithin (optional)

1 teaspoon MCT oil or extra-virgin coconut oil

Rounded ¼ teaspoon Gluccie

1½ to 2 cups ice

2 tablespoons (½ scoop) unflavored Pristine Whey Protein Powder

FOR THE BABY SMOOTHIE

½ cup cold water or unsweetened nut milk

¼ teaspoon chaga extract (I use VitaJing Herbs brand)

¼ teaspoon pure vanilla extract

1 teaspoon Super Sweet Blend

2 pinches Mineral Salt

⅛ teaspoon ground cinnamon

1 to 2 black peppercorns, or a little ground black pepper (optional)

2 teaspoons Integral Collagen

2 doonks Sunfower Lecithin (optional)

½ teaspoon MCT or extra-virgin coconut oil

Generous ⅛ teaspoon Gluccie

¾ cup ice

1 tablespoon unflavored Pristine Whey Protein Powder

SERENE CHATS: *I know not all of you will have chaga extract lying around, so enjoy all the other shake and smoothie recipes in this chapter and just skip this one if you don't want to purchase it online. But for those interested in a superboosted immune system, join me and indulge in a smoothie with the deep earthy flavor of chaga—a mushroom from the birch tree forests in the Sayan Mountains of Siberia—that has been traditionally enjoyed for thousands of years. Chaga is king of medicinal mushrooms. It boosts energy while easing mild tension. It promotes detoxification and supports healthy digestion. It powerfully bolsters the immune system and strengthens respiratory health. It balances blood sugar levels and helps curb the desire to constantly snack.*

1. Put all the ingredients (except the ice and whey) in a blender and blend until smooth. Add the ice and blend again. Add the whey and blend to creamy whipped chai-flavored perfection.

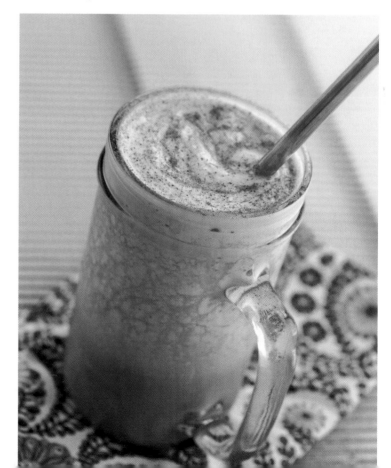

whipped piña colada shake

(E)

SINGLE SERVE

FOR THE BIGGIE SHAKE

1 teaspoon extra-virgin coconut oil

½ cup unsweetened cashew or
almond milk

½ cup water

¾ cup frozen pineapple pieces

2 tablespoons plain 0% Greek yogurt
or 1% cottage cheese (optional)

½ teaspoon Natural Burst pineapple
extract*

½ teaspoon Natural Burst coconut
extract (optional, for a piña colada
effect)*

1½ tablespoons (1 scoop) Integral
Collagen (optional)

1½ to 2 teaspoons Super Sweet
Blend*

Generous ¼ teaspoon Gluccie*

3 pinches Mineral Salt

1 to 1½ cups ice

2 tablespoons (½ scoop) unflavored
Pristine Whey Protein Powder*
(or 4 tablespoons if you omit the
collagen)

FOR THE BABY SHAKE

½ teaspoon extra-virgin coconut oil

¼ cup unsweetened cashew or
almond milk

¼ cup water

Generous ⅓ cup frozen pineapple
pieces

1 rounded tablespoon plain
0% Greek yogurt or 1% cottage
cheese (optional)

¼ teaspoon Natural Burst pineapple
extract

¼ teaspoon Natural Burst coconut
extract (optional, for a piña colada
effect)*

2 teaspoons Integral Collagen
(optional)

¾ to 1 teaspoon Super Sweet Blend*

Generous ⅛ teaspoon Gluccie*

1 to 2 pinches Mineral Salt

½ to ¾ cup ice

1 tablespoon unflavored Pristine Whey
Protein Powder* (or 2 tablespoons if
you omit the collagen)

You'll feel like you are on a tropical island while sipping this
delightfulness. If you don't have coconut extract, don't worry
about it. This is still a great pineapple drink.

1. Add all the ingredients (except the ice and whey protein)
   to a blender and blend well. Add the ice and blend until
   smooth. Add the whey and blend for 10 seconds more.

* FOR NSI: USE GROCERY STORE ON-PLAN SWEETENER AND EXTRACTS, SUB XANTHAN
GUM FOR THE GLUCCIE, AND FIND AN ON-PLAN WHEY PROTEIN (SEE PAGE 43).

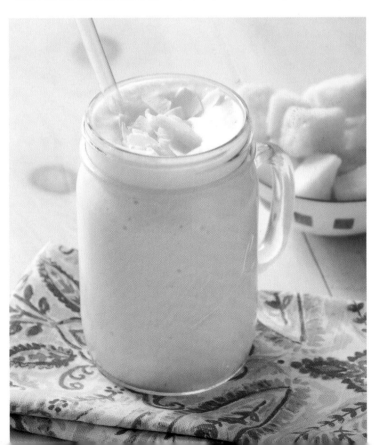

SECRET SHAKES

PEARL CHATS: Serene had this crazy idea to put okra in smoothies in the *Trim Healthy Mama Cookbook*. She called them Secret Big Boy Smoothies. Who would be nuts enough to ever make them, I wondered. It's one thing to disguise okra in soups, but in a shake? I'd never tasted one and the whole idea of the word "okra" combined with the word "smoothie" sounded Skeeery! But she insisted we put them in the book and kept yelling in her Serene voice, "Okra heals your gut and has incredible slimming powers. And my shakes are big and yummy. Ladies will love them!!!!!"

I thought I was right at first, because after the cookbook came out it was like crickets chirping when it came to feedback on those recipes . . . a bunch of silence. I assumed people were being polite. You know . . . if you can't say something nice, don't say anything at all. But then some of our bravest Trim Healthy Mamas announced they'd summoned the nerve to try them and that they were delicious. Soon they started posting pictures all over Facebook of their creamy okra smoothies. Next thing you know we were hearing about how these drinks were helping Mamas out of weight loss stalls and causing stubborn weight to finally melt! More and more people got brave enough to try, and suddenly blenders everywhere were whizzing okra every morning. Okra challenges were born! Mamas challenged each other to have an okra shake every day. Now, nobody blinks when okra smoothies are mentioned. It's the new THM normal.

So . . . I guess Serene proved me wrong and I, too, am now one of those crazy women who puts okra in her shakes. The key is you gotta blend the heck out of the okra so there is not one speck left showing its green self. Once it is completely creamified, you know your shake is going to rock your taste buds and roll your pounds off!

The following five recipes are all new, and all feature okra.

mocha secret big boy

FP

SINGLE SERVE

FOR THE BIGGIE SMOOTHIE

1 cup brewed coffee, cooled

1 cup frozen diced okra (you can start out with just ¾ cup to get used to it)

2 tablespoons unsweetened cocoa powder

1 teaspoon extra-virgin coconut oil, or 1 to 2 teaspoons MCT oil

½ teaspoon pure vanilla extract or coffee extract

3 generous pinches Mineral Salt

1 tablespoon Super Sweet Blend*

1½ tablespoons (1 scoop) Integral Collagen (optional)

¼ teaspoon Sunflower Lecithin (optional)

12 to 16 large ice cubes

2 tablespoons (½ scoop) unflavored Pristine Whey Protein Powder* (or 4 tablespoons if omitting the collagen)

FOR THE BABY SMOOTHIE

½ cup brewed coffee, cooled

½ cup frozen diced okra

1 tablespoon unsweetened cocoa powder

½ teaspoon extra-virgin coconut oil, or 1 teaspoon MCT oil

¼ teaspoon pure vanilla extract or coffee extract

1 to 2 generous pinches Mineral Salt

1½ teaspoons Super Sweet Blend*

2 teaspoons Integral Collagen (optional)

⅛ teaspoon Sunflower Lecithin (optional)

6 to 8 large ice cubes

1 tablespoon unflavored Pristine Whey Protein Powder* (or 2 tablespoons if omitting the collagen)

This is modeled after the original Secret Big Boy, which was an FP and has the most slimming power if you are trying to push through a stall. This new version uses coffee for the perfect all-in-one pick-me-up breakfast, lunch, or afternoon snack.

1. Place all the ingredients (except the ice and whey protein) in a blender and blend until very smooth. You want all the okra completely broken down first, so blend like a blending fool! Add the ice and blend well again. You may have to stop the blender and stir a couple times or add the ice slowly until it is broken down. Add the whey and blend for 10 to 20 seconds more. Taste and adjust the flavors if needed to "own it!"

NOTE: You can use chocolate Pristine Whey Protein in this shake in place of unflavored. If you do, omit the sweetener and only use half the cocoa. Taste at the end to see if more sweetener is needed or not.

* FOR NSI: USE A GROCERY STORE ON-PLAN SWEETENER AND WHEY PROTEIN (SEE PAGE 43).

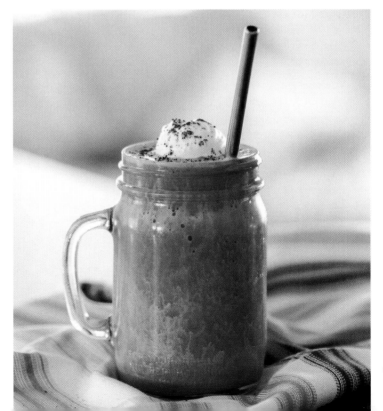

gingerbread secret big boy ⒻⓅ

SINGLE SERVE

FOR THE BIGGIE SMOOTHIE
1 or 2 rooibos tea bags
½ cup just off the boil water
1 cup cold water
1 cup frozen diced okra
1 teaspoon MCT oil or extra-virgin coconut oil
½ teaspoon pure vanilla extract
3 generous pinches Mineral Salt
3½ teaspoons Super Sweet Blend*
¼ teaspoon ground ginger
½ teaspoon ground cinnamon
¼ teaspoon ground allspice
⅛ teaspoon ground nutmeg
⅛ teaspoon blackstrap molasses (optional)
1½ tablespoons (1 scoop) Integral Collagen (optional)
¼ teaspoon Sunflower Lecithin (optional)
12 to 16 large ice cubes
2 tablespoons (½ scoop) unflavored Pristine Whey Protein Powder* (or 4 tablespoons if omitting the collagen)

OPTIONAL TOPPING
1 tablespoon THM Baking Blend
¼ teaspoon ground cinnamon
¾ teaspoon Super Sweet Blend*
½ teaspoon butter

FOR THE BABY SMOOTHIE
1 rooibos tea bag
¼ cup just off the boil water
½ cup cold water
½ cup frozen diced okra
½ teaspoon MCT oil or extra-virgin coconut oil
¼ teaspoon pure vanilla extract
1 to 2 pinches Mineral Salt

1 to 2 teaspoons Super Sweet Blend*
⅛ teaspoon ground ginger
¼ teaspoon ground cinnamon
⅛ teaspoon ground allspice
2 doonks grated nutmeg
2 doonks blackstrap molasses (optional)
2 teaspoons Integral Collagen (optional)
⅛ teaspoon Sunflower Lecithin
6 to 8 large ice cubes
1 tablespoon unflavored Pristine Whey Protein Powder*
Optional topping (halved) listed for Biggie smoothie

Another new Secret Big Boy for you, caffeine-free and with all the warming spices of gingerbread!

1. Brew the tea bag(s) in the boiled water for 5 minutes, then discard them. Add the tea to a blender along with all the other ingredients (except the ice cubes and whey protein) and blend until very smooth. You want all the okra completely broken down first, so blend like a maniac! Add the ice and blend well again. You may have to stop the blender and stir a couple times or add the ice slowly until it is broken down. Add the whey and blend for 10 to 20 seconds more. Taste and adjust the flavors if needed to "own it!"

2. Make the optional topping. Squish up all the topping ingredients into crumbles and top the smoothie.

* FOR NSI: USE A GROCERY STORE ON-PLAN SWEETENER AND WHEY PROTEIN (SEE PAGE 43).

milk chocolate truffle secret shake

S

SINGLE SERVE

FOR THE BIGGIE SHAKE

¾ to 1 cup frozen diced okra

1 cup unsweetened cashew or
    almond milk

1 tablespoon unsweetened cocoa
    powder

1 tablespoon Super Sweet Blend*
    (or 2 tablespoons or so of Gentle
    Sweet, which tastes amazing for
    newbies)

¼ cup 1% cottage cheese

2 tablespoons heavy cream

3 pinches Mineral Salt

¼ teaspoon Gluccie*

1½ to 2 cups ice

3 tablespoons unflavored Pristine
    Whey Protein Powder*

FOR THE BABY SHAKE

⅓ cup frozen diced okra

½ cup unsweetened cashew or
    almond milk

1½ teaspoons unsweetened cocoa
    powder

1½ teaspoons Super Sweet Blend*
    (or 1 tablespoon Gentle Sweet)

2 tablespoons 1% cottage cheese

1 tablespoon heavy cream

1 to 2 pinches Mineral Salt

⅛ teaspoon Gluccie*

¾ to 1 cup ice

1 tablespoon unflavored Pristine
    Whey Protein Powder*

Tastes like the creamy inside of a chocolate truffle . . . mmmm.

1. Put the okra and nut milk in a blender and blend until smooth. We mean blend like a mighty warrior until not one speck of okra is left floating! Add all the other ingredients (except the ice and whey protein) and blend again. Add the ice and blend until smooth. Add the whey and blend until whippy.

NOTE: You can use chocolate Pristine Whey Protein Powder in place of unflavored. If you do, omit the sweetener and cocoa, but taste at the end as you may need just a little sweetener to taste.

* FOR NSI: USE A GROCERY STORE ON-PLAN SWEETENER AND SUB XANTHAN GUM FOR THE GLUCCIE. FIND AN ON-PLAN WHEY PROTEIN (SEE PAGE 43).

peanutty, chocolaty, banana-y secret shake   Ⓔ

SINGLE SERVE

FOR THE BIGGIE SHAKE

1 cup unsweetened almond or cashew milk

¾ cup frozen diced okra

1 small or ½ large banana

2 tablespoons Pressed Peanut Flour*

1½ tablespoons unsweetened cocoa powder

½ teaspoon Natural Burst banana extract*

1 tablespoon Super Sweet Blend*

3 to 4 generous pinches Mineral Salt

¾ teaspoon sugar-free natural-style peanut butter

¼ teaspoon Gluccie*

1 generous cup ice

3 tablespoons unflavored Pristine Whey Protein Powder*

FOR THE BABY SHAKE

½ cup unsweetened almond or cashew milk

¼ to ⅓ cup frozen diced okra

¼ to ½ large banana

1 tablespoon Pressed Peanut Flour*

2 teaspoons unsweetened cocoa powder

¼ teaspoon Natural Burst banana extract*

1½ teaspoons Super Sweet Blend*

1 to 2 pinches Mineral Salt

½ teaspoon sugar-free natural-style peanut butter

⅛ teaspoon Gluccie*

½ cup ice

1 tablespoon unflavored Pristine Whey Protein Powder*

This shake is so smooth and silky, it is hard to believe it is an E and doesn't contain a bunch of fat. It is a great way to get healthy carbs into your life to keep your metabolism revving.

1. Put the nut milk and okra in a blender and blend until perfectly smooth with no green floating okra business to be seen. Add all the other ingredients (except the ice and whey protein) and blend again. Add the ice and blend until smooth. Add the whey and blend until whipped.

NOTE: You can use chocolate Pristine Whey Protein Powder. If you do, omit the sweetener and pull the cocoa back to 2 teaspoons for the Biggie size. Taste at the end, as you may need a little sweetener depending on your sweet tooth.

* FOR NSI: USE A GROCERY STORE SUGAR-FREE DEFATTED PEANUT FLOUR, EXTRACT, AND ON-PLAN SWEETENER. SUB XANTHAN GUM FOR THE GLUCCIE. FIND AN ON-PLAN WHEY PROTEIN (SEE PAGE 43).

tropical secret smoothie

E

SINGLE SERVE

FOR THE BIGGIE SMOOTHIE

1 cup unsweetened cashew or
   almond milk

⅓ cup frozen diced okra

¾ cup frozen mango chunks

1 tablespoon Super Sweet Blend*

½ teaspoon Natural Burst coconut
   extract or pure vanilla extract

3 pinches Mineral Salt

¼ teaspoon Gluccie*

10 ice cubes

4 tablespoons (1 scoop) unflavored
   Pristine Whey Protein Powder*

FOR THE BABY SMOOTHIE

½ cup unsweetened cashew or
   almond milk

3 tablespoons frozen diced okra

⅓ cup frozen mango chunks

1½ teaspoons Super Sweet Blend*

¼ teaspoon Natural Burst coconut
   extract or pure vanilla extract

1 to 2 pinches Mineral Salt

⅛ teaspoon Gluccie*

5 ice cubes

1 tablespoon unflavored Pristine
   Whey Protein Powder*

1. Put the nut milk and okra in a blender and blend with utmost vigor until perfectly smooth. Add all the other ingredients (except for the ice and whey protein) and blend again until the mango is smooth. Add the ice and blend until it is broken down. Add the whey and blend again for 10 to 20 seconds.

* FOR NSI: USE A GROCERY STORE ON-PLAN SWEETENER AND SUB XANTHAN GUM FOR THE GLUCCIE. FIND AN ON-PLAN WHEY PROTEIN (SEE PAGE 43).

GUT-HEALING SHAKES AND SMOOTHIES

The following five shakes are all designed with unique ingredients to help soothe inflamed guts and settle painful digestive issues. You won't find Gluccie or xanthan gum thickening these shakes as those can sometimes be a little harsh for troublesome tummies. Gelatin does a beautiful job of thickening while healing your gut lining at the same time. If your tummy doesn't do well using whey protein, you can sub with a mix of egg white protein mixed with collagen and still get a reasonably creamy result. Many of these recipes call for kefir, which is a wonderful addition for problematic tummies, as it adds "good bugs" to your gut. You can use store-bought kefir or Serene's recipe for kefir on page 459. If you don't have kefir or need to be dairy-free, just use unsweetened cashew or almond milk or water.

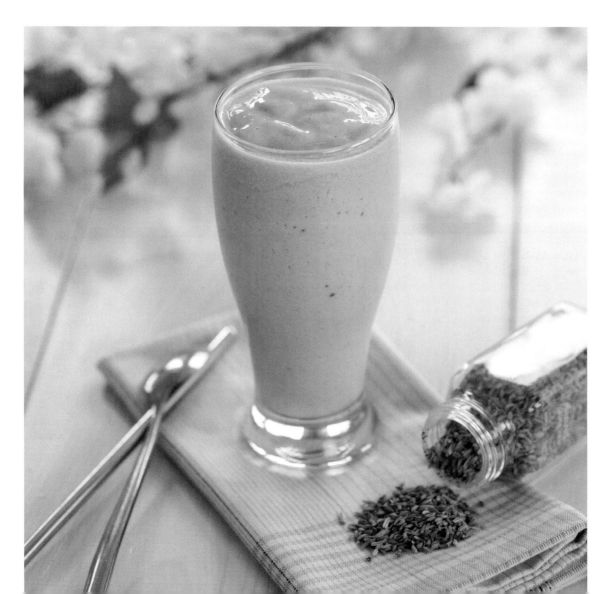

fennel 'n' figs feel better shake   Ⓔ

SINGLE SERVE

FOR THE BIGGIE SHAKE

4 dried figs, rinsed well

½ cup water, for soaking figs

1½ teaspoons Just Gelatin

½ cup just off the boil water

2 teaspoons fennel seeds, or
  2 fennel tea bags

1 teaspoon MCT oil or extra-virgin
  coconut oil

½ cup plain low-fat kefir,
  unsweetened cashew or almond
  milk, or cold water

⅛ teaspoon Sunflower Lecithin
  (optional)

1½ tablespoons (1 scoop) Integral
  Collagen

4 pinches Mineral Salt

½ teaspoon pure vanilla extract

2 to 3 doonks Pure Stevia Extract
  Powder

2 cups ice

2 tablespoons (½ scoop) unflavored
  Pristine Whey Protein Powder

FOR THE BABY SHAKE

2 dried figs, rinsed well

¼ cup water, for soaking figs

¾ teaspoon Just Gelatin

¼ cup just off the boil water

1 teaspoon fennel seeds, or 1 fennel
  tea bag

½ teaspoon MCT oil or extra-virgin
  coconut oil

¼ cup plain low-fat kefir or cold
  water

2 doonks Sunflower Lecithin
  (optional)

2 rounded teaspoons (½ scoop)
  Integral Collagen

2 pinches Mineral Salt

¼ teaspoon pure vanilla extract

1 to 2 doonks Pure Stevia Extract
  Powder

½ to 1 cup ice

1 tablespoon unflavored Pristine
  Whey Protein Powder

Tastes like a Fig Newton but oh so healthy for you! Fennel and figs are two known digestive aids and together perform like a dynamite duo. Hmmm . . . maybe the word "dynamite" doesn't work well when we are talking digestion and thinking daisy fresh underwear, so let's change that to "delicate duo," shall we? Fresh figs are a lovely E fruit but are hard to find year-round and are expensive, and the dried fruit is seldom eaten on the THM plan. What to do, what to do? No worries, if you soak dried figs overnight and let them reabsorb their water content, they work beautifully in this E smoothie. The soaking releases some of the fruit sugars from the figs into the water so they are easier on your blood sugar. The flavor combination of figs and fennel is something you must try . . . amazing!

1. Soak the figs in the ½ cup water overnight (or for several hours).

2. Once you're ready to make your shake, stir the gelatin into the boiled water. Add the fennel seeds (or tea bags) and steep for 5 to 10 minutes. Strain through a fine-mesh sieve into a bowl and stir in the oil.

3. Drain the figs, discard the water, and place the figs in a blender. Add the fennel tea, kefir, lecithin (if using), collagen, salt, vanilla, and stevia. Blend until the figs are completely smooth. Add the ice and blend again. Add the whey and blend to perfection. Taste and adjust the flavors to "own" your figginess.

minty tummy-soother shake

SINGLE SERVE

FOR THE BIGGIE SHAKE

1½ teaspoons Just Gelatin

½ cup just off the boil water

2 mint tea bags

1 teaspoon MCT oil or extra-virgin coconut oil

½ cup plain kefir (see Note)

½ cup frozen diced okra

Small handful of fresh spinach or 1 tablespoon frozen

⅛ teaspoon Sunflower Lecithin

1½ tablespoons (1 scoop) Integral Collagen

3 pinches Mineral Salt

2 teaspoons Super Sweet Blend, or more to taste

¼ to ½ teaspoon pure mint extract (optional)

1 to 1½ cups ice

2 tablespoons (½ scoop) unflavored Pristine Whey Protein Powder

FOR THE BABY SHAKE

¾ teaspoon Just Gelatin

¼ cup just off the boil water

1 mint tea bag

½ teaspoon MCT oil or extra-virgin coconut oil

¼ cup plain kefir (see Note)

¼ cup frozen diced okra

A few fresh spinach leaves

2 doonks Sunflower Lecithin

2 teaspoons Integral Collagen

1 to 2 pinches Mineral Salt

1 teaspoon Super Sweet Blend, or more to taste

⅛ to ¼ teaspoon pure mint extract (optional)

½ to ¾ cup ice

1 tablespoon unflavored Pristine Whey Protein Powder

When your tummy is all in knots you need to give it a minty hug. Mint calms and soothes an agitated gut. But hey . . . even if your gut feels fine, this tastes delish and has great slimming powers. (While this recipe does have okra, it wants to hang out here in the Gut-Healing section.)

1. Put the gelatin in the boiled water and stir until dissolved. Add the tea bag(s) and brew for about 5 minutes. Remove the tea bag(s), squeezing them, then add the oil.

2. Pour the tea mixture into a blender. Add the kefir, okra, spinach, lecithin, collagen, salt, sweetener, and mint extract (if using). Blend like a superhero so all the okra and spinach are totally smooth. Add the ice and blend again until it is broken down. Add the whey and whip it all until smooth. Taste and adjust the flavors to "own it."

NOTE: Low- or nonfat kefir will keep this smoothie in FP mode because only ½ cup is used (in full cup amounts, we consider store-bought, nonfat kefir E). Consider your smoothie an S if you use full-fat kefir (yummy). If you don't have kefir or are dairy-free, use water or unsweetened nut milk.

* FOR DF: OMIT WHEY PROTEIN AND SUB WITH EGG WHITE OR PEA PROTEIN. OMIT KEFIR; SEE NOTE ABOVE ON WHAT TO SUB FOR KEFIR.

chamomile cuddle shake

(E)

SINGLE SERVE

FOR THE BIGGIE SHAKE

2 chamomile tea bags
½ cup just off the boil water
1½ teaspoons Just Gelatin
1 teaspoon MCT oil or extra-virgin coconut oil
½ cup plain low-fat kefir, unsweetened cashew or almond milk, or cold water
½ large banana or 1 small banana, (frozen banana makes an even creamier smoothie)
⅛ teaspoon Sunflower Lecithin (optional)
1½ tablespoons (1 scoop) Integral Collagen
3 to 4 pinches Mineral Salt
½ teaspoon pure vanilla extract
¼ teaspoon Natural Burst banana extract (optional)
2 to 3 doonks Pure Stevia Extract Powder, or more to taste
2 cups ice
2 tablespoons (½ scoop) unflavored Pristine Whey Protein Powder

FOR THE BABY SHAKE

1 chamomile tea bag
¼ cup just off the boil water
¾ teaspoon Just Gelatin
½ teaspoon MCT oil or extra-virgin coconut oil
¼ cup plain low-fat kefir, unsweetened cashew or almond milk, or cold water
⅓ large banana
2 doonks Sunflower Lecithin (optional)
2 rounded teaspoons (½ scoop) Integral Collagen

2 pinches Mineral Salt
¼ teaspoon pure vanilla extract
⅛ teaspoon Natural Burst banana extract (optional)
1 to 2 doonks Pure Stevia Extract Powder, or more to taste
1 cup ice
1 tablespoon unflavored Pristine Whey Protein Powder

Remember Peter Rabbit? He had to have a dose of chamomile tea for his aching tummy. Chamomile's famous folklore medicine is no fairy tale. The oils derived from chamomile's daisy-like flowers quiet muscle spasms and soothe inflamed mucous membranes in the gut. Chamomile is also a powerful infection fighter and helps fight all hosts of cancers, especially thyroid cancer. Bananas are also on the simple list of home remedies for easing digestive complaints. Their pectin helps with bowel troubles and their potassium helps balance electrolytes. Be sure your banana is ripe, otherwise the unripened starches can bother a troubled tummy.

1. Brew the tea in the boiled water for about 5 minutes. Remove the tea bag(s) and stir in the gelatin. Add the oil. Pour this into a blender and add all the other ingredients (except the ice and whey protein) and blend until smooth. Add the ice and blend again. Add the whey and whip into a yummy tummy cuddle.

bloat be gone smoothie

FP

SINGLE SERVE

FOR THE BIGGIE SMOOTHIE

2- to 4-inch piece fresh ginger (depending upon how much moonshine-type kick you can handle, but we love using the whole 4 inches)

½ cup cool water

½ cup plain low-fat kefir* (best not to use full fat here due to inclusion of apple) or unsweetened cashew or almond milk

1 medium cucumber, peeled and chopped into chunks

½ small green apple or ¼ large green apple, chopped into chunks

1 teaspoon MCT oil

⅛ teaspoon Sunflower Lecithin

1½ tablespoons (1 scoop) Integral Collagen

2 pinches Mineral Salt

3 doonks Pure Stevia Extract Powder

1 tablespoon Baobab Boost Powder (optional)

Juice of ½ lemon

2 cups ice

1 generous teaspoon Just Gelatin

1 tablespoon cool water, for the gelatin

1 tablespoon just off the boil water, for the gelatin

FOR THE BABY SMOOTHIE

1- to 2-inch piece fresh ginger

¼ cup cool water

¼ cup plain low-fat kefir* or unsweetened nut milk

½ medium cucumber, peeled and chopped into chunks

¼ small green apple, chopped

½ teaspoon MCT oil

2 doonks Sunflower Lecithin

This recipe is designed to nuke . . . we mean "cuke" your bloated tummy troubles away. Wake up and have the Biggie smoothie as your breakfast. It is filling and delicious in a feisty, yet creamy sort of way. This is the one smoothie in this chapter that *must* be consumed alone. Don't eat other foods with it. It is medicine for your body, so allow it to work its healing. You don't have to chug it down . . . sip on it if you like, then after a couple hours, if you can't finish it, leave some for a later snack. If you feel like you need another full shake for lunch for more intense cleansing, go ahead and do a half-day cleanse. Have a regular afternoon snack and dinner, as you don't need to do this longer than a half day.

Cucumbers are alkaline, hydrating, and full of cleansing fiber. They contain multiple B vitamins that ease the stress we too easily wear all over our bodies, especially in our tummies. Ginger is the king of anti-inflammatories and it helps pop those gas bubbles that swirl and churn and make you feel like a bloated goat. Apples and baobab are full of pectin, which helps get the peristaltic action of your digestive system moving along. When there is a traffic jam in the ol' colon we need a little pectin to clear the road (or should we say . . . the load).

1. Choose your level of ginger boldness (don't be afraid, go for it!) and blend it with the cool water in a blender on low for about 30 seconds—not on high or the fiber will become so much a part of the liquid that you cannot strain it out. (If making the Baby size of this drink you will have to blend the ginger with both the kefir and water, otherwise your blender won't have enough liquid to blend.)

2. Strain the liquid through a fine-mesh sieve into a small bowl. Grab the strained ginger pulp and give it a squeeze into the bowl to harvest all the medicinal goodness.

3. Rinse the blender and place the strained ginger juice into it along with the kefir, cucumber, apple, MCT oil, lecithin, collagen, salt, stevia, baobab powder (if using), lemon juice, and ice. Blend until perfectly smooth.

4. Combine the gelatin and cool water in a mug and stir to dissolve. Add the boiled water and stir again. Add to the blender and blend again until whipped.

2 rounded teaspoons (½ scoop)
  Integral Collagen

Pinch of Mineral Salt

1 or 2 doonks Pure Stevia Extract
  Powder

½ tablespoon Baobab Boost
  Powder (optional)

Squeeze of fresh lemon

1 cup ice

½ teaspoon Just Gelatin

2 teaspoons cool water, for the
  gelatin

1 tablespoon just off the boil water,
  for the gelatin

NOTE: You'll notice this recipe does not include whey protein. A few rare people tend to bloat with whey protein and this smoothie is anti-bloat, so let's leave it out this time. You get some protein with the kefir and gelatin, but it is okay to sometimes have meals with a little less protein. This is designed to be a cleansing smoothie rather than a building smoothie.

LAST NOTE: Since this is an FP smoothie, you are not using a full apple. Give the rest of the apple pieces to the children or put them in a baggie with lemon juice for later.

* FOR DF: USE NUT MILK OR WATER.

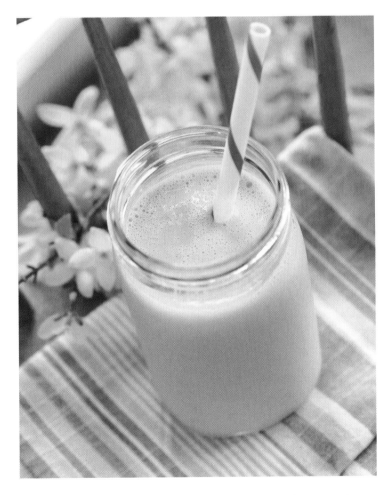

cobbler calmer shake

FOR THE BIGGIE SHAKE

1½ teaspoons Just Gelatin

½ cup just off the boil water

2 chamomile tea bags

2 tablespoons old-fashioned rolled oats

1 teaspoon MCT oil or extra-virgin coconut oil

½ cup plain low-fat kefir, unsweetened cashew or almond milk, or cold water

⅛ teaspoon Sunflower Lecithin (optional)

1½ tablespoons (1 scoop) Integral Collagen

3 pinches Mineral Salt

2 teaspoons Super Sweet Blend, or more to taste

1 teaspoon pure vanilla extract

Generous ¼ teaspoon ground cinnamon or apple pie spice

1 small apple, coarsely cut

1 tablespoon Baobab Boost Powder (optional)

1½ to 2 cups ice

2 tablespoons (½ scoop) unflavored Pristine Whey Protein Powder

FOR THE BABY SHAKE

¾ teaspoon Just Gelatin

¼ cup just off the boil water

1 chamomile tea bag

1 tablespoon old-fashioned rolled oats

½ teaspoon MCT oil or extra-virgin coconut oil

¼ cup plain low-fat kefir, unsweetened almond or cashew milk, or cold water

2 doonks Sunflower Lecithin (optional)

2 rounded teaspoons (½ scoop) Integral Collagen

1 to 2 pinches Mineral Salt

1 teaspoon Super Sweet Blend, or more to taste

½ teaspoon pure vanilla extract

Generous ⅛ teaspoon ground cinnamon or apple pie spice

½ small apple, coarsely cut

1½ teaspoons Baobab Boost Powder (optional)

1 cup ice

1 tablespoon unflavored Pristine Whey Protein Powder

Get all the scrumptiousness of an apple cobbler in a creamy, tummy-calming shake. Once again chamomile stars in the show here to soothe tummy woes and build up your immune system. If you are not a hot tea person, shakes are the new way to get your chamomile in! Let every sip fill your energy bank, calm your tummy, heal your body, and satisfy your love of apple-icious desserts.

1. Stir the gelatin into the boiled water until dissolved. Add the tea bag(s) and oats and brew for about 5 minutes so the oats can soften. Remove the tea bag(s), squeezing them, and stir in the oil.

2. Pour into a blender and add the rest of the ingredients (except the ice and and whey protein) and blend until smooth. Add the ice and blend again. Add the whey, blend again, and enjoy the apple-iciousness.

QUICKIE KEFIR SMOOTHIES

You got twenty seconds? You got a meal! The following two recipes are delicious filling drinks with plenty of protein to be a quick run-out-the-door meal for breakfast (or perhaps a light lunch). Kefir floods your gut with healthy probiotics and nourishes your body in countless ways. There is an option to use either 1 or 2 cups kefir here. If you choose to use just 1 cup kefir, that leaves you room for adding more food to your meal if you feel you need it. If choosing to use 2 cups kefir, you have plenty of fuel in your meal so no need to add more food. Each option gives a different smoothie result, so find your own favorite.

NOTE: *The Quickie Kefir Smoothies will be E, FP, or S, depending on what kefir you choose.* Store-bought kefir should always be low-fat as it still contains some carbs, so if using store-bought kefir, your smoothie will be a light E. Homemade kefir using the double-fermented recipe from page 459 will be FP if using fat-free milk and S if using whole milk.

chocolate quickie kefir smoothie   **E**, **FP**, OR **S**

SINGLE SERVE

Option 1: 2 cups plain kefir, store-bought or homemade double-fermented (page 459)
Option 2: 1 cup plain kefir plus 1 cup ice
1 scoop chocolate Pristine Whey Protein Powder

OPTIONAL ADD-IN
½ teaspoon maca powder, such as Sunfood Maca Extreme

This chocolate probiotic smoothie is chock-full of all those good bugs you want your tummy to catch. Once again, this is an incredible smoothie just with kefir and whey protein; adding maca is up to you.

1. Blend everything until smooth. Don't whizz and whizz if using the no-ice option, just blend for about 10 seconds.

strawberry quickie kefir smoothie

E, FP, OR S

SINGLE SERVE

Option 1: 2 cups plain kefir,
store-bought or homemade
double-fermented (page 459)

Option 2: 1 cup plain kefir plus
1 cup ice

1 scoop strawberry Pristine Whey
Protein Powder

OPTIONAL ADD-ONS

Juice of ½ lemon (store-bought
kefir isn't very zingy so this gives
a tart burst)

1 tablespoon Baobab Boost Powder

½ teaspoon maca powder, such as
Sunfood Maca Extreme

SERENE CHATS: *If you love strawberries and creamy drinks are your "thang," then this recipe will become your fast favorite for an insanely quick breakfast or lunch on the go. Really, you only have two main ingredients here and the smoothie is great just using those. I do use the add-ons listed, but I've always been a "throw in more and more options" sort of gal. You don't have to do that.*

1. Blend everything smooth. Don't whizz and whizz if you opt for the no-ice option. You don't want to make it poofy. Just blend for 10 seconds. Quick and yum!

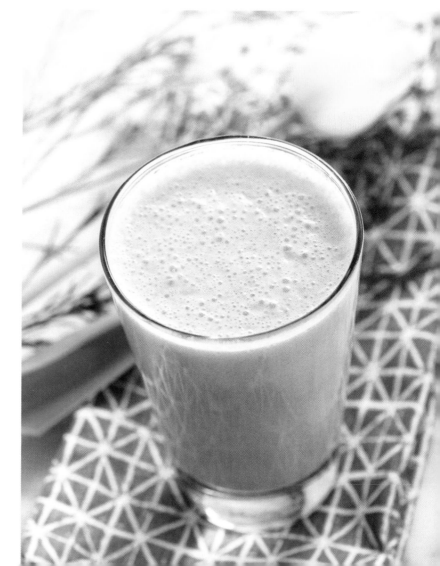

SNACK-SIZE SMOOTHIES

The following two smoothies are not big enough for a full meal but are perfect for an afternoon delight.

beet it creamy smoothie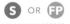

½ cup Beautiful Beet Kvass
  (page 461)
1 cup plain kefir (see Note)
1 doonk Pure Stevia Extract Powder
  (optional)
½ cup ice (optional)

This pink 'n' pretty drink is a probiotic delicacy. It's a mixture of two powerfully healing and renowned fermented elixirs and will rock your gut world. There's gonna be a partaay . . . good bugs are getting ready to dance in your belly!

1. Place the kvass, kefir, and stevia in a blender and blend until smooth. Pour into a tall glass as is or pour over ice and enjoy.

NOTE: This will be an FP if using low-fat kefir and S if using whole-milk kefir.

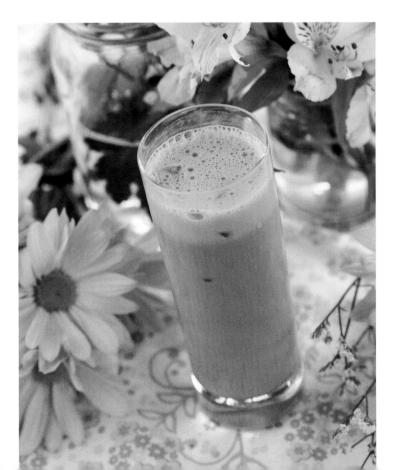

mexican papaya sister smoothie

1 cup fresh or frozen papaya
(see Note)

1 teaspoon black papaya seeds
(optional, but work up to more if
you can as they kill parasites)

1 cup plain low-fat kefir

Juice of 1 lemon

A doonk or two Pure Stevia Extract
Powder (optional)

1 to 2 tablespoons Baobab Boost
Powder (optional)

Big smile (Vange says it's not
optional)

We recently went to Mexico to celebrate the twenty-fifth wedding anniversary of our sister Vange and her husband, Howard. Vange knows how to enjoy life to the MAX . . . we mean to the SUPER POWER OF MAXIMUM! She literally milks the joy out of every second of life. Her favorite food is papaya and in Mexico with papaya everywhere, Vange felt like she was in seventh heaven. It catapulted her jubilant expressive living to another realm. We were so entertained watching her enjoy Mexico with papayas everywhere, we didn't need any other entertainment.

If you can't beat 'em you join 'em, right? We very much enjoy papayas, too, but Vange felt we were lacking enthusiasm. She took it upon herself to train us in properly celebrating them. She made us partake of them while oohing and aahing and heralding their gorgeous goodness. She made us drizzle fresh lemon or lime all over and even chew on their seeds and we *had* to have our best and hugest smiles on. She even packed us "to go" cups filled with papaya from the breakfast buffets and shoved them in our faces when we looked a little tired tearing around the back streets of Mexico in our rental van. This recipe is a tribute to our wild but wonderful, red-headed big sister, Vange.

Quick health highlights on papaya: The bright color gives a hint at its healthy powers. Papaya contains special phytonutrients, antioxidants, and digestive enzymes that have a remarkable effect both internally and externally. It is a gentle fruit on blood sugar so a wonderful Trim Healthy Mama E option. It is no wonder Christopher Columbus loved it so much he called it the "fruit of the angels."

P.S. Try to find Mexican papayas and not the varieties from Hawaii. Mexican papayas are non GMO, and the Hawaiian variety sadly are contaminated with genetically modified strains.

1. Blend everything up smooth and gorgeous and pour into a beautiful cup.

NOTE: If you can't find papaya, then we like cantaloupe as a substitute. But it is our little secret and we won't tell Vange!

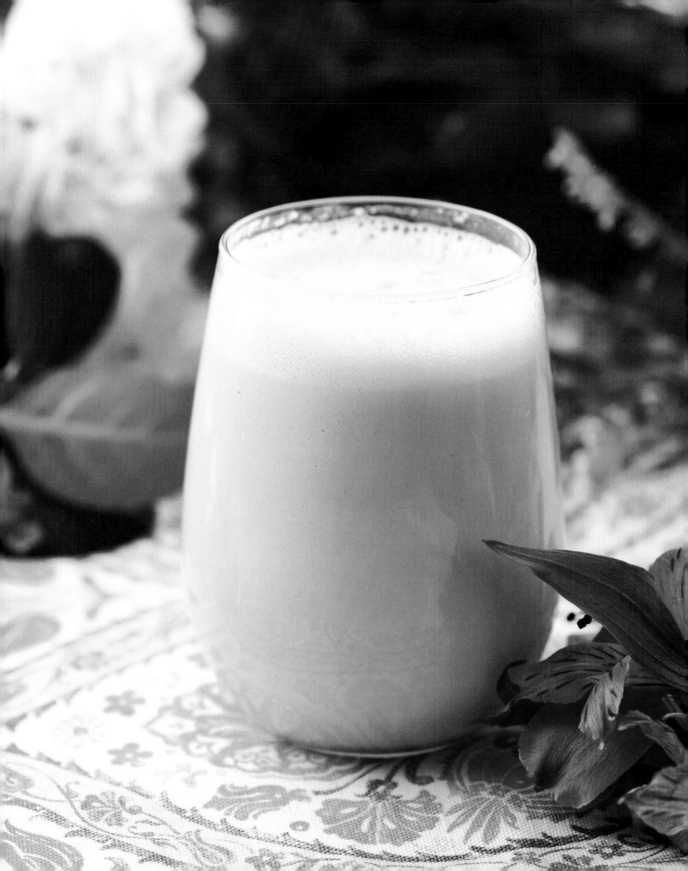

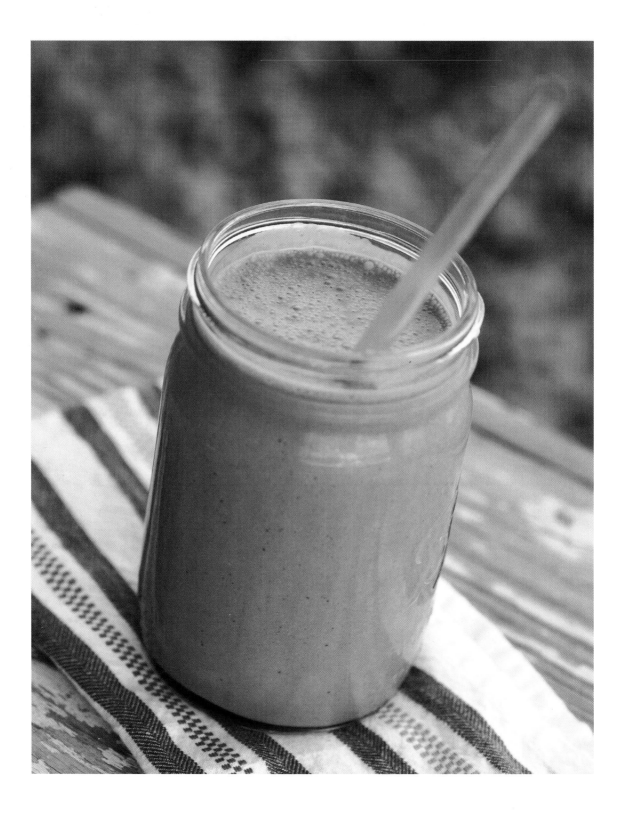

yuck yum bitty

SINGLE OR DOUBLE SERVE

SERENE CHATS: *And now for the last smoothie of the book. We dare you to do the Yuck Yum Bitty! I say "we" because I have proudly got my Drive-Thru Sue, normal-taste-bud sissy Pearl on my side with this one. She is the one who told me it is soooo Yuck Yum!! This smoothie is called a Bitty because there is a bitter note to it that at first makes you wrinkle your nose, but you grow to like it over time, then you love it, then you crave it . . . then it is your forever favorite drink! Pearl literally steals this from my blessed hands!*

Everywhere we go I take my Bitty as a meal or snack to fall back on. Whether we are recording for our podcast, at the THM office for a meeting, writing together for our books, at the airport, in Pearl's MESSY van (she drives me everywhere), I always pull it out from my diaper bag and save my own day. It's my perfect GTPAM (go-to plan-ahead meal) for our beautifully chaotic lives. If I'm rushing out the door I can throw it together in a few seconds and know I have a Super Purist healthy and satisfying meal or backup plan for if we are only around junk food. You see, this thing is a cross between a drink and food. To me, it is like a hearty meal in a mason jar. It is not cold and icy like other smoothies; it actually tastes best at room temperature in my opinion, right out of my bag. You can literally eat it with a spoon if you make the thickened version, no straws required.

Pearl, of course, never plans ahead and always wants a sip or a bite of mine when she is starving on days when we have business meetings and the guys at the office want Chinese food for the umpteenth time in a row. Of course, that one sip goes from one to twenty-one. She always starts with the word "yuck" but keeps on chowing down and very soon changes it to "yum . . . YUM!!!" You see this Bitty is so uniquely yum that it almost has a little yuck. But the yuck is intriguingly exciting and delicious. There is suspense and victory in every swallow. It's a thriller of a drink, an awesome mouthful experience where you get to push against the normal boundaries of yum and see how far you can go without falling into the pit of yuck! Want to try some? This is all part of the dare.

To be honest, I never planned on sharing the recipe for this Bitty with the whole wide world. It is kind of like a personal blankie with my own "goobers" on it and I didn't think anyone else would really get it, so I never thought of it as cookbook material. I really don't like overly sweet foods, so I designed the Bitty to achieve the very flavor pinnacle of how I enjoy my smoothies . . . a little tart . . . a little earthy . . . a lot creamy, with a deep base note of antioxidant-rich bitter cocoa. But on one of our podcasts Pearl opened up her trap about the crazy smoothie I was drinking (and that she was stealing) and it was suddenly public. I thought people would listen and shudder and that would be that, but shockingly we had so many Mamas write in wanting the recipe for the "Yuck Yum Bitty." Those e-mails just keep a-coming— our listeners keep demanding this drink!

It rocks my world, I kid you not, and I could eat/drink it for breakfast, lunch, and dinner (with some salads and a few of my Trimmy Bisque soups thrown in for a now and then change-up). In this busy season of book writing I can sip and keep working away (I know it's naughty to not relax and eat at the table, but sometimes life throws a curve ball and you gotta keep truckin'). So rather than derailing to sugar when life gets chaotic, how about letting the Yuck Yum be your lifeline, too!

This recipe, when mixed with the chia seeds, swells up into a big quart of wonderful Yuck Yum stuff. I throw in all the superfoods I ever get for treats from my husband and for birthdays and Christmas and blend them with cocoa, tart homespun kefir, and berries. The chia-thickened version is usually enough for a couple of small meals or snacks for me. I usually just eat it slowly until I am satisfied and put the rest away for a snack later in the day. It stays great in the fridge or in your bag. You can divide it from the beginning into two separate jars, but you don't have to. The thickened version can be enjoyed with a spoon and is especially delightful when you want to eat rather than drink your meal. That is Pearl's favorite.

P.S. My body thrives on my double-fermented, pasture-fed raw-milk kefir. I almost always have this as a filling S, using full-fat kefir, but I seem to burn it like rocket fuel and it keeps me Trim. There may be some of you who will not be able to down it with as much abandon as I can. We all have different genetic metabolisms and certain foods, like dairy, work better for some of us than others. Keep in touch with your weight loss or maintenance progress and see if the S Bitty is something you can have regularly or just occasionally. Perhaps try the FP version described in the Note or the Coconut Yuck Yum Bitty (opposite) if the full-fat dairy stalls you.

BUILD A YUCK YUM BITTY IN FOUR OR FIVE ITTY-BITTY STEPS:

1 YUCK YUM BITTY BASE

2 cups plain double-fermented kefir (page 459), see Note

1 to 2 tablespoons unsweetened cocoa powder

1 to 2 tablespoons Baobab Boost Powder (optional, but preferred, as it gives vitamic C and a wonderful tart flavor)

Large handful of frozen raspberries or frozen or fresh cranberries in season

1 to 2 doonks Pure Stevia Extract Powder (don't make it too sweet or it's NOT a true Bitty; you'd have to call it Yum Yum Bitty)

2 YUCK YUM BITTY PROTEINS (pick 1, or pick 2 and halve them)

1 scoop unflavored Pristine Whey Protein Powder (you can use chocolate or strawberry pristine whey, but if you do, don't add the stevia)

1 scoop Integral Collagen

1 scoop fermented pea protein (I use Nutrasumma plain Fermented Pea Protein)

3 YUCK YUM BITTY SUPERFOOD FATS
(leave out or pick 1; see Note)

1 to 2 tablespoons hemp seeds

1 tablespoon ground flax seeds

1 to 2 tablespoons cold-pressed flax oil (from a refrigerated black bottle)

1 tablespoon MCT oil

4 YUCK YUM BITTY SUPERFOOD SPICES AND POWDERS (pick 1 to 3 choices; cinnamon is great if you prefer to keep things simple)

1 teaspoon ground cinnamon

1 teaspoon matcha tea

½ teaspoon maca powder

½ teaspoon chaga extract (I use VitaJing Herbs brand)

½ to 1 teaspoon ashwaghanda root powder (such as Terrasoul Superfoods brand)

½ teaspoon amla powder

1 teaspoon lúcuma powder

5 YUCK YUM BITTY THICKENERS
(leave out or pick 1)

4 tablespoons whole soaked chia seeds with 1 cup water (if using chia, don't use another superfood fat)

1½ teaspoons Just Gelatin (with 2 tablespoons cool water and 2 tablespoons just off the boil water for blooming)

1. If using the chia seeds for thickening, make them ahead of time by putting them in 1 cup water for a few hours or overnight (I usually keep a jar or 2 of this soaked chia in the fridge, ready for Yuck Yum Bitty making). If using gelatin to thicken, dissolve it first in the cold water, stir, and then add the boiled water.

2. Place your Bitty Base ingredients in a blender and before you "press play," pick your protein choice, and ask yourself if you want the option of an added superfood fat. Throw those items in along with your choice of superfood spices or powders and blend until creamy. If using gelatin, blend it in at the end. If using chia, stir the gel in after blending; it will create a tapioca pearl–like consistency and is super hydrating and wonderful.

NOTE: Store-bought kefir is not really fermented enough if using this as an S recipe like I usually do. You need a double-fermented kefir when in S mode, so if you want to use store-bought kefir, leave it out of the fridge overnight to double-ferment. You can make this an FP smoothie by using homemade kefir from skim milk or using store-bought low-fat kefir that you leave out for another ferment. Consider your Bitty an E if you use low-fat kefir from a store and don't do a second ferment. For these FP or E versions, don't add an extra fat option and thicken with the gelatin rather than the chia seeds.

COCONUT YUCK YUM BITTY Ⓢ

SINGLE OR DOUBLE SERVE

COCONUT BITTY BASE
1 cup coconut kefir (page 460)
1 cup water
1 to 2 tablespoons unsweetened cocoa powder
1 to 2 tablespoons Baobab Boost Powder (optional)
1 large handful frozen raspberries or frozen or fresh cranberries in season

If you are one of our dairy-free Mamas, our sister Vange has got you covered. She can't drink dairy kefir so she makes coconut kefir. Here is her version of the Yuck Yum Bitty. Only the base ingredients are different. All the add-ons are the same, including proteins, fats, and thickeners, but this will always be an S. Make it the same way as for the original Yuck Yum Bitty.

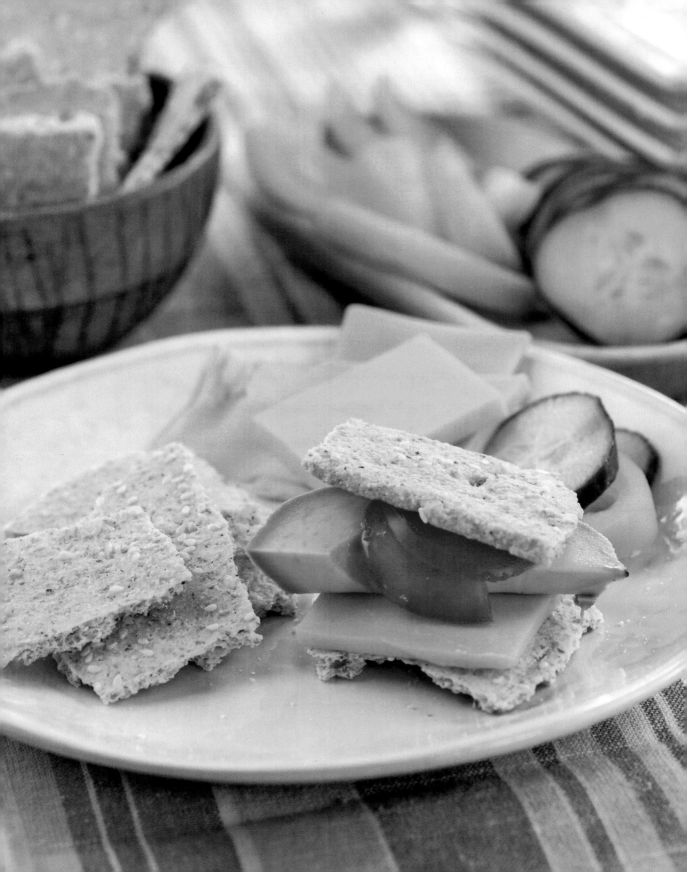

Crackers, Crusts, Toppings & More

Beauty Blend Recipes:

Crackers, Crusts, Cookies, Cereal & More

SERENE CHATS: *The following recipes are all made from a core blend of dry ingredients that are abundantly rich in beautifying and restoring glycine and proline amino acids for your skin and hair, thanks to the combination of both gelatin and collagen. We call this mix Beauty Blend; however, it aids more than your beauty; it also fortifies your immune system and soothes achy joints. Now you can celebrate crackers, cookies, cereals, blondies, pizza, and pie crusts all while enhancing rather than destroying your body's healthy vigor and glow.*

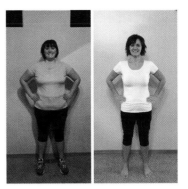

Today is my one year trim-aversary! What an awesome journey the last year has been. It has been full of ups and downs and lots of learning. I am so grateful I decided to take the plunge and start this program. I am happy to say goodbye to that fifty pounds and to say hello to feeling comfortable in my skin again. This plan has blessed both me and my family. I had one of my daughters join me, and she was able to shed a few unwanted pounds, and now my husband has decided to join me. I'm excited to see the plan work for him.

If you're feeling discouraged, I would just encourage you to keep going and give yourself the needed grace that comes with trying to improve the way you're eating. With my food, I try to keep things really simple. My favorite breakfast is just two eggs, fried in butter. For lunch, I really enjoy eating a chef salad with diced ham and hard-boiled eggs with lots of veggies added, a small sprinkle of cheese, and an on-plan ranch dressing. I also really enjoy the Just Like Campbell's Tomato Soup (from the first cookbook) with an on-plan grilled cheese. I eat a lot of leftovers at lunch time. There are so many simple dinners I enjoy. As far as snacks go, I love having stevia-sweetened yogurt with an apple for an E. It's supereasy and so tasty. I don't make a lot of desserts, but I usually eat a square (sometimes two) of 86% cacao chocolate every day. I love chocolate and can't go without it!

My biggest tip for newbies is to just be consistent with the plan. Give yourself grace when you eat off-plan, and try again in three hours. I have found that with this mentality, even when I went off-plan on purpose it never derailed me as has happened in the past. Also, be patient with yourself and your weight loss. There were many times when my weight loss stalled, but I just continued to follow the plan and I always started losing again. This is definitely a marathon, not a sprint. And take your measurements! There were many times I didn't see the number on the scale move, but the number on the tape measure had definitely gone down. Take pictures as well. It is so amazing and satisfying to see the changes that occur along the way. Also, make sure to set small, attainable goals throughout your weight-loss journey. That way you can celebrate victories all along the way.

I am truly grateful to have found this plan. It has changed the way I look at food and has given me something I am happy to stick with. I am so grateful to finally feel comfortable in my skin again. And that was my ultimate goal. I wanted to be able to look in the mirror and feel good about the way I looked and feel like my outside finally matched who I was on the inside. —**KARI S.**

beauty blend graham crackers
or savory sesame crackers

FP OR **S**

MULITPLE SERVE

½ cup THM Baking Blend

1 tablespoon Just Gelatin

3 tablespoons (2 scoops) Integral Collagen

1 teaspoon aluminum-free baking powder

FOR THE GRAHAM VERSION

3 pinches Mineral Salt

2 tablespoons Gentle Sweet

2 tablespoons butter*

¾ cup egg whites (carton or fresh)

1 teaspoon pure vanilla extract

FOR THE SAVORY SESAME VERSION

6 pinches Mineral Salt

½ to ¾ teaspoon garlic and/or onion powder

2 teaspoons toasted sesame oil

4 teaspoons butter*

¾ cup egg whites (carton or fresh)

Dried parsley flakes for sprinkling

Sesame seeds, for sprinkling

(ONE-SIXTH OF THE RECIPE IS FP, MORE BECOMES A VERY LIGHT S)

These crackers snap and crunch with a light and beautiful crisp. You get two for one with this adaptable, easy peasy recipe. The mildly sweet graham version of this cracker is perfect used as wafers for desserts or in every way you would use a graham cracker. If you prefer a sweeter graham cracker, then add a couple doonks of Pure Stevia Extract to the recipe below, but don't add more Gentle Sweet. That adds too much moisture to the recipe somehow and they won't crisp as well . . . much trial and error taught us that. You can get creative by adding ¾ teaspoon cinnamon and/or ginger to make gingersnap-style cookies/crackers, but don't underestimate the simple delicious addictiveness of this original recipe.

The savory version is perfect for topping with cheese or avocado and tomato or with any of the dips (pages 518 to 524) or even for nachos (page 303). The crackers also can be crumbled into soups or on top of salads for that crunch fix we all desire. If you don't enjoy the flavor of sesame, leave the oil out and use only butter (see Savory Crackers, below).

1. Preheat the oven to 300°F. Line an extra-large 11½ x 17½-inch rimmed baking sheet with parchment paper or use 2 smaller baking sheets.

2. Put the Baking Blend, gelatin, collagen, and baking powder in a food processor and pulse to combine.

3. **FOR THE GRAHAM VERSION:** Pulse in the salt and Gentle Sweet. Add the butter and pulse a few times to coat with flour. Add the egg whites and vanilla and blend for another few seconds. Take the blade out of the processor and stir the ingredients well (or blend all in a bowl with a stick blender). Pour directly onto the baking sheet and spread out with the back of a spatula or with water-moistened fingers. Spread as thinly as possible to cover almost the entire sheet. Think very thin crackers (they rise a little). If using the 1 large baking sheet, leave only about ½ inch on all sides uncovered.

   FOR THE SAVORY SESAME VERSION: Pulse in the salt and garlic and/or onion powder. Add the sesame oil and butter and pulse a few times to coat with flour. Add the egg whites and blend for another few seconds. Take the blade out of the processor and stir the ingredients well (or blend all in a bowl with a stick blender). Spread on the baking sheet as

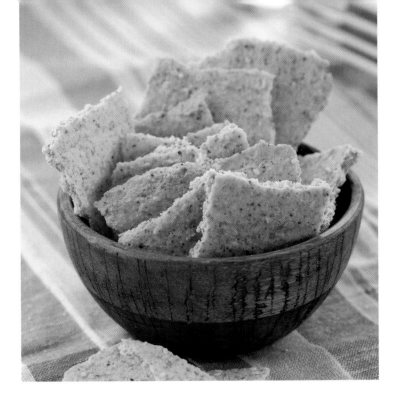

directed for the graham version. Sprinkle with parsley flakes and sesame seeds.

4. Bake for 20 minutes, then reduce the oven temperature to 170°F and keep in the oven for another 2 to 3 hours. Turn the oven off and let cool in the oven. Once cooled, break into rustic-shaped crackers (or you can choose to score before baking into rectangular shapes). Store in a zippy bag to keep snappin' fresh (zippies in the freezer keep them their snappiest).

VARIATION

SAVORY CRACKERS: This is a version without sesame, which is great for Fast Nachos or Tostadas (page 303). Omit the sesame oil and increase the total amount of butter to 2 tablespoons. Omit the sprinkled sesame seeds. Bake as directed. Break them into smaller pieces for nachos or much larger shapes to use as a tostada base.

NOTE: There is very little prep to these crackers, just a longish oven time. If you work during the day, best to make this recipe in the evening or over the weekend. Or you can cook for the 20 minutes before you go to bed, then let them crisp all night at 170°F while you sleep.

* FOR DF: USE COCONUT OIL IN PLACE OF BUTTER.

no moo cheesecake–stuffed cookie sammies
S

MULTIPLE SERVE

Dough from Beauty Blend Graham
   Crackers (page 504)*
No Moo Cream Cheese (page 441)

1. Preheat the oven to 300°F. Line an extra-large baking sheet with parchment paper

2. Make the dough and spread it on the baking sheet as directed, but score the dough into shapes after spreading it out. Bake as directed.

3. Once cooled, break into scored shapes, stuff with the "cream cheese," then freeze the cookie sandwiches. You can eat them frozen or, if you prefer, thawed in the fridge.

* FOR DF: USE COCONUT OIL IN PLACE OF BUTTER IN CRACKERS.

DF FRIENDLY

beauty blend thin and crispy pizza crust
FP

MAKES 2 LARGE CRUSTS (HALVE INGREDIENTS TO MAKE JUST 1 PIZZA)

1 cup THM Baking Blend
2 tablespoons Just Gelatin
6 tablespoons (4 scoops) Integral
   Collagen
¼ to ½ teaspoon Mineral Salt
2 teaspoons aluminum-free baking
   powder
4 tablespoons (½ stick) butter*
1 teaspoon Italian seasoning
½ teaspoon garlic powder
   (optional)
½ teaspoon onion powder
   (optional)
1½ cups egg whites (carton or
   fresh)

(ONE-TWELFTH OF THE RECIPE IS FP, BUT
S ONCE COMBINED WITH TOPPINGS.)

1. Preheat the oven to 300°F. Line 2 rimmed baking sheets with parchment paper.

2. Put the Baking Blend, gelatin, collagen, salt, baking powder, Italian seasoning, garlic powder (if using), and onion powder (if using) in a food processor and pulse to combine. Add the butter and pulse a few times to coat with flour. Add the egg whites and blend for another few seconds. Take the blade out of the food processor and stir the ingredients well. (Or blend all in a bowl with a stick blender.)

3. Spread the mixture out very thinly on the baking sheets. Bake for 40 minutes, then turn off the oven and let cool slowly in the turned-off oven.

4. Top with your favorite pizza toppings and broil until the cheese is bubbling.

* FOR DF: USE COCONUT OIL IN PLACE OF BUTTER.

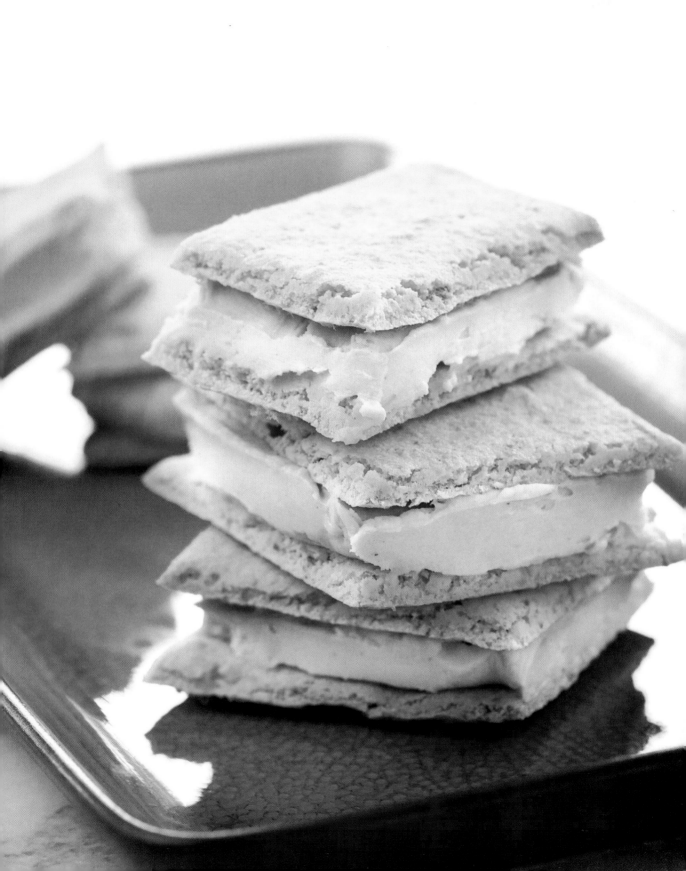

beauty blend base pie crust

FP OR S

MULTIPLE SERVE

Coconut oil cooking spray or butter,
   for the pie plate
⅓ cup THM Baking Blend
¾ teaspoon Just Gelatin
2 tablespoons Integral Collagen
¾ teaspoon aluminum-free baking
   powder
2 pinches Mineral Salt
1 tablespoon Gentle Sweet
1 tablespoon plus 1 teaspoon
   butter*
½ cup egg whites (carton or fresh)
¾ teaspoon pure vanilla extract

(ONE-SIXTH OF THE RECIPE IS FP,
MORE BECOMES A VERY LIGHT S.)

This is a great pie base to use sometimes as it is lighter than our Traditional Pie Crust (page 408). Although delicious, you don't want to use heavy crusts all of the time. Take out the sweetener, add a dash more salt, and it also makes a good savory base for a quiche (see the variation below). You should know ahead of time that this crust won't press into the sides of your pie plate as it is more of a wet mixture than most pie crusts before baking. It is only a base for the bottom of your pie. It has the same ingredients as the Beauty Blend Graham Crackers (page 504), but in a smaller quantity so your crust doesn't get too thick.

1. Preheat the oven to 300°F. Spray a 9-inch pie plate with coconut oil or grease with butter.

2. Put the Baking Blend, gelatin, collagen, baking powder, salt, and sweetener in a food processor and pulse to combine. Add the butter and pulse a few times to coat with flour. Add the egg whites and vanilla and blend for another few seconds. Take the blade out of the food processor and stir the ingredients well. (Or blend all in a bowl with a stick blender.)

3. Scrape the mixture into the pie plate and spread it out with a spatula. Bake for 20 minutes, then turn off the oven and let the crust cool slowly in the turned-off oven. Once cooled, add your pie filling.

VARIATION

SAVORY BEAUTY BLEND PIE CRUST: Omit the sweetener and the vanilla and increase the salt to 4 pinches.

* FOR DF: USE COCONUT OIL IN PLACE OF BUTTER.

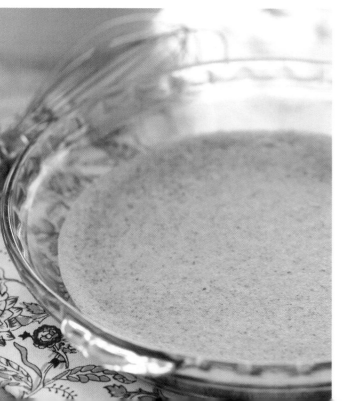

beauty blend cereal

FP OR S

MULTIPLE SERVE

½ cup THM Baking Blend

1 tablespoon Just Gelatin

3 tablespoons (2 scoops) Integral Collagen

1 teaspoon aluminum-free baking powder

3 pinches Mineral Salt

2 tablespoons Gentle Sweet

2 tablespoons butter*

¾ cup egg whites (carton or fresh)

1 teaspoon pure vanilla extract

1 teaspoon ground cinnamon (optional)

Unsweetened almond milk and Gentle Sweet, for serving

Fresh blueberries and slivered or chopped almonds, for serving (optional)

(ONE-SIXTH OF THE RECIPE IS FP, WITHOUT NUTS; MORE BECOMES A VERY LIGHT S, BUT IF YOU ADD NUTS, THIS WILL BE AN S.)

SERENE CHATS: *Missing cereal? Welcome it back! This is reminiscent of Grape-Nuts. As written, this cereal is only mildly sweet; we tried to add more sweetener to it but then it wouldn't crisp and crunch as well. You'll want to add a rounded teaspoon or more of Gentle Sweet to your bowl once you have poured in your unsweetened nut milk. That gives the perfect, sweet cereal result and you'll happily crunch and slurp your bowl down. My husband loves this stuff and not just for breakfast. He gets hangry at night and this is a lovely lighter option for a late-night snack if you don't stuff too many nuts in it.*

1. Preheat the oven to 300°F. Line an extra-large 11½ x 17½-inch rimmed baking sheet with parchment paper.

2. Put the Baking Blend, gelatin, collagen, baking powder, salt, and sweetener in a food processor and pulse to combine. Add the butter and pulse a few times to coat with flour. Add the egg whites, vanilla, and cinnamon (if using) and blend for another few seconds. (Or blend all in a bowl with a stick blender.)

3. Pour directly onto the baking sheet and spread out with the back of a spatula. You want to spread it as thinly as possible to cover almost the entire sheet, think thin cracker depth. Leave only about ½ inch on all sides that is not covered.

4. Bake for 20 minutes, then reduce the oven temperature to 170°F and keep in the oven for another 2 to 3 hours. Turn the oven off and let cool in the turned-off oven. Once cooled, break up the crackers into chunks, then place in a food processor. Pulse until they turn into little crunchy pellets (similar to Grape-Nuts) and store in a zippy bag.

5. Once ready to eat, pour into a bowl, then douse with unsweetened almond milk, adding a teaspoon or so of Gentle Sweet for added sweetness, if needed. The addition of a handful of blueberries and almonds rocks this cereal bowl into a yummy breakfast taste bud party.

* FOR DF: USE COCONUT OIL IN PLACE OF BUTTER.

beauty blend cookie pizza

MULTIPLE SERVE

½ cup THM Baking Blend

1 tablespoon Just Gelatin

3 tablespoons (2 scoops) Integral Collagen

1 teaspoon aluminum-free baking powder

¼ cup Gentle Sweet plus 1 tablespoon Super Sweet (if you don't have Super Sweet just use 3 tablespoons Gentle Sweet plus 3 doonks Pure Stevia Extract Powder)

½ teaspoon Mineral Salt

4 tablespoons (½ stick) butter

2 tablespoons ghee (clarified butter)

¾ cup egg whites (carton or fresh)

1½ teaspoons pure vanilla extract

½ teaspoon Natural Burst butter extract

½ cup Trim Healthy Chocolate Chips or chopped 85% chocolate

Optional smattering: chopped walnuts, pecans, macadamia nuts, or shredded unsweetened coconut

This is one giant yummy, crunchy cookie that you can break off into delicious pieces, a favorite with children.

1. Preheat the oven to 300°F and line an extra-large cookie sheet with parchment paper.
2. Put the Baking Blend, gelatin, collagen, baking powder, sweeteners, and salt in a food processor and pulse to combine. Add the butter and ghee and pulse a few times to coat with flour. Add the egg whites, vanilla, and butter extract and blend for another few seconds. Take the blade out of the food processor and stir in the chocolate chips and chopped nuts (if using). (Or blend all the ingredients except the chocolate chips and nuts in a bowl with a stick blender, then stir them in.)
3. Spread out thinly on the baking sheet and bake for 40 minutes, then reduce the oven temperature to 170°F and keep in the oven for another 2 to 3 hours. Turn the oven off and let cool in the turned-off oven.

beauty blend chewy coconut cookies ⓢ

1 cup shredded unsweetened coconut

½ cup THM Baking Blend

1 tablespoon Just Gelatin

3 tablespoons (2 scoops) Integral Collagen

1 teaspoon aluminum-free baking powder

½ teaspoon Mineral Salt

3 to 4 tablespoons Gentle Sweet

1 tablespoon Super Sweet Blend, or 3 to 4 doonks Pure Stevia Extract Powder

4 tablespoons (½ stick) butter

1 tablespoon ghee (clarified butter)

¾ cup egg whites (carton or fresh)

1 teaspoon pure vanilla extract

½ to ¾ teaspoon Natural Burst butter extract

Trim Healthy Chocolate Chips or 85% chocolate, melted (optional)

SERENE CHATS: *These are yummy as is or decorated with swirls of melted chocolate and left to harden again in the fridge. Nonsweeties like me will prefer only 2 tablespoons of Gentle Sweet and 2 teaspoons Super Sweet, but Pearl said I needed to give the option of more. She's bossy like that.*

1. Preheat the oven to 300°F. Grease a baking sheet.

2. Put the coconut, Baking Blend, gelatin, collagen, baking powder, salt, and sweeteners in a food processor and pulse to combine. Add the butter and ghee and pulse a few times to coat with flour. Add the egg whites, vanilla, and butter extract and blend for another few seconds. Take the blade out of the food processor and stir the ingredients well. (Or blend all the ingredients in a bowl with a stick blender.)

3. Refrigerate the mixture for a bit so the gelatin can firm up the dough. Once the dough is firm, drop spoonfuls onto the prepared baking sheet and bake for 40 minutes, then turn off the oven and allow to cool in the turned-off oven. (For ultimate chewiness, after 40 minutes of baking at 300°F, reduce the oven temp to 170°F and bake for a couple more hours, then allow to cool in the turned-off oven.)

4. Melt the chocolate (if using) in a heat-safe bowl over a small pot of water on medium-high heat. Dip half of each cookie in some melted chocolate or drizzle the chocolate over the cookies.

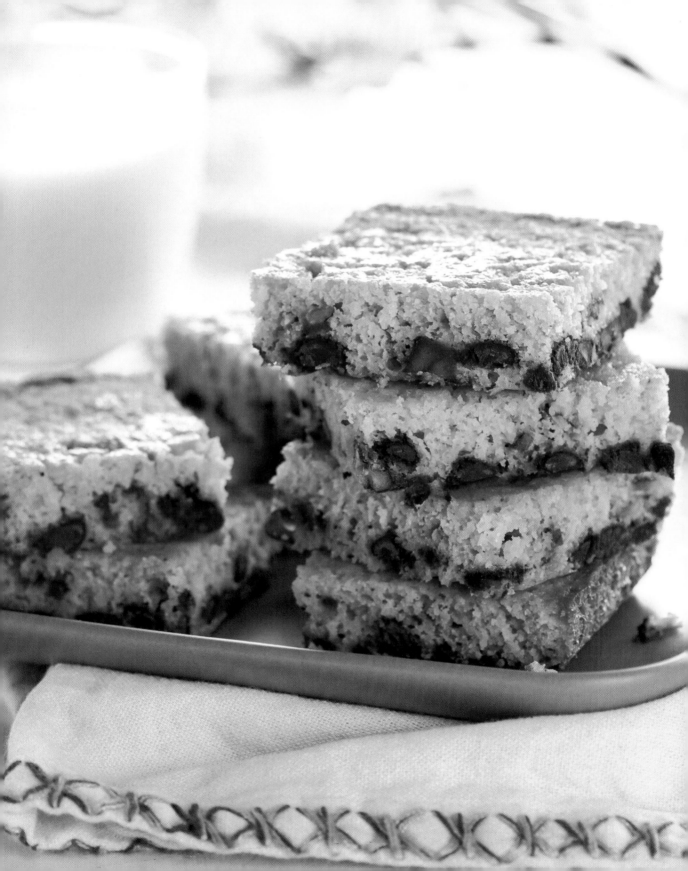

beauty blend blondies

S

MULTIPLE SERVE

½ cup THM Baking Blend

1 tablespoon Just Gelatin

3 tablespoons (2 scoops) Integral Collagen

1 teaspoon aluminum-free baking powder

¼ cup Gentle Sweet

1 tablespoon Super Sweet, or 3 to 4 doonks Pure Stevia Extract Powder

½ teaspoon Mineral Salt

4 tablespoons (½ stick) butter

2 tablespoons ghee (clarified butter)

¾ cup egg whites (carton or fresh)

1½ teaspoons pure vanilla extract

½ to ¾ teaspoon Natural Burst butter extract

1 tablespoon plain 0% Greek yogurt

⅓ cup Trim Healthy Chocolate Chips or chopped 85% chocolate

Optional smattering: chopped walnuts, pecans, or macadamia nuts

1. Preheat the oven to 300°F. Grease an 8-inch square baking dish.

2. Put the Baking Blend, gelatin, collagen, baking powder, sweeteners, and salt in a food processor and pulse to combine. Add the butter and ghee and pulse a few times to coat with flour. Add the egg whites, vanilla, butter extracts, and yogurt and blend for another few seconds. Take the blade out of the food processor, add the chocolate chips and optional nuts, and stir well. (Or blend all the ingredients except the chocolate chips and nuts in a bowl with a stick blender, then stir them in.)

3. Spread the batter into the prepared dish. Bake for 40 minutes, then turn off the oven and allow to cool in the turned-off oven. (For chewier brownies, after 40 minutes of baking at 300°F, reduce the oven temp to 170°F and bake for another hour, then allow to cool in the turned-off oven.)

DF FRIENDLY

BEAUTY BLEND COOKIE BREAD

MULTIPLE SERVE

SERENE CHATS: *Slice this yummy little loaf into cookie slices! My kids devour these! This is similar to the blondies—but without the yogurt, you have a DF-friendly recipe.*

1. Omit the yogurt and add 1 more tablespoon egg whites. Make the batter as for the blondies, then put the batter into a medium-size bread tin and bake in the same way as Beauty Blend Blondies. Cut into cookie slices.

* FOR DF: USE COCONUT OIL IN PLACE OF BUTTER.

Sauces, Dressings, Dips & Other Odds and Ends

To all our Drive-Thru Sues: Yes, store-bought dressings such as ranch or blue cheese or creamy Italian can be used on plan. But they are usually far from superfoody. More often than not, they contain a bunch of hydrogenated soybean oil along with long lists of other not so great ingredients. But we know . . . you don't always want to make your own dressing and we want you to eat lots of salads, so sometimes just pouring on a bit of store-bought ranch keeps you sane. That's fine, just try to avoid dressings with more than trace amounts of sugar. Best to water down full-fat store-bought dressings just a bit, or a better option is to buy yogurt-based dressings such as Bolthouse Farms brand (look for dressings with no more than 2 carbs).

We'd also love you to start making Deep S instant dressings. Just pour extra-virgin olive oil or MCT oil over your plate of greens, then top with your choice of vinegar (we use apple cider vinegar and/or balsamic with no more than 2 grams of carbs), then shake on salt, pepper, and optional Gentle Sweet and a little green can Parmy cheese. Takes you 30 seconds and is a slimming way to go!

Included in this chapter are some awesome homemade dressings, some of which are FP (but don't taste like it). You don't have to make them as soon as you start your THM journey, but once you have your feet wet and aren't feeling so overwhelmed, give them a try. They contain superfood fats and other immune-boosting ingredients to make sure your dressings boost your health rather than drag it down. Please also try the awesome dips and sauces in this chapter. And please don't miss the Quirky Jerky recipe hidden away at the end of this chapter because we didn't know where else to put it.

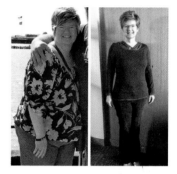

Two years ago, my doctor told me that if I did not bring my blood sugar A1C number down I would have to go on diabetes medicine. I did not want that because there is a family history of heart disease and diabetes in my family. A lady at my church had lost weight. I asked her how she did it, and she told me about Trim Healthy Mama. I work at a library, so I checked out the book, never knowing that it would change my life! After being on the plan for two months, I went back to my doctor and had bloodwork done again to check my A1C number for blood sugar. My doctor was very happy because my number had gone from 7.8 to 5.3! She told me whatever you are doing, DON'T STOP!

I have now lost eighty pounds and am in maintenance mode. I no longer take prescription medicine for high blood pressure and I am no longer prediabetic. I have just started the Workins Exercise DVDs with Serene and Pearl and love them! My husband joined me on plan and has lost forty pounds. Thank you, Trim Healthy Mama, for giving me a future!

–DANA H.

basic pancake syrup

FP

MAKES ABOUT 1½ CUPS

1 cup water
2½ to 3 tablespoons Gentle Sweet*
½ teaspoon Natural Burst maple extract
½ teaspoon Natural Burst butter extract
1 to 2 pinches Mineral Salt
¼ teaspoon Gluccie*

We brought this over from *Trim Healthy Mama Cookbook* because it is so handy, easy, and wonderful, we couldn't leave it out for all our new-to-planners in this book. Pair it with Blender Freezer Waffles (page 336) or any of the pancakes or waffles in the Blood Sugar–Balancing Breakfasts chapter.

1. Put all the ingredients (except the Gluccie) in a small saucepan and bring to a simmer over medium heat. Reduce the heat to medium-low, whisk in the Gluccie a little at a time (keep whisking like crazy so it doesn't clump). Allow to simmer for a couple minutes.

* FOR NSI: USE A GROCERY STORE ON-PLAN SWEETENER, GROCERY STORE EXTRACTS, AND SUB XANTHAN GUM FOR THE GLUCCIE.

perfect pizza sauce

FP

MAKES JUST OVER 1½ CUPS

1 (14.5-ounce) can crushed tomatoes
1 doonk Pure Stevia Extract Powder, or ½ to ¾ teaspoon Super Sweet Blend*
½ teaspoon onion powder
¾ teaspoon garlic powder
¾ to 1 teaspoon dried oregano
½ teaspoon paprika
½ teaspoon Mineral Salt
⅛ teaspoon black pepper

This can be used in any recipe in this book that calls for a 14-ounce jar of pizza sauce. It yields very close to the same amount (maybe a tad more). You can put it in a squirt bottle, too, for topping all sorts of things.

1. Mix all the ingredients well with a whisk or blend with a stick blender (or in a stand blender). Store in the refrigerator for all your pizza sauce needs.

* FOR NSI: USE A GROCERY STORE ON-PLAN SWEETENER.

easiest mayo

S

MULTIPLE SERVE

½ cup avocado oil

½ cup MCT oil (or ¾ cup avo oil and ¼ cup MCT oil if your digestive system is still adjusting to large amounts of MCT oil)

Juice of 1 large lemon, or 2 tablespoons bottled lemon juice

½ teaspoon Mineral Salt

1 large egg

1 teaspoon Nutritional Yeast or mellow miso (yellow or white)

1 tablespoon liquid whey or kefir water, drained from homemade kefir or store-bought plain yogurt with active cultures (optional; see Note)

OPTIONAL SEASONINGS (ONE OR ALL)

¼ teaspoon black pepper

¼ teaspoon garlic powder

1 teaspoon onion powder

¼ to ½ teaspoon mustard powder or wasabi powder

SERENE CHATS: *Store-bought mayo is on-plan, but as the purist of our sister team I have to point out that while it can be included, it is far from optimum. If you want my frank opinion, I'd say most store-bought mayo is a horrible GMO cocktail of hydrogenated soybean oil. Pearl would argue and go on about how although not a superfood, it doesn't raise blood sugar. Then she'll tell me that most of you don't have the time or energy to make everything homemade and if we force you to you'll just quit! Quitting is way worse for your health than eating store-bought mayo, she'll say. I agree on that point, but this won't take you more than a couple minutes and you'll reap so many benefits replacing the store-bought stuff with it. I know I've given you other mayos in other books, but this one won't let you down.*

This recipe uses a combination of MCT oil and avocado oil. I avoid olive oil in my mayo because the flavor is too overpowering. MCT oil is virtually flavorless and very silky, and not only revs the thermogenic temperature of your body to kick fat to the wayside, but it is the ultimate brain fuel and the quickest energy jolt possible. Avocado oil is smooth, mellow, and mild and I use it to cut the MCT oil as too much MCT oil too soon can give some of us folks the runs . . . as in run to the bathroom! Too much will sure clean you out! When you slowly work up to a larger amount, this problem goes away, but I think a mixture of these two delicious oils makes the perfect mayo.

While we have sung the praises of MCT oil in our books, avocado oil has its own special merits. It mostly consists of the much acclaimed oleic acid, an omega-9 fatty acid. Not only is avo oil resistant to oxidation, so it does not become rancid as quickly as other vegetable oils, it helps speed cell regeneration and wound healing, combats microbial infections, reduces inflammation internally and externally, and prevents flare-ups of many autoimmune diseases.

1. You will need a stick blender for this recipe. One of those cheap, handheld doobiwhackers will do. Place all the ingredients in a jar large enough to fit all your ingredients and your blender.

2. Immerse the blender into the mixture and start blending at the bottom of the jar. Blend until smooth while slowly lifting the blending stick higher in the mixture. It should only take a minute to make the yummiest fat-burning mayo ever.

NOTE: While not necessary, this addition makes the mayo last longer and imparts extra-healthy enzymes.

kickin' dippin' sauce, dip, or dressing   FP

LARGE FAMILY SERVE (OR MULTIPLE SINGLE SERVES)

½ to 1 dried habanero (or 1 dried milder chili pepper for heat babies)

2 tablespoons yellow miso

3 tablespoons Nutritional Yeast

½ teaspoon onion powder

⅛ teaspoon garlic powder

1 teaspoon dried oregano

¼ teaspoon chipotle powder

¼ teaspoon ground cumin

1 tablespoon finely grated Pecorino Romano or Parmesan (optional)

1 to 2 teaspoons apple cider vinegar (depending on your love of zing)

½ cup just off the boil water

¾ cup canned fire-roasted diced tomatoes (most of the juice drained)

Dash of mesquite liquid smoke

1 tablespoon coconut oil, red palm oil, or MCT oil

½ cup 1% cottage cheese, for creamy version (optional)

SERENE CHATS: *This is an addictive sauce that has so many uses in my home. I keep heaps of the creamy version in the fridge (quadruple amounts) and put it on our table for almost every meal. My spice-loving kids scarf it down. It amps up protein and is a great flavorful addition to the side of your plate no matter what meal you are eating. Dip some of your food into it and your whole meal starts kickin'! If your children are not as spice loving as mine, don't use the habanero. Try a dried mild chili pepper.*

The cottage cheese is completely optional here. It makes the sauce creamy, but I originally created this sauce without cottage cheese and it has so many uses that way, too. You can drizzle the non–cottage cheese version over meats and veggies before baking or swirl it over brown rice or smear it in any sandwich or wrap. It is even great over salad for a dressing! Everything tastes better with it. I also keep some of the original cottage-cheese-less version of this sauce in a squirt bottle in my fridge—do that and none of your meals will lack for flavor.

1. Blend all the ingredients with a stick blender (you can use a stand blender, but it's way easier with the stick version). Done!

NOTE: Purists might like to add a little kefir or yogurt whey water (about 2 tablespoons) when making this sauce and leave the sauce out for an afternoon to let it ferment. This will inoculate it with probiotics and not only rev up the health offering it brings but also enable a longer refrigerator life.

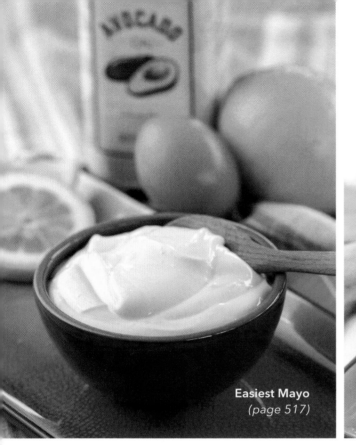

Easiest Mayo
(page 517)

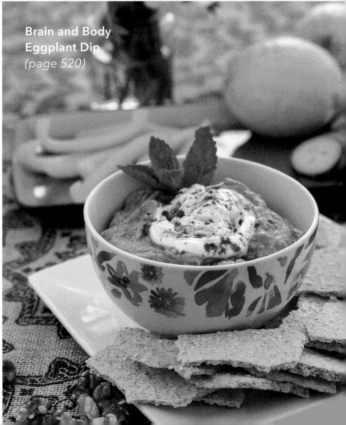

**Kickin' Dippin' Sauce,
Dip, or Dressing**
(opposite)

Perfect Pizza Sauce
(page 516)

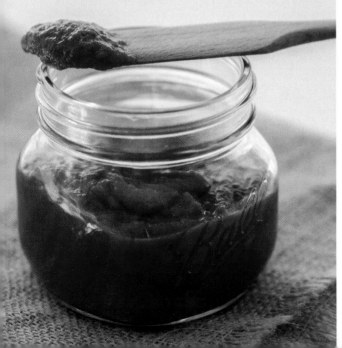

**Brain and Body
Eggplant Dip**
(page 520)

brain and body eggplant dip

FP OR S

3 small eggplants (or 2 bigger ones, but smaller taste better)
1 tablespoon MCT oil or avocado oil
½ large onion, diced
2 garlic cloves, minced (3 or 4 for garlic freaks like Serene)
2 teaspoons dried crushed mint
1½ to 3 tablespoons (1 to 2 scoops) Integral Collagen
2 teaspoons Mineral Salt
⅛ teaspoon black pepper
⅛ teaspoon cayenne pepper (optional)
¾ cup plain 0% Greek yogurt or plain low-fat kefir (or full-fat kefir for S)

ABSOLUTELY DIVINE S OPTIONS
2 additional tablespoons MCT oil
½ cup walnuts

OPTIONAL GARNISHES
Fresh mint leaves
Sumac powder or paprika

SERENE CHATS: *You'll eat this for the yum factor, but there's a lot more than just yum going on here. Eggplant is rich in fiber but low in calories and satiates the appetite. It does this by powerfully regulating your blood sugar and inhibiting your hunger hormone ghrelin through high amounts of both soluble and insoluble fiber. Suffering from foggy thinking? Eggplant can help. It has a substance called nasunin, which studies show inhibits detrimental behavior in the brain. The dark purple color means it is teaming with phytonutrients that boost mental health and cognitive activity. It wields a fierce axe against the free radicals that scavenge your brain and cause neural degeneration. Eggplant delivers oxygen-rich blood to the brain, which helps neural pathways flourish and stimulates memory and analytic thought. It is also an abundant source of potassium, which is known as a vasodilator and widens blood vessels to the brain. I chose to add MCT oil because it is ultimate brain fuel and has even been clinically studied to reverse dementia. This dip is brain food on steroids! By adding a scoop or two of our grass-fed collagen powder we amp up this beautifying, body-repairing food. Let's dig in and feast our brain and bodies strong!*

Dip on-plan breads and crackers—such as Beauty Blend Savory Sesame Crackers (page 504)—or crudités into it or use it as a side.

1. Preheat the oven to 400°F.

2. Wash the eggplants and prick them in a few places with a fork. Bake on a large baking sheet for 30 to 40 minutes. Be sure not to burn the skin, as that contains many of the brain nutrients. Remove from the oven, slice them open, and let them cool for 15 to 20 minutes (you can bake them the day before, but this dip is lovely served warm and fresh).

3. Heat 1 tablespoon MCT oil in a small skillet over medium heat. Add the onion and garlic and sauté until translucent. Remove from the heat, add the dried mint, and stir well.

4. Cut off the caps of the eggplant, coarsely chop the flesh, and place in a food processor. Add the minty onions and garlic, collagen, salt, pepper, and cayenne (if using) and process until creamy. If making the S option, add the extra oil while processing and pulse the walnuts at the end so they are chewy morsels.

5. Place this mixture in a serving bowl and stir in the yogurt or kefir. Garnish with fresh mint leaves if desired and a dash of sumac powder or paprika for a red splash of color.

cauliflower hummus

MULTIPLE SERVE

1 (16-ounce) bag frozen cauliflower, or 3 to 4 cups fresh florets

2 tablespoons MCT oil, extra-virgin olive oil, or avocado oil (or choose 2 and use 1 tablespoon of each)

3 tablespoons tahini (sesame paste), or almond butter in a pinch

4 to 6 garlic cloves, minced

Juice of 1 lemon

Mineral Salt and black pepper

1 or 2 teaspoons extra-virgin olive oil, for drizzling

Enjoy this creamy dip with Beauty Blend Savory Sesame Crackers (page 504), cut veggies, or well toasted Wonderful White Blender Bread (page 242).

1. Steam the cauliflower until tender. Transfer it to a food processor and add the oil, tahini, garlic, lemon juice, and salt and black pepper to taste (be generous, you need plenty of these seasonings) and process until completely smooth. Taste and adjust . . . need more salt and pepper? More lemon? Own the flavors, then pour into a bowl and drizzle the olive oil over the top.

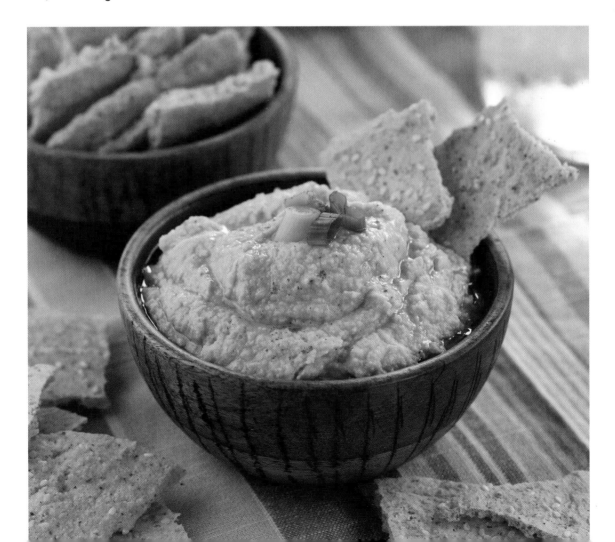

fiery fermented hot sauce

FP

MULTIPLE SERVE

1 medium to large tomato, quartered

6 to 10 rainbow mini peppers, coarsely chopped

1 to 3 habaneros (jalapeños for wussies . . . sorry)

2 teaspoons Mineral Salt

1 teaspoon yellow miso

½ cup apple cider vinegar, or more to taste

2 teaspoons onion powder

¼ to ½ teaspoon garlic powder, or 1 to 2 garlic cloves, minced

½ teaspoon Gluccie

3 to 4 tablespoons Nutritional Yeast

Optional (see Note):

1 to 2 tablespoons fresh liquid whey (harvested from homemade kefir or yogurt or from the top of store-bought plain yogurt with live cultures)

SERENE CHATS: *Fire up those taste buds and that metabolism . . . this is totally yumzers, mates! At my home, when we run out of this stuff we groan and whine until we make it again. Everything gets kicked up a notch in flavor and fire with a drizzle of this awesomeness on top. What's better is that it's loaded with live enzymes, superfoods, and nutrition. That store-bought stuff made from white vinegar, corn, and probably GMO pales in comparison.*

1. Blend everything well in a blender until smooth. Bottle it up with a cap or put it in a lidded jar (I use old store-bought hot sauce bottles). If you added the whey, then leave it on your counter for a day or overnight to establish some good bugs. Store in the fridge.

NOTE: If you leave out the liquid whey, you must refrigerate the mixture straightaway.

cottage citrus dip

FP WITH **E** OPTION

MULTIPLE SERVE

2 cups 1% cottage cheese

Juice of ½ large lemon, 1 small lemon, or 1 lime

Juice of ¼ orange (only for E; see Note)

1 tablespoon water

1 to 2 tablespoons Baobab Boost Powder (optional)

With only two main ingredients, this is a cinch and adds just the right touch to make so many of your meals more awesome! Put it on the side of E meals that need a bit more oomph or are just begging for fresh, zingy flavor; or add to any meal that needs a bit more protein. It pairs beautifully with Loaves and Fishes Bake (page 130). While the Baobab Boost Powder is optional here, it makes this dip incredible. If you are on a tight budget and want to conserve baobab, use just 1 tablespoon instead of 2 and omit the water. Also, try the herby variation below (an FP for Ranch lovers).

1. Mix all the ingredients with a stick blender until smooth (or process in a food processor).

NOTE: We don't usually include fruit juice on-plan, but this is just a little bit paired with heaps of protein.

VARIATION

COTTAGE HERBY DIP: For an herby variation, blend or process the cottage cheese until smooth. Omit the citrus juice and baobab powder. Add in 1 teaspoon dried dill, 2 teaspoons dried parsley, and 1 finely diced green onion or a smattering of fresh chives.

karate chop kale pesto **S**

LARGE FAMILY SERVE OR MULTIPLE SINGLE SERVES (HALVE IF YOU DESIRE)

4 cups super packed down fresh kale (all kale works, but baby kale is awesie!)

3 tablespoons extra-virgin olive oil (if using this pesto in a cooked dish, replace with 2 tablespoons MCT oil)

Juice of ½ lemon

6 tablespoons water

1 cup grated Parmesan cheese (refrigerated pre-grated or home-grated on the smallest grater hole size), or ½ cup powder-style Parmesan cheese (from the green can)

½ to ¾ cup walnuts

1 teaspoon Mineral Salt (or more to taste if you are a salty head)

½ teaspoon black pepper

2 to 4 garlic cloves, minced (to taste)

1 tablespoon Nutritional Yeast

3 tablespoons Baobab Boost Powder (optional, but preferred)

½ cup 1% cottage cheese (optional, for a creamy version; we suggest trying the original version first)

Optional: 2 to 3 tablespoons fermented whey liquid (from the top of your Greek yogurt) or plain kefir (see Note)

The problem with making traditional pesto is that unless you are blessed to have basil in season in your own garden, it is hard and expensive to come by in amounts large enough for a decent batch of pesto. Kale is everywhere these days, but if you are like us you have a giant bag in your fridge that you planned to use in a recipe and didn't get a chance.

This recipe is the perfect answer for kale that needs to be used now before it goes to waste. It is quick to make, and freezes and thaws beautifully. The handiness of kale is not the only reason we use it for this pesto. Kale is trendy these days for good reason—it is one of the most nutrient-dense foods in existence. This recipe doesn't just give you a little dose of kale, it literally packs it up to your gills in such a delicious and tantalizing way that you won't even realize the enormity of greens you are eating until you feel your health buzzing! You just might find yourself doing cool karate chop moves alone in the kitchen like a superhero with all your newfound energy. Kale is very low in oxalates, so it is safe to eat in large amounts without worrying about overdoing. Oxalates are an acidic substance found in some foods that can cause inflammation and pain for certain people, so nothing we want to overdo.

Kale has high amounts of vitamin C and, combined with Baobab Boost Powder (another super C source you can read about on page 42), this pesto is a true beauty food. Vitamin C is necessary to synthesize collagen in your body and is the key to making all your supplemental collagen get to work restoring structure to your bones, joints, organs, skin, hair, and teeth.

Slather this pesto on pizza crusts (see page 252), dip in on-plan crackers such as Savory Sesame Crackers (page 504) and crudités, sauté it with Troodles (zucchini noodles) or konjac noodles (see page 43), or dip sprouted-grain or sourdough crusts into it for a healthy Crossover treat. Dig in by the spoon if you want, but do yourself a favor and just eat it for goodness sake!

1. Place the kale in a large bowl. Adding only a few handfuls at a time to a food processor, process the kale with a little of the oil, lemon juice, or water for each batch (the little bit of liquid helps keep the processor blades going). Once all the kale is processed along with all the water, oil, and lemon juice, add the Parmesan, walnuts, salt, pepper, garlic, nutritional yeast, baobab powder (if using), cottage cheese

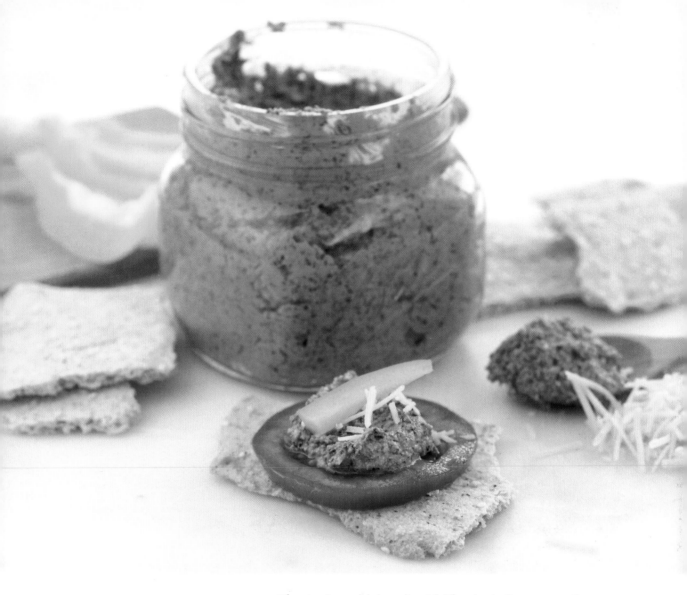

(if using), and whey liquid (if using). Process until super smooth.

NOTE: The option of adding the liquid whey (from the top of your Greek yogurt) or kefir adds a probiotic infusion that will inoculate your pesto. Leave it out on the countertop for an afternoon after making it and then refrigerate it from then on. This will not only add a boost to its health benefits, but prolong the life of your pesto and allow you to enjoy it longer.

P.S. FROM SERENE: I had a bumper crop of arugula one year and used it to make this yummy pesto. Arugula tastes amazing as a pesto green because its sharp, astringent punch is similar in strength to basil.

Salad Dressings

SERENE CHATS: *I am sending this rant over to Pearl and I hope she puts it in the book. I have to keep a watch on her because she tends to "accidentally" leave some of my rants out. So here goes . . . salads can be the healthiest food in the world OR THEY CAN BE DESTROYED! Pouring poisonous hydrogenated GMO soybean oil laced with corn syrup, preservatives, and other unpronounceables makes those delicious tender greens downright scary (keep that last sentence in, Pearl! . . . I'm watching you, no softening it to your Drive-Thru ways).*

The following are delicious dressings that are made from a base of core Trimmy ingredients. You learned about those in my Trimmy Bisque soups (pages 162 to 195). These dressings are creamy, superfoody, and pumped with beautifying collagen protein. Drive-Thru Sue's listen up here . . . these are super-duper quick to Trimmy up. Yes, you're still a Trim Healthy Mama if you use some store-bought ranch dressing now and then. I sure am not going to make you feel bad because you are making baby steps, but as you get your feet wetter in the journey you won't feel so overwhelmed, and trying one of these dressings will be fun rather than a chore. We have created a Trimmy knockoff of many beloved classic dressings and thrown in a crazy one just for sheer flavor adventure. Drizzle and dazzle your salad life!

NOTE: Most of these Trimmy dressings use a little gelatin in the mix for superfood thickening. This way they have less need for fats and calories so they can qualify as FP or light S. You can use the dressings immediately after making, but the thick and creamy texture is achieved after a night in the refrigerator. Give them a good shake or a little stir before serving. If you prefer thinner dressings, always feel free to thin with a little water.

LONG LIFE TRIMMY DRESSING TRICK: Add a couple tablespoons fresh liquid kefir (preferably from raw kefir) or drained from the top of store-bought plain yogurt with active cultures. You can also choose to use a tablespoon of plain store-bought kombucha or plain KeVita (a brand of kefir water). Inoculating your dressing in this manner and leaving it on the counter for an afternoon before refrigerating will extend its ability to stay fresh for a lot longer.

ranch trimmy dressing

FP WITH S OPTION

MULTIPLE SERVE (MAKES CLOSE TO 2 CUPS)

1 teaspoon Just Gelatin

2 tablespoons cool water

2 tablespoons just off the boil water

1 to 2 garlic cloves, minced

1 teaspoon Mineral Salt

¼ teaspoon black pepper

2 teaspoons onion powder

1 tablespoon rice vinegar

1 teaspoon Dijon mustard

¼ teaspoon Sunflower Lecithin

3 tablespoons MCT oil

1½ tablespoons (1 scoop) Integral
Collagen

4 tablespoons (1 scoop) unflavored
Pristine Whey Protein Powder*

1 cup plain 0% Greek yogurt*

1 teaspoon dried dill

3 tablespoons dried parsley flakes

2 green onions, diced ultrafine, or a
handful of finely diced fresh chives

SERENE CHATS: *A FUEL PULL RANCH DRESSING, PEOPLE! YES, I'M YELLING! THIS IS GOOD NEWS.*

1. Put the gelatin and the 2 tablespoons cool water in a 1-cup measuring cup and stir until the gelatin dissolves. Add the boiled water and stir again. Add enough cool water to come to the 1-cup line, then pour into a blender.

2. Add the garlic, salt, black pepper, onion powder, vinegar, mustard, lecithin, MCT oil, and collagen. Trimmy it up with a good blend. Add the whey protein and blend for 3 to 5 seconds more. Turn the blender off and gently stir in the yogurt, herbs, and green onions. Pour into a jar. This dressing can be used immediately, but it has the best texture after being refrigerated for a day to let the gelatin thicken properly.

* FOR DF: DAIRY-FREE FOLK CAN REPLACE THE YOGURT WITH A LARGE HASS AVOCADO AND A SQUEEZE OF LEMON JUICE AND/OR A TABLESPOON OR 2 OF BAOBAB POWDER. THE AVOCADO VERSION WILL OF COURSE BE AN S. ALSO OMIT WHEY PROTEIN.

DF

honey-mustard trimmy dressing

S

MULTIPLE SERVE (MAKES ABOUT 1½ CUPS)

1 teaspoon Just Gelatin

2 tablespoons cool water

2 tablespoons just off the boil water

⅓ cup plus 1 tablespoon Dijon
mustard

⅓ cup plus 1 tablespoon apple
cider vinegar

⅓ cup Gentle Sweet

1¼ teaspoons Mineral Salt

3 tablespoons MCT oil

1½ tablespoons (1 scoop)
Integral Collagen

1 tablespoon Baobab Boost Powder
(optional)

⅛ teaspoon Sunflower Lecithin

1. Put the gelatin in a 1-cup measuring cup with the 2 tablespoons cool water and stir to dissolve. Add the boiled water and stir again. Add enough cool water to come up to ½ cup. Pour into the blender.

2. Add all the remaining ingredients and Trimmy it up with a good blend. Pour into a jar.

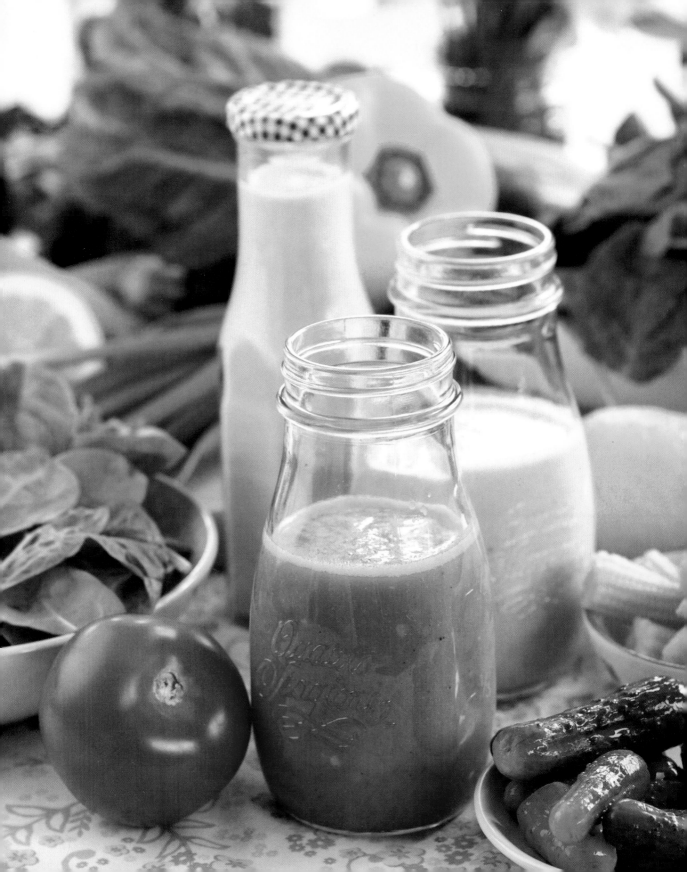

thousand island trimmy dressing ⒻⓅ

MULTIPLE SERVE (MAKES ABOUT 1½ CUPS)

1 teaspoon Just Gelatin
2 tablespoons cool water
2 tablespoons just off the boil water
3 tablespoons MCT oil
3 tablespoons tomato paste
3 tablespoons apple cider vinegar
3 tablespoons Gentle Sweet
1 teaspoon Mineral Salt
¼ teaspoon black pepper
1½ tablespoons (1 scoop)
   Integral Collagen
⅛ teaspoon Sunflower Lecithin
1 to 2 tablespoons finely diced
   sweet onion
2 tablespoons finely diced pickles

Unbelievably, yes . . . a creamy Thousand Island dressing that is an FP!

1. Put the gelatin and the 2 tablespoons cool water into a 1-cup measuring cup and stir to dissolve. Add the boiled water and stir again. Add enough cool water to come up to 1 cup. Pour this gelatin/water mix into a blender and blend for a few seconds.

2. Add the MCT oil, tomato paste, vinegar, sweetener, salt, black pepper, collagen, and lecithin and Trimmy to perfection with a nice blend. Pour into a jar and add the onion and pickles.

caesar trimmy dressing Ⓢ

MULTIPLE SERVE (MAKES CLOSE TO 2 CUPS)

½ cup MCT oil
3 tablespoons extra-virgin olive oil
¼ cup fresh lemon juice
½ cup water
6 teensy anchovy fillets (packed in
   olive oil)
1 teaspoon Dijon mustard
1 teaspoon Mineral Salt
¼ teaspoon black pepper
1 teaspoon Nutritional Yeast
1½ tablespoons (1 scoop) Integral
   Collagen
1 to 2 garlic cloves, minced
3 tablespoons finely grated fresh
   Parmesan cheese (lightly packed
   to measure), or use powder-style
   Parmy (from the green can) and
   don't pack down
1 tablespoon Baobab Boost Powder
   (optional)
⅛ teaspoon Sunflower Lecithin

1. Place all the ingredients in a blender and blend until smooth and creamy. Pour into a jar.

tahini trimmy dressing

S

MULTIPLE SERVE (MAKES CLOSE TO 2 CUPS)

1 teaspoon Just Gelatin
2 tablespoons cool water
2 tablespoons just off the boil water
½ cup tahini (sesame paste)
5 tablespoons apple cider vinegar
3 tablespoons soy sauce or tamari
1 to 2 large garlic cloves, minced
1 tablespoon miso (yellow or white)
½ teaspoon black pepper
½ teaspoon Mineral Salt
1 teaspoon onion powder
½ teaspoon garlic powder
1 tablespoon Gentle Sweet, or 1 or
   2 doonks Pure Stevia Extract
   Powder
1½ tablespoons (1 scoop)
   Integral Collagen
2 tablespoons Baobab Boost
   Powder (optional)
⅛ teaspoon Sunflower Lecithin
1 tablespoons dried parsley flakes
3 green onions, finely diced
   (optional)

Tahini is a delicious sesame seed paste that makes the most wonderful dressing. Usually though, sesame seed dressings are very heavy in fat and calories. This is a much lighter S than most sesame dressings so you can pour more on!

1. Put the gelatin in a 1-cup measuring cup. Add the 2 table-spoons cool water and stir to dissolve. Add the boiled water and stir it again. Add enough additional cool water to come up to 1 cup. Pour it into a blender and add another ½ cup cool water. Blend this gelatin/water mix for a few seconds.

2. Add the tahini, vinegar, soy sauce, garlic, miso, black pepper, salt, onion powder, garlic powder, sweetener, collagen, baobab powder, and lecithin. Trimmy everything smooth and creamy with a nice blend. Pour into a jar and add the parsley flakes and green onions.

italian trimmy dressing   ⓕⓟ

MULTIPLE SERVE (MAKES ABOUT 1½ CUPS)

1 teaspoon Just Gelatin

2 tablespoons cool water

2 tablespoons just off the boil water

3 tablespoons balsamic vinegar

¼ cup apple cider vinegar

1 tablespoon Gentle Sweet

3 tablespoons Baobab Boost
Powder (not optional; it helps
thicken and keep it FP)

1 teaspoon Mineral Salt

¼ teaspoon black pepper

1 to 2 garlic cloves, minced

1 teaspoon onion powder

3 tablespoons MCT oil

1½ tablespoons (1 scoop) Integral
Collagen

⅛ teaspoon Sunflower Lecithin

3 tablespoons powder-style
Parmesan cheese (from the
green can)

2 tablespoons very finely diced red
bell pepper

1 tablespoon dried onion flakes

1½ tablespoons dried parsley flakes

2 teaspoons dried basil

2 teaspoons dried oregano

1. Put the gelatin and the 2 tablespoons cool water into a 1-cup measuring cup and stir to dissolve. Add the boiled water and stir again. Add enough cool water to come up to 1 cup. Pour this gelatin/water mix into a blender and blend for a few seconds.

2. Add the vinegars, sweetener, baobab powder, salt, black pepper, garlic, onion powder, MCT oil, collagen, and lecithin. Trimmy it up with a nice blend.

3. Pour it into a jar and stir in the Parmesan, bell pepper, onion flakes, parsley flakes, basil, and oregano. Stir well.

greek trimmy dressing

MULTIPLE SERVE (MAKES ABOUT 1½ CUPS)

1 teaspoon Just Gelatin

2 tablespoons cool water

2 tablespoons just off the boil water

¼ cup olive oil

¼ cup MCT oil

⅛ teaspoon Sunflower Lecithin

1½ tablespoons (1 scoop) Integral Collagen

¼ cup balsamic vinegar or apple cider vinegar

Juice of 2 lemons

3 garlic cloves, minced

1 teaspoon Mineral Salt

¼ teaspoon black pepper

2 tablespoons Baobab Boost Powder (optional)

½ to 1 tablespoon Gentle Sweet (use the larger amount if using apple cider vinegar)

20 Kalamata olives, diced super fine

½ cup finely crumbled feta cheese (no thick chunks, just rice-size pieces)

2 tablespoons dried parsley flakes

1. Put the gelatin and the 2 tablespoons cool water into a 1-cup measuring cup and stir to dissolve. Add the boiled water and stir again. Add enough cool water to come up to 1 cup. Pour this gelatin/water mix into a blender and blend for a few seconds.

2. Add the olive oil, MCT oil, lecithin, collagen, vinegar, lemon juice, garlic, salt, black pepper, baobab powder (if using), and sweetener. Trimmy smooth with a good blend.

3. Pour into a jar and stir in the olives, feta, and parsley flakes.

crazy kombucha trimmy dressing

MULTIPLE SERVE (MAKES CLOSE TO 2 CUPS)

1 teaspoon Just Gelatin

2 tablespoon cool water

2 tablespoons just off the boil water

1 cup plain kombucha (or a flavor that melds with the smoky chili flavors of this dressing . . . mint or berry wouldn't work; you know what I mean)

3 tablespoons MCT oil

1½ tablespoons (1 scoop) Integral Collagen

⅛ teaspoon Sunflower Lecithin

1 teaspoon Mineral Salt

¼ teaspoon black pepper

Juice of 2 large limes

¼ teaspoon chipotle powder

½- to 1-inch chunk red jalapeño, for hotties, or the same amount of red bell pepper, for regulars

1 teaspoon onion powder

1 teaspoon Dijon mustard (optional)

2 tablespoons Baobab Boost Powder

½ teaspoon mesquite liquid smoke

1 teaspoon cumin seeds

2 tablespoons powder-style Parmesan cheese (from the green can)

2 teaspoons dried oregano

SERENE CHATS: *This dressing is not your normal or traditional tasting condiment. It kicks and smokes and gets a hold of your taste buds in a surprisingly addictive way. The first taste is ummmmm . . . . and the second taste registers awesome. Don't bother making it if you don't like trying new things. This is a rugged adventure to uncharted flavor land. It rocks drizzled over tuna that's bedded on sprouted-grain or artisan sourdough toast. It keeps really well in the fridge due to its high probiotic content, and the flavors just keep getting better. Any courageous foodies wanna give it a go?*

1. Put the gelatin and cool water into a cup and stir to dissolve. Add the boiled water and stir again. Set aside to cool so that when adding it to the kombucha it doesn't kill the live enzymes.

2. Place the kombucha, MCT oil, collagen, lecithin, salt, black pepper, lime juice, chipotle powder, jalapeño or bell pepper, onion powder, mustard (if using), baobab powder, and liquid smoke in a blender and blend until creamy. Reduce the speed to low, open the lid, and while the blender is whizzing, pour in every drop of the gelatin mix, then cover and blend again on high for 10 seconds.

3. Add the cumin seeds and blend for just a few seconds (you don't want these seeds perfectly smooth but not large and scratchy either . . . just flavorful chewy flecks).

4. Pour the dressing into a jar and stir in the Parmesan and oregano.

quirky jerky

S

2 pounds lean grass-fed beef or venison (Drive-Thru Sue's can use lean ground turkey)

2 large carrots, grated

2 large celery stalks, finely diced

2 green onions, finely diced (optional)

1 cup diced fresh cranberries or raspberries

½ cup walnuts (or any kind of nut), finely diced

½ cup flax seeds or chia seeds

½ cup sesame seeds, hulled hemp seeds, or any other favorite seeds

3 tablespoons Nutritional Yeast

1¼ teaspoons Mineral Salt (salt lovers will want another ¼ teaspoon)

1½ teaspoons cumin seeds (optional)

½ to 1 teaspoon ground cumin (use the larger amount if you don't use the cumin seeds)

1 teaspoon onion powder

1 teaspoon chipotle powder or chili powder

½ teaspoon garlic powder

½ teaspoon red pepper flakes (reduce to ¼ teaspoon if scared of spice)

⅛ teaspoon cayenne pepper (reduce to just a doonk if scared of spice)

3 tablespoons apple cider vinegar

½ teaspoon mesquite liquid smoke (1 full teaspoon for smoke lovers)

SERENE CHATS: *This jerky is REAL FOOD FOR ON THE GO. This AIN'T no plastic, fake food, processed jerky stick! This here is whole-food protein along with veggies and healthy fat from seeds, all slow-baked with the perfect fusion of spice and crispness, no dehydrator needed. It is quirky because the texture is a little different from regular jerky since it is slow-baked rather than dried, but we've grown to prefer this sort of jerky now. If you have to rush off to work in the mornings, it is best to make this on the weekend or on your days off, as it has a long, low bake time.*

Go ahead and throw a couple pieces into your purse in a baggie for true nourishment and satiety while out and about, or dip a piece or two in your favorite on-plan dip like Kickin' Dippin' Sauce (page 518). We call this the perfect natural snack!

1. Preheat the oven to its lowest setting (around 170°F) and preferably on a convection setting if you have it. Line 2 large baking sheets with parchment paper or grease 2 large pizza stones.

2. Mix everything up well with your hands in a large bowl. Spread the mixture super thin by squishing and spreading it flat with your hands on the baking sheets or stones.

3. Bake all night (7 to 8 hours). In the morning, flip the sheets of jerky and keep baking another 3 to 4 hours, or until the jerky is incredibly crispy. Turn the oven off and let the jerky cool inside the turned-off oven.

4. Break the jerky up into snack bar–size pieces. Store in zippy bags in the freezer for the long term. This keeps them super crispy and yumzers.

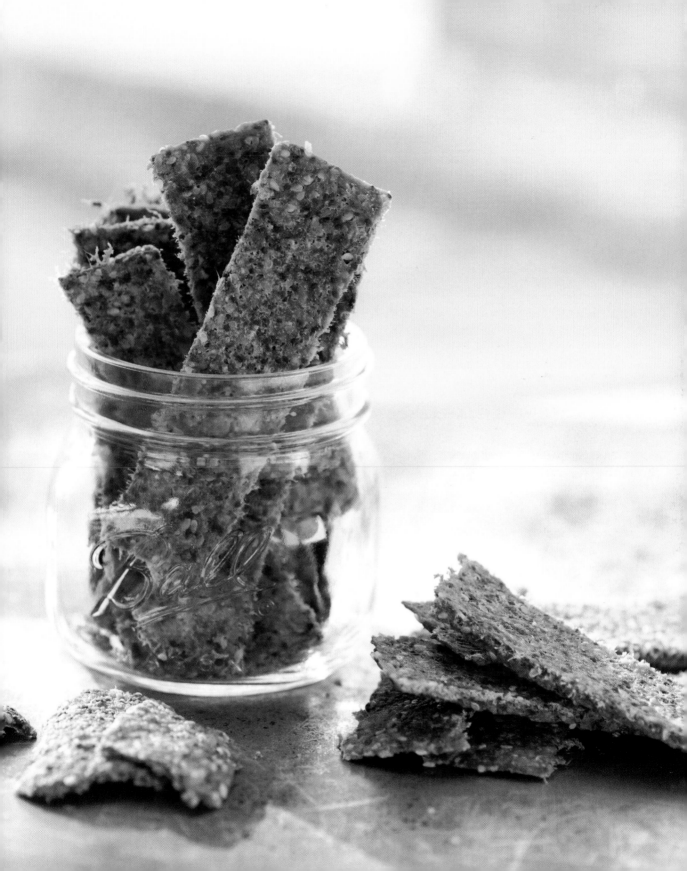

Appendix

THE MEAL RECAP

THE SATISFYING (S) MEAL

1. More fat, less carbs (anchored with protein)

2. Keep grains, sweet potatoes, and most fruits away from **S** meals

BUILD AN S MEAL

- Choose your protein (lean or fatty meat or fish, whole eggs, and egg whites).
- Add fats as desired.
- Add optional Fuel Pull foods like nonstarchy veggies, berries, and cultured dairy.

TIPS

- Good fats can also include egg yolks, butter, red meat, coconut oil, and red palm oil, in addition to extra-virgin olive oil, nuts, and avocados.
- Nonstarchy veggies can be any vegetable that is not a root vegetable (such as potato, sweet potato, or carrot) or corn.
- Nuts are also allowed in moderation.

S-Friendly Meats: All meats and fish, both fatty or lean (grass-fed is best but not mandatory)

S-Friendly Eggs: Whole eggs and egg whites

S-Friendly Dairy: Heavy cream; half-and-half; butter; all cheeses; sour cream; double-fermented kefir; both full-fat and reduced-fat forms of cottage cheese, ricotta cheese, feta cheese, and paneer; plain Greek yogurt, both 0% (stick to half cup as dessert or full cup for main protein) and full-fat; Laughing Cow Creamy Light Swiss cheese wedges (for non-purists)

S-Friendly Veggies: All nonstarchy veggies. Don't go overboard with tomatoes, onions, peas, butternut squash, and acorn squash. Small amounts of carrots can be squeezed in here and there.

S-Friendly Fruit: Up to 1 cup of all kinds of berries (except blueberries—keep those to ½ cup); lemons and limes

S-Friendly Nuts and Seeds: Raw or roasted seeds or nuts in moderation, nut butters without sugar in moderation, nut and seed flours in moderation

S-Friendly Condiments: Most cold-pressed oils; mayo; mustard; horseradish sauce; vinegar; salad dressings with 2 grams of carbs or less; olives; nutritional yeast; all broth and stock prepared without sugar, spices, and seasonings; unsweetened cocoa powders; sugar-free ketchup; sugar-free hot sauce, extracts

S-Friendly Grains and Beans: Keep these foods away from your **S** meals, with the exception of very small garnish amounts to be used occasionally.

S-Friendly Healthy Specialty Items: Pristine Whey Protein Powder (www.trimhealthy mama.com); Integral Collagen (www.trimhealthymama.com); Just Gelatin (www.trim healthymama.com); Trim Healthy Mama Baking Blend (www.trimhealthymama .com); Pressed Peanut Flour (www.trimhealthymama.com); Gluccie (www.trim healthymama.com); plan-approved sweeteners (www.trimhealthymama.com); Baobab Boost Powder (www.trimhealthymama.com); Not Naughty or Trim Healthy Noodles or Not Naughty Rice (www.trimhealthymama.com); Trim Healthy Chocolate Chips (www.trimhealthymama.com); chocolate or a square or two of 85% dark chocolate; 100% cacao baker's chocolate; unsweetened nut milks such as almond, cashew, coconut, or flax seed

S-Friendly "Personal Choice" Items: Joseph's low-carb pita or lavash bread, low-carb tortillas, fat-free Reddi-wip, Laughing Cow Creamy Light Swiss cheese wedges, Dreamfields pasta (limit to once a week)

THE ENERGIZING (E) MEAL

1. More healthy carbs, less fat (anchored with protein)
2. Your carbs include fruit, sweet potatoes, beans/legumes, and gentle whole grains like oatmeal or quinoa.

BUILD AN E MEAL

- Choose your lean protein.
- Add your carb (fruit, gentle whole grains, beans/legumes, or sweet potatoes).
- Add minimal fat (roughly 1 teaspoon); nuts and seeds are only used in garnish amounts.
- Add optional Fuel Pull foods like nonstarchy veggies and berries and optional lean dairy.

TIPS

- Keep carbs to palm-size portions.
- MCT oil has the lowest amount of calories, so occasionally you can use 2 teaspoons with your **E** meal.
- Don't make corn your go-to grain.

E-Friendly Meat: All lean meats, chicken breast, tuna packed in water, salmon (look for less than 5 grams of fat), all other fish (not fried), venison, turkey breast, lean ground turkey or chicken (96% to 99% lean), lean deli meats (natural brands are best); ground meats with higher fat levels can be browned, drained, then rinsed well with hot water and used in **E** meals in up to 4-ounce portions

E-Friendly Egg Sources: Egg whites

E-Friendly Dairy: 0% plain Greek yogurt, low-fat or nonfat regular plain yogurt, plain low-fat or nonfat kefir, 1% cottage cheese (2% should be fine for purists who cannot find a suitable 1%), low-fat ricotta cheese (up to ¼ cup), skim mozzarella cheese (in small amounts), reduced-fat or 2% hard cheeses (small sprinkles only)

E-Friendly Grains: Brown rice (up to ¾ cup cooked serving); quinoa (up to ¾ cup cooked serving); whole barley (up to ¾ cup cooked serving); farro (up to ¾ cup cooked serving); oatmeal (up to 1¼ cups cooked serving); whole-grain bread in sprouted, artisan sourdough, or dark rye form (2-piece servings); sprouted tortilla (1 large tortilla); sprouted whole-grain flours; sprouted whole-grain pasta; 4 Light Rye, Fiber, or Flax Seed Wasa crackers or 2 to 3 Multi-Grain, Hearty, Sourdough, or Whole Grain Wasa crackers (most Ryvita crackers are **E**-friendly, too); popcorn (4 to 5 cups of popped kernels spritzed with 1 teaspoon fat); baked blue corn chips

E-Friendly Fruit: All fruits in moderate quantities, e.g., 1 apple, 1 orange, 1 peach, 1 generous slice of cantaloupe; all berries in liberal quantities; use dried fruits very sparingly

E-Friendly Beans and Legumes: All beans and legumes, including lentils and split peas—stick to 1 cup densely packed cooked, but more can be eaten when liquid is involved, i.e., chili or lentil soup

E-Friendly Veggies: All veggies except potatoes; enjoy sweet potatoes (1 medium) and carrots, both raw and cooked

E-Friendly Oils: 1 teaspoon oil (exception of occasional 2 teaspoons MCT oil)

E-Friendly Nuts: Limit nuts to garnish amounts or 1 teaspoon nut butters

E-Friendly Condiments: Mustard, horseradish sauce, hot sauce, low-fat dressings, mayo (up to 1 teaspoon), soy sauce/tamari/Bragg liquid aminos/coconut aminos, all vinegars, all spices without sugar, unsweetened cocoa powder, extracts, nutritional yeast, all skimmed stock and broth (prepared without sugar)

E-Friendly Healthy Specialty Items: Pristine Whey Protein Powder (www.trimhealthy mama.com), Integral Collagen (www.trimhealthymama.com), Just Gelatin (www.trimhealthymama.com), Pressed Peanut Flour (www.trimhealthymama.com), Baobab Boost Powder (www.trimhealthymama.com), Gluccie (www.trimhealthymama .com), plan-approved sweeteners (www.trimhealthymama.com), Trim Healthy Mama Baking Blend (www.trimhealthymama.com), Not Naughty or Trim Healthy Noodles or Rice (www.trimhealthymama.com), unsweetened nut milks (avoid coconut milk for **E** meals)

E-Friendly "Personal Choice" Items: Joseph's low-carb pita or lavash bread (fruit, beans, or sweet potatoes will be needed for a proper **E** meal), low-carb tortillas (fruit, beans, or sweet potatoes will be needed for a proper **E** meal), fat-free Reddi-wip, Laughing Cow Creamy Light Swiss cheese wedges, Dreamfields pasta (limit to once a week; another carb source will be needed), light Progresso soups (another carb source will be needed)

FUEL PULLS

These are lighter foods that round out your plates and make your **S** and **E** meals complete (although they can be occasional full meals). They have low amounts of both fats and carbs.

BUILD A FUEL PULL MEAL
- Choose your lean protein; limit meat to 3 to 4 ounces.
- Add minimal fat (roughly 1 teaspoon).
- Add other Fuel Pulls to your plate: generous nonstarchy veggies, moderate berries, and optional lean dairy.

TIPS
- Limit nuts to garnish amounts or 1 teaspoon nut butters.
- Examples of nonstarchy veggies: asparagus, broccoli, cabbage, cauliflower, cucumber, eggplant, mushrooms, jicama, tomatoes, yellow squash, zucchini, sugar snap peas, okra, onions, green onions, leeks, parsley, all leafy greens, radishes, spaghetti squash, pumpkin, chestnuts, baby Chinese corn
- Fuel Pulls shine as slimming snacks and desserts and help you avoid accidental Crossovers.

Fuel Pull-Friendly Meat: All lean meats in 3- to 4-ounce portions, chicken breast, tuna packed in water, salmon (look for less than 5 grams of fat), all other fish (not fried), venison, turkey breast, lean ground turkey or chicken (96% to 99% lean), lean deli meats (natural brands are best), ground meats with higher fat levels can be browned, drained, then rinsed well with hot water and used in FP meals in 3- to 4-ounce portions

Fuel Pull-Friendly Egg Sources: Egg whites

Fuel Pull-Friendly Dairy: 0% plain Greek yogurt, double-fermented nonfat kefir, 1% cottage cheese, low-fat ricotta cheese (up to ¼ cup), skim mozzarella cheese (in small amounts), reduced-fat 2% hard cheeses (small sprinkles only)

Fuel Pull-Friendly Veggies: All nonstarchy veggies. Avoid potatoes, corn, sweet potatoes, and parsnips.

Fuel Pull-Friendly Fruit: Up to 1 cup of all kinds of berries, lemons, and limes can be used, but keep blueberries to ½ cup.

Fuel Pull–Friendly Grains and Beans: 2 Light Rye, Fiber, or Flax Seed Wasa crackers or 2 Sesame Ryvita crackers; up to ¼ cup beans or oats occasionally (not in every Fuel Pull meal)

Fuel Pull–Friendly Oils: 1 teaspoon oil (exception of occasional 2 teaspoons MCT oil)

Fuel Pull–Friendly Condiments: Mustard; horseradish sauce; hot sauce; low-fat dressings; mayo (up to 1 teaspoon); soy sauce/tamari/Bragg liquid aminos/coconut aminos; all vinegars; all sugar-free spices; unsweetened cocoa powder; skimmed broth or stock prepared without sugar, extracts

Fuel Pull–Friendly Healthy Specialty Items: Pristine Whey Protein Powder (www.trimhealthymama.com), Integral Collagen (www.trimhealthymama.com), Just Gelatin (www.trimhealthymama.com), Gluccie (www.trimhealthymama.com), Baobab Boost Powder (www.trimhealthymama.com), plan-approved sweeteners (www.trimhealthymama.com), Trim Healthy Mama Baking Blend (www.trimhealthymama.com), Pressed Peanut Flour (www.trimhealthymama.com), Not Naughty or Trim Healthy Noodles or Rice (www.trimhealthymama.com), unsweetened nut milks (avoid coconut milk for FP)

Fuel Pull–Friendly "Personal Choice" Items: Joseph's low-carb pita or lavash bread, low-carb tortillas, fat-free Reddi-wip, Laughing Cow Creamy Light Swiss cheese wedges, light Progresso soups (avoid chowder versions)

CROSSOVERS (XO)

Crossovers merge the two fuels of fats and carbs for healthy tandem fueling. They keep to the **E** guidelines of carbs and add as many fats as desired.

BUILD A CROSSOVER MEAL

- Choose your protein (lean or fatty meat or fish, whole eggs or egg whites, or cultured dairy products).
- Add fats as desired (even if your protein source contains fat, other fats can be added).
- Add your carb in **E**-meal-safe amounts (fruit, gentle whole grains, beans/legumes, or sweet potatoes).
- Add optional Fuel Pull foods to your plate (nonstarchy veggies, berries, and cultured dairy).

TIPS

1. People with extremely high metabolisms and healthy growing children will do well with mostly Crossover meals.

2. Pregnant and nursing women, as well as Maintenance Mamas, will benefit from including some Crossover meals.

S HELPERS (SH)

Add a little carb to your **S** meal for pleasure's sake, but not enough that it becomes a Crossover.

TIP

People who may not be used to eating meals with lower amounts of carbs, or people who suffer with hypoglycemia, may at first need **S** Helpers to help their bodies gently adapt to the pure **S** meal. Children with weight issues can use S helpers to gently trim down.

SAME FOODS LIST AS S MEALS (WITH THESE ADDITIONAL OPTIONS):

⅓ to ½ cup quinoa

¼ cup brown rice

⅓ to ½ cup oatmeal

⅓ to ½ cup beans or lentils

½ piece of fruit like an apple or orange

½ medium sweet potato

1 piece of whole-grain sprouted, dark rye, or artisan sourdough bread toast

½ sprouted-grain wrap or low-carb tortilla

S, E, and FP Index

S MEALS

SAVORY MAINS AND SIDES

FAMILY THEME NIGHTS

HANGRY MEALS FOR ONE

E MEALS

FP MEALS

Index